Handbook of Pediatric Eye and Systemic Disease

W0091931

Handbook of Pediatric Eye and Systemic Disease

Edited by

Kenneth W. Wright, MD
Director, Wright Foundation for Pediatric Ophthalmology
Director, Pediatric Ophthalmology, Cedars-Sinai Medical
Center, Clinical Professor of Ophthalmology, University of
Southern California—Keck School of Medicine, Los Angeles,
California

Peter H. Spiegel, MD
Focus On You, Inc., Palm Desert, California
Inland Eye Clinic, Murrieta, California
Children's Eye Institute, Upland, California

Lisa S. Thompson, MD
Attending Physician, Stroger Hospital of Cook County,
Chicago, Illinois

Illustrators
Timothy C. Hengst, CMI
Susan Gilbert, CMI
Faith Cogswell

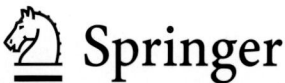 Springer

Kenneth W. Wright, MD
Director, Wright Foundation for
    Pediatric Ophthalmology
Director, Pediatric Ophthalmology,
    Cedars-Sinai Medical Center,
Clinical Professor of
    Ophthalmology, University of
    Southern California—Keck School
    of Medicine
Los Angeles, CA
USA

Peter H. Spiegel, MD
Focus On You, Inc.
Palm Desert, CA
Inland Eye Clinic,
Murrieta, CA
Children's Eye
    Institute
Upland, CA
USA

Lisa S. Thompson, MD
Attending Physician
Stroger Hospital of Cook County
Chicago, IL
USA

Library of Congress Control Number: 2005932934

ISBN 10: 0-387-27927-X   e-ISBN 0-387-27928-8
ISBN 13: 978-0387-27927-5

Printed on acid-free paper.

Printed in China   (BS/EVB)

9 8 7 6 5 4 3 2 1

springer.com

Preface

Pediatric ophthalmology is a broad field encompassing many diverse topics including embryology, chromosomal abnormalities, neurology, crainio-facial abnormalities, systemic diseases, retina disease, and strabismus. This variety makes pediatric ophthalmology interesting and intellectually stimulating, but at the time somewhat daunting. The handbook series is designed to give the practitioner an easy to understand, succinct yet detailed reference on various subjects related to pediatric ophthalmology.

The *Handbook of Pediatric Eye and Systemic Disease* is a practical resource on the diagnosis and management of eye disorders associated with pediatric systemic disease. A concise but comprehensive description of ocular manifestations of pediatric systemic disease is presented. These chapters are designed to be reader-friendly. They are organized with clear sub-headings that allow the readers to quickly find their area of interest such as *systemic characteristics*, *ocular findings*, or *treatment*. Excellent color photographs and diagrams illustrate the clinical points and help with disease recognition. Extensive use of tables and information boxes simplify and summarize complex topics. Each chapter is fully referenced to provide evidence-based practice guidelines and further in-depth reading. The last chapter is a compendium of hundreds of systemic diseases and chromosomal abnormalities that affect the eye. In this compendium are thorough lists of both systemic and ocular findings for each disease. This is an excellent aid to diagnosing syndromes based on the characteristics of the eye abnormality.

Another important use of the *Handbook of Pediatric Eye and Systemic Disease* is patient and family education. Parents are rightfully concerned about the effects of systemic disease on their child's eyes. Information, including diagrams and photographs from the handbook about the eye manifestations of systemic disease, can be shared with the families. This important information is often lacking in general texts on ophthalmology and pediatrics.

I hope you will find the *Handbook of Pediatric Eye and Systemic Disease* to be an invaluable adjunct to your pediatric practice.

Kenneth W. Wright, MD

Contents

Contributors

J. Bronwyn Bateman, MD

Nancy Chernus-Mansfield, MA

Cynthia S. Cook, DVM, PhD

Alissa A. Craft, MD

Maya Eibschitz-Tsimhoni

Roger K. George, MD

Natalie C. Kerr, MD, FACS, FAAP

Lois J. Martyn, MD

Marilyn T. Miller, MD

Maria A. Musarella, MD

Anna Newlin, MS, CGC

Enikö Karman Pivnick, MD

Kathleen K. Sulik, PhD

Elias I. Traboulsi, MD

R. Christopher Walton, MD

Kenneth W. Wright, MD

Embryology

Cynthia S. Cook, Kathleen K. Sulik, and Kenneth W. Wright

DIFFERENTIATION OF GERM LAYERS AND EMBRYOGENESIS

After fertilization of the ovum within the uterine tube, cellular mitosis results in formation of a ball of 12 to 16 cells, the morula. A fluid-filled cavity within this embryonic cell mass forms, resulting in a transformation into a blastocyst that begins to penetrate the uterine mucosa on approximately the sixth day postfertilization. The cells of the blastocyst continue to divide with the cells of the future embryo proper (embryoblast) accumulating at one pole. The cells of the primitive embryoblast differentiate into two layers, the *epiblast* and the *hypoblast*. These two cellular layers bridge the central cavity of the blastocyst, thus dividing the blastocyst into the amniotic cavity and the yolk sac (Fig. 1-1).

During the third week of gestation, the two-layered embryoblast transforms into a trilaminar embryo as central epiblast cells invaginate between the epiblast and hypoblast layers. Invagination of central epiblast cells creates a longitudinal groove through the midline of the caudal half of the epiblast, the *primitive streak*. This invagination of epiblast cells is termed *gastrulation* (Fig. 1-2A,B). Invaginating epiblast cells differentiate to form the *mesodermal* germ layer, which spreads out to fill the space between the epiblast and hypoblast. Gastrulation proceeds in a cranial to caudal progression and continues through the fourth week of human gestation. These invaginating epiblast cells displace the hypoblast cells to form the *endoderm*. The epiblast cells therefore give rise to all three definitive germ layers: *ectoderm*, *mesoderm*, and *endoderm* (Fig. 1-2C).

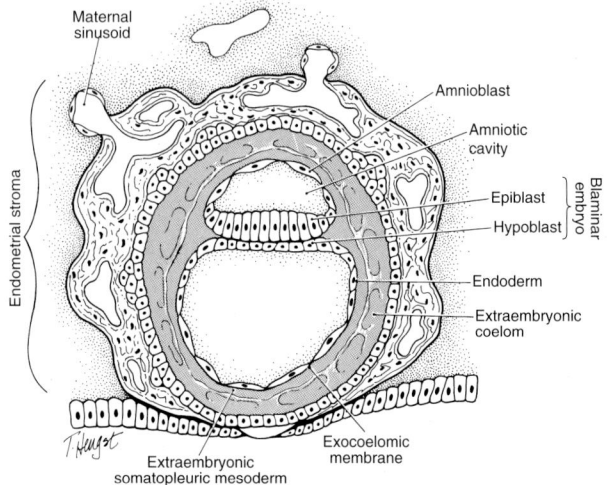

FIGURE 1-1. Drawing of a human blastocyst (12 days gestation) that has penetrated the maternal endometrium. An embryoblast has formed that consists of two cell layers: the epiblast above and the hypoblast below.

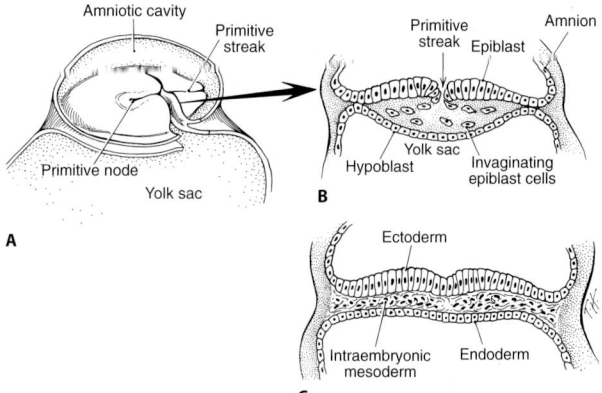

FIGURE 1-2A–C. (A) Drawing of a 17-day-old embryo in gastrulation stage (dorsal view) with the amnion removed. **(B)** Cross section of a 17-day-old embryo through the primitive streak. The primitive streak represents invagination of epiblast cells between the epiblast and hypoblast layers. Note the epiblast cells filling the middle area to form the mesodermal layer. **(C)** Cross section of the embryo at the end of the third week shows the three definitive germ layers: ectoderm, mesoderm, and endoderm.

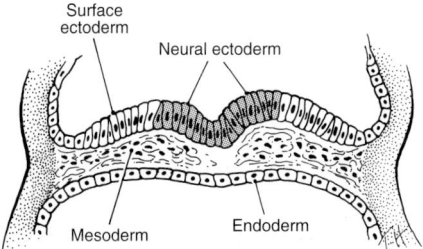

FIGURE 1-3. Drawing of an 18-day-old embryo sectioned through the neural plate. Note that the ectoderm in the area of the neural groove (*shaded cells*) has differentiated into neural ectoderm whereas the ectoderm on each side of the neural groove remains as surface ectoderm (*clear white cells*).

Toward the end of gastrulation, the ectoderm anterior to the primitive streak differentiates into columnar *neural ectoderm*; this expands, forming the *neural plate* from which the brain develops (Figs. 1-3, 1-4). Neural ectoderm on each side of the central neural groove expands to form bilateral elevations called the *neural folds* (Fig. 1-5). A central valley in the enlarging neural plate is called the *neural groove*. Ectoderm at the lateral margins of the neural plate has the flat, hexagonal morphology typical of *surface ectoderm* (Figs. 1-5, 1-6). By 21 days of human

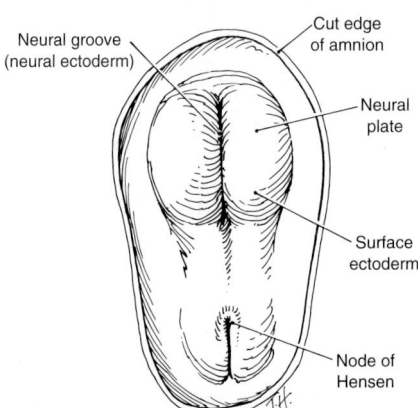

FIGURE 1-4. Drawing of dorsal aspect of embryo at 18 days gestation showing neural groove and enlarging neural plate.

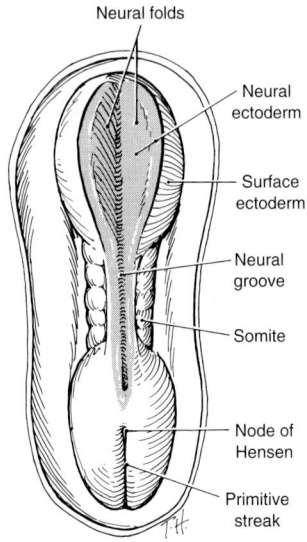

Neural folds

Neural ectoderm

Surface ectoderm

Neural groove

Somite

Node of Hensen

Primitive streak

FIGURE 1-5. Dorsal view of a human embryo at 20 days gestation. The neural plate transforms into two neural folds on each side of the neural groove. The neural groove in the middle of the embryo is *shaded* to represent neural ectoderm; the *unshaded* surface of the embryo is surface ectoderm.

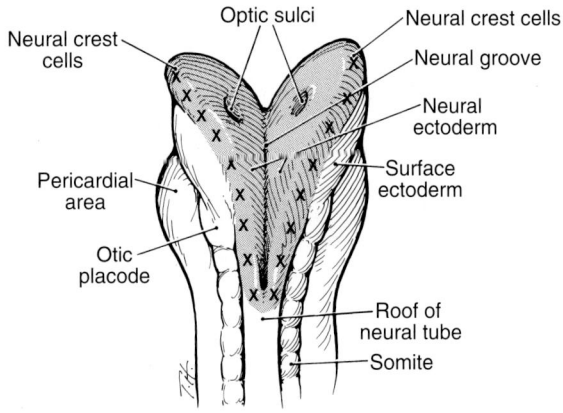

Optic sulci

Neural crest cells

Neural crest cells

Neural groove

Neural ectoderm

Surface ectoderm

Pericardial area

Otic placode

Roof of neural tube

Somite

FIGURE 1-6. Drawing of 21-day-old embryo (dorsal view) showing the enlarging cephalic neural folds, which are separate and have not yet fused. The central neural folds have fused to form the neural tube. The neural tube, groove, and facing surfaces of the large neural folds are made up of neural ectoderm; surface ectoderm covers the rest of the embryo. Neural crest cells (*X*) are found at the junction of the neural ectoderm and surface ectoderm. Neural crest cells migrate beneath the surface ectoderm spreading throughout the embryo and specifically to the area of the optic sulci. Neural ectoderm, *dark shading*; surface ectoderm, *white*; neural crest cells, *cross-hatched area*. The neural groove is still open at this point, and somites have formed along the lateral aspect of the neural tube.

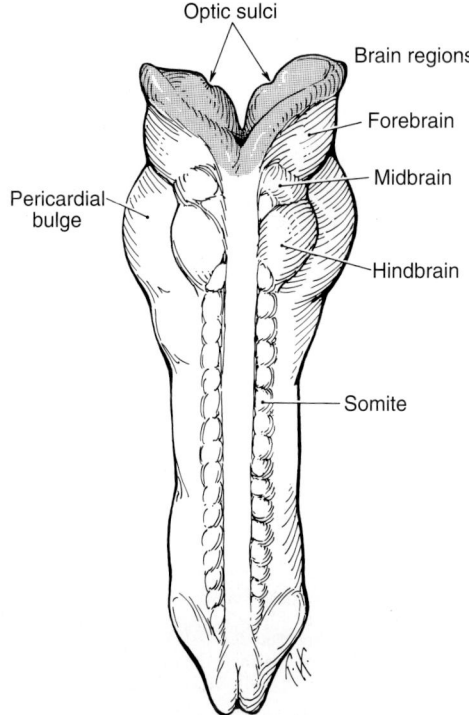

FIGURE 1-7. Drawing of approximately 23-day-old embryo, dorsal view, showing partial fusion of the neural folds. Brain vesicles have divided into three regions: forebrain, midbrain, and hindbrain. Note that the facing surfaces of the forebrain neural folds are lined with neural ectoderm (*shaded cells*) but the majority of the embryo is covered by surface ectoderm (*clear white*). On the inside of both forebrain vesicles is the site of the optic sulci (optic pits). The neural crest cells that will populate the region around the developing optic vesicles originate from the midbrain region.

gestation, while the neural tube is still open, the first sign of the developing eye is seen. The *optic sulci* or *optic pits* develop as invaginations on the inner surface of the anterior neural folds (Figs. 1-6, 1-7, 1-8). During expansion of the optic sulci, the central aspect of the neural folds approach each other and fuse, creating the longitudinal *neural tube.* Fusion of the neural folds

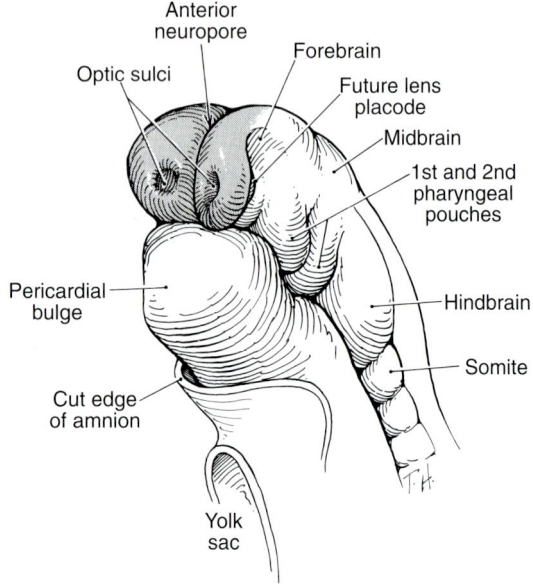

Anterior neuropore

Optic sulci

Forebrain

Future lens placode

Midbrain

1st and 2nd pharyngeal pouches

Pericardial bulge

Hindbrain

Somite

Cut edge of amnion

Yolk sac

FIGURE 1-8. Drawing of anterior view of embryo at similar stage to Figure 1-7 (23 days) shows the optic sulci on the inside of the forebrain vesicles. *Shaded area*, neural ectoderm. The optic sulci evaginate and expand toward the surface ectoderm as the neural tube closes anteriorly. (From Webster WS, Lipson AH, Sulik KK. Am J Med Genet 1988;31:505–512, with permission.)

is initiated in the region of the future neck and proceeds along the midline in both caudal and cranial directions. Following closure of the neural tube, the neural ectoderm and optic sulci are internalized, and the embryo is then covered by surface ectoderm (Fig. 1-7).

Neural Crest Cell Development

As the neural folds elevate and approach each other, a specialized population of mesenchymal cells, the *neural crest cells*, emigrate from the junction of the neural and surface ectoderm (see Fig. 1-6). Progenitor cells in the neural folds are multipotent, with potential to form multiple ectodermal derivatives, including epidermal, neural crest, and neural tube cells. These cells are induced by interactions between the neural plate and epidermis. The competence of the neural plate to respond to inductive interactions changes as a function of embryonic age.[92] These stellate cells migrate peripherally beneath the surface ectoderm to spread throughout the embryo and surround the area of the developing optic sulci. Neural crest cells play an important role in eye development, as they are the precursors (anlage) to major structures, including cornea stroma, iris stroma, ciliary muscle, choroid, sclera, and orbital cartilage and bone (Table 1-1).[55,64] The patterns of neural crest emergence and emigration correlate with the segmental disposition of the developing brain.[72] Migration and differentiation of the neural crest cells are influenced by the hyaluronic acid-rich extracellular matrix and the optic vesicle basement membrane.[17] This acellular matrix is secreted by a surface epithelium as well as the crest cells and forms a space through which the crest cells migrate. Fibronectin secreted by the noncrest cells forms the limits of this mesenchymal migration.[65] Interactions between the migrating neural crest and the associated mesoderm appear to be essential for normal crest differentiation.[76,77]

TABLE 1-1. Embryonic Origins of Ocular Tissues.

Neural ectoderm (optic cup)
  Neural retina
  Retinal pigment epithelium
  Pupillary sphincter and dilator muscles
  Posterior iris epithelium
  Ciliary body epithelium
  Optic nerve

Neural crest (connective tissue)
  Corneal endothelium
  Trabecular meshwork
  Stroma of cornea, iris, and ciliary body
  Ciliary muscle
  Choroid and sclera
  Perivascular connective tissue and
    smooth muscle cells
  Meninges of optic nerve
  Orbital cartilage and bone
  Connective tissue of the extrinsic
    ocular muscles
  Secondary vitreous
  Zonules

Surface ectoderm (epithelium)
  Corneal and conjunctival
    epithelium
  Lens
  Lacrimal gland
  Eyelid epidermis
  Eyelid cilia
  Epithelium of adnexa glands
  Epithelium of nasolacrimal duct

Mesoderm (muscle and vascular
    endothelium)
  Extraocular muscle cells
  Vascular endothelia
  Schlemm's canal endothelium
  Blood

Somite Development

During the development and closure of the neural groove, paraxial mesoderm increases in the center of the embryo to form *somites* (see Figs. 1-5, 1-6). The somites increase in number to approximately 40, and eventually this paraxial mesoderm becomes mesenchyme that, in turn, develops into connective tissue, cartilage, muscle, and bone for the trunk and extremities. The neural segmentation pattern appears to be dependent on the underlying mesoderm. In the region of the brain rostral to the developing inner ear, the mesodermal segments are called *somitomeres*, whereas segments caudal to this level are somites.[72,75] The somitomeres are mesodermal in origin and give rise to the myoblasts of the extraocular muscles and vascular endothelium in and around the eye. Unlike the trunk and extremities, orbital bone and ocular connective tissue are derived from neural crest cells, not mesoderm.

It is important to point out that *mesenchyme* is a broad term for any embryonic connective tissue, whereas mesoderm specifically relates to the middle embryonic layer. At one time the middle embryonic layer (the mesoderm) was thought to be responsible for most of the ocular and adnexal tissues. Embryologic studies have shown that mesoderm plays a relatively small role in the development of head and neck mesenchyme and is probably responsible only for the striated muscle of the extraocular muscles and vascular endothelium. With respect to the ocular development and development of the head and neck, most of the mesenchyme or connective tissue comes from the neural crest cells (see Table 1-1).

OPTIC VESICLE AND OPTIC CUP

As the neural folds progressively fuse in a cranial direction, dilation of the closed neural tube occurs to form the "brain vesicles." By 3 weeks, these vesicles undergo neural segmentation and form the specific parts of the brain, that is, *forebrain* (prosencephalon), *midbrain* (mesencephalon), and *hindbrain* (rhombencephalon) (see Fig. 1-7). Surface ectoderm covers the outside of the forebrain, and neural ectoderm lines the inner or facing surfaces of the paired forebrain vesicles from which the eyes develop (Figs. 1-8, 1-9). The *optic sulci* develop as bilateral evaginations of neural ectoderm on the facing surfaces of the

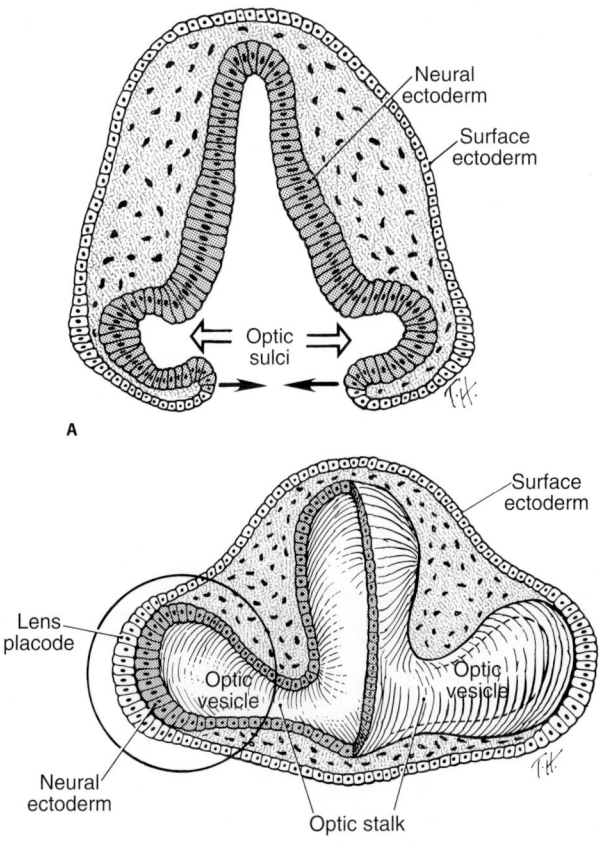

B

FIGURE 1-9A–B. (A) Drawing of a cross section through forebrain and optic sulci of 23- to 26-day-old embryo, during the period of neural tube closure. The optic sulci are lined by neural ectoderm (*shaded cells*); the surface of the forebrain is covered with surface ectoderm (*clear white cells*). As the optic sulci (neural ectoderm) evaginate towards the surface ectoderm (hollow arrows), the edges of the brain vesicles move together to fuse, thus closing the neural tube (*solid arrows*). **(B)** Drawing of a cross section through a 26-day-old embryo at the level of the optic vesicle. The neural tube has closed, the surface ectoderm now covers the exterior of the forebrain, and the neural ectoderm is completely internalized. The surface ectoderm cells overlying the optic vesicles thicken to form the early lens placode. (From Cook CS, Sulik KK. Scanning Electron Microsc 1986;III:1215–1227, with permission).

forebrain vesicles. Expansion of the optic sulci toward the surface ectoderm and fusion of the forebrain vesicles create the *optic vesicles* (Figs. 1-9, 1-10) by approximately day 25 to 26 (embryo size, 3 mm). Closure of the neural tube and expansion of the optic vesicles occur through the mechanical influences of the cytoskeletal and extracellular matrix and localized proliferation and cell growth.[91]

The mesencephalic neural crest cells populate the region around the optic vesicle and ultimately give rise to nearly all the connective tissue structures of the avian eye, and the same can be presumed for the mammalian eye (see Table 1-1).[55,64] An external bulge indicating the presence of the invaginating optic vesicle can be seen at approximately 25 days human gestation (see Fig. 1-9). The optic vesicle appears to play a significant role in the induction and size determination of the palpebral fissure and orbital and periocular structures.[56]

At approximately 27 days gestation, the surface ectoderm that is in contact with the optic vesicle thickens to form the *lens placode* (Figs. 1-9, 1-10, 1-11). The lens placode and underlying neural ectoderm invaginate through differential growth (Fig. 1-10). The invaginating neural ectoderm folds onto itself as the optic vesicle collapses, creating a double layer of neural

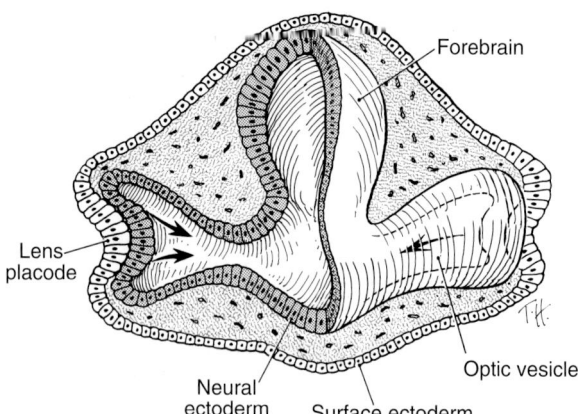

FIGURE 1-10. Drawing of a transection through a 28-day-old embryo shows invaginating lens placode and optic vesicle (*arrows*), thus creating the optic cup. Note the orientation of the eyes 180° from each other; this corresponds to the SEM view shown in Figure 1-12C.

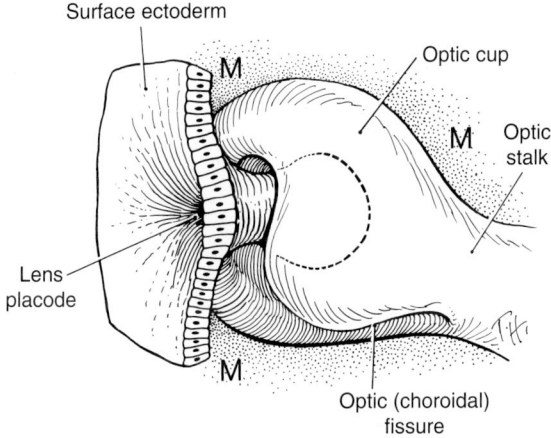

A

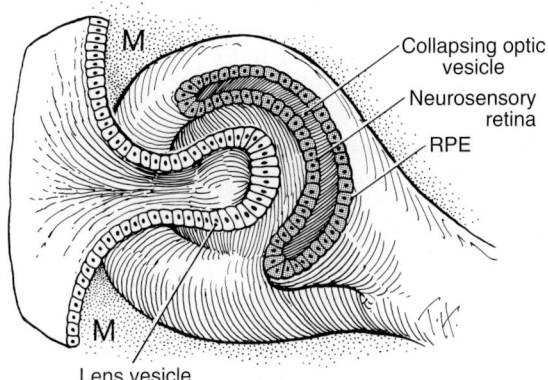

B

FIGURE 1-11A,B. Drawings show the formation of the lens vesicle and optic cup. Note that the optic fissure is present as the optic cup is not yet fused inferiorly. Mesenchyme (*M*) surrounds the invaginating lens placode. The optic stalk is continuous with the forebrain. Note that the optic cup and optic stalk are neural ectoderm. *RPE*, retinal pigment epithelium.

ectoderm, the *optic cup* (Fig. 1-11). The optic cup will eventually differentiate into *neurosensory retina* (inner layer) and *retinal pigment epithelium* (RPE) (outer layer) (Fig. 1-11). Local apical contraction[112] and physiological cell death[91] have been identified during invagination of the lens placode and formation of the optic cup. In the mouse embryo, Msx2, a homeobox-containing transcription factor, is expressed only in the cells of the optic cup that are destined to become neural retina. In vitro Msx2 has been shown to suppress RPE differentiation and may be involved in the initial patterning of the optic cup.[48] Abnormal differentiation of the outer layer of the optic cup to form aberrant neural retina has been demonstrated in several mutant mouse strains.[21,26,109] The area of future retinal differentiation demonstrates the greatest concentration of vimentin (a cytoskeletal protein) in the optic cup.[53] Regionally, within the optic cup, spatial orientation is predicted by expression of the transcription factor, vax2, which defines the ventral region (area of the optic fissure).[10] The PAX6 gene has been demonstrated within cells of neural ectodermal origin (optic cup and, later, in the ciliary body and retina), surface ectoderm (lens), and neural crest (cornea).[74] The widespread distribution of this gene supports its involvement in many stages of ocular morphogenesis.

The Optic Fissure

Invagination of the optic cup occurs in an eccentric manner with formation of a seam, the *optic fissure*, inferiorly (Figs. 1-11, 1-12). The optic fissure is also known as the *embryonic fissure* or *choroidal fissure*. Mesenchymal tissue (of primarily neural crest origin) surrounds and is within the optic fissure and optic cup, and at 5 weeks the *hyaloid artery* develops from mesenchyme in the optic fissure. This artery courses from the *optic stalk* (precursor to the optic nerve) through the optic fissure to the developing lens (Fig. 1-12). The lens vesicle separates from the surface ectoderm at approximately 6 weeks, the same time as closure of the optic fissure. Closure of the optic cup occurs initially at the equator with progression anteriorly and posteriorly.

Once the fissure has closed, secretion of primitive aqueous fluid by the primitive ciliary epithelium establishes intraocular pressure (IOP), which contributes to expansion of the optic cup.[15,29] Experimental studies have shown that placement of a capillary tube into the vitreous cavity of a chick eye reduces the IOP and markedly slows growth of the eye.[29] Histological

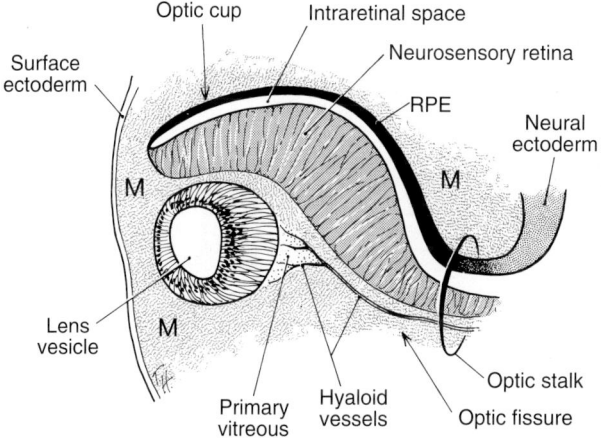

FIGURE 1-12. Drawing of cross section at approximately 5 weeks gestation through optic cup and optic fissure. The lens vesicle is separated from the surface ectoderm. Mesenchyme (*M*) surrounds the developing lens vesicle; the hyaloid artery is seen within the optic fissure. (From Cook CS, Sulik KK. Scanning Electron Microsc 1986;III:1215–1227, with permission.)

examination of these intubated eyes demonstrated proportional reduction in size of all the ocular tissues except the neural retina and the lens, which were normal in size for the age of the eye. The retina in these eyes was highly convoluted and filled the small posterior segment. Thus, it may be concluded that growth of the neural retina occurs independently of that of the other ocular tissues. Experimental removal of the lens in the eye does not alter retinal growth.[30] Growth of the choroid and sclera appear to be dependent upon IOP, as is folding of the ciliary epithelium.[12] Failure or late closure of the optic fissure prevents the establishment of normal fetal IOP and can therefore result in *microphthalmia* associated with *colobomas*, that is, colobomatous microphthalmia (see Ocular Dysgenesis later in this chapter).

Figure 1-13 shows a diagram of the eye at the end of the seventh week and after optic fissure closure. At this stage, the neurosensory retina and pigment epithelium are in apposition, the optic nerve is developing, and the lens has separated from the cornea, thus forming the anterior chamber. Mesenchymal tissue

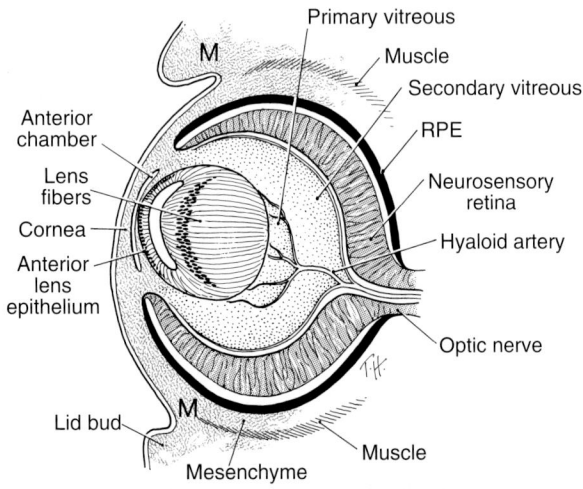

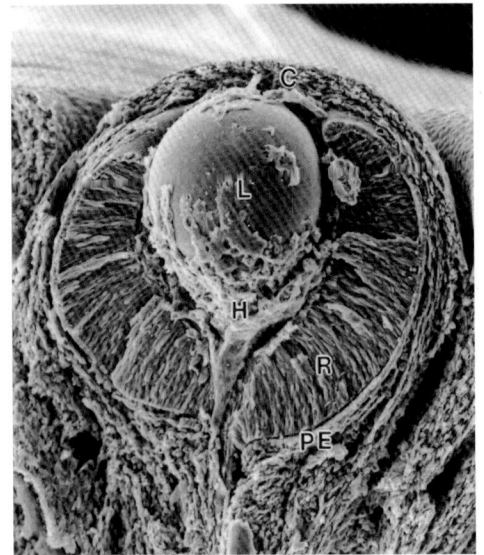

FIGURE 1-13. Overview at the 7th week of gestation. The developing eye is surrounded by mesenchyme of neural crest origin. (From Sulik KK, Schoenwolf GC. Scanning Electron Microsc 1985;IV:1735–1752, with permission.)

(neural crest cell origin) around the primitive retina develops into the choroid and sclera. Peripheral to the developing globe are linear accumulations of myoblasts (mesodermal origin) that are anlagen of the extraocular muscles. The eyelids are small buds above and below the developing eye. The hyaloid vasculature courses from the primitive optic nerve to the posterior lens capsule.

LENS

Thickening of the lens placode can be seen on gestational day 27 in the human (see Fig. 1-10). Before its contact with the optic vesicle, the surface ectoderm must become competent to respond to lens inducers. It then receives inductive signals from the anterior neural plate, so that it gains a "lens-forming bias" specified for lens formation. Complete lens differentiation requires both inductive signals from the optic vesicle and an inhibitory signal from head neural crest to suppress any residual lens-forming bias in head ectoderm adjacent to the lens.[38] In the chick, a tight extracellular matrix-mediated adhesion between the optic vesicle and the surface ectoderm has been described.[47,57,69] This anchoring of the mitotically active surface ectoderm results in cell crowding, cell elongation, and formation of the thickened placode.[119] Adhesion between the optic vesicle and the lens placode is thought to ensure alignment of the lens in the visual axis.[15] Although adhesion between the optic vesicle and surface ectoderm exists, electron microscopic studies have demonstrated that there is no direct cell contact.[22,49,108] The basement membranes of the optic vesicle and the surface ectoderm remain separate and intact throughout the contact period. Experimental studies have demonstrated a requirement for functional PAX6 gene in both the optic vesicle and surface ectoderm to mediate lens placode induction.[23] The BMP4 gene, which is present only in the optic vesicle, is also required for lens induction.[35]

The lens placode invaginates forming the hollow lens vesicle (Figs. 1-11, 1-12). The size of the lens vesicle is determined by the area of contact of the optic vesicle and the surface ectoderm. Lens vesicle detachment from the surface ectoderm occurs on day 33 (7–9 mm) and is the initial event leading to the formation of the chambers of the eye. This process of separation is accompanied by active migration of epithelial cells out of the keratolenticular stalk or junction,[37] cellular necrosis, and basement membrane breakdown.[36] Although apoptosis (programmed cell death) is a normal feature of lens vesicle separation, excessive and persistent cell death is associated with aphakia in the lap mouse mutant.[8]

Induction of a small lens vesicle that fails to undergo normal separation from the surface ectoderm is one of the characteristics of teratogen-induced anterior segment malformations described in animal models.[24,28,81,102] In the mouse mutant (dyl), this failure of lens vesicle separation is caused by a mutation in the FoxE3 gene that promotes survival and proliferation while preventing differentiation of the lens epithelium.[18] AP-2 transcription factors also influence lens vesicle separation as well as causing mis-expression of PAX6 and MIP26 genes.[109] Anterior lenticonus, anterior capsular cataracts, and anterior segment dysgenesis with keratolenticular adhesions (Peters' anomaly) may result from faulty keratolenticular separation. Further discussion of anterior segment dysgenesis follows. Arrest of lens development at the lens stalk stage results in aphakia in mutant mice (ak mutation). In addition to aphakia, affected eyes exhibit absence of a pupil and abnormalities in the iris, ciliary body, and vitreous.[40,41]

The hollow lens vesicle consists of a single layer of epithelial cells with cell apices directed toward the center of the sphere. Following detachment from the surface ectoderm, the lens vesicle is surrounded by a basal lamina, the future lens capsule. Abnormalities in this basement membrane may result in involution of the lens vesicle, resulting in later aphakia.[8] At approximately 37 days gestation, *primary lens fibers* form from elongation of the posterior lens epithelium of the lens vesicle (Fig. 1-14).[51] The retinal anlage promotes primary lens fiber formation in the adjacent lens epithelial cells. Experimental in vivo rotation of the lens vesicle in the chick eye by 180° results in elongation of the lens epithelial cells nearest the presumptive retina, regardless of the orientation of the transplanted lens.[31] Thus, the retina develops independently from the lens although the lens appears to rely upon the retina for cytodifferentiation. In the mouse, the Prox1 and Maf genes have been demonstrated to mediate lens fiber elongation.[88,110] As these posterior epithelial cells lengthen to fill the lumen of the lens vesicle, they lose their nucleus and most organelles.[14] Upregulation of lens-specific proteins, CP49 and CP95, is demonstrated after closure of the lens stalk.[51] The primitive lens filled with primary lens fibers is the *embryonic lens nucleus*. After the epithelial cells

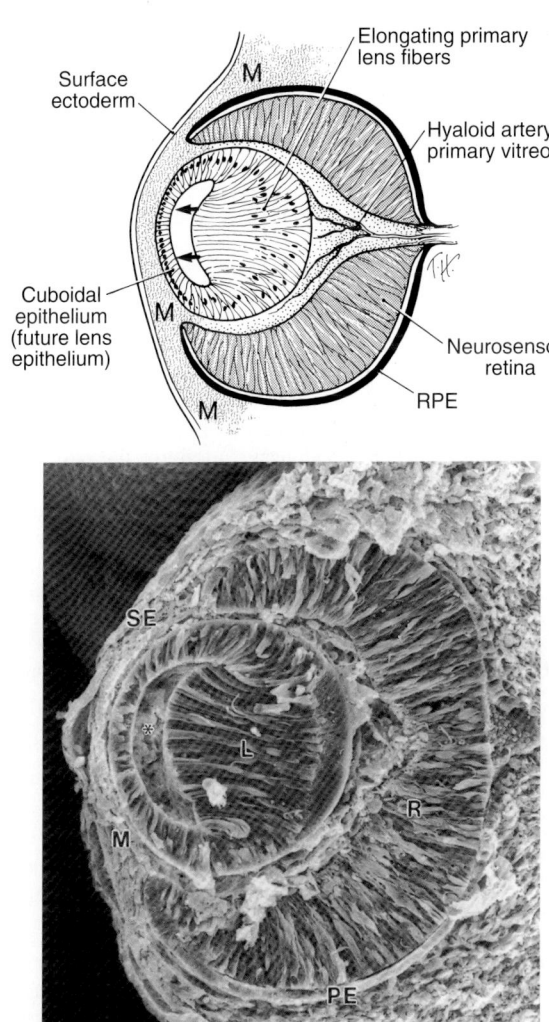

FIGURE 1-14. Formation of the embryonic lens nucleus and primary lens fibers at approximately 7 weeks. Note that mesenchyme (*M*) of neural crest origin surrounds the optic cup. The posterior lens epithelial cells (located nearest the developing retina, *R*) elongate, forming the primary lens fibers (*L*). The anterior epithelium remains cuboidal and becomes the anterior epithelium in the adult. The optic fissure is now closed.

of the posterior lens elongate to form the fibers of the embryonal nucleus, they eventually separate from the posterior capsule; therefore, there is an absence of epithelial cells on the posterior capsule. In the adult, the embryonic nucleus is the central round, slightly dark sphere inside the Y sutures. There are no sutures within the embryonal nucleus. The lens fibers have extensive interdigitations with a relative absence of extracellular space. Anterior lens epithelial cells (nearest the corneal anlage) remain cuboidal and become the permanent lens epithelium, which is mitotic throughout life, giving rise to future secondary fetal and adult cortical lens fibers.

After the embryonic nucleus is formed, *secondary lens fibers* develop from anterior epithelial cells to form the fetal nucleus. The anterior epithelial cells migrate to the periphery of the lens (lens equator), where they elongate and differentiate into lens fibers. This region of the lens is called the *lens bow*. These secondary lens fibers elongate anteriorly and posteriorly around the embryonic nucleus to meet at the anterior and posterior poles of the lens (Fig. 1-15). The lens fibers exhibit surface interdigitations with relative lack of extracellular space. Unlike more mature cortical lens fibers that have tapered ends, these fetal lens fibers (secondary lens fibers) have blunt tips, so when they meet they form a faint adherence or "suture." This meeting of the secondary lens fiber ends results in two Y sutures, the anterior upright Y suture and the posterior inverted Y suture

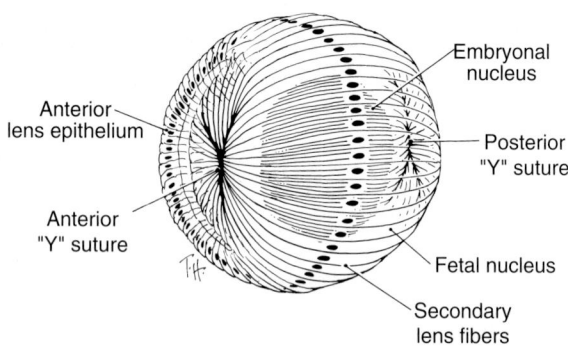

FIGURE 1-15. Diagram of secondary lens fibers and Y sutures. Secondary lens fibers elongate at the equator to span the entire lens, from the anterior Y suture to the posterior Y suture. The anterior Y suture is upright and the posterior Y suture is inverted.

(Fig. 1-15). The fetal nucleus consists of the secondary lens fibers and can be clinically identified as that part of the central lens that is inside the Y sutures but outside the embryonic nucleus. The lens differentiates under the influence of many growth factors, including FGF, IGF, PDGF, and TGF, and genes become active encoding cytoskeletal proteins (filensin, phakinin, vimentin, nestin), structural proteins (crystallins), and membrane proteins.[39,118] Abnormal initiation and differentiation of secondary lens fibers have been demonstrated in the Cat2 and Cat3 mutant mouse strains. These eyes exhibit abnormalities limited to the lens, unlike the aphakia mutant eyes, which have malformations of the anterior segment and vitreous and folding of the retina.[40]

At birth, the lens is almost entirely made up of lens nucleus with minimal lens cortex. Lens cortex continues to develop from the anterior epithelial cells postnatally and throughout life. Congenital cataracts that occur as a result of abnormal formation of primary or secondary lens fibers would be expected to be localized in the nuclear region between the Y sutures. Abnormal lens vesicle separation from the surface ectoderm would be associated with defects in anterior epithelium or lens capsule and may cause anterior polar cataracts. Incomplete regression of the pupillary membrane can be associated with (secondary) anterior lens opacities. A defect of the surface ectoderm or basement membrane could result in cataracts associated with anterior or posterior lenticonus.

Tunica Vasculosa Lentis

The lens receives nutrition and blood supply from the *hyaloid artery*, a branch of the primitive ophthalmic artery. The hyaloid artery first enters the eye through the optic fissure (see Fig. 1-12) and then becomes incorporated into the center of the optic nerve as the optic fissure closes. The hyaloid vessels form a network around the posterior lens capsule and then anastomose anteriorly with the network of vessels in the pupillary membrane (Fig. 1-16). The pupillary membrane consists of vessels and mesenchyme that overlie the anterior lens capsule (see Development of Anterior Segment). This hyaloid vascular network that forms around the lens is called the *tunica vasculosa lentis*. The hyaloid vasculature reaches its greatest development at approximately 10 weeks gestation. The tunica vasculosa lentis and hyaloid artery regress during the end of the fourth month of

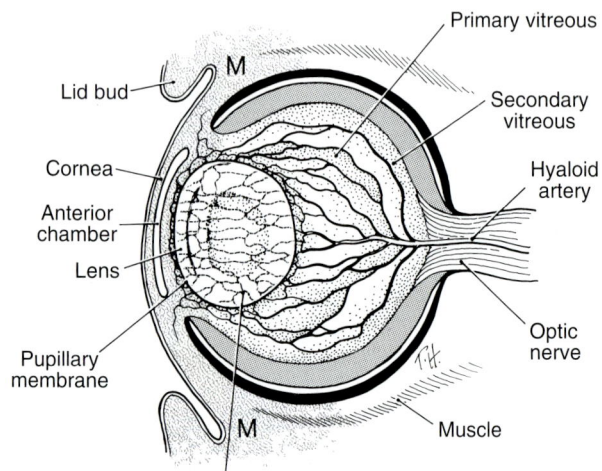

FIGURE 1-16. Drawing of a 2-month-old fetal eye shows the hyaloid vascular system and tunica vasculosa lentis.

gestation. The clinical lens anomaly, *Mittendorf's dot*, is a small (1–2 mm) area of fibrosis on the posterior capsule and is probably a manifestation of incomplete regression of the hyaloid artery where it attaches to the posterior capsule. The regression of the pupillary membrane begins during the sixth month and is usually complete by the eighth month. *Persistent pupillary membranes* result from incomplete regression. These iris strands may connect to an anterior polar cataract (Fig. 1-17) or area of corneal endothelial fibrosis.

CORNEA AND ANTERIOR CHAMBER

The anterior margins of the optic cup advance beneath the surface ectoderm and its subjacent mesenchyme following lens vesicle detachment at approximately day 33 of gestation. The surface ectoderm overlying the optic cup and lens represents the presumptive *corneal epithelium*; it secretes a thick matrix producing the *primary cornea stroma*.[43] This acellular material consists of collagen fibers, hyaluronic acid, and glycosaminoglycans. Neural crest cells migrate between the surface ectoderm and

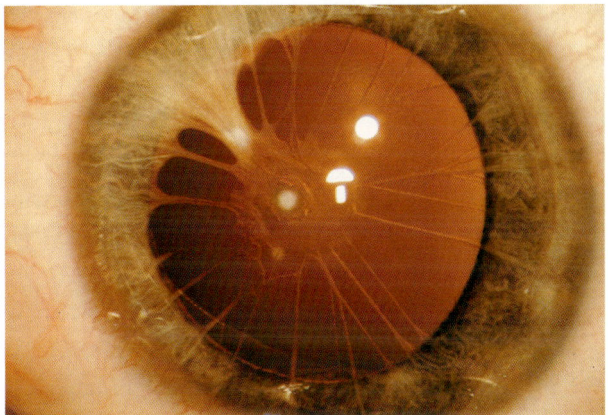

FIGURE 1-17. Photograph of persistent pupillary membrane with small central anterior polar cataract.

optic cup using the basal lamina of the lens vesicle as a substrate or scaffold.[11] Hydration of hyaluronic acid helps to create the space for cellular migration.[105] This loosely arranged neural crest cell-derived mesenchyme initially fills the future anterior chamber and gives rise to the corneal stroma, corneal endothelium, the anterior iris stroma, the ciliary muscle, and most of the structures of the iridocorneal angle. Separation of the corneal mesenchyme (neural crest cell origin) from the lens (surface ectoderm origin) results in formation of the anterior chamber. Mesenchymal tissue surrounds the lens and forms the tunica vasculosa lentis and is continuous anteriorly with the pupillary membrane. Capillaries within the tunica vasculosa lentis anastomose with the hyaloid vascular system. The vascular endothelium appears to be the only component of the anterior segment that is of mesodermal origin, as even the vascular smooth muscle cells and pericytes are of neural crest origin.[55,64]

The anterior corneal stroma remains acellular and gives rise to *Bowman's membrane*, which underlies the corneal epithelium. Although the corneal epithelium is of surface ectodermal origin, Bowman's membrane is a condensation of anterior corneal stroma that is of neural crest cell origin. Type I collagen fibrils and fibronectin secreted by the developing keratocytes (neural crest cell origin) form the secondary corneal stroma. Subsequent dehydration of the corneal stroma results in loss of much of the fibronectin and a 50% reduction in thickness of the stroma.[44,65] The endothelium plays an important role in the dehydration of the stroma. Patches of endothelium become confluent during the early part of the fourth month of gestation and develop zonulae occludentes at their apices by the middle of the fourth month of gestation.[115] By the sixth month of gestation, *Descemet's membrane* and *endothelium* are structurally and functionally present and, at this time, the cornea achieves relative transparency. Proteoglycans containing keratan sulfate chains play a role in generating and maintaining corneal transparency.[34]

IRIS AND CILIARY BODY

The two layers of the optic cup (neural ectoderm origin) consist of an inner nonpigmented layer and an outer pigmented layer. Both the pigmented and nonpigmented epithelia of the iris and ciliary body develop from the anterior aspect of the optic cup whereas the retina develops from the posterior optic cup. The optic vesicle is organized with all cell apices directed to the center of the vesicle (see Figs. 1-10, 1-11). During optic cup invagination, the apices of the inner and outer epithelial layers become adjacent. Thus, the cells of the optic cup are oriented apex to apex.

A thin periodic acid–Schiff-(PAS) positive basal lamina lines the inner aspect (vitreous side) of the nonpigmented epithelium and retina (inner limiting membrane). At approximately 4.5 months, both the pigmented and nonpigmented epithelial cells show apical cilia that project into the intercellular space. There is also increased prominence of Golgi complexes and associated vesicles within the ciliary epithelial cells.[12] These changes and the presence of "ciliary channels" between apical surfaces probably represent the first production of aqueous humor.[113]

The iris develops by an anterior growth of the optic cup. The iris stroma develops from the anterior segment mesenchymal tissue of neural crest cell origin. The iris epithelium, including the pupillary sphincter and dilator muscles, originates from the neural ectoderm of the optic cup.[51,62,63,104] The smooth muscles of the pupillary sphincter and dilator muscles represent the only muscles in the body of neural ectodermal origin. In avian species, however, the pupillary muscles are striated and originate from stromal mesenchymal (neural crest) cells that migrate into the muscle bundles to become skeletal muscle cells.[116,117]

The ciliary body develops as the neuroectoderm of the anterior optic cup folds, and underlying mesenchyme differentiates into the ciliary muscles. Tertiary vitreous in the area of the ciliary body folds develops into lens zonules.

IRIDOCORNEAL ANGLE

Iridocorneal angle maturation begins during the 15th week of gestation through a combination of processes.[85–87] Differential growth of the vascular tunic results in posterior movement of the iris and ciliary body relative to the trabecular meshwork and exposure of the outflow pathways.[4] *Schlemm's canal* is identified during the 16th week.[114] There is gradual cellular rearrangement and mesenchymal atrophy, as well as enlargement of numerous large spaces, until they become confluent with the anterior chamber.[98] The corneal trabeculae enlarges and the corneal endothelium covering the angle recess regresses. The discontinuity of the cellular layer covering the angle and the many lacunae present in late gestation may be correlated with the normal development of an increase in the outflow facility of aqueous humor. It may be speculated that, if the splitting and rebuilding of the endothelial membrane lining of the early iridocorneal angle is arrested, a block to normal outflow may result. Persistence of the endothelial (Barkan's) membrane has been postulated to be of significance in the pathogenesis of congenital glaucoma.[13,42,61,68,70,111] Postnatal remodeling of the drainage angle is associated with cellular necrosis and phagocytosis by macrophages, resulting in opening of the spaces of Fontana (clefts in the trabecular meshwork) and outflow pathways.[86,87]

Studies using staining for neuron-specific enolase (NSE) indicate that, although most of the structures of the iridocorneal angle are of neural crest origin, the endothelial lining of Schlemm's canal (like the vascular endothelium) is mesodermal.[1,78]

CHOROID AND SCLERA

Both the choroid and the sclera are of neural crest origin. The anterior sclera forms as a condensation of mesenchymal tissue that is continuous with the cornea (see Fig. 1-13). This condensation progresses posteriorly toward the optic nerve and, by approximately 12 weeks, the mesenchymal condensation has enveloped the optic nerve. The lamina cribrosa consists of mesenchymal cells that have penetrated the optic nerve. The cornea and sclera are derived from the same mesenchymal tissue, except for the corneal epithelium, which is of surface ectoderm origin.

The choroid is a highly vascular pigmented tissue that develops from mesenchymal tissue (neural crest) surrounding endothelial blood spaces (mesoderm). The blood spaces organize and give rise to the embryonic choriocapillaris at approximately 2 months of gestation.[16,45,80] At approximately 4 months, the choriocapillaris connects with the short posterior arteries and joins with the outer venous layer and the four vortex veins. Outside the choriocapillaris, multiple anastomoses between arterioles and venules occur, thus forming the fetal choroid plexus.

RETINA

The retina develops from neural ectoderm, with the retinal pigment epithelium (RPE) developing from the outer layer of the optic cup and the neurosensory retina developing from the inner layer of the optic cup (Figs. 1-11, 1-12, 1-13, 1-14, 1-18). As with the ciliary epithelium, invagination of the optic vesicle causes the apices of the inner nonpigmented layer to be directed

FIGURE 1-18A–C. (A) At approximately 38 days, the hyaloid vasculature surrounds the lens (*L*) with capillaries that anastomose with the tunica vasculosa lentis. Axial migration of mesenchyme forms the corneal stroma and endothelium (*C*). The retina (*R*) is becoming stratified while the pigment epithelium (*PE*) remains cuboidal. (B) By day 41, the retina has segregated into inner (*IN*) and outer (*ON*) neuroblastic layers. The ganglion cells are the first to differentiate, giving rise to the nerve fiber layer (*arrowhead*). The pigment epithelium has become artifactually separated from the neural retina in this specimen. (From Cook CS, Sulik KK. Scanning Electron Microsc 1986;III:1215–1227, with permission.) (C) Differentiation of the retina progresses from the central to the peripheral regions. At this time, the inner (*IN*) and outer (*ON*) neuroblastic layers are apparent at the posterior pole but, peripherally, the retina consists of outer nuclear and inner marginal zones. Between the inner and outer neuroblastic layers is a clear zone, the transient fiber layer of Chievitz. *PE*, pigment epithelium; *arrowhead*, nerve fiber layer. (From Cook CS, Sulik KK. Scanning Electron Microsc 1986;III:1215–1227, with permission.)

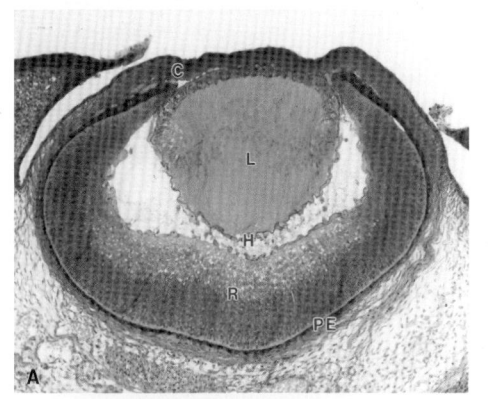

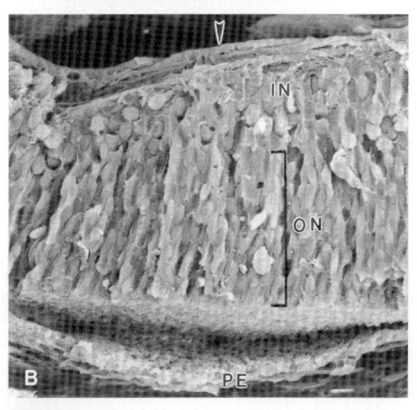

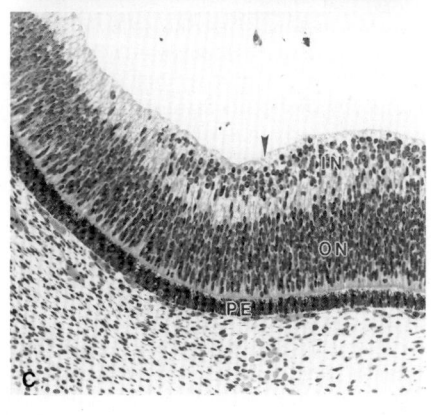

outward, to face the apices of the outer pigmented layer, which are directed inward. Thus, the apices of these two cell layers are in direct contact. Primitive RPE cells are columnar, but by 5 weeks they change shape to form a single layer of cuboidal cells that exhibit the first pigment granules in the embryo. Bruch's membrane, the basal lamina of the RPE, is first seen during this time (optic cup stage) and becomes well developed by 6 weeks when the choriocapillaris is starting to form. By 4 months, the RPE cells take on a hexagonal shape on cross section and develop microvilli that interdigitate with projections from photoreceptors of the nonpigmented layer.

By the sixth week postfertilization, the nonpigmented inner layer of the optic cup differentiates into an outer nuclear zone and an inner marginal zone. Cell proliferation occurs in the nuclear zone with migration of cells into the marginal zone. This process forms the inner and outer neuroblastic layers (Fig. 1-18B,C), separated by their cell processes, which make up the transient fiber layer of Chievitz. With further realignment of cells, this layer is mostly obliterated by 8 to 10 weeks gestation. The ganglion cells of the inner neuroblastic layer are the first to differentiate (7th week), giving rise to a primitive nerve fiber layer (Fig. 1-18B,C, arrow).

By the 16th week, mitosis has nearly ceased and retinal differentiation commences, as does synaptic contact between retinal neurons.[99] Cellular differentiation progresses in a wave from inner to outer layers and from central retina to peripheral retina (Fig. 1-18C). The ganglion cells give rise to a more defined nerve fiber layer that courses to the developing optic nerve. Cell bodies of the Mueller and amacrine cells differentiate in the inner portion of the outer neuroblastic layer; bipolar cells are found in the middle of the outer neuroblastic layer, with horizontal cells and photoreceptors maturing last, in the outermost zone of the retina.[99] Early in development, retinal cells demonstrate neurite regeneration in vitro. This regenerative capability decreases with age and is lost postnatally in the rat at a time that corresponds to the time of eye opening and retinal maturation (equivalent to the eighth month of human gestation).[106] Thy-1, the most abundant surface glycoprotein found in the retina, is primarily associated with ganglion cells and appears to regulate neurite outgrowth.[97]

Macular differentiation occurs relatively late, beginning in the sixth month.[46] First, multiple rows of ganglion cells accumulate in the central macular area. At this time, the immature cones are localized in the central macular area while the rods develop in the periphery. At 7 months, the inner layers of the retina (including ganglion cells) spread out to form the central macular depression or primitive fovea. The cones in the foveal area elongate, allowing denser cone populations and enhanced foveal resolution. These changes in foveal cones continue until after birth. At birth, the fovea is fairly well developed and consists of a single row of ganglion cells, a row of bipolar cells, and a horizontal outer plexiform layer of Henle. It is not until several months postpartum that the ganglion cells and bipolar cells completely vacate the fovea centralis.

Retinal Vasculature

The fetal ophthalmic artery is a branch of the internal carotid artery and terminates into the hyaloid artery. The hyaloid artery enters the optic cup via the optic fissures and stalk (developing optic nerve) (see Fig. 1-12). At approximately 6 weeks gestation, the ophthalmic artery becomes entrapped in the optic cup as the optic fissure closes. The portion of the hyaloid artery within the optic stalk eventually becomes the central retinal artery, while the more terminal parts of the hyaloid artery arborize around the posterior aspect of the developing lens. The hyaloid artery gradually atrophies and regresses as branches of the hyaloid artery become sporadically occluded by macrophages.[52,54] Regression of the hyaloid vasculature is usually complete by the fifth month of human gestation. *Bergmeister's papilla* represents a remnant of the hyaloid vasculature that does not regress; this is a benign anomaly consisting of a small fibrous glial tuft of tissue that emanates from the center of the optic disc.

The hyaloid vasculature is the primary source of nutrition to the embryonic retina. Regression of the hyaloid vasculature serves to stimulate retinal vessel angiogenesis. Spindle-shaped mesenchymal cells from the wall of the hyaloid vein at the optic disc form buds that invade the nerve fiber layer during the fourth month of gestation.[6] Subsequently, solid cords of mesenchymal cells within the inner retina canalize and contain occasional red blood cells at approximately 5 months gestation. In situ differentiation of craniofacial angioblasts has been demonstrated in avian species using polyclonal antibodies to quail endothelial cells.[75] Vascular budding and further differentiation form the deeper capillary network in the retina.[73] The primitive capillaries have laminated walls consisting of mitotically active cells secreting basement membrane.[95] Those cells in direct contact with the bloodstream differentiate into endothelial cells while the outer cells become pericytes. Tissue culture experiments have demonstrated that the primitive capillary endothelial cells are multipotent and can redifferentiate into fibroblastic, endothelial, or muscle cells, possibly illustrating a common origin of these different tissue types.[6] Pigment epithelium derived factor (PEDF) has been demonstrated to inhibit angiogenesis of the cornea and vitreous. Inadequate levels may play a permissive role in ischemia-driven aberrant vascularization.[33]

The central retinal artery grows from the optic nerve to the periphery, forming the temporal and nasal retinal arcades. By approximately 5 months, the retinal arcades have progressed to the equator of the eye. At this time, the long and short posterior ciliary arteries are well developed, with the long posterior artery supplying the anterior segment and the short posterior artery supplying the choroid. The retinal arteries grow from the optic nerve toward the ora serrata and reach the nasal periphery first (by 8 months).[73] Even at birth, however, there is usually a crescent of avascular retina in the temporal periphery. The fact that a newborn infant has an immature temporal retina without complete vascularization may explain why there have been scattered cases of retinopathy of prematurity in full-term infants. Oxygen affects angiogenesis and seems to play a role in stimulating and retarding vessel growth.[83] In immature kitten retinas, increased oxygen concentration causes atrophy and regression of capillaries whereas hypoxia increases capillary arborization.[79] Endothelial cell growth is also promoted by low oxygen tension, and endothelial growth is inhibited by high oxygen tension.[7] *Vasoendothelial growth factor (VEGF)* both stimulates and maintains normal vessel growth to the peripheral retina. High oxygen downregulates VEGF, stopping the normal process of peripheral vascularization.[2,58,84] These findings give rise to the hypothesis that retinopathy of prematurity (ROP) is secondary to initial increased oxygen concentration, which results in inhibition or retraction of peripheral capillary networks (*vasoobliteration*).[5] This lack of peripheral capillary network subsequently results in retinal hypoxia increased VEGF then secondary endothelial cell growth and neovascularization (i.e., ROP).[82] There is evidence that strict curtailment of O_2 dose early in a premature infants course reduces the incidence of severe ROP.[112a]

VITREOUS

The primary vitreous first appears at approximately 5 weeks gestation and consists of the hyaloid vessels surrounded by mesenchymal cells, collagenous fibrillar material, and macrophages (see Fig. 1-12). Most of the mesenchymal cells are of neural crest origin. The secondary vitreous forms at approximately 8 weeks at the time of fetal fissure closure (see Fig. 1-13).[9] It circumferentially surrounds the primary vitreous containing the hyaloid vessels. The secondary vitreous consists of a gel containing compact fibrillar network, primitive hyalocytes, monocytes, and a small amount of hyaluronic acid.[19] Primitive hyalocytes produce collagen fibrils that expand the volume of the secondary vitreous. At the end of the third month, the tertiary vitreous forms as a thick accumulation of collagen fibers between the lens and optic cup (Fig. 1-19). These fibers are called the marginal bundle of Drualt. Drualt's bundle has a strong attachment to the inner layer of the optic cup and is the precursor to the vitreous base and lens zonules. The early lens zonular fibers appear

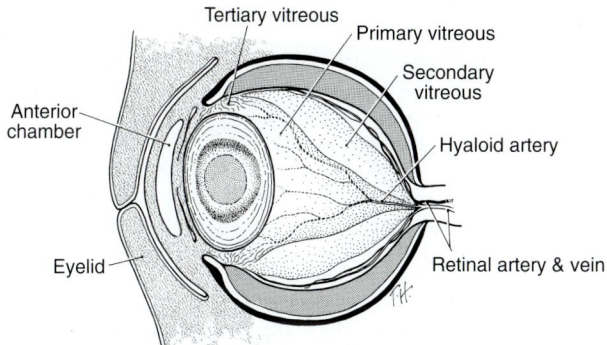

FIGURE 1-19. Drawing of cross section of a 10-week-old eye shows the primary vitreous, secondary vitreous, and tertiary vitreous. The primary vitreous includes the hyaloid artery and associated matrix; it extends centrally from the optic nerve to the retrolental space. The secondary vitreous surrounds the primary vitreous; it has less vasculature and is clearer than the primary vitreous. The tertiary vitreous forms between the lens equator and the area of the ciliary body; the lens zonules develop within the fibrillar matrix in this. Note that eyelids are fused at this stage.

to be continuous with the inner limiting membrane of the non-pigmented epithelial layer covering the ciliary muscle. Toward the end of the fourth month of gestation, the primary vitreous and hyaloid vasculature atrophies to a clear, narrow central zone, *Cloquet's canal*. Apoptosis occurs during hyaloid vessel regression.[51] Persistence of the primary vitreous and failure of the posterior tunica vasculosa lentis to regress can result in *persistent hyperplastic vitreous* (PHPV). PHPV consists of a fibrovascular membrane that extends from the optic nerve along the hyaloid remnant and covers the posterior capsule of the lens. During the fifth month of gestation, an attachment forms between the ciliary body and the lens (*Weiger's ligament,* or capsulohyaloidal ligament). Later in development, at approximately 5 to 6 months, the hyaloid system completely regresses and the hyaloid artery blood flow ceases. At birth, Cloquet's canal persists as an optically clear zone emanating from the optic nerve to the back of the lens. Cloquet's canal is a remnant of primary vitreous. Most of the posterior vitreous gel at birth is secondary vitreous with the vitreous base and zonules representing tertiary vitreous.

OPTIC NERVE

The optic stalk is the initially hollow structure connecting the optic vesicle with the forebrain. At approximately 6 weeks gestation, axons from developing ganglion cells pass through vacuolated cells from the inner wall of the optic stalk. Emanating from the center of the primitive nerve is the hyaloid artery. A glial sheath forms around the hyaloid artery. As the hyaloid artery regresses, a space between the hyaloid artery and the glial sheath enlarges. Bergmeister's papilla represents a remnant of these glial cells around the hyaloid artery. The extent of the Bergmeister's papilla is dependent on the amount of hyaloid and glial cell regression. Glial cells in this area migrate into the optic nerve and form the primitive optic disc. The glial cells around the optic nerve and the glial part of the lamina cribrosa come from the inner layer of the optic stalk, which is of neural ectoderm origin. Later, there is development of a mesenchymal (neural crest cell) portion of the lamina cribrosa. By the third month, the optic nerve shifts nasally as the temporal aspect of the posterior pole enlarges. The *tissue of Kuhnt*, which circumferentially surrounds the intraocular part of the optic nerve and acts as a barrier between the optic nerve and retina, comes from glial tissue in the region of the disc and mesenchyme from nearby developing retinal vasculature. Myelinization of the optic nerve starts at the chiasm at about 7 months gestation and progresses toward the eye. Normally, myelinization stops at the lamina cribrosa at about 1 month after birth. At birth, the myelin is thin, with the layers of myelin increasing into late childhood.

Myelinated nerve fibers occur if the myelinization continues past the lamina cribrosa (Fig. 1-20). The best explanation as to why myelinization passes the lamina cribrosa is the presence of heterotopic oligodendrocytes or glial cells within the retinal nerve fiber layer. This concept contrasts with the theory that there is a congenital defect in the lamina cribrosa that allows myelinization to progress into the retina. Autopsy studies of myelinated nerve fibers have failed to show a defect in the lamina cribrosa; therefore, myelinated nerve fibers most probably represent ectopic myelinization.[100,101] Myelinization of the nerve fibers is often associated with high myopia and amblyopia. Patients with this disorder should be aggressively treated by correcting the refractive error and initiating occlusion

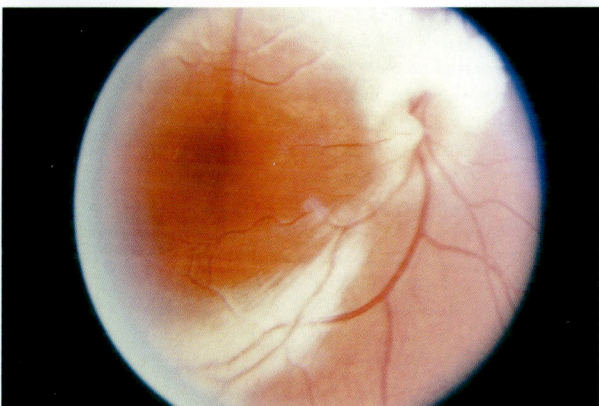

FIGURE 1-20. Photograph of myelinated nerve fibers emanating from the disc. Myelinated nerve fibers will cause a local scotoma; however, in the macular and foveal region, their presence does not usually preclude good central vision.

therapy of the sound eye to treat the amblyopia, as good visual outcome can be achieved even when there is macular involvement.[103]

EYELIDS

The eyelids develop from surface ectoderm that gives rise to the epidermis, cilia, and conjunctival epithelium. Neural crest cell mesenchyme gives rise to deeper structures including the dermis and tarsus. The eyelid muscles, orbicularis and levator, are derived from mesoderm. By 6 weeks of gestation, the upper and lower eyelid buds are visible (see Fig. 1-15). They come from mesenchymal accumulations called frontonasal (upper lid) and maxillary (lower lid) processes. The lid folds grow together and elongate to cover the developing eye. Upper and lower lids fuse together at approximately 10 weeks. By 6 months gestation, glandular structures and cilia develop, and the lids gradually separate.

EXTRAOCULAR MUSCLES

The extraocular muscles arise from mesoderm in somitomeres (preotic mesodermal segments), with the primitive muscle cone first appearing at 5 to 7 weeks gestation (Fig. 1-13). The oculo-motor innervated muscles originate from the first and second somitomeres, the superior oblique muscle from the third somit-omere, and the lateral rectus muscle from the fifth somito-mere.[77] The motor nerves to the extraocular muscles grow from the brain to the muscle and innervate the mesodermal conden-sation at approximately 1 month.

The extraocular muscles develop from local mesenchyme (mesodermal origin) in situ within the orbit, rather than from anterior growth of surrounding mesoderm, as had been an earlier hypothesis. Additionally, muscles do not grow from the orbital apex anteriorly; rather, the insertion, belly, and origin develop simultaneously.[93,94] The orbital axes rotate from the early stages of optic cup development to adulthood.

OCULAR DYSGENESIS

Syndromes of ocular dysgenesis are summarized in Table 1-2.

Microphthalmia

Studies of ocular malformations induced by teratogen exposure have been helpful in identifying sensitive periods during development. Microphthalmia and anophthalmia may result from insult at a number of developmental stages. Acute exposure to teratogens during early gastrulation stages results in an overall deficiency of the neural plate with subsequent reduction in size of the optic vesicle. This aberration results in microphthalmia, which may be associated with a spectrum of secondary malformations including anterior segment dysgenesis, cataract, and PHPV.[24,27,28] Deficiency in size of the globe as a whole is often associated with a corresponding small palpebral fissure. Because the fissure size is determined by the size of the optic vesicle (most likely during its contact with the surface ectoderm), support is provided for a malformation sequence beginning at the time of formation of the optic sulcus or optic vesicle.

Failure or late closure of the optic fissure prevents the establishment of normal fetal IOP and can result in microphthalmia associated with colobomas, that is, colobomatous microphthalmia (Fig. 1-27). This syndrome may be associated with orbital (or eyelid) cysts (Fig. 1-28). It is important to recognize that delay in closure of the fissure during a critical growth period may result in inadequate globe expansion. However, if the fissure eventually closes, it may be difficult to distinguish between colobomatous and noncolobomatous microphthalmia. In colobomatous microphthalmia, the optic vesicle size is initially normal and a normal-sized palpebral fissure would be expected, whereas with microphthalmia that results from a primary abnormality in the neural plate and optic sulci, the palpebral fissure would be small.

Optic Fissure Closure Anomalies (Coloboma)

Colobomas represent an absence of tissue that may occur through abnormal fusion of the optic fissure, which normally closes at 4 to 5 weeks gestation. Colobomas may occur anywhere along the optic fissure and can affect the iris, choroid,

TABLE 1-2. Summary of Syndromes of Ocular Malformations.

Syndrome	Microphthalmia	Anterior segment dysgenesis	Ocular coloboma	Glaucoma
CHARGE	+		+	
Meckel's	+		+ Uveal	
Rubenstein–Taybi			+	
Basal cell nevus syndrome			+ Iris	
Cat's eye		+	+	
Axenfeld-Rieger's Autosomal dominant iridogoniodysgenesis		+		+ Gonio-dysgenesis
Nail patella		Iris hypoplasia Ciliary body hypoplasia		
Branchiootorenal		+		Cataract
Microphthalmia	+	+/−	+/−	+/−
Peters' anomaly	+/−	+		

TABLE 1-2. (continued)

Other ocular abnormalities	Nonocular anomalies	Genetics (mice)	Genetics (human)
	Choanal atresia Growth retardation Genital hypoplasia Ear anomalies (deafness) Hypospadias		+/− X-linked autosomal recessive
	Heart defect Renal/hepatic disease Occipital encephaloceles Microcephaly Hydrocephaly Cleft palate		Autosomal recessive condition mapped to chromosome 17q21-q24
Cataract Ptosis	Mental retardation Broad fingers and toes Short stature Cardiac anomalies Renal anomalies		Translocation involving chromosome 2p13.3 and 16p13.3
Strabismus Cataract	Hypertelorism Basal cell nevus Cleft lip/palate Mental retardation Anal atresia Preauricular skin tags Renal anomalies		CECR1 on 9q22.3-q31 22q11
Iris hypoplasia	Craniofacial Dental defects Hypertelorism	FoxC1 FoxC2 Mfl (mice)	FKHL7 gene 6p24-p25
		Lmx1B	Chromosome 9
Branchial arch	anomalies Ear anomalies Renal anomalies	EYA1 17 Ccnf	16p13.3 14q32
Anterior lenticonus; cataract	Craniofacial Heart defects Dwarfism Syndactyly	Cat4a on chromosome 8	RIEG1 on chromosome 4q25

(continued)

TABLE 1-2. Summary of Syndromes of Ocular Malformations. (continued)

Syndrome	Microphthalmia	Anterior segment dysgenesis	Ocular coloboma	Glaucoma
Renal/coloboma		Optic disc coloboma		
Cyclopia/holo-procecephaly	+/–	+/–	+/–	+/–
Leber's congenital amaurosis				
Septooptic dysplasia				
Rieger's anterior segment dysgenesis		+		
Aniridia	+/–	+	+/–	+
Goldenhar's oculoauriculovertebral	+	Upper lid coloboma		

Source: NIH Online Mendelian Inheritance in Man: www3.ncbi.nlm.nih.gov/

macula, and optic nerve (Figs. 1-21, 1-22, 1-23). Colobomas are often associated with microphthalmia (colobomatous microphthalmia) or, less frequently, orbital or eyelid cysts (Fig. 1-22). Because the optic fissure closes first at the equator of the eye, and then in a posterior and anterior direction, colobomas are most frequently found at the two ends of the optic fissure, that is, iris and optic nerve. When the optic nerve is involved in the coloboma, vision is usually affected, in some cases causing blindness. Optic nerve colobomas may be associated with basal encephaloceles, which also represent a failure of fissure closure.[59,85] Large choroidal colobomas may be associated with posterior pole staphylomas, causing macular disruption and poor vision. Occasionally, a line of choroidal colobomas occur along the fetal fissure area with skip areas (Fig. 1-23). Isolated iris colobomas usually do not affect visual acuity unless there is an associated refractive error. Typical iris colobomas occur infer-

TABLE 1-2. (continued)

Other ocular abnormalities	Nonocular anomalies	Genetics (mice)	Genetics (human)
	Renal anomalies	19 Pax2	PAX2 on 10q24.3-q25.1
Cyclopia	Holopro-cencephaly		Sonic hedgehog (SHH) on 7q36 HPE12on 1q22.3
Cataract pigmentary retinopathy Keratoconus	Central blindness Mental retardation	3 Rpe65	CRX Autosomal recessive RPE65 on 1p31
Optic disc hypoplasia	Growth hormone deficiency	14Hesx1	Autosomal recessive HESX1 on 3p21.1-3p21.2
Cataract ± Corneal opacity		Fra-2	Autosomal dominant 4q28-q31(PAX6), PITX3 on 10q25
Cataract Foveal hypoplasia	Wilm's tumor	2Sey	Autosomal dominant PAX6 on 11p13
Epibulbar dermoid	Ear malformations Facial asymmetry Vertebral anomalies		Autosomal dominant GHS on 7p

onasally along the location of the optic fissure whereas atypical iris colobomas are not associated with abnormal fissure closure and can occur elsewhere. Atypical iris colobomas usually have an intact iris root (Fig. 1-24).

Differentiation of choroidal and iris stroma is determined by the adjacent structures of the optic cup: the iris epithelium, anteriorly, and the future retinal pigment epithelium, posteriorly. In animals exhibiting primary abnormalities in differentiation of the outer layer of the optic cup, anterior and posterior segment colobomas are seen in a very specific distribution associated with the iris epithelium or RPE defects,[25,26] and this is the most likely explanation for atypical uveal colobomas. The term lens coloboma is actually a misnomer, as this defect results from a lack of the zonular pull in the region of the coloboma rather than regional hypoplasia of the lens. Ciliary body colobomas are often associated with abnormal lens shape or subluxation or both.

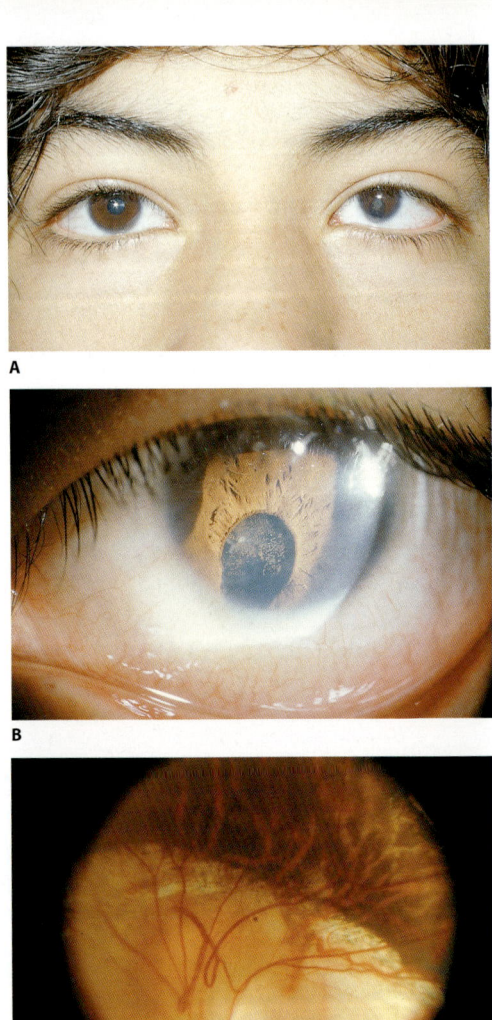

FIGURE 1-21A–C. **(A)** Photograph of patient with left colobomatous microphthalmia and normal right eye. **(B)** Slit lamp view of the iris coloboma left eye. Note the pigment on anterior capsule of the lens. **(C)** Optic nerve coloboma of left eye with inferior choroidal coloboma that extended anteriorly to meet the iris coloboma seen in **(B)**.

Colobomatous microphthalmia with eyelid cyst syndrome may be unilateral or bilateral (see Fig. 1-28). Colobomatous cysts form from the inner layer (neuroectoderm) of the optic cup as it grows out of the persistent opening of the optic fissure. The lower lid cyst contains primitive vitreous contents that were not enclosed within the eye because the optic fissure did not close. The cyst has a stalk that connects to the microphthalmic eye. For those who are unaware of the syndrome, the lid cyst is often mistaken as an abnormal eye located in the lid.

Dermoids and Dermolipomas

Dermoids are choristomas (histologically normal tissue in an abnormal location) and are thought to represent arrest or inclusions of epidermal and connective tissues (surface ectoderm and neural crest cells). They may be associated with abnormal closure of the optic fissure. This collection of epidermal and connective tissue can occur at the limbus (limbal dermoid), in the conjunctiva (dermolipoma), and subcutaneously in and around the orbit. The most common location of subcutaneous periorbital dermoid cysts is the superotemporal and superonasal quadrants of the orbital rim. These dermoids are usually found attached to bone, associated with a cranial suture.

Limbal dermoids are similar to subcutaneous dermoid cysts and consist of epidermal tissue and, frequently, hair (Fig. 1-25). Corneal astigmatism is common in patients with limbal dermoids. Astigmatisms greater than $+1.50$ are usually associated with meridional and anisometropic amblyopia. Removal of limbal dermoids is often indicated for functional and cosmetic reasons, but the patient should be warned that a secondary scar can recur over this area. Limbal dermoids can involve deep corneal stroma, so the surgeon must take care to avoid perforation into the anterior chamber.

Dermolipomas (lipodermoids) are usually located in the lateral canthal area and consist of fatty fibrous tissue (Fig. 1-26). They are almost never a functional or cosmetic problem and are best left alone. If removal is necessary, only a limited dissection should be performed to avoid symblepharon and scarring of the lateral rectus. Unfortunately, restrictive strabismus with limited adduction frequently occurs after removal of temporal dermolipomas.

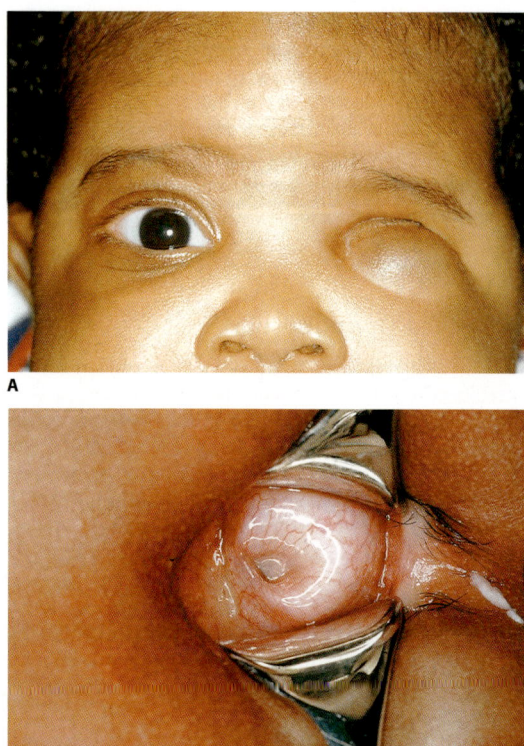

FIGURE 1-22A–B. (A) Photograph of 6-month-old with colobomatous microphthalmia and orbital cyst anomaly. Note the left lower eyelid cyst causing a mass in the lower lid, left blepharophimosis (small lids and narrow lid fissure), and apparently normal right eye. **(B)** Desmarres retractors open the eyelids in an attempt to expose the microphthalmic left eye. The only remnant of eye that could be seen externally was a small dimple just nasal to the lid retractors.

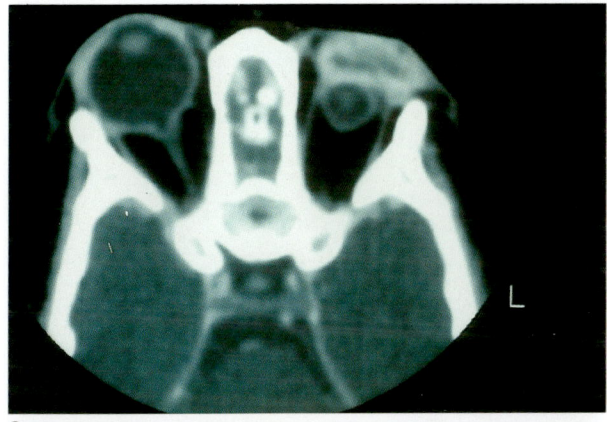

C

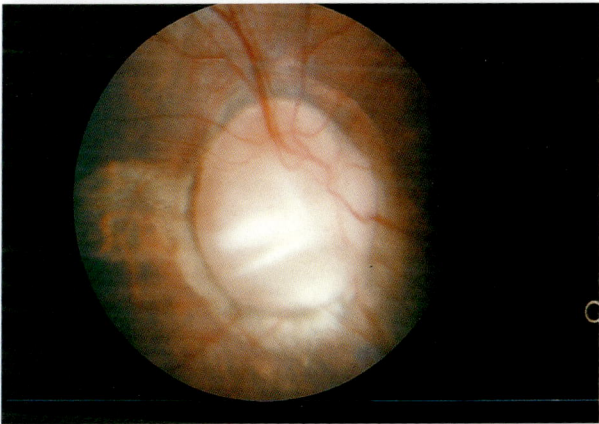

D

FIGURE 1-22C–D. (C) CT scan shows the presence of a left microph-thalmic eye, left lower lid cyst, and right optic nerve coloboma. At the time of surgery to remove the cyst, a stalk was found connecting the cyst to the microphthalmic eye. **(D)** Fundus photograph of optic nerve, right eye (good eye). Note the presence of a large optic nerve coloboma. This was an isolated optic nerve coloboma; the right eye was otherwise normal.

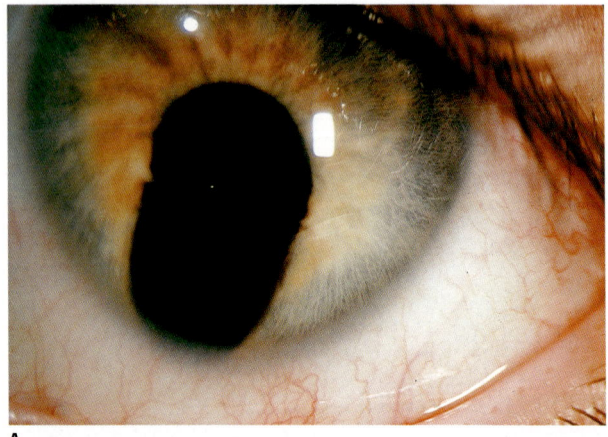

A

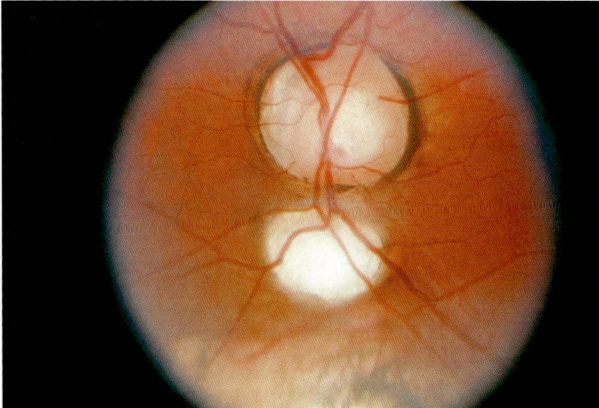

B

FIGURE 1-23A,B. Patient with iris (**A**) and choroidal and optic nerve (**B**) colobomas in typical inferior location. Note the choroidal skip lesion inferior to the disc.

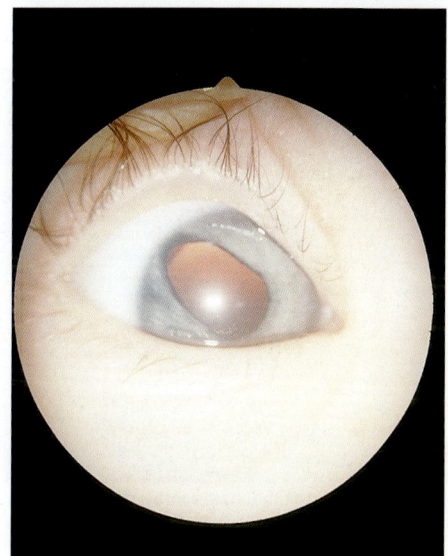

FIGURE 1-24. Photograph of ectropion uvea caused by peripheral anterior stromal membrane pulling the pupillary margin forward, exposing posterior pigment epithelium. Note there is an associated corectopia and dyscoria. The appearance of the eccentric pupil could be classified as an atypical iris coloboma. This is not a true coloboma because of the location and the presence of an intact iris root.

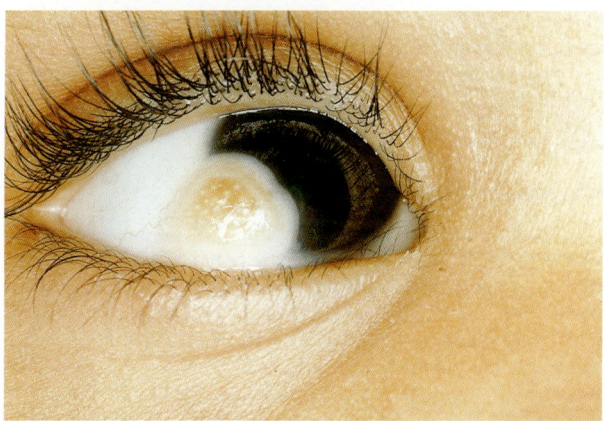

FIGURE 1-25. Isolated limbal dermoid at inferotemporal limbus, right eye. Hair cilia emanates from the center of the lesion. These limbal dermoids are often associated with large astigmatisms and can cause astigmatic, anisometropic amblyopia.

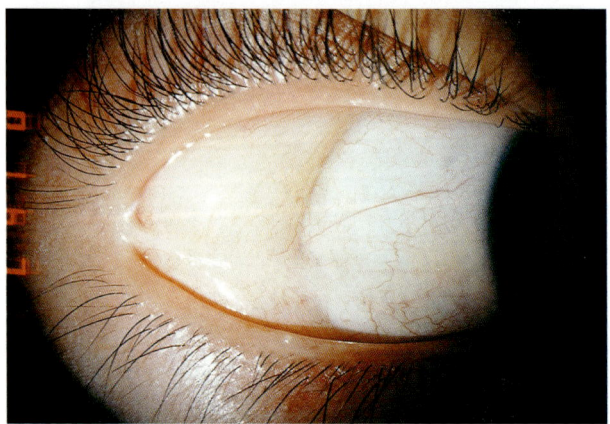

FIGURE 1-26. Dermolipoma in lateral canthal area, right eye. These are benign; however, if removed, can cause restrictive strabismus and fat adherence syndrome.

Goldenhar's syndrome (oculoauriculovertebral dysplasia) is a clefting anomaly of the first brachial arch and is associated with neural crest cell abnormalities. Goldenhar's syndrome is characterized by the combination of epibulbar dermoids (dermolipomas and limbal dermoids), ocular coloboma (Fig. 1-27), incomplete cryptophthalmos or lid colobomas, preauricular skin tags, vertebral anomalies, and, sporadically, with heart and pulmonary defects.

Cryptophthalmos

Cryptophthalmos is a congenital failure of lid and eye separation and development. In most cases, cryptophthalmos is inherited as an autosomal recessive trait, which may include mental retardation, cleft lip or palate, cardiac anomalies, or genitourinary abnormalities. The eyelids may be colobomatous, with the colobomatous lid fusing with the peripheral cornea or conjunctiva (incomplete cryptophthalmos; Fig. 1-27). Complete cryptophthalmos is a total absence of normal eyelids and lid fold, with the eye covered by skin that is adherent to an abnormal cornea. The cornea is often thin, being replaced by a

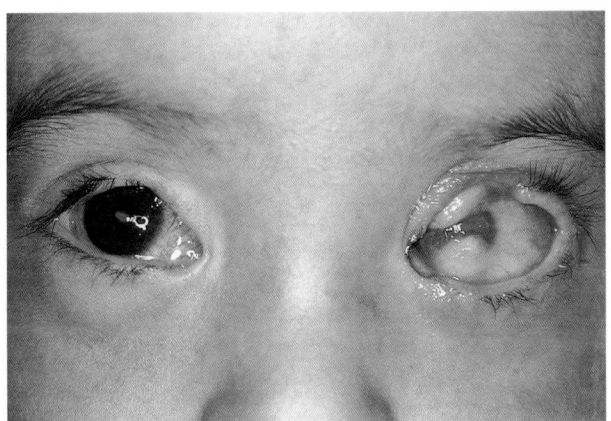

A

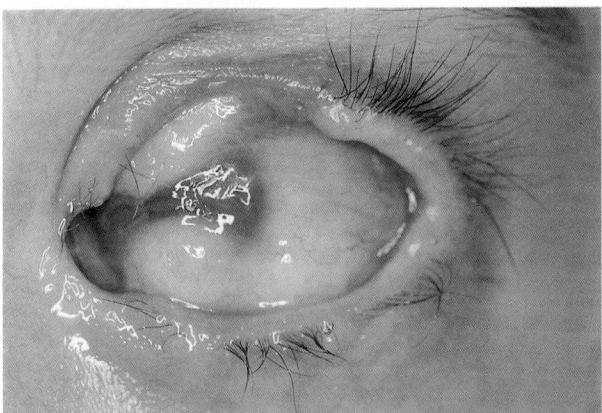

B

FIGURE 1-27A,B. (A) Photograph of a patient with Goldenhar's syndrome and incomplete cryptophthalmos of left eye. Cryptophthalmos consists of fusion of the upper lid to the cornea of the left eye. In addition to cryptophthalmos, patient has bilateral upper lid colobomas and left inferior limbal dermoid. **(B)** Close-up view of the left eye shows upper lid coloboma and cryptophthalmos with upper lid adhesion to the cornea and conjunctiva and inferior dermoid cyst.

fibrovascular tissue rather than clear cornea. The anterior segment is often abnormal, having a small or absent lens and anomalies of the iris or ciliary body. When associated with microphthalmia and anterior segment dysgenesis, this developmental abnormality is initiated at the optic vesicle stage with secondary effects on neural crest and surface ectoderm. In the rare cases where the globe and anterior segment are normal, cryptophthalmos could be caused by an abnormality in surface ectoderm.

Cornea Plana

Cornea plana is a failure of the cornea to steepen relative to the curvature of the globe and normally occurs between the third and fourth month of gestation. This failure to steepen results in a relatively flat cornea. Cornea plana can be associated with other anterior segment anomalies (Fig. 1-28) or inherited as an autosomal dominant or recessive trait.

Sclerocornea

Sclerocornea is a condition in which the junction between the cornea and sclera is indistinct. Additionally, the cornea appears

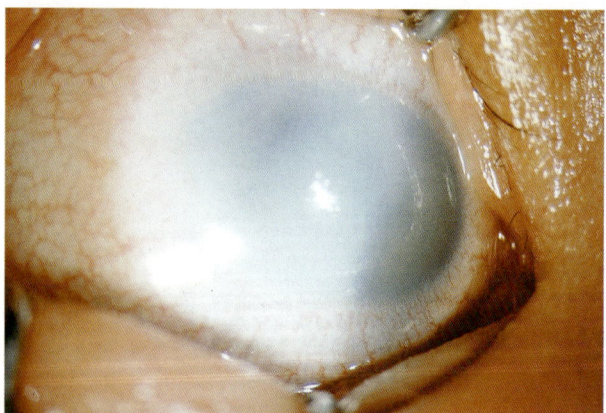

FIGURE 1-28. Photograph of congenital corneal opacity involving the temporal half of the cornea. Handheld slit lamp examination revealed iris strands to the cornea, flat peripheral cornea, and a blending of sclera and cornea in the periphery. The diagnosis is anterior chamber dysgenesis syndrome, including sclerocornea, cornea plana, and Peter's anomaly.

to be relatively small, as the limbal cornea is replaced by a mixture of cornea and scleral tissue.[67] Sclerocornea may be associated with other anomalies such as microphthalmia, coloboma, and anterior chamber dysgenesis (Fig. 1-28).

Anterior Segment Dysgenesis

Human anterior segment dysgenesis encompasses a broad spectrum of malformations including posterior embryotoxon, anterior displacement of Schwalbe's line, Axenfeld's anomaly (anterior displacement of Schwalbe's line associated with peripheral iris strands to Schwalbe's line), Peters' anomaly (central corneal opacity with absence of Descemet's membrane and endothelium in the area of the opacity), Rieger's anomaly (iris stromal hypoplasia with pseudopolycoria and iridocorneal attachments), or other combinations of iridocorneal or iridolenticular adhesions associated with various anterior segment anomalies. Congenital glaucoma is frequently associated with anterior segment dysgenesis syndromes.

Because most of the structures of the ocular anterior segment are of neural crest origin, it is tempting to incriminate this population of cells as being abnormal in differentiation or migration in cases of anterior segment dysgenesis. This theory has received widespread support and has resulted in labeling these conditions as "ocular neurocristopathie," particularly when other anomalies exist in tissues that are largely derived from neural crest cells (e.g., Rieger's syndrome; craniofacial connective tissue and teeth). There are several arguments in opposition to this theory. First, the neural crest is a predominant cell population of the developing craniofacial region including the eye. In fact, the number of tissues that are not neural crest derived is smaller than those which are (see Table 1-1). Thus, most malformations of this region would be expected to involve neural crest tissues, which may reflect their ubiquitous distribution rather than their common origin. The normal development of the choroid and sclera (also of neural crest origin) in anterior segment dysgenesis argues against a primary neural crest anomaly. Second, the neural crest is an actively migrating population of cells that is influenced by adjacent cell populations, and the perceived anomaly of neural crest tissue may be a secondary effect in many cases.

It is also important to recognize that, although much of the maturation of the iridocorneal angle occurs during the third trimester, much earlier events may influence anterior segment development. Anterior segment dysgenesis syndromes that are characterized primarily by axial deficits in corneal stroma and endothelium accompanied by corresponding malformations in the anterior lens capsule and epithelium (Peters' anomaly) most likely represent a manifestation of abnormal keratolenticular separation. The spectrum of malformations included in Peters' anomaly can be induced by teratogen exposure in mice at a time corresponding to the third week postfertilization in the human, just before optic sulcus invagination. Alternative theories for the pathogenic mechanism leading to Peters' anomaly, namely, intrauterine infection or anterior displacement of the lens or iris diaphragm, fail to explain the relatively localized axial defects.

Other anterior segment dysgenesis syndromes are characterized by more peripheral iridocorneal angle malformations and may represent malformations that are initiated somewhat later in gestation. These syndromes are often accompanied by absent or abnormal lining of Schlemm's canal, which is of mesodermal origin. In posterior polymorphous dystrophy and iridocorneal endothelial syndromes, the primary anomalies appear to be associated with the corneal endothelium and its basement membrane, both neural crest derivatives. Abnormal-appearing collagen within the trabecular meshwork has been identified in all these syndromes. Its significance is unknown; however, it may relate to neural crest abnormality.

Gene mutations that affect ocular neural crest cell populations and result in anterior segment dyogenesis have been identified. Of particular note is a genetic form of Rieger's syndrome caused by mutation in a homeobox transcription factor, PITX2.[3] In-situ hybridization in mice has shown that mRNA encoded by this gene is localized in the periocular mesenchyme.

Congenital Glaucoma

Although glaucoma may accompany any of the anterior segment syndromes described previously, elevated intraocular pressure (IOP) is usually not present at birth, in contrast to true congenital glaucoma. Earlier theories described the gonioscopic presence of a "Barkan's membrane" covering the trabecular meshwork in eyes with congenital glaucoma. Most histological examinations of affected eyes have failed to demonstrate such a membrane. Studies have revealed anterior displacement of the ciliary body and iris base, representing the immature conformation seen in fetuses during the second trimester. In the absence of other malformations, these cases of congenital (and juvenile) glaucoma most likely represent arrested maturation and remodeling of the iridocorneal angle, which occur during the last trimester.

Pupillary Anomalies

Corectopia is defined as an eccentric location of the pupil, which may be normal or malformed (Fig. 1-29). The pupil may have an abnormal shape (dyscoria) and not be in line with the lens. Corectopia may be associated with corresponding ectopia of the lens that may or may not be in line with the ectopic pupil. Colobomas can be mistaken as eccentric pupils, but true colobomas lack peripheral iris whereas corectopia has an intact peripheral iris. *Ectopia lentis et pupillae* is the eccentric location of both the lens and pupil, which may be eccentric together and in line or, more commonly, displaced in opposite directions (Fig. 1-29).

Polycoria is a condition in which there are many openings in the iris that result from local hypoplasia of the iris stroma and pigment epithelium. True polycoria actually is a condition in which there is more than one pupil and the multiple pupils all have a sphincter and the ability to contract. Most cases of

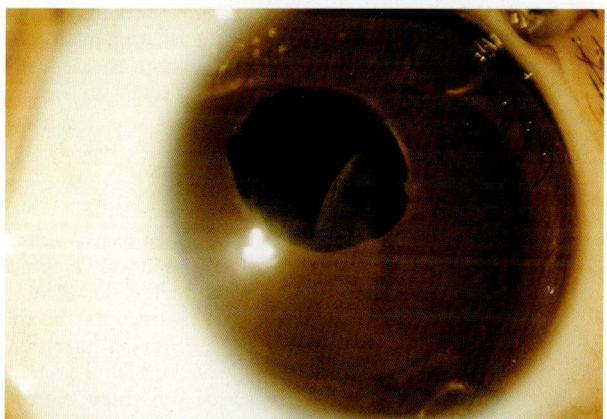

FIGURE 1-29. Photograph of corectopia associated with iris hypoplasia and ectopia lentis. Note that the corectopia is the opposite direction to the ectopia lentis.

polycoria, however, are actually pseudopolycoria as only one of the pupils is the true pupil with an iris sphincter muscle. Therefore, in almost all clinical situations, the correct term is *pseudopolycoria*. Iris stromal hypoplasia, in the absence of an iris epithelium defect, represents a defect in neural crest cell migration and development.

Ectropion uvea (congenital) is iris pigment epithelium that is present at the pupillary margin and on the anterior iris stroma, most likely caused by an exuberant growth of neural ectoderm over the iris stromal mesenchyme. It can also be caused by iris stromal atrophy or congenital fibrosis of the anterior iris stroma that contracts and everts the pupillary margin to expose the pigment epithelium. This last mechanism also results in corectopia (see Fig. 1-24).

Persistent Hyperplastic Primary Vitreous

Persistent hyperplastic primary vitreous (PHPV) relates to an abnormality in the regression of the primary vitreous in the hyaloid artery and is usually associated with microphthalmia. It is also referred to as persistent fetal vasculature. A fibrovascular stalk emanates from the optic nerve and attaches to the posterior capsule. The retrolenticular vascular membrane covers the posterior half of the lens and usually extends to attach to the ciliary processes. With time, the retrolenticular membrane contracts, pulling the ciliary processes centrally. If the lens and membrane are not removed, secondary glaucoma may occur. Early surgery (lensectomy and anterior vitrectomy) is indicated to prevent amblyopia and to maintain integrity of the eye.

Retinal Dysplasia

Disorganized differentiation of the retina is often seen as a component of multiple ocular malformation syndromes. The inner optic cup may continue to proliferate in a microphthalmic eye, leading to folds and rosettes. The retina is dependent on the underlying retinal pigment epithelium for normal differentiation. Expression of cyclin-dependent kinase inhibitor protein, p27(Kip1), precedes withdrawal of retinal cells from the cell cycle, leading to terminal differentiation. Displacement of p27(Kip1)-deficient Müller glia into the photoreceptor layer is associated with experimental retinal dysplasia.[66]

Malformation Complexes Involving the Eye, Brain, and Face

It is not surprising, considering that the eye is an extension of the brain, that developmental abnormalities of the eye and brain frequently are concurrent. Among the most severe brain malformations are those involving abnormal closure of the neural tube or severe forebrain midline reduction abnormalities. These malformations are frequently accompanied by anophthalmia, microphthalmia, anterior chamber cleavage abnormalities, or abnormal ocular placement (hypertelorism or hypotelorism, synophthalmia). Animal models have provided information regarding the developmental basis for a number of these malformation complexes. Because many of the relevant ocular abnormalities have been discussed earlier, the remainder of this chapter focuses on dysmorphogenesis of the brain and face.

Development of the forebrain and the midportion of the face above the oral cavity are intimately related. The olfactory (nasal) placodes become distinguishable on the frontolateral aspects of the frontonasal prominence during the fourth week of gestation. The thickened olfactory ectoderm is initially part of the anterolateral rim of the anterior neural folds. As the frontonasal prominence develops, elevations (termed the medial and lateral nasal prominences) form around the olfactory epithelium. As their name implies, the nasal prominences develop into the nose. The lower portions of the medial nasal prominences also contribute to the upper lip and form the portion of the alveolar ridge that contains the upper four incisors as well as the associated part of the hard palate that is termed the primary palate. On each side of the developing face, fusion of the medial nasal prominence with the lateral nasal prominence and the maxillary prominence of the first visceral arch is required for normal formation of the upper lip. As previously mentioned, neural crest cells are a predominant contributor to craniofacial development and provide, among other components, the skeletal and connective tissues of the face. This function is in contrast to the majority of the skull, whose progenitor populations are mesodermal.

The maxillary prominence, the tissue of which is primarily neural crest derived, is located below the developing eye and contributes to the lower eyelid. The upper lid is associated with the lateral nasal prominence as well as other tissues of the frontonasal prominence. Lid colobomas might be expected to occur at sites between the various growth centers that contribute to the eyelids. In addition to its maxillary component, the first visceral arch is made up of a mandibular subunit that contributes to the lower jaw and part of the external ear. The mandibular portion of the first arch has significant mesodermal progenitor cells in addition to those of neural crest origin.

Holoprosencephaly, Synophthalmia, and Cyclopia

Formation of a single median globe (cyclopia) or two incomplete (and apparently) fused globes (synophthalmia) may occur by two different mechanisms. Experimental studies in amphibian embryos have demonstrated "fate maps" identifying the original location of the ectodermal tissue that will form the globes as a single bilobed area which crosses the midline in the anterior third of the trilaminar embryonic disc. An early failure in separation of this single field could result in formation of a single median globe or two globes that appear to be "fused" which, in reality, have failed to fully separate. Later, in gestation, loss of the midline territory in the embryo could result in fusion of the ocular fields that were previously separated. This loss of midline territory is seen in holoprosencephaly (a single cerebral hemisphere).[96] Mutation in a number of different human genes can cause holoprosencephaly. Among the genes identified are sonic hedgehog (SHH), the protein product that is expressed at early stages of embryogenesis in the ventral midline of the forebrain and the subjacent tissue. SHH mutation results in holoprosencephaly type 3.[90] Mutation in other genes that are conserved in the animal kingdom, including SIX3 (the Drosophila sine oculis homeobox gene) and ZIC2, a homolog of the Drosophila odd-paired gene, are also associated with holoprosencephaly (HPE).[20,107]

Acute exposure of rodent embryos to teratogens at gastrulation stages of embryogenesis can result in the spectrum of malformations associated with holoprosencephaly. Loss of progenitor populations in the median aspect of the developing forebrain epithelium or its underlying mesoderm cause the subsequent dysmorphogenesis. Selective loss of the midline-associated tissues results in abnormally close approximation of the olfactory placodes and tissue deficiencies in the medial nasal prominence derivatives. At the mild end of the spectrum is a facial phenotype characteristic of fetal alcohol syndrome (Fig. 1-30A,B). Midline deficiencies can be so severe that the nose is

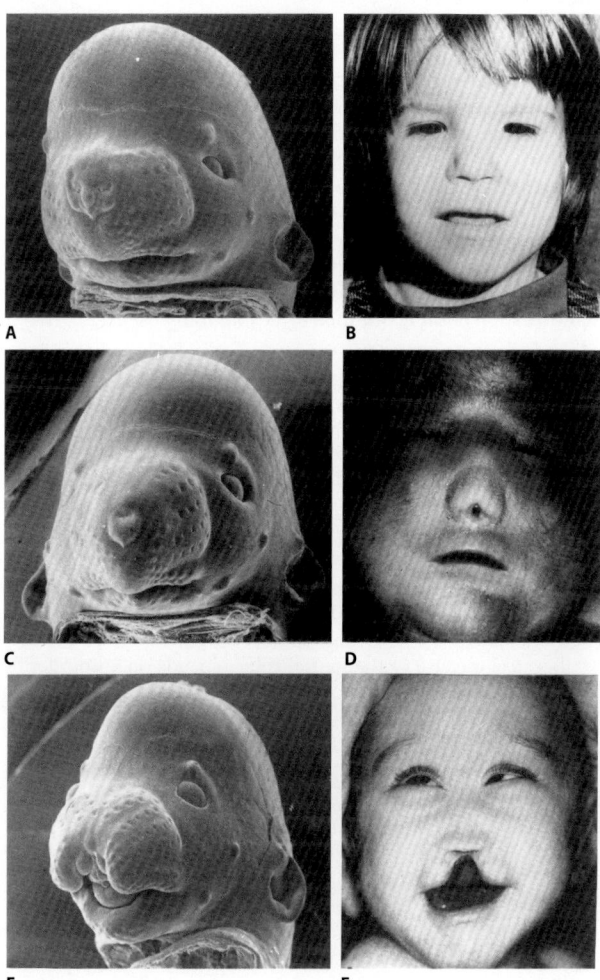

FIGURE 1-30A–F. Abnormally close proximity of the nasal placodes and subsequent deficiency in medial nasal prominence development results in the development of a small nose and a long upper lip (from nose to mouth) with a deficient philtrum. Variable degrees of severity of effect in ethanol-exposed mouse fetuses results in phenotypes comparable to those in humans with fetal alcohol syndrome (**A,B**), cebocephaly (**C,D**), and premaxillary agenesis (**E,F**). (From Siebert JR, Cohen MM Jr, Sulik KK. Holoprosencephaly: an overview and atlas of cases. New York: Wiley-Liss, 1990, with permission.)

derived from two conjoined nasal placodes, and lateral nasal prominences and hypotelorism is marked (Fig. 1-30C,D). Deficiencies that involve not only the anterior midline region but also the neural crest cells that contribute to the maxillary prominences (i.e., the crest cells derived from the mesencephalic neural folds) appear to be the basis for the premaxillary agenesis malformation complex illustrated in Figure 1-30E,F. In some rodent models, as in humans, mandibular deficiencies can also occur in conjunction with upper midface abnormalities, yielding the malformation complex termed *agnathia-holoprosencephaly*.

Exencephaly (Anencephaly) and Encephalocele

Although based on experimental evidence in animal models, most open neural tube defects (exencephaly, or anencephaly) result from failure of the neural tube to close, and some may be accounted for by postclosure rupture. Animal models have also illustrated that encephaloceles may be the result of abnormal closure. For example, delayed closure of the anterior neuropore appears to result in a rather tenuous closure with abnormally thin neuroepithelium and subsequent frontonasal encephalocele.

Because closure of the neural tube depends on a number of factors including the presence of normal neuroepithelium and its underlying mesenchyme and extracellular matrix, the types of and targets for insult that could result in failure of closure are also multiple. One of the most vulnerable periods for insult resulting in exencephaly in rodent embryos occurs before elevation of the cranial neural folds, when the embryos have approximately four to eight somite pairs (corresponding to the end of the third and beginning of the fourth week postfertilization in the human). At this time, premigratory neural crest cells appear to be particularly vulnerable to insult, their loss resulting in mesenchymal deficiency as well as interruption of the neuroepithelial integrity.[60]

Frontonasal Dysplasia

Median facial clefts with accompanying hypertelorism (frontonasal dysplasia) occur in widely varying degrees of severity. Animal models indicate that teratogen-induced distension (resulting from excessive fluid accumulation) of the neural tube shortly after the time of closure can account for some forms of frontonasal dysplasia.[32] Also of interest is an animal model resulting from a transgenically induced mutation.[71] The rather unusual phenotype results from delayed closure of the anterior neural folds and abnormal separation of the olfactory placodes from the rim of the neural plate.

References

1. Adamis AP, Molnar ML, Tripathi BJ, Emmerson MS, Stefansson K, Tripathi RC. Neuronal-specific enolase in human corneal endothelium and posterior keratocytes. Exp Eye Res 1985;41:665–668.
2. Aiello LP. Vascular endothelial growth factor. 20th-century mechanisms, 21st-century therapies. Investig Ophthalmol Vis Sci 1997; 38:1647–1652.
3. Alward WLM, Semina EV, et al. Autosomal dominant iris hypoplasia is caused by a mutation in the Rieger syndrome (RIEG/PITX2) gene. Am J Ophthalmol 1998;125:98–100.
4. Anderson DR. The development of the trabecular meshwork and its abnormality in primary infantile glaucoma. Trans Am Ophthalmol Soc 1981;79:458–485.
5. Ashton N. Oxygen and the growth and development of retinal vessels. In vivo and in vitro studies. Am J Ophthalmol 1966;62: 412–435.
6. Ashton N. Retinal angiogenesis in the human embryo. Br Med Bull 1970;26:103.
7. Ashton N, Tripathi B, Knight G. Effect of oxygen on the developing retinal vessels of the rabbit. I. Anatomy and development of the retinal vessels of the rabbit. Exp Eye Res 1972;14:214.
8. Aso S, Tashiro M, Baba R, Sawaki M, Noda S, Fujita M. Apoptosis in the lens anlage of the heritable lens aplastic mouse (lap mouse). Teratology 1998;58:44–53.
9. Balazs EA, Toth LZ, Ozanics V. Cytological studies on the developing vitreous as related to the hyaloid vessel system. Graefes Arch Klin Exp Ophthalmol 1980;213:71.
10. Barbieri AM, Lupo G, et al. A homeobox gene, vax2, controls the patterning of the eye dorsoventral axis. Proc Natl Acad Sci USA 1999;96:10729–10734.
11. Bard J, Hay E, Meller S. Formation of the endothelium of the avian cornea: a study of cell movement in vivo. Dev Biol 1975;42:334.
12. Bard J, Ross A. The morphogenesis of the ciliary body of the avian eye. Dev Biol 1982;92:87–96.
13. Barkan O. Pathogenesis of congenital glaucoma. Am J Ophthalmol 1955;40:1–11.
14. Beebe D, Compart P, Johnson M, Feagans D, Feinberg R. The mechanism of cell elongation during lens fiber cell differentiation. Dev Biol 1982;92:54–59.

15. Beebe DC. Ocular growth and differentiation factors. New York: Wiley, 1985.

16. Berson D. The development of the choroid and sclera in the eye of the foetal rat with particular reference to their developmental interrelationship. Exp Eye Res 1965;4:102.

17. Blankenship TN, Peterson PE, Hendrickx AG. Emigration of neural crest cells from macaque optic vesicles is correlated with discontinuities in its basement membrane. J Anat 1996;188:473–483.

18. Blixt A, Mahlapuu M, Aitola M, Pelto-Huikko M, Enerback S, Carlsson P. A forkhead gene, FoxE3, is essential for lens epithelial proliferation and closure of the lens vesicle. Genes Dev 2000;14: 245–254.

19. Bremer FM, Rasquin F. Histochemical localization of hyal-uronic acid in vitreous during embryonic development. Investig Ophthalmol Vis Sci 1998;39:2466–2469.

20. Brown SA, Warburton D, et al. Holoprosencephaly due to mutations in ZIC2, a homologue of Drosophila odd-paired. Nat Genet 1998;20:180–183.

21. Bumsted KM, Barnstable CJ. Dorsal retinal pigment epithelium differentiates as neural retina in the microphthalmia (mi/mi) mouse. Investig Ophthalmol Vis Sci 2000;41:903–908.

22. Cohen A. Electron microscopic observations of the developing mouse eye. I. Basement membranes during early development and lens formation. Dev Biol 1961;3:297–316.

23. Collinson JM, Hill RE, West JD. Different roles for Pax6 in the optic vesicle and facial epithelium mediate early morphogenesis of the murine eye. Development (Camb) 2000;127:945–956.

24. Cook C. Experimental models of anterior segment dysgenesis. Ophthal Paediatr Gen 1989;10:33–46.

25. Cook C, Burling K, Nelson E. Embryogenesis of posterior segment colobomas in the Australian shepherd dog. Prog Vet Comp Ophthalmol 1991.

26. Cook CS, Generoso WM, Hester D, Peiffer RL Jr. RPE dysplasia with retinal duplication in a mutant mouse strain. Exp Eye Res 1991;52:409–415.

27. Cook CS, Nowotny AZ, Sulik KK. Fetal alcohol syndrome. Eye malformations in a mouse model. Arch Ophthalmol 1987;105: 1576–1581.

28. Cook CS, Sulik KK. Keratolenticular dysgenesis (Peters' anomaly) as a result of acute embryonic insult during gastrulation. J Pediatr Ophthalmol Strabismus 1988;25:60–66.

29. Coulombre A. The role of intraocular pressure in the development of the chick eye. J Exp Zool 1956;133:211–225.

30. Coulombre AJ, Coulombre JL. Lens development. I. Role of lens in eye growth. J Exp Zool 1964;156:39.

31. Coulombre JL, Coulombre AJ. Lens development IV. Size, shape and orientation. Investig Ophthalmol 1969;8:251–257.

32. Darab DJ, Minkoff R, Sciote J, Sulik KK. Pathogenesis of median facial clefts in mice treated with methotrexate. Teratology 1987;36: 77–86.

33. Dawson DW, Volpert OV, et al. Pigment epithelium-derived factor: a potent inhibitor of angiogenesis. Science 1999;285:245–248.

34. Dunlevy JR, Beales MP, Berryhill BL, Cornuet PK, Hassell JR. Expression of the keratan sulfate proteoglycans lumican, keratocan and osteoglycin/mimecan during chick corneal development. Exp Eye Res 2000;70:349–362.

35. Furuta Y, Hogan BLM. BMP4 is essential for lens induction in the mouse embryo. Genes Dev 1998;12:3764–3775.

36. Garcia-Porrero JA, Collado JA, Ojeda JL. Cell death during detachment of the lens rudiment from ectoderm in the chick embryo. Anat Rec 1979;193:791–804.

37. Garcia-Porrero JA, Colvee E, Ojeda JL. The mechanisms of cell death and phagocytosis in the early chick lens morphogenesis. A scanning electron microscopy and cytochemical approach. Anat Rec 1984;208:123.

38. Grainger RM, Henry JJ, Saha MS, Servetnick M. Recent progress on the mechanisms of embryonic lens formation. Eye 1992;6:117–122.

39. Graw J. Genetic aspects of embryonic eye development in vertebrates. Dev Genet 1996;18:181–197.

40. Graw J. Cataract mutations and lens development. Prog Retin Eye Res 1999;18:235–267.

41. Grimm C, Chatterjee B, et al. Aphakia (ak), a mouse mutation affecting early eye development: fine mapping, consideration of candidate genes and altered Pax6 and Six3 gene expression pattern. Dev Genet 1998;23:299–316.

42. Hansson HA, Jerndal T. Scanning electron microscopic studies on the development of the iridocorneal angle in human eyes. Investig Ophthalmol 1971;10:252–265.

43. Hay E. Development of the vertebrate cornea. Int Rev Cytol 1980; 63:263.

44. Hay ED, Revel JP. Fine structure of the developing avian cornea. In: Wolsky A., Chen P (eds) Monographs in developmental biology. Basel: Karger, 1969.

45. Heimann K. The development of the choroid in man. Choroidal vascular system. Ophthalmol Res 1972;3:257.

46. Hendrickson A, Kupfer C. The histogenesis of the fovea in the macaque monkey. Investig Ophthalmol 1976;15:746.

47. Hendrix RW, Zwaan J. Changes in the glycoprotein concentration of the extracellular matrix between lens and optic vesicle associated with early lens differentiation. Differentiation 1974;2: 357.

48. Holme RH, Thomson SJ, Davidson DR. Ectopic expression of Msx2 in chick retinal pigmented epithelium cultures suggests a role in patterning the optic vesicle. Mech Dev 2000;91:175–187.

49. Hunt H. A study of the fine structure of the optic vesicle and lens placode of the chick embryo during incubation. Dev Biol 1961;3: 175–209.

50. Imaizumi M, Kuwabara T. Development of the rat iris. Investig Ophthalmol 1971;10:733.

51. Ireland ME, Wallace P, et al. Up-regulation of novel intermediate filament proteins in primary fiber cells: an indicator of all vertebrate lens fiber differentiation? Anat Rec 2000;258:25–33.

52. Ito M, Yoshioka M. Regression of the hyaloid vessels and pupillary membrane of the mouse. Anat Embryol 1999;200:403–411.

53. Iwatsuki H, Sasaki K, Suda M, Itano C. Vimentin intermediate filament protein as differentiation marker of optic vesicle epithelium in the chick embryo. Acta Histochem 1999;101:369–382.

54. Jack RL. Regression of the hyaloid vascular system. An ultrastructural analysis. Am J Ophthalmol 1972;74:261.

55. Johnston M, Noden D, Hazelton R, Coulombre J, Coulombre A. Origins of avian ocular and periocular tissues. Exp Eye Res 1979;29: 27–43.

56. Jones K, Higgonbottom M, Smith D. Determining the role of the optic vesicle in orbital and periocular development and placement. Pediatr Res 1980;14:703–708.

57. Karkinen-Jaaskelainen M. Permissive and directive interactions in lens induction. J Embryol Exp Morphol 1978;44:167–178.

58. Klagsbrun M, Moses MA. Molecular angiogenesis. Chem Biol 1999;6:217–224.

59. Koenig S, Naidich T, Lissner G. The morning glory syndrome associated with sphenoidal encepyhalocele. Ophthalmology 1982; 89:1368–1373.

60. Kotch LE, Sulik KK. Experimental fetal alcohol syndrome: proposed pathogenic basis for a variety of associated facial and brain anomalies. Am J Med Genet 1992;44:168–176.

61. Kupfer C, Kaiser-Kupfer M. New hypothesis of developmental anomalies of the anterior chamber associated with glaucoma. Trans Ophthal Soc UK 1978;98:213–215.

62. Lai YL. The development of the dilator muscle in the iris of the albino rat. Exp Eye Res 1972;14:203.

63. Lai YL. The development of the sphincter muscle in the iris of the albino rat. Exp Eye Res 1972;14:196.

64. Le Lievre C, Le Dourin N. Mesenchymal derivatives in the neural crest. Analysis of chimaeric quail and chick embryos. J Embryol Exp Morphol 1975;34:125.

65. LeDourin N. The neural crest. Cambridge: Cambridge University Press, 1982.

66. Levine EM, Close J, Fero M, Ostrovsky A, Reh TA. p27(Kip1) regulates cell cycle withdrawal of late multipotent progenitor cells in the mammalian retina. Dev Biol 2000;219:299–314.

67. March W, Chalkley T. Sclerocornea associated with Dandy–Walker cyst. Am J Ophthalmol 1974;78:54–57.

68. Maumenee A. The pathogenesis of congential glaucoma: a new theory. Am J Ophthalmol 1959;827–859.

69. McKeehan M. Cytological aspects of embryonic lens induction in the chick. J Exp Zool 1951;31–64.

70. McMenamin PG. Human fetal iridocorneal angle: a light and scanning electron microscopic study. Br J Ophthalmol 1989;73:871–879.

71. McNeish JD, Thayer J, Walling K, Sulik KK, Potter SS, Scott WJ. Phenotypic characterization of the transgenic mouse insertional mutation, legless. J Exp Zool 1990;253:151–162.

72. Meier S. The distribution of cranial neural crest cells during ocular morphogenesis. Prog Clin Biol Res 1982;82:1–15.

73. Michaelson IC. The mode of development of the vascular system of the retina with some observations on its significance for certain retinal diseases. Trans Ophthalmol Soc UK 1948;68:137–180.

74. Nishina S, Kohsaka S, et al. PAX6 expression in the developing human eye. Br J Ophthalmol 1999;83:723–727.

75. Noden D. Vertebrate craniofacial development: the relation between ontogenetic process and morphological outcome. Brain Behav Evol 1991;38:190–225.

76. Noden D. Periocular mesenchyme: neural crest and mesodermal interactions. In: Tasman W, Jaeger E (eds) Duane's foundations of clinical ophthalmology. Hagerstown: Lippincott, 1993:1–23.

77. Noden DM. The embryologic origins of avian craniofacial muscles and associated connective tissues. Am J Anat 1983;168:257–269.

78. Nucci P, Tredici G, Manitto MP, Pizzini G, Brancato R. Neuron-specific enolase and embryology of the trabecular meshwork of the rat eye: an immunohistochemical study. Int J Biol Markers 1992;7:253–255.

79. Oshima K, Ishikawa T. Effects of oxygen on developing vessels in the kitten retina. Nippon Ganka Gakkai Zasshi 1975;79:813.

80. Ozanics V, Rayborn ME, Sagun D. Observations on the ultrastructure of the developing primate choroid coat. Exp Eye Res 1978;26:25.

81. Ozeki H, Shirai S. Developmental eye abnormalities in mouse fetuses induced by retinoic acid. Jpn J Ophthalmol 1998;42:162–167.

82. Patz A. Current concepts of the effects of oxygen on the developing retina. Curr Eye Res 1984;3:159–163.

83. Patz A, Hoeck L, DeLaCruz E. Studies on the effect of high oxygen administration in retrolental fibroplasia: nursery observations. Am J Ophthalmol 1952;27:1248–1253.

84. Pierce EA, Foley Ed, Smith LE. Regulation of vascular endothelial growth factor by oxygen in a model of retinopathy of prematurity. Arch Ophthalmol 1996;114:1219–1228.

85. Pollock J, Newton T, Hoyt W. Transsphenoidal and transethmoidal encephaloceles: a review of clinical and roentgen features in 8 cases. Radiology 1968;90:442–452.

86. Reme C, D'Epinay SL. Periods of development of the normal human chamber angle. Doc Ophthalmol 1981;51:241.

87. Reme C, Urner U, Aeberhard B. The development of the chamber angle in the rat eye. Graefe's Arch Clin Exp Ophthalmol 1983;220: 139–153.

88. Reme C, Urner U, Aeberhard B. The occurence of cell death during the remodelling of the chamber angle recess in the developing rat eye. Graefe's Arch Clin Exp Ophthalmol 1983;221:113–121.

89. Ring BZ, Cordes SP, Overbeek PA, Barsh GS. Regulation of mouse lens fiber cell development and differentiation by the Maf gene. Development (Camb) 2000;127:307–317.

90. Roessler E, Belloni E, et al. Mutations in the human Sonic Hedgehog gene cause holoprosencephaly. Nat Genet 1996;14:357–360.

91. Schook P. A review of data on cell actions and cell interactions during the morphogenesis of the embryonic eye. Acta Morphol Neerl Scand 1978;16:267–286.

92. Selleck MA, Bronner-Fraser M. The genesis of avian neural crest cells: a classic embryonic induction. Proc Natl Acad Sci U S A 1996;93:9352–9357.

93. Sevel D. Reappraisal of the origin of human extraocular muscles. Ophthalmology 1981;88:1330.

94. Sevel D. The origins and insertions of the extraocular muscles: development, histologic features, and clinical significance. Trans Am Ophthalmol Soc 1986;84:488–526.

95. Shakib M, De Oliveira F. Studies on developing retinal vessels. X. Formation of the basement membrane and differentiation of intra-mural pericytes. Br J Ophthalmol 1966;50:124–133.

96. Siebert JR, Cohen MM Jr, Sulik KK, Shaw C, Lemire R. Holoprosencephaly: an overview and atlas of cases. New York: Wiley-Liss, 1990.

97. Simon PD, McConnell J, et al. Thy-1 is critical for normal retinal development. Brain Res Dev Brain Res 1999;117:219–223.

98. Smelser GK, Ozanics V. The development of the trabecular meshwork in primate eyes. Am J Ophthalmol 1971;71:366.

99. Spira AW, Hollenberg MJ. Human retinal development. Ultrastructure of the inner retinal layers. Dev Biol 1973;31:1–21.

100. Straatsma B, Foos R, Heckenlively J, Christensen R. Myelin-ated retinal nerve fibers: clinicopathologic study and clinical correla-tions. Excerpta Med 1978;32:36.

101. Straatsma B, Foos R, Heckenlively J, Taylor G. Myelinated retinal nerve fibers. Am J Ophthalmol 1981;91:25–38.

102. Stromland K, Miller M, Cook C. Ocular teratology. Surv Ophthal-mol 1991;35:429–446.

103. Summers C, Romig L, Lavoie J. Unexpected good results after therapy for anisometropic amblyopia associated with unilateral peripapillary myelinated nerve fibers. J Pediatr Ophthalmol Strabismus 1991;28:134–136.

104. Tamura T, Smelser GK. Development of the sphincter and dilator muscles of the iris. Arch Ophthalmol 1973;89:332.

105. Toole B, Trelstad R. Hyaluronate production and removal during corneal development in the chick. Dev Biol 1971;26:28.

106. Tsai RK, Sheu MM, Wang HZ. Capability of neurite regeneration of rat retinal explant at different ages. Kao Hsiung I Hsueh Ko Hsueh Tsa Chih 1998;14:192–196.

107. Wallis DE, Roessler E, et al. Mutations in the homeodomain of the human SIX3 gene cause holoprosencephaly. Nat Genet 1999;22:196–198.

108. Weiss P, Jackson S. Fine structural changes associated with lens determination in the avian embryo. Dev Biol 1961;532–554.

109. West-Mays JA, Zhang J, et al. AP-2alpha transcription factor is required for early morphogenesis of the lens vesicle. Dev Biol 1999;206:46–62.

110. Wigle JT, Chowdhury K, Gruss P, Oliver G. Prox1 function is crucial for mouse lens-fibre elongation. Nat Genet 1999;21:318–322.

111. Worst J. Congenital glaucoma. Remarks on the aspect of chamber angle, ontogenetic and pathogenetic background, and mode of action of goniotomy. Investig Ophthalmol 1968;7:127–134.

112. Wrenn JT, Wessels NK. An ultrastructural study of lens invagination in the mouse. J Exp Zool 1969;171:359.

112a. Hong PH, Wright KW, Fillafer S, Sola A, Chow LC. Strict Oxygen Management is Associated with Decreased Incidence of Severe ROP, Presented ARVO, 2002.

113. Wulle K. The development of the productive and draining system of the aqueous humor in the human eye. Adv Ophthalmol 1972:296–355.

114. Wulle KG. Electron microscopic observations of the development of Schlemm's canal in the human eye. Trans Am Acad Ophthalmol Otolaryngol 1968;72:765.

115. Wulle KG, Ruprecht KW, Windrath LC. Electron microscopy of the development of the cell junctions in the embryonic and fetal human corneal endothelium. Investig Ophthalmol 1974;13:923.

116. Yamashita T, Sohal G. Development of smooth and skeletal muscle cells in the iris of the domestic duck, chick and quail. Cell Tissue Res 1986;244:121–131.

117. Yamashita T, Sohal G. Embryonic origin of skeletal muscle cells in the iris of the duck and quail. Cell Tissue Res 1987;249:31–37.

118. Yang J, Bian W, Gao X, Chen L, Jing N. Nestin expression during mouse eye and lens development. Mech Dev 2000;94:287–291.

119. Zwaan J, Hendrix RW. Changes in cell and organ shape during early development of the ocular lens. Am J Zool 1973;13:1039–1049.

2

Breaking the News: The Role of the Physician

Nancy Chernus-Mansfield

Janet and Marc thought their life was as close to perfection as any family's life could be. Married for 8 years, they had one daughter, Missy, age 5, and Brian, age 3 months, their long-awaited son. At Brian's 3-month routine well-baby checkup, the pediatrician remarked that Brian might have strabismus because his eyes appeared to turn in and weren't "working together," as Janet later described it. The pediatrician was very reassuring, however, and told Marc and Janet that he would like the baby to be examined by a pediatric ophthalmologist "just to be on the safe side." Marc had recently started a new and more responsible job so it was decided that Janet would take Brian for the eye examination herself, to minimize the amount of time Marc was away from the office.

Thursday, July 14, began like many others for Janet. She got Missy off to kindergarten, kissed Marc goodbye, and packed up for the day's outing, an eye doctor's appointment. Preparing a 3-month-old to meet a new doctor was a challenge for Janet. She wanted Brian not only to look his best but to be his most alert and charming self.

When Janet arrived for the appointment, everything seemed easy enough. She filled out the routine medical information and was brought into the examining room. The doctor came in, introduced himself, and asked Janet some questions about Brian's development and about the pregnancy. As Brian was being examined, Janet began to feel twinges of anxiety. Brian was screaming. For the doctor to get a good look at his eyes, he explained to Janet that he would have to put a speculum in Brian's eyes to keep them open and in position. Unprepared for the papoose board they placed him on, or for the torturous-looking instrument the doctor used, Janet was becoming extremely upset. Finally the examination was complete, or so Janet thought. The doctor said he couldn't give a diagnosis, however, without some additional tests. Janet didn't understand. Why would crossed eyes require additional tests? The doctor would not comment. He told Janet he wanted more information and would arrange for her to go across the street to a facility that could do the tests. Quickly, Janet called her neighbor to make arrangements for Missy to be picked up from kindergarten. Although she was feeling upset by the morning's examination, Janet thought it best not to call and alarm Marc because she thought the doctor was probably just being thorough.

Janet took Brian across the street to the laboratory where they did electrophysiological tests. Fortunately, Brian had fallen asleep and the flashing lights and electrodes did not seem to bother him. The person who did the tests did not give Janet any information. He told her to return to her physician's office.

When Janet entered the doctor's office this time, she was feeling very apprehensive. She was ushered into the doctor's office, instead of an examining room. After about 15 long minutes, the doctor appeared. He sat down behind his desk, took out Brian's chart, and began to speak. From what Janet can remember, he said something like this: "The test confirmed what I have suspected. Your baby has a condition known as Leber's congenital amaurosis. This condition affects the optic nerves and, from my experience, I believe he is totally blind. There is no treatment. I am sorry. I wish you and your family the best of luck."

Janet can't remember what happened after that. She has no memory of her drive home, of picking up Missy, or of calling Marc. What she does remember is feeling that her life, Brian's life, Marc's life, and Missy's life were over. Nothing would ever be the same again.

Thursdays were busy days for Jack Smith, M.D. He had private patients in the morning and clinic patients all afternoon. At 38, he had achieved his dream of becoming a successful pediatric ophthalmologist. He had always had an interest in ophthalmology but, after his pediatric rotation, he decided that pediatric ophthalmology was a truly exciting field. Jack felt lucky that his wife of 12 years was always supportive of him and that all three of his children, Jack Jr., 10, Jennifer, 8, and Jason, 6, seemed happy and were proud of their dad. He enjoyed the challenge of his work in his private office as well as his research and teaching at the medical school. He had developed a particular interest in treating strabismus and had become the leading specialist in his area.

After arriving at his office, Jack surveyed his schedule and buzzed Karen, his "right arm," to send in the first patient. As he entered the examining room he saw Janet, an attractive thirtyish woman, gazing lovingly at her infant. Jack suspected that the baby had strabismus. The call from the pediatrician was brief, and indicated nothing out of the ordinary. Jack introduced himself and began the examination. Almost immediately he could feel a knot beginning in his stomach as he noted the presence of a nystagmus. By the time the baby was papoosed and the speculum was in place, he was really concerned. He thought, "Maybe it won't be as bad as I think it is; wait for the ERG." He would feel his discomfort build as he told Janet he wanted some additional tests. "No need to alarm her at this point," he thought. So he sent Janet across the street and proceeded to see the many other children waiting for their examinations.

At 11:45 A.M., the call came from the electrophysiology lab. Jack's suspicions were confirmed: Leber's—a totally blind baby. In 45 minutes he would be face-to-face with Janet. This was the only part of his practice he dreaded—giving bad news. What should he tell her? He wished he knew. "Does anyone?" he wondered. "I will just give her the facts. There's no way to sugarcoat this," he thought. Nothing had prepared him to break people's hearts.

Jack doesn't remember the details of Janet's reaction. He knew, of course, that she was extremely upset. Primarily, though, he felt overwhelming helplessness. None of his hard-won expertise could fix this baby; no patching, no surgery, no nothing. All Jack could do was hope that this family had the strength to cope with the diagnosis. The thought came, "If it was one of my kids, what would I do?" He dismissed that thought quickly. It was too painful. "I'm getting morbid; probably most of the kids do great, and their parents can handle their problems." At least Jack wanted to think so. He loved being a pediatric ophthalmologist because he could really help kids. It was so satisfying to see a child who had amblyopia, for example, and to know that with patching the child's vision would be assured. He didn't really know that much about what happened to the few blind children he had encountered. They seemed okay, but, Jack thought, to be fully honest, they were the patients with whom he spent the least time. There was, after all, nothing he could do for them.

Yet that day he couldn't shake the feeling of discomfort as he continued to see patients. His mind kept returning to Janet and the pain on her face. What would life be like for her and for her family? Janet seemed shocked when she heard the diagnosis, but she was very quiet. She hadn't said very much or even asked any questions other than, "Are you sure there is nothing that can be done?" He had said "No." Maybe, he thought in retrospect, just saying "no" was too brusque. He hated to admit there was nothing more he could do and that he was unable to offer further hope. Maybe he should have said more. Is there something else he could have done for her? He just didn't know.

PARENTAL REACTIONS TO THE DIAGNOSIS OF BLINDNESS

The impact of blindness on all family members is tremendous. Before the birth of any baby, we all have dreams and expectations about what the future holds. Expecting a child is a special time for most parents. Mothers and fathers love their baby long before it is born. They love the baby because they project onto their child all their dreams, fantasies, and expectations. For many parents, their hopes are realized when a healthy child is born. But for a moment try to imagine all these expectations and dreams destroyed by hearing the doctor say, "Your baby is blind." Parents are devastated. They experience a blow that is totally shattering. As Pearl Buck said when learning her daughter was mentally retarded, "All the joy of my life was gone."

Author Renee Nastoff, the parent of a child with a disability, eloquently described her pain when she wrote, "I fight the unseen enemy. I have reason for revenge but nothing against which to vent my outrage. My child is held hostage by a cruel twist of fate. Only a parent can comprehend the frustration of fighting an attacker that can't possibly be hurt. It is in the air all around me every moment of my life, overshadowing all decisions about my child, crushing and destroying the simple parental right to dream—about Little League, college, marriage, grandchildren. I can feel the enemy now, its fingers tightening at my throat, forcing what I thought were controlled tears. Sometimes it loosens its painful clasp, but never does it desert its hold on my life. I can't kill this stranger, and I can't break away. Yet it tries to force the very spirit of life from me. It will remain with me forever."

A parent experiences one of life's most devastating losses when a child is born with a disability. What the parent has lost is the anticipated perfect child—that very-much-loved-and-dreamed-of child to whom they have already become attached. Surprisingly, the degree of the baby's impairment is not always the crucial factor in determining the parent's reactions. The most important determinant is the parent's dreams for that child. Loss is the hardest thing that we, as human beings, experience. It is not an uncommon event that affects only certain people, nor is loss merely defined as death of a loved one. It actually touches each of us many times and in many ways in our lifetime. Loss shatters the dreams that are the most basic to a person's existence. Major losses with which we are all familiar include divorce, death, or illness. However, less profound losses can include the loss of physical attractiveness, career recognition, money, etc. The significance of the loss varies for each person and depends on how meaningful that particular loss is to the individual's identity. Loss is a common human experience cutting across all socioeconomic lines. The loss of the expected perfect baby is a major trauma in a family's life. The kinds of feelings that parents have in response to their child's visual impairment may be confusing to them. Feelings of shock, helplessness, fear, denial, depression, sadness, anger, guilt, disappointment, and uncertainty are natural and occur with intensity. Many parents have called this time a "mourning period" because the feeling of sadness is so acute. As one mother said: "I felt like my perfect baby had died and I had a different baby— a blind one." Another parent said, "I was so confused. What I expected to be the happiest time of my life turned out to be the saddest."

Grieving is a normal and spontaneous reaction to loss, but in our culture this normal reaction is often regarded as abnormal. Society may view people who are grieving appropriately as though they are behaving inappropriately. Grieving is the process that enables human beings to deal with loss. Yet parents report that the expression of their grief often cuts them off from the very support they need. As one father said, "I haven't cried since I was 12, but now whenever anyone asks about my son, I start to cry. I know that I make people uncomfortable and they often try to avoid me." This father's expression of his feelings is a healthy response that will eventually enable him to cope with his grief. It is part of the process of detaching from the child he wished for and forming an attachment to his actual child.

Another important and universal reaction parents express is an overwhelming need to understand the reason for their child's impairment. Parents say:

"The question 'why' is always in the back of my mind. Am I to blame?"

"When I was pregnant, I moved the furniture."

"There were various medications I was taking for my asthma. I often wonder, 'Was the medicine the cause of my baby's handicap?' "

"When I was pregnant with John, I couldn't quit work. We had no insurance, and I sometimes think maybe I could have taken it easier and should not have worried about the money. When I'm alone I start blaming myself."

It is natural for parents to look for reasons to explain their child's blindness. When a painful event occurs, it is human nature to feel that perhaps we could bear the pain better if we would understand why it happened, if we could make sense of something so senseless. When people feel lost, they want a road map, and answers seem to provide the needed map. For some people, medical explanations are helpful; for others, religious beliefs provide comfort; but for the vast majority of parents, there are no satisfying answers that relieve the pain or diminish the feeling that "life is not fair." Most of us have a deep sense of justice and fairness, and it is terribly hard to think that something this tragic can happen without a reason. Some fortunate families who are religious believe that, although they don't understand why, God has a purpose and this helps them cope with their child's disability. Many parents never find a reasonable explanation. People find it hard to think that a catastrophic disability happens randomly or that the world could be so chaotic that who or what a person is, or does, is of no consequence. Most of us grow up believing that justice prevails, that bad things happen to bad people and good things happen to good people. Reconciling this view with one's own life is very difficult for all of us. A physician once said, in helping a family deal with this issue: "Often people think that, because they took drugs in high school or had a teenage abortion, they may be responsible for the child's disability. I reassure my patients that all of us can find fault with ourselves in reviewing our lives. However, I tell parents that their previous behaviors have nothing to do with their child's disability. It is simply a random event, and they were unlucky. I find that my patients are very relieved when I reassure them about these issues."

Most parents do begin to cope quickly and in tandem with grieving. Although parents love their disabled child and make the necessary adjustments, their lives are never the same. The pain comes and goes forever.

BREAKING THE NEWS: THE ROLE OF THE PHYSICIAN

Physicians are often unaware the their role has a direct effect on the family's adaptation process. The way the physician presents the diagnosis to the family is crucial. For the rest of their lives, parents will remember not just what they were told, but the way in which it was communicated by the physician.

The following ingredients are necessary in a successful doctor–patient or doctor–parent interaction: consideration, truth, clarity, awareness, compassion, trust, accessibility, and professional kindness.

Consideration

Always sit down when talking to a family. Sit down in a private place, with no spectators. Do not appear rushed, even though you may have a waiting room full of patients. Look directly at the parents, make eye contact, and do not write or dictate into a recorder as you are talking. Try not to be interrupted when giving bad news; the family needs your undivided attention. During the diagnostic process, don't think out loud. This causes unnecessary anxiety. Don't talk with other medical personnel in front of the family; this can be accomplished before or after you have finished explaining the diagnosis. Above all, treat people as you would like to be treated in a like situation.

Truth

It is understandably difficult for the physician to give bad news. It is best to be direct, but not blunt. As one physician said, "There are many ways to say the same thing: truth doesn't mean brutality. Your face can stop a clock—when I'm with you, time stands still." Although both statements convey the same cognitive information, the emotional impact is significantly different.

Clarity

Give information using plain language. When parents are anxious, it interferes with understanding. Often physicians use medical jargon to protect themselves in this time of stress. Physicians must give the information clearly and directly. Sometimes in their discomfort, doctors unconsciously resort to excessive discussion or speculation about the disease or use too much intellectual discourse. This is not helpful to the family.

Awareness

Be aware of how the family is feeling. Acknowledge your own feelings as well. Recognize how you feel as a doctor giving a diagnosis for which there is no cure. Remember that the family is frightened and in more pain than you are and think about how the news is affecting them. Often physicians talk about disease or body parts to depersonalize the information and to depersonalize the enormity of the task of giving a difficult diagnosis.

Compassion

Allow yourself to feel compassion for your patient, for their parents, and for yourself. Compassion will not distort the professional relationship. Rather, your concern and discomfort about the diagnosis can be helpful to a family. Even if you are ill at ease or uncomfortable, the human connection your feelings can create may help the family to cope. Your expression, body language, and tone of voice are important. Your words will be etched forever in the memory of the family.

Trust

Parents must trust you not only as a physician who is medically competent, but as someone that they can count on to help them in this critical period. They must trust you to be honest at all times. Parents must also be able to trust that you recognize their pain and sorrow and will not abandon them.

Accessibility

Because of the emotional impact of the diagnosis, parents need to be able to talk with you more than once. Often it is helpful to leave the room for a period of time after the initial diagnosis

United Cerebral Palsy Association
7 Penn Plaza, Suite 804
New York, NY 10001
800/USA-1UCP
212/268-6655

CHARGE Syndrome

CHARGE Accounts
c/o Quota Club
2004 Parkade Blvd.
Columbia, MO 65202
314/442-7604

Chronic Illness

N.O.R.D.
National Organization for Rare Disorders
P.O. Box 8923
New Fairfield, CT 06812
http://www.rarediseases.org

Magic Foundation
(Optic Nerve Hypoplasia)
1327 N. Harlem Ave.
Oak Park, IL 60302
709/383-0808
http://www.magicfoundation.org

Parents of Chronically Ill Children
1527 Maryland St.
Springfield, IL 62702
217/522-6810

Deaf/Blind

John Tracy Clinic
806 West Adams Blvd
Los Angeles, CA 90007
800/522-4582

Hydrocephalus

Hydrocephalus Association
2040 Polk St., Box 342
San Francisco, CA 94109
415/776-4713

Hydrocephalus Support Group
c/o Kathy McGowan
6059 Mission Rd., #106
San Diego, CA 92108
619/282-1070

National Hydrocephalus Foundation
22427 S. River Rd.
Joliet, IL 60436
815/467-6548

Lawrence Moon Bardet Biedl Syndrome

Lawrence Moon Bardet Biedl Syndrome Network
18 Strawberry Hill
Windsor, CT 06095
203/688-7880

Marfan Syndrome

National Marfan Foundation
382 Main St.
Port Washington, NY 10050
516/883-8712

Mental Retardation

Association for Retarded Citizens of the U.S.
500 E. Border St., Suite 300
Arlington, TX 76010
817/261-6003

Neurofibromatosis

National Neurofibromatosis Foundation
141 Fifth Ave., Suite 7-S
New York, NY 10010
800/323-7938
212/460-8980

Visual Impairments

American Foundation for the Blind
15 West 16th St.
New York, NY 10011
800/AF-BLIND (232-5463)
212/620-2043

American Printing House for the Blind
1839 Frankfort Ave.
P.O. Box 6085
Louisville, KY 40206-0085
502/895-2405

Association for Macular Diseases
210 East 64th St.
New York, NY 10021
212/655-3007

The Institute for Families of Blind Children
P.O. Box 54700
Mailstop #111
Los Angeles, CA 90054-0700
323/669-4649

National Association for the Visually Impaired
P.O. Box 317
Watertown, MA 02272-0317
800/562-6265
Fax: 617/972-7444
(Some areas have a state organization as well; NAPVI can direct
the parent)

National Organization for Albinism and Hypopigmentation
(NOAH)
155 Locust St., Suite 1016
Philadelphia, PA 19102
800/473-2310
215/545-2322

Parents and Cataract Kids (PACK)
c/o Geraldine Miller
P.O. Box 73
Southeastern, PA 19399
215/352-0719

Retinoblastoma International
4650 Sunset Blvd., M.S. 88
Los Angeles, CA 90027
323/669-2299
www.retinoblastoma.net

New England Retinoblastoma Support Group
603 Fourth Range Road
Pembroke, NH 03275

General Resources

The Family Resource Coalition
230 N. Michigan Avenue
Suite 1625, Dept. W
Chicago, IL 60601
(Identification of parent support groups all over the country)

Reaching Out: A Directory of National Organizations Related to Maternal and Child Health
38th and R Streets, NW
Washington, DC 20057
202/625-8400

Team of Advocates for Special Kids
100 W. Cerritos Ave.
Anaheim, CA 92805
714/533-8275

Other National Toll-Free Numbers:

American Council of the Blind 800/424-8666
Better Hearing Institute 800/424-8576
Epilepsy Information Line 800/332-1000
Cystic Fibrosis Foundation 800/344-4823
Downs Syndrome 800/221-4602
Easter Seal Society 800/221-6827
Health Information Clearinghouse 800/336-4797
Spina Bifida 800/621-3141
Fragile X Foundation 800/835-2246
American Kidney Fund 800/835-8018
National Information Center for Orphan Drugs and Rare Disease 800/336-4797
Sickle Cell Association 800/421-8453
Retinitis Pigmentosa (RP) Association International 800/344-4877
Local School Districts or State Departments of Special Education

Search on the Internet for most current information.

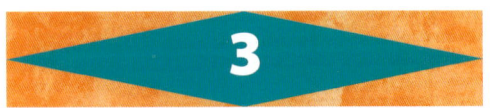

Chromosomal Anomalies and the Eye

J. Bronwyn Bateman

BASIC CONCEPTS OF CHROMOSOMAL DISEASE

Deoxyribonucleic acid (DNA) is the fundamental unit that directs the orchestration of cellular function and transmits traits from one generation to the next. It is a self-reproducing macromolecule that determines the composition of proteins within the cell. The gene is a sequence of DNA that encodes for a single, specific protein or regulates the expression of a gene; just as the DNA is arranged as beads on a necklace, the genes (specific segments of DNA) are similarly aligned. The information contained in the DNA is transcribed to ribonucleic acid (RNA), an intermediary template, which is, in turn, translated to the specific protein. The DNA of functional genes is arranged in exons and introns; exonic sequences are transcribed into RNA, and the intronic sequences are removed. Sequence variation is considerably greater for the introns. The nuclear genes and other untranslated DNA are organized as chromosomes, discrete organelles within the nucleus. The majority of the DNA of a cell is arranged as chromosomes within the nucleus; a small percentage of DNA is within the mitochondria in the cytoplasm of the cell and primarily orchestrates oxidative metabolism. Different species of animals and plants have different numbers of chromosomes; for example, a mouse has 40 and a tomato 24. Humans have 23 pairs, of which 2, an X and a Y, determine gender. Each nucleated cell of the organism has the same DNA as every other cell unless a mutation or chromosomal anomaly has occurred after conception.

Humans are diploid organisms with two sets of each chromosome and, therefore, two sets of each gene, one member of each pair being inherited from a parent; the X and Y chromosomes are the exception as they are structurally different but paired. An individual is homozygous for a gene pair if the DNA sequence of each is identical and is heterozygous (or a hetererozygote) if the sequences differ. Alternative forms of a gene are called alleles; a null allele is one in which a protein is not evident. Many enzymatic deficiencies are inherited as autosomal recessive diseases; the heterozygote shows no evidence of the disease because one chromosome is normal and 50% activity of the enzyme is functionally adequate. Many autosomal dominant disorders are caused by mutations of structural genes. Autosomal dominant disorders are manifest with only one chromosome abnormal (heterozgote) because all structural building blocks must be normal to build a normal structure. If a portion of chromosome is missing, the deleted genes are not transcribed or, if adjacent to the deletion, a gene may be transcribed abnormally. Conversely, if a portion of a chromosome is duplicated, the genes within the duplicated region are transcribed, resulting in an abundance of protein or, as occurs with deletions, the adjacent genes may be transcribed abnormally.

DNA consists of 2 strands of nucleotides, each with a base, a pentose (five-carbon) sugar (deoxyribose in the case of DNA), and a phosphoric acid; RNA has a similar structure with the exception of the base uracil instead of cytosine. The 2 strands of nucleotides are bound together at each base forming a complementary sequence of base pairs. Hydrogen bonding between the bases adenine (A, a purine) from one strand and thymine (T, a pyrimidine) from the other or guanine (G, a purine) and cytosine (C, pyrimidine) maintain the alignment of the two strands. The tertiary structure of the double strand makes the classic double helix. Because the pairing of A with T and G with C is essential to the secondary and tertiary structure, the two strands are complementary.

The precise order of the base pairs within the exons of a gene determines the amino acid sequence of the protein it encodes. For each amino acid, a triplet of DNA bases (a codon) provides the information for the amino acid of the protein, and some amino acids are represented by more than one codon. For example, the amino acid phenylalanine is encoded by either of the triplets uracil-uracil-uracil or uracil-uracil-cytosine. Protein sequence can be determined on the basis of the DNA sequence.

Some of the chromosomal DNA may be repetitive, and such sequences are transcribed; the evolutionary significance is unknown.

"Genetic" defects occur at many different molecular levels. Single gene defects may be produced by a *single gene mutation*, an alteration of the DNA sequence or a deletion or duplication of DNA within a single gene, which causes a change of one or more amino acids of the protein product. Point mutations of functional significance to the organism usually occur within an exon or exon–intron boundary or in a regulatory sequence. Mutations of single genes are the basis of Mendelian inheritance patterns including autosomal recessive, autosomal dominant, and X-linked. *Chromosomal abnormalities* encompass deletions (loss) or duplications (additional) of larger regions of DNA and alter the function of more than one gene; such abnormalities, if sufficiently large, may be identified under the microscope. The term cytoplasmic or *mitochondrial inheritance* was coined to describe diseases such as Leber optic atrophy, which are passed from a mother to offspring but not from the father to his progeny because sperm have few mitochondria. Such diseases are caused by abnormalities of the mitochondrial DNA. Last, *multifactorial inheritance* is poorly understood and difficult to prove scientifically; it is defined as a genetic predisposition to a disease with the manifestations or expression of the disease being influenced by environmental factors in either the intrauterine or postnatal period.

During the process of cell replication (mitosis), nuclear DNA is duplicated and each daughter cell receives the same information as the parent unless a mutation or chromosomal anomaly occurs. The process of gamete (spermatozoa or ova) formation (meiosis) involves a halving of the number of chromosomes. During meiosis, a single cell forms four gametes (ova or sperm), each of which has half the number of chromosomes (haploid), and therefore genes, of the parent cell. Crossing-over (exchange of DNA) between homologous chromosomes (a pair with the same gene loci in the same order) probably occurs during the replication process, and genetic material is exchanged. This process reorganizes the alleles on a chromosome and increases genetic variability. Errors may occur in the duplicative process of mitosis or meiosis and result in somatic and germinal defects, respectively. During fertilization, two haploid cells fuse to form a diploid cell with the normal number of chromosomes. A germinal defect in a gene or chromosome is present in all cells of the body and is caused by an error in one or both of the gametes. Alternatively, a chromosomal abnormality may occur relatively early in gestation, resulting in a portion of cells with the defect; termed *mosaicism*, the condition is usually defined by the percentage of abnormal cells and/or the cell types associated with the abnormality. Rarely, the testicles or ovaries, may exhibit mosaicism with some cell lines containing a mutation of a gene or chromosomal aberration.

A phenotype is the physical, biochemical, and physiological features of an individual as determined by genotype (genetic constitution). A similar phenotype may occur as a result of different gene defects or chromosomal abnormalities and is termed *genetic heterogeneity*. Examples of genetic heterogeneity are common in ophthalmology. Retinitis pigmentosa is an important ophthalmic disease exhibiting genetic heterogeneity, as this disease may be inherited by different gene defects; as an autosomal dominant, an autosomal recessive, or an X-linked recessive disorder. Within the category of autosomal dominant retinitis pigmentosa, mutations of rhodopsin and peripherin proteins have been identified as the basis of the disease. Similarly, different chromosomal anomalies may result in overlap of phenotypic features. Thus, classification of diseases is most reliably made on the basis of specific chromosomal abnormalities.

Chromosomes may be studied under the microscope by arresting the progression of the mitotic (duplicative) process. Using this technique (Karyotyping) the chromosomes can be visualized under the microscope and the specific chromosomal identification can be made on the basis of length and by using stains such as trypsin-Giemsa (G banding) (Fig. 3-1),[320] quinacrine mustard (Q banding),[45] "reverse" (following controlled denaturation by heat, followed by Giemsa staining), silver (stains nucleolar organizing regions), and C banding (the centromere and regions with heterochromatin stain). All methods identify bands or specific regions and are useful for studying the specific structure of a chromosome. The number of chromosomes can be counted and the bands of each studied for deletions, duplications, and other anomalies. Chromosomes were initially classified by size and given numbers when banding permitted identification. Relatively new techniques for arresting the progression of mitosis earlier in the cell cycle have been developed. In the late prophase or early metaphase stage of

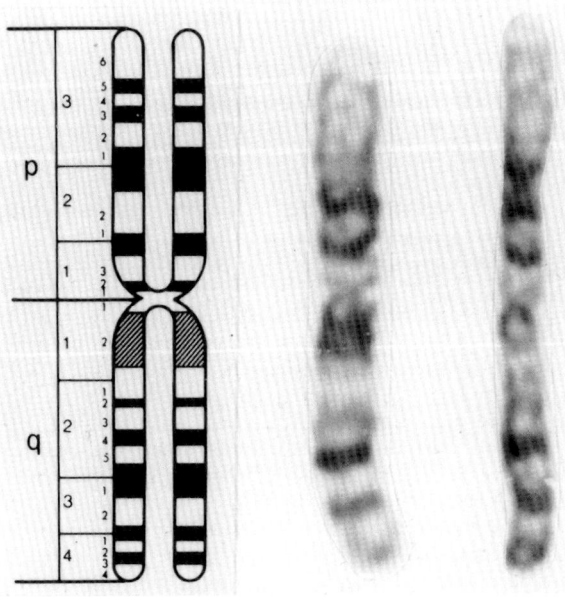

A   **B**   **C**

FIGURE 3-1A-C. Chromosome 1. **(A)** Diagrammatic representation of G (Geimsa) bands. **(B)** Metaphase banding pattern. **(C)** Early metaphase (high-resolution) banding pattern. (Courtesy of Dr. R.S. Sparkes.)

mitosis, the chromosomes are longer and less condensed, permitting identification of more bands; therefore, smaller deletions or duplications can be detected by analyzing the chromosomes in these stages. This "extended" analysis, called high-resolution banding, is more time consuming but is particularly useful if a specific chromosomal anomaly is suspected (Fig. 3-1). Techniques have been developed to identify duplicated or missing portions of chromosomes using DNA probes of known chromosomal location with fluorescent in situ hybridization (FISH). The probes may be specific for a chromosomal region (single-copy cosmid) (Fig. 3-2) or represent sequences on an entire chromosome (Fig. 3-3).

In 1956, Tjio and Levan identified the correct number of human chromosomes as 46[351]; previously, the total had been

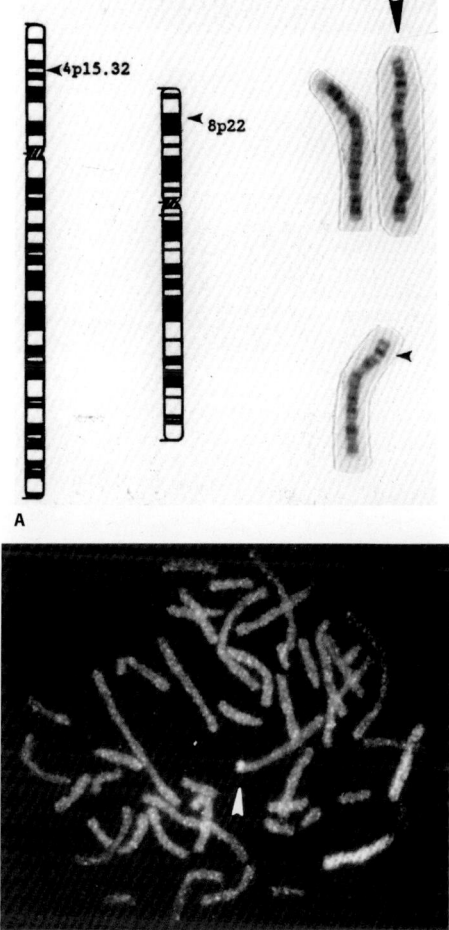

FIGURE 3-2. Fluorescent in situ hybridization (FISH) technique. **Left:** (A) Idiogram of chromosomes 4 and 8 demonstrates a translocation with suspected breakpoints at 4p15.32 and 8p22 (arrows). (B) Partial karyotype of normal and abnormal (arrow) chromosomes 4. An example of a normal chromosome 8 with the suspected breakpoint of 8p22 (arrow) is *below*. This karyotype described as 46,XY,−4,+der(4t)(4;8)(p15.32;p22) de novo is from a patient with Wolf–Hirschorn syndrome and represents a deletion of the chromosome 4p and, presumably, a duplication of chromosome 8p (partial trisomy). (Courtesy of Laurel Estabrooks, Ph.D.) **Right:** The 4;8 translocation illustrated by chromosome 8-specific paint probes. Specific chromosome 8 paint probes hybridize to the two copies of normal chromosome 8 (entire chromosome has hybridized to the paint probes) and to an additional segment on the distal short arm of chromosome 4 (*arrow*). (Courtesy of Dr. L. Estabrooks.)

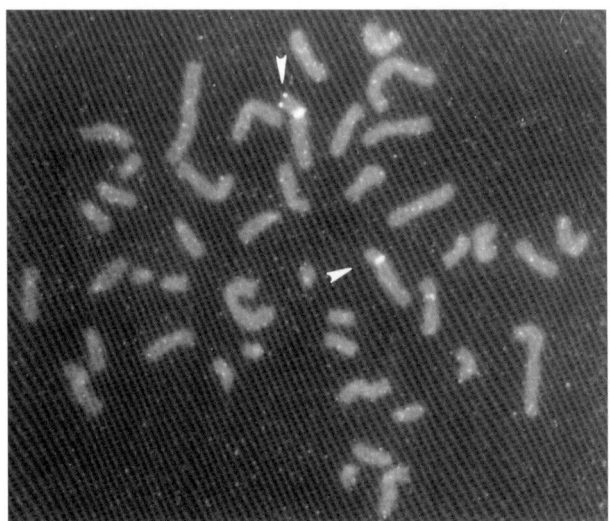

FIGURE 3-3. FISH technique. Cosmid probes specific for the distal region of chromosome 4p illustrate a deletion of chromosome 4p; one *arrow* indicates the hybridized region of the normal chromosome 4 and the other *arrow* indicates the region of the short arm of chromosome 4 with the deletion and without hybridization. A "repeat probe" specific for the centromeric region of chromosome 4 is used to identify the chromosome 4 pair (hybridized region at site of constriction of chromosome). (Courtesy of Dr. L. Estabrooks, with permission.)

believed to be 48. The normal human chromosome complement consists of 22 pairs of autosomes and 1 pair of gender-determining chromosomes (XY for male and XX for female), divided into groups on the basis of length and centromeric position. The short arm of a chromosome is termed "p" and the long arm "q," and any portion may be duplicated or deleted. In 1960, the initial Denver classification was developed at a meeting in Colorado, based on the overall length and centromeric position; seven groups, labeled A through G, were created. In 1971, the Paris nomenclature was created and banding further identified each chromosome. Chromosomes 1, 2, and 3 constitute group A; 4 and 5, group B; 6 to 12 and X, group C; 13 to 15, group D; 16 to 18, group E; 19 and 20; group F; and 21, 22, and Y, group G.

In the late 1950s, the first chromosomal aberrations were identified as an abnormal number of chromosomes. The basis of

Turner's syndrome (monosomy X),[97] Klinefelter's syndrome (a male with one Y chromosome and more than one X chromosome),[165] and Down's syndrome (trisomy 21)[194] (Fig. 3-2) was established shortly after the publication of Tjio and Levan.[351] Many other chromosomal diseases have since been delineated. Chromosomal studies are now a major diagnostic tool in the evaluation of children with congenital malformations and developmental delay. Approximately 1 in every 200 liveborn children and more than half of spontaneous abortions carry a chromosomal abnormality.

Most numerical chromosomal anomalies originate during gametogenesis and are caused by nondisjunction or anaphase lag. During the first meiotic division, homologous, duplicated chromosomes pair and then segregate with each migrating to opposite poles independently; two cells, each with 23 randomly duplicated chromosomes, are the result. A second division of the duplicated chromosomes follows. Failure of separation of homologous chromosomes may occur in the first division or failure of chromatid separation of the duplicated chromosomes may occur in the second. In either case, complementary gametes with 24 chromosomes (1 present in duplicate) and 22 chromosomes (1 missing) may result. If the former is fertilized by a normal gamete (23 chromosomes), the zygote would have 47 chromosomes, 1 being present in triplicate (trisomy); if the latter, the zygote would have 45 chromosomes with 1 missing (monosomy). An abnormal number of chromosomes is termed *aneuploidy*. The autosomal trisomies compatible with term gestation are those of chromosomes 13, 18, and 21, all of which are associated with mental retardation, dysmorphic features, and malformations. Trisomies of other chromosomes that are usually lethal in utero are identified in spontaneous abortions or may result in a live birth if occurring in a mosaic form. Autosomal monosomy is usually lethal, although monosomies of chromosomes 21 and 22 have been reported.

Nondisjunction of sex-determining chromosomes results in less severe phenotypic consequences. Monosomy X is the basis of Turner's syndrome, and females with XXX and XXXX have been identified. Males with XXY and XYY are not uncommon, and increasing numbers of X and Y to XXXXY or XXYY have been reported (Klinefelter's syndrome). If nondisjunction occurs after fertilization, mosaicism results. Cell lines with trisomies or monosomies may persist in the fetus or individual. The diagnosis of mosaicism requires chromosomal analysis of more than one tissue type. In general, cells with autosomal monosomies are nonviable, but monosomy of chromosomes 9, 21, 22, and X may persist.

The second group of clinically recognizable chromosomal syndromes is deletions or missing portions of a chromosome, called partial monosomies; the total number of chromosomes is normal. Most result from a break in a chromosome, usually of a terminal portion with subsequent loss from the cell. If the deletion was de novo in an egg or sperm, only a single child in a family is expected to have the chromosomal abnormality. Deletions also may be inherited as the unbalanced form of a translocation for which a normal parent has an abnormal but balanced chromosome constitution (see following) or may occur sporadically as a result of an abnormality of one of the germ cells (Fig. 3-4). Many partial deletions occur frequently enough that each is considered a syndrome. Ring chromosomes are formed when the ends of chromosome break and form a ring; clinical variation is considerable. There is loss of chromatin (DNA) from both

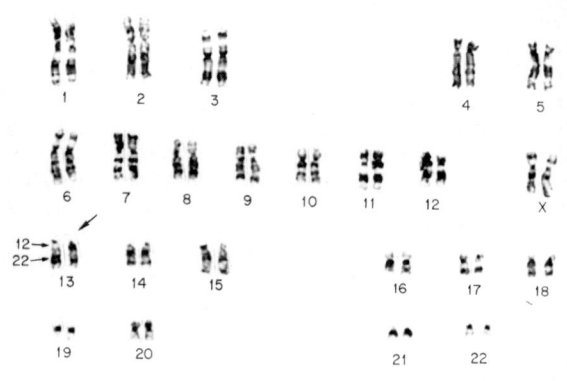

FIGURE 3-4. Deletion 13q. Karyotype of a patient with mental retardation and retinoblastoma caused by an interstitial deletion of the long arm of chromosome 13. The deleted material extends from bands q14 through q22 (46,XX,13q−) as depicted by *small arrows* on the normal left chromosome 13. The *large arrow* identifies the deleted chromosome 13. (Courtesy of Dr. R.S. Sparkes.)

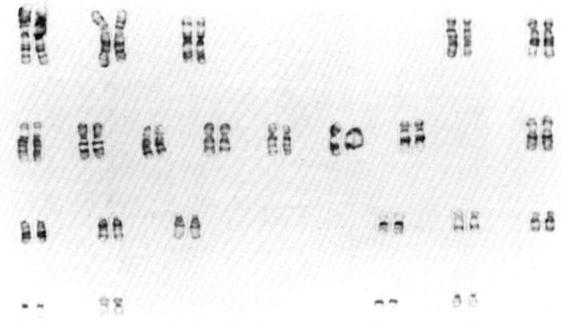

FIGURE 3-5. Ring chromosome 11. Karyotype of a patient with mild mental retardation, short stature, and behavioral problems. (Courtesy of Dr. R.S. Sparkes.)

ends, and affected children may resemble those with simple deletions of the same chromosome (Fig. 3-5).

The third general group is defined by a duplication of a portion of a chromosome, called partial trisomy. The FISH technique may provide the source; if small, the origin of the "extra" chromosomal DNA may be difficult to determine. Partial duplications may be caused by an extra piece of a chromosome, resulting in an increase in the total number of chromosomes (aneuploidy), or by the attachment of duplicated material to another chromosome.

The fourth general category is translocation. DNA may be transferred from one chromosome to another, a translocation; if no genetic material is lost, the translocation is balanced (Fig. 3-6). The first identified human translocations were centric fusions between two acrocentric chromosomes (centromere near one end of the chromosome), which reduced the chromosome count by one; nonessential DNA on the short arms was lost, and the affected individual was apparently normal. Some chromosomes are predisposed to this type of translocation in which the two long arms of a chromosome are fused at or near the centromere with loss of all or a portion of the two short arms; such a translocation between bi-armed chromosomes is termed Robertsonian (Fig. 3-7). Most of the translocations causing

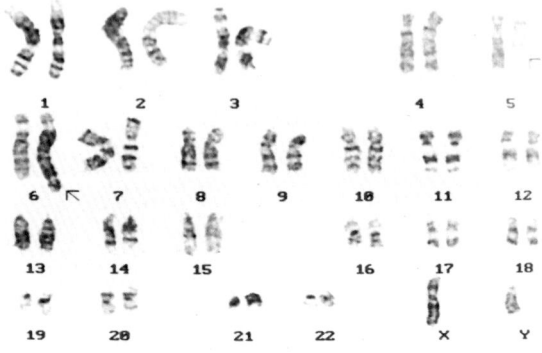

FIGURE 3-6. Translocation. Karyotype of a patient with a translocation between the long arms of chromosomes 5 and 6, as identified by the *arrows*. The break on the chromosome 5 is at band q13 and that of chromosome 6 is q23. This patient is described as has 46,XY,t(5;6)(q13;q23). (Courtesy of Dr. R.S. Sparkes.)

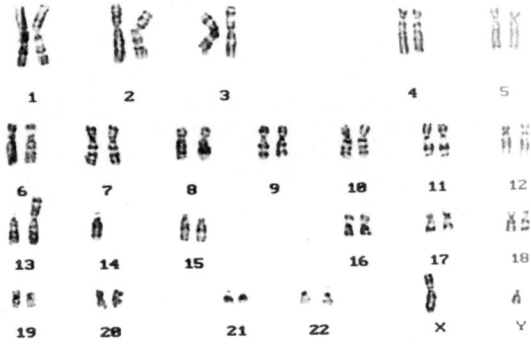

FIGURE 3-7. Robertsonian translocation. Karyotype of a male carrier of a Robertsonian translocation involving chromosomes 13 and 14. This patient has 45 chromosomes and is described as having 45,XY,t(13q,14q). (Courtesy of Dr. R.S. Sparkes.)

Down's syndrome (trisomy 21) are caused by Robertsonian translocations. Carriers of reciprocal translocations are usually clinically normal and are detected because of unbalanced offspring; such carriers may produce a child with multiple anomalies or have a history of fetal wastage.

A nomenclature system has been adopted to describe the human chromosome complement and indicate departures from normalcy. An extra or missing chromosome or a piece of a chromosome is indicated by a plus (+) or a minus (−), respectively; thus, 47,XX+21 is a female with trisomy 21. A female with a partial trisomy of the long arm of chromosome 3 would be described as 46,XX,3q+. A female with an interstitial deletion of the long arm of one chromosome 13 would be depicted as 46,XX,13q− (see Fig. 3-4). A male with a translocation in whom DNA has been transferred from the long arm of one chromosome 5 with a breakpoint at band 13 to the long arm of one chromosome 6 with a breakpoint at band 23 and visa versa without apparent loss of DNA would be described with a "t" as 46,XY,t(5;6)(q13;q23) (see Fig. 3-6). The ring chromosome is depicted as "r," and the structure may be unstable. For example, a ring of chromosome 11 would be described as 11r (Fig. 3-5).

Chromosomal analysis is required for definitive diagnosis of any anomaly. Case reports of familial translocations, deletions, and duplications in which identification of structural abnormalities using chromosomal banding techniques have led to the delineation of many syndromes of partial monosomy (deletion) or partial trisomy (duplication).

Many identifiable chromosomal syndromes exhibit ocular manifestations, and the most common include hypertelorism, epicanthus, up- or downward slanting of the palpebral fissures, blepharoptosis, strabismus, and microphthalmia. However, these features are not specific, and any or all structures of the eye may be abnormal in a patient with a chromosomal anomaly. The most common manifestation with the potential for visual impairment is *microphthalmia*, a malformation in which the anteroposterior diameter and volume of the eye are reduced; it is a relatively common malformation, occurring in 0.22 in 1000 live births, and has been reported to be associated with a variety of chromosomal anomalies.[148] A *coloboma* of the uvea (iris in or choroid in Fig. 3-8) is caused by incomplete closure of the fetal fissure; the "typical" position is inferior to nasal. Incomplete closure of the fetal fissure can cause a spectrum of malforma-

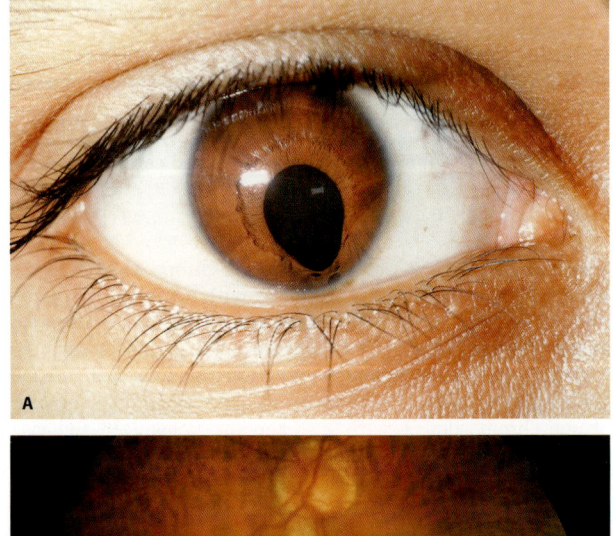

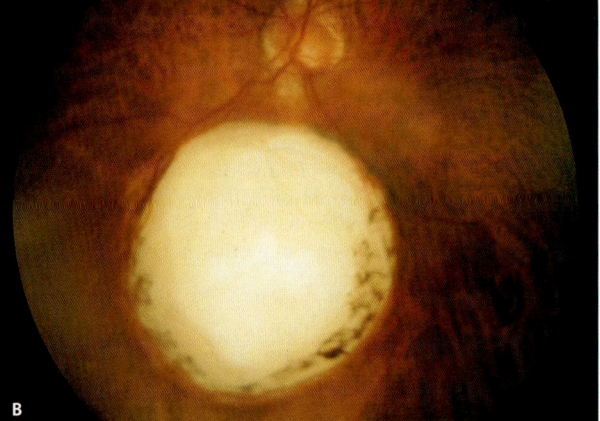

FIGURE 3-8. Coloboma of the iris (*A*) and of the choroid/retina (*B*).

tions ranging from an iris coloboma or microcornea to clincial anophthalmia. The prevalence of coloboma of the eye has been reported to be 0.26 per 1000 births.[148] Any chromosomal defect associated with a colobomatous ocular malformation should be considered to be associated with a malformation within this spectrum. Table 3-1 summarizes the chromosomal anomalies that have been reported in association with colobomatous and

TABLE 3-1. Chromosomal Aberrations in Colobomatous Microphthalmia.

Duplications

1q+	(Pan et al. 1977)[257]
2q+	(Cotlier et al. 1977)[61]
3q+	(Fryns et al. 1978; van Essen et al. 1991)[118]
4q+	(Wilson et al. 1970)[389]
5p+	(Carnevale et al. 1982)[43]
7q+	(Vogel et al. 1973)[371]
8q+	(Fujimoto et al. 1975)[122]
9p+	(Rethore et al. 1977)[282]
9p+q+	(Schwanitz et al. 1977)[317]
10p+	(Cantu et al. 1975)[41]
13q+	(Hsu et al. 1977)[160]
22q+	(Walknowska[72a] et al. 1977)

Deletions

2q–	(Frydman et al. 1989[104]; Young et al. 1983[404]; Fryns et al. 1977)[116]
3q–	(Alvarado et al. 1987)[8]
4p–	(Wilcox et al. 1978)[382]
4r	(Carter et al. 1969)[44]
5p–	(Schwartz et al. 1968)[318]
6r	(Moore et al. 1973; Salamanca-Gomez et al. 1975; Peeden et al. 1983)[262a,347a]
7q–	(Taysi and Burde 1982)
10q–	(Shapiro et al. 1985)[323]
11q–	(Ferry et al. 1981[94a]; Bialasiewicz et al. 1987)[25]
13q–	(O'Grady et al. 1974)[249a]
13r	(Saraux et al. 1970)
17p–	(Stratton et al. 1986)[339]
18p–	(Kuchle et al. 1991)[188]
18q–	(Schinzel et al. 1975)[309]
18r	(Yanoff et al. 1970)[400]

Trisomies

8	(Rutzler et al. 1974)[298]
13	(Cogan and Kubara 1964)[57]
18	(Mullaney 1976)
22	(Antle et al. 1990)[12]

Triploidy (Cogan 1971)

Tetraploidy (Scarbrough et al. 1984)[304]

Duplications

2p+	(Mayer et al. 1978; Nagano et al. 1980)[219]
3p+	
4p+	(Gonzalez et al. 1977)[136]
4q+	(Bonfante et al. 1979)[29]
6p+	(Smith and Pettersen 1985)[329]
7p+	(Milunsky et al. 1989)[231]
9p+	(Allderdice et al. 1983)[6]
9q+	(Allerdice et al. 1983)[6]
10q+	(Yunis et al. 1976)[410a]
14q+	(Raoul et al. 1975)[296]
15q+	(Cohen et al. 1975)[58]
17p+	(Feldman et al. 1982)[93]

Deletions

1q–	(Watson et al. 1986)[375]
6p–	(Sachs et al. 1983)[299]

Trisomy

9	(Sutherland et al. 1976; Kaminker et al. 1985; Williams et al. 1985; Levy et al. 1989; Sandoval et al. 1999)[173,200,303,344,385]

TABLE 3-2. Chromosomal Rearrangements with Cyclopia and Synophthalmia.

Trisomy	
13	(Howard 1977)[156]
18	(Lang and Alfi 1976)[191]
Duplications	
3p+	(Gimelli et al. 1985)[129]
Deletions	
11q−	(Helmuth et al. 1989)[149]
18r	(Cohen et al. 1972)
18p−	(Nitowksi et al. 1966; Faint and Lewis 1964)

noncolobomatous forms of microphthalmia; Table 3-2 describes the association with synophthalmia/cyclopia.

All forms of microscopically identifiable chromosomal deletions, duplications, or aneuploidies are associated with some element of mental retardation with the exception of some X-chromosomal anomalies. Chromosomal analysis may be appropriate for diagnostic purposes for patients with mental, developmental, or growth retardation and two or more congenital anomalies.

Prenatal diagnosis of chromosomal and some single gene disorders can be performed by either traditional amniocentesis or chorion villus sampling, a technique that can be performed as early as the eighth week after conception. The indications include "advanced" maternal age, a parent being a carrier of a balanced chromosomal rearrangement, a previously affected child or relative, or a fetal anomaly detected by ultrasonography. Although clinically significant structural ocular anomalies such as hypo- or hypertelorism and microphthalmia/anophthalmia have been detected prenatally, they are usually detected in association with other fetal anomalies. Some prenatally determined ocular anomalies, such as congenital cataracts, have rarely been detected before the third or late second trimester.

Mental retardation occurs in most of the genetic syndromes in this chapter so this chapter does not include mental retardation in the description of the chromosomal anomalies unless it is unique or not evident.

TRISOMY SYNDROMES

Trisomy 8

Trisomy of chromosome 8 only occurs in a mosaic form in live births. Many organ systems may be involved in the disorder. The facial features are characteristic with a prominent forehead, broad-based nose, everted upper lip, high-arched and/or cleft palate, stretched lingual frenulum, micrognathia, and large, dysplastic ears with a prominent antihelix. The neck is short and broad; the trunk of the body tends to be long and thin. Skeletal anomalies include structural and numerical vertebral abnormalities, spina bifida, scoliosis, pectus carinatum, absent patellae, and hip abnormalities. Renal and ureteral anomalies and cardiac defects are common. Ophthalmic features include hypertelorism, downward slanting of the palpebral fissures, strabismus, blepharoptosis, blepharophimosis, corneal opacities, cataracts, heterochromia of the irides, and colobmatous microphthalmia.[11,37,99,238,266,282,284,298,373]

Trisomy 9

Trisomy 9 is rare in live births; most cases are mosaic. Microcephaly and intrauterine growth retardation are consistent features. Facial features include micrognathia, low-set ears, and a broad-based nose with a bulbous tip. Skeletal abnormalities are consistently present and include fixed or dislocated large joints, hypoplastic or displaced bones, and hand anomalies; genital and renal anomalies may occur. Ophthalmic features include up- or downslanting of the palpebral fissures, narrow palpebral fissures, hypertelorism, epibulbar dermoid, corneal opacities, enophthalmos, and microphthalmia.[72,91,173,200,202,212,281,303,344,385]

Trisomy 10

Trisomy 10 is rare and occurs only in the mosaic state in live births. Affected individuals experience failure to thrive, have developmental delay, and die early in life. General features include a high forehead; dysplastic, large ears; retrognathia, a long slender trunk; marked plantar and palmar furrows; and cardiopathy. Nonspecific ophthalmic manifestations include hypertelorism, mongoloid eye slant and blepharophimosis.[69]

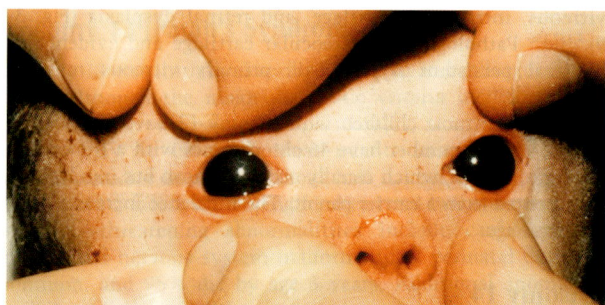

FIGURE 3-10. Trisomy 18. The corneas are enlarged as a result of glaucoma. (Courtesy of Eric A. Wulfsberg, M.D.)

ciliary processes, breaks in the iris sphincter, posterior subcapsular cataract, and retinal pigment epithelial alterations.[133,294]

Trisomy 18 is caused by the presence of an extra chromosome 18; rarely, an unbalanced translocation may cause the syndrome. The incidence increases with maternal age.

Trisomy 21 (Down's Syndrome)

The most common trisomy among live births is chromosome 21 or Down's syndrome, deriving its eponym from Langdon Down, who first described the clinical features in 1866.[79] Systemic findings include hypotonia; brachycephaly; a large protruding tongue; small nose with a low, small bridge; small, poorly defined ears; short, thick neck; stubby hands with a single palmar crease; clinodactyly of fifth digit with hypoplasia of mid-digital phalanges; short, stubby feet with a wide gap between first and second toes; and cardiac malformations. Affected individuals have a higher incidence of leukemia. Males are usually sterile; females, on occasion, are fertile.[280]

The ocular features include epicanthus, upward slanting of the palpebral fissures, myopia, strabismus, nystagmus, blepharitis, ectropion of the eyelids, keratoconus, *Brushfield spots* of the irides, infantile glaucoma, congenital or acquired cataracts, and an increased number of retinal vessels crossing the disc margin.[42,46,130,322,353] The pathological features include focal condensation or hyperplasia of the iris in the region of the Brushfield spots, choroidal congestion, elongation of the ciliary processes, and focal hyperplasia of the retinal pigment epithelium.[130,131]

Most affected children have 47 chromosomes with an extra chromosome 21.[194] About 5% have 46 chromosomes with a translocation involving chromosome 13, 14, or 15, with 14 being most frequent, or a Robertsonian translocation involving either chromosome 21 or 22 (G group), with 21 being most frequent. The translocation may be inherited from a phenotypically normal parent with 45 chromosomes. There are no clinical differences between children with Down's syndrome caused by trisomy 21 or by a translocation. The overall incidence of Down's syndrome is 1 in 700 live births and is age dependent. The risk increases with increasing maternal age. The recurrence risk for parents of a child with Down's syndrome is about 1% if both parents have normal chromosomes. In the event of a parental translocation, the risk is higher if the mother is the carrier; in the rare case of a 21;21 translocation in a parent, all the offspring will have Down's syndrome (see Fig. 3-7).

Mosaicism for trisomy 21 is common. The clinical manifestations vary from a normal phenotype to that of typical Down syndrome.

Trisomy 22

Trisomy 22 causes severe growth and developmental retardation, craniofacial anomalies including microcephaly, arhinencephalon, depressed nasal bridge with a flat nose, preauricular skin tags, dysplastic ears, and high arched or cleft palate, and micrognathia; other features include cardiac, pulmonary, and gastrointestinal malformations. Individuals with partial or mosaic trisomy 22 have been well described; trisomy 22 in a live birth is rare.

Ophthalmic manifestations epicanthus, hypertelorism, up- or downward slanting of the palpebral fissures, blepharoptosis, strabismus, synophrys, cataract, dislocated lenses, optic nerve hypoplasia, colobomatous microphthalmia, and persistent hyperplastic primary vitreous.[12,306,326,372,380]

MONOSOMY SYNDROMES

Monosomy 21

Complete or partial deletion of chromosome 21 causes prenatal growth retardation and craniofacial anomalies including microcephaly, prominent nose, downturned corners of the mouth, micrognathia, and cleft lip and/or palate. Death results from recurrent respiratory infections and gastrointestinal illness. Ophthalmic features include epicanthus, downward slanting of the palpebral fissures, Peters' anomaly of the anterior segment, cataracts, and microphthalmia.[107,263,291,392]

Monosomy 22

Complete absence or deletion of chromosome 22 causes pre- and postnatal growth retardation, microcephaly, hypotonia, and seizures. Additional features include a flat nasal bridge, bifid uvula, and large, low-set ears. Cardiac anomalies may be evident. Deletions including the pericentric region may result in the DiGeorge anomalad with absent or hypoplastic thymus, absent or hypoplastic parathyroids, and great and conotruncal cardiac malformations; skeletal and limb deformities may also be evident. Ophthalmic features include epicanthus, hypertelorism, upward slanting of the palpebral fissures, and blepharoptosis.[71,175,376]

DELETIONAL SYNDROMES

Deletion 1q

Partial monosomy of the long arm of chromosome 1 is rare. Affected individuals have microcephaly, sparse and fine hair, a round face with a carp-shaped mouth and distinctive lower lip, cardiac malformations, and hypoplastic nails. Ophthalmic features include up- or downward slanting of palpebral fissures, epicanthus, hypertelorism, strabismus, blepharoptosis, synophrys, and microphthalmia.[1,171,210,228,375]

Deletion 2q

Partial monosomy of the long arm of chromosome 2 is characterized by relatively nonspecific findings including microcephaly, thin nasal bridge and a short upturned nose, low-set and/or dysplastic ears, micrognathia, and cleft or arched palate; additional features include cardiac and lung malformations, cystic gonads, and digital anomalies. The ophthalmic manifestations include downslanting of the palpebral fissures, epicanthus, narrow palpebral fissures, thick eyebrows and lashes, blepharoptosis and blepharophimosis, corneal opacities, cataracts, optic nerve hypoplasia, nystagmus, and colobomatous microphthalmia.[104,116,234,275,404]

Deletion 3p

Partial monosomy of the short arm of chromosome 3 is characterized by a coarse, triangular face, micrognathia, broad and flat nose, long philtrum, and low-set and/or dysplastic ears; additional features include pectus excavatum and digital anomalies including syndactyly. Ophthalmic manifestations include hypertelorism, epicanthus, downturned and narrow palpebral fissures, synophrys, blepharoptosis, and optic atrophy.[167,241]

Deletion 3q

Partial monosomy of the long arm of chromosome 3 is extremely rare. Features include microcephaly, growth retardation, an unusual facial appearance with cleft lip/palate, cardiac malformations, and clubfeet. Ophthalmic features include narrow palpebral fissures, epicanthus, blepharophtosis, strabismus, cataract, and colobomatous microphthalmia.[8,9,123,368]

Deletion 4p (Wolf–Hirschhorn Syndrome)

The physical findings in partial deletion of the short arm of chromosome 4 (see Fig. 3-3) include microcephaly, seizures, prominent glabella, midline scalp defects, preauricular dimple, cleft lip/palate or high arched palate, deformed nose, hemangiomas, hydrocephalus, and undescended testes and hypospadias in males.[393] Colobomatous microphthalmia is common as is hypertelorism, epicanthus, and downward slanting of the palpebral fissures and strabismus; blepharoptosis, corneal opacities (Peters' anomaly), the anterior segment abnormalities of Rieger's anomaly, and cataracts may occur.[185,218,382]

Deletion 4q

Deletion of the long arm of chromosome 4 results in two distinctive syndromes depending on the location of the deleted material. Terminal deletions are associated with postnatal macrocephaly and the following facial features: dysplastic ears, short nose with a flat nasal bridge, midface hypoplasia, cleft lip and/or palate, and micrognathia. Additional manifestations include skeletal anomalies, cardiac, renal, gastrointestinal, and genital anomalies. Seizures may be evident, and life span is usually very short. Ophthalmic features include hypertelorism, epicanthus, laterally displaced inner canthi, up- or downward slanting of the palpebral fissures, and features of Williams syndrome including stellate irides.[166,232,352]

The manifestations of an interstitial deletion of the long arm of chromosome 4 are less well defined. The features include dysplastic ears, micrognathia, and skeletal anomalies. Reported ophthalmic features include hypertelorism, epicanthus, downward slanting of the palpebral fissures, strabismus, prominent supraorbital ridges, and Rieger's anomaly.[22,54,203,232]

Ring 4

Ring 4 is a rare chromosomal abnormality characterized by microcephaly, micrognathia, a rounded broad nose, and malformed ears. Colobomatous microphthalmia and/or blepharoptosis may be evident.[45,222]

Deletion 5p (Cri du Chat Syndrome)

Lejeune and his colleagues[195] originally described the syndrome due to the partial deletion of the short arm of chromosome 5. Affected individuals have a low birth weight and are hypotonic; the neonatal growth rate is slow. The catlike cry is most noticeable in infancy and is attributable to an abnormality in structure of the larynx. Findings include microcephaly with a round face, micrognathia, low-set ears, and cardiac malformations. Ophthalmic features include a up- or downward slanting of the palpebral fissures, hypo- or hypertelorism, epicanthus, blepharoptosis, myopia, reduced tear production, strabismus with or without reduced abduction, cataracts, glaucoma, tortuous retinal vessels, foveal hypoplasia, optic atrophy, and colobomatous microphthalmia.[33,77,88,157,211,245,383]

Deletion 5q

Deletion of the long arm of chromosome 5 is characterized by high-arched palate and low-set and/or dysplastic ears; additional features include tracheal narrowing and a sacral dimple. Ophthalmic features include strabismus and blepharoptosis.[211]

Deletion 6p

Partial monosomy of the short arm of chromosome 6 is an uncommon chromosomal abnormality with nonspecific general features. Ophthalmic manifestations include hypertelorism, downslanting of the palpebral fissures, epicanthus, strabismus, Peters anomaly, and microphthalmia.[255,278,299,414]

Deletion 6q

Partial monosomy of the long arm of chromosome 6 is a rare chromosomal anomaly characterized by neonatal hypotonia, dolichocephaly, a small, high forehead, facial asymmetry, and a long thorax with truncal obesity and small hands and feet. Ophthalmic features include upslanting and/or narrowing of palpebral fissures and epicanthus.[109,364,399]

Ring 6

The features of ring 6 are nonspecific with a consistent pattern of growth retardation, microcephaly, malformed or low-set ears, micrognathia, and a flat nasal bridge. Ophthalmic features include hypertelorism, epicanthus, downslanting of the palpebral fissures, strabismus, blepharoptosis, micro- or megalocornea, posterior embryotoxon, Rieger anomaly, aniridia, glaucoma, optic atrophy, albinoid fundi, nystagmus, and colobomatous microphthalmia.[52,177,199,236,300]

Deletion 7p

Monosomy of the short arm of chromosome 7 is characterized by craniofacial features of craniosynostosis with scaphocephaly and trigonocephaly, glossoptosis, limitation of joint movements, camptodactyly, cardiac malformations, renal hypoplasia, and hypoplastic external genitalia. Ophthalmic features include hypotelorism and "prominent eyes."[102]

Deletion 7q

Monosomy of the long arm of chromosome 7 is characterized by structural abnormalities of the face including a broad nasal bridge with a stubby nose, a large mouth with an everted lower lip and downturned corners, low-set and malformed ears, and skeletal abnormalities such as short hands and feet, clubfeet, and lobster-claw deformities. Hydrocephalus with cortical atrophy and/or seizures may be evident. The specific features of the syndrome are a function of the missing portion of the long arm of chromosome 7.

Individuals with a deletion of the terminal region of chromosome 7 (q3) have the following, relatively consistent features: developmental delay, growth retardation, hypotonia, unusual facial appearance with a broad nasal bridge and bulbous nasal tip, microcephaly, holoprosencephaly, cleft lip and/or palate, anomalous auricles, single transverse palmar creases, genital anomalies in males, abnormal electroencephalogram, and ocular abnormalities. Most terminal deletions extend from the q32 or the q35 bands; the specific breakpoint does not differentiate the two clinically. Generally, affected fetuses or individuals have some ocular abnormality with nonspecific findings such as epicanthus, hypertelorism, and upward slanting of the lids being the most common; synophrys, strabismus, glaucoma, colobomatous microphthalmia, and optic nerve atrophy may occur.[35,174,249,335,361,405] Friedrich and colleagues reported an individual with optic atrophy and a coloboma of the optic nerve who had a terminal deletion from the 7q32 region.[102] Reynolds and colleagues described a child with a more distal deletion from the 7q34 region who had colobomatous microphthalmia, corneal opacification with vascularization, posteriorly subluxed lenses, and a falciform fold of the retina.[283]

McMorrow and colleagues reported an infant with bilateral anophthalmia and other malformations associated with an interstitial deletion of the long arm of chromosome 7 from the q21.1 to q36.1 bands.[224] Absence of the adrenal glands has been reported in monosomy q1 and q3 (distal deletions).

Life span appears to be longer for monosomy 7q2 as compared to monosomy 7q1 and distal deletions. Ophthalmic manifestations of an interstitial deletion of the q2 band include hypertelorism, epicanthus, and downslanting of the palpebral fissures in monosomy 7q1[267]; hypertelorism, epicanthus, and short, upslanting palpebral fissures.[215,405]

Deletion 8p

Monosomy of the short arm of chromosome 8 in band 2 is characterized by microcephaly with a narrow head and high forehead, protruding occiput, a flat nasal bridge with a short nose, a short neck, micrognathia, a broad chest with wide-set and hypoplastic nipples, cardiac malformations, and, in males, hypospadias, cryptorchidism, and testicular hypoplasia. Ophthalmic manifestations include hypertelorism, epicanthus, downslanting of the palpebral fissures, strabismus, and nystagmus.[27,34,253,279]

Deletion 9p

Monosomy of the short arm of chromosome 9 causes craniofacial anomalies including trigonocephaly, a flattened nasal bridge, short nose, anteverted nares, long philtrum, small mouth, and micrognathia; the ears are low set with small lobes and hypoplastic helices. The internipple distance is increased, the metacarpals short, and the nails dysplastic. Genital hypoplasia occurs in both males and females. Ophthalmic features include up- and downward slanting of the palpebral fissures, epicanthus, hypertelorism, strabismus, blepharoptosis, exophthalmos, and congenital glaucoma.[2,75,125,246,281,297,369,403,404]

Deletion 10p

Deletion of the short arm of chromosome 10 is uncommon. Affected individuals have growth retardation and microcephaly. Facial features include frontal bossing, low nasal root, anteverted nares, micrognathia, dysplastic ears, and a short neck. Wide-spaced nipples and cardiac and genitourinary malformations may also occur. Ophthalmic features include hypertelorism, downslanting and/or narrowing of the palpebral fissures, epicanthus, strabismus, blepharoptosis, and corneal opacities.[84,141,182,343]

Deletion 10q

Monosomy of the long arm of chromosome 10 causes low birth weight, hypotonia, and microcephaly. Affected individuals may have brachycephaly, a broad and prominent nasal bridge, a small nose with anteverted nostrils, low-set and large ears, a prominent upper lip, and short neck; cleft lip/palate and micrognathia may be evident. Additional features include growth retardation, skeletal anomalies including clinodactyly, syndactyly, an abnormal chest with wide-spaced nipples, and delayed bone age. Ophthalmic features include hypertelorism, up- or downward slanting and narrowing of the palpebral fissures, scant lashes, strabismus, and colobomatous microphthalmia.[51,86,201,227,323,347,362,378,395,413]

Deletion 11p

The constellation of aniridia, retardation (mental), and genitourinary anomalies has been associated with a predisposition to Wilms' tumor and is termed the WAGR syndrome. Deletion of the short arm of chromosome 11 involving the 11p13 band accounts for most cases[21,286,330,374]; one patient has had aniridia and Wilms tumor without a microscopically detectable deletion.[285] Aniridia may be associated with other ocular malformations including cataract, glaucoma, corneal dystrophies, and macular hypoplasia. Genitourinary malformations appear to be more common in males and include cryptorchidism, hypospadias, and pseudohermaphroditism; renal anomalies may be present. Microcephaly, cardiac malformations, and polydactyly have been reported. Although Wilms' tumor has been the embryonal tumor usually associated with this syndrome, benign gonadoblastoma has also been reported.[374]

The deletion may occur de novo or as a consequence of meiotic events in a normal carrier parent. The gene for catalase has been mapped in the proximity of the aniridia locus in band p13 on the short arm of chromosome 11,[172] and the activity of this enzyme is reduced in the presence of some deletions.[21,240]

All children with aniridia and this deletion should be followed carefully by abdominal ultrasound to facilitate early detection of Wilms' tumor.

Deletion 11q

Individuals with a partial deletion of the long arm chromosome 11 have growth retardation and craniofacial features including trigonocephaly, microcephaly, a short, broad nose with a depressed bridge, and a carp-shaped mouth. Affected individuals may have malformations of the heart or kidney. Ophthalmic features include hypertelorism, epicanthus, up- or downward slanting of the palpebral fissures, strabismus, blepharoptosis, Peters' anomaly, colobomatous microphthalmia, and cyclopia.[21,25,110,149,226,235,250,308,345]

Ring 11

Ring formation of chromosome 11 has features similar to deletion of the long arm. Features include microcephaly with a flat occiput and musculoskeletal anomalies. Ophthalmic features include hypertelorism, epicanthus, up- or downward slanting of the palpebral fissures, narrow palpebral fissures, strabismus, blepharoptosis, microcornea, anterior segment dysgenesis, and a stellate pattern of the iris (see Fig. 3-5).[62,66,248,254]

Deletion 12p

Deletion of the short arm of chromosome 12 causes moderate to severe developmental delay with microcephaly and characteristic facial features including a long-pointed nose, micrognathia, and low-set, large ears. Other manifestations include cryptorchidism and micropenis in males. Ophthalmic features include hypertelorism, epicanthus, downward sloping of the palpebral fissures, strabismus, synophrys, sclerocornea, optic atrophy, and probably glaucoma.[28,178,282,296]

Ring 12

Ring formation of chromosome 12 causes growth retardation, cafe-au-lait spots, pectus excavatum, hypothyroidism, and glandular hypospadias. Ophthalmolgic features include strabismus.[258]

Deletion 13q

Partial monosomy for chromosome 13 caused by either deletion of part of the long arm or ring 13 results in similar phenotypes including microcephaly and trigonocephaly; facial features include a prominent bridge of the nose; small chin; large, low-set, malformed ears; and facial asymmetry (see Fig. 40-4). Other features include absent or hypoplastic thumbs, cardiac and renal malformations, anal atresia, and features of Noonan syndrome; males may have hypospadias and undescended testes. Ophthalmic findings of interstitial deletions of 13q include hypertelorism, up- or downward slanting and/or narrow palpebral fissures, epicanthus, strabismus, blepharoptosis, cataract, retinoblastoma, Rieger syndrome, and colobomatous microphthalmia.[5,187,214,243,245,252,290,336,339,348,387]

The retinoblastoma gene is located in band 14 of the long arm of chromosome 13 and has become a prototype for the study of the hereditary predisposition to cancer. The initial evidence for the location of the gene came from children who had mental retardation, dysmorphic features, and retinoblasoma associated with a deletion in the long arm of chromosome 13[332,412]; approximately 6% of children with a retinoblastoma have been shown to have a detectable deletion in the same regions.[36] The autosomal dominant form of the disease was later localized to the same region by the identification of linkage with esterase D,[333] a red cell enzyme that had been previously mapped to the same region on the long arm of chromosome 13.[334] Assay of esterase D may be a method for identification of small deletions.[63] Thereafter, Benedict and colleagues[23] demonstrated homozygosity for the locus (inactivation or both alleles) in tumor cell lines supporting a recessive pattern on a cellular level. The gene has been cloned,[103,126,193] and risk assessment is greatly improved.[48,142,381] Prenatal diagnosis may be possible for families with a germinal mutation or a balanced translocation.

Ring 13

See deletion 13q.

Deletion 14q

Partial deletion of the long arm of chromosome 14 is associated with dysmorphic facial features including a round face, hypertrichosis with thick eyebrows, a short nose with a flat root and bulbous tip; long philtrum, and micrognathia; dolicho- and brachycephaly may be evident. Ophthalmic features include epicanthus, narrow palpebral fissures, strabismus, synophrys, blepharoptosis, and glaucoma.[159,247,357,399,401]

Ring 14

Ring formation of chromosome 14 causes growth delay and craniofacial abnormalities including micro- and dolicocephaly, high forehead, bulbous nasal tip, large, low-set ears, high-arched palate, micrognathia, thin upper lip, downturned corners of the mouth, and a short neck with skin folds; other manifestations include seizures, widely spaced nipples, cardiac malformations, pigmentary abnormalities including cafe-au-lait spots and viteligo, and simian creases of the hands. Ophthalmic features include hypertelorism, epicanthus, downslanting of the palpebral fissures, and alterations of the retinal pigmental epithelium.[32,158,205,314]

Deletion 15q

Deletion of the q11–13 region of the long arm of chromosome 15 causes either the Angelman or Prader–Willi syndrome. Angelman syndrome is caused by deletion of the maternally derived chromosome 15, generally, bands q11.3 through q13. The syndrome is characterized by absent speech, seizures, and a puppet-like jerky gait. Prader–Willi syndrome is characterized by hypotonia, obesity with an onset in early childhood, hypogonadism, and small hands and feet; deletion of band q11.3 of the paternally derived chromosome 15 is the basis of the syndrome. In both, ocular hypopigmentation is evident.[76,209,265]

Ring 15

A ring formation of chromosome 15 is characterized by growth retardation, microcephaly, acromicria, and micrognathia; other features include cardiac, renal, and skeletal malformations; cafe au lait spots; and gonadal hypoplasia. Ophthalmic features include hypertelorism, strabismus, nystagmus, and retinal depigmentation.[38,109,192,397]

Deletion 16q

Deletion of the long arm of chromosome 16 causes growth retardation, hypotonia, and craniofacial malformations including a high forehead, large anterior fontanel, prominent metopic suture, diastasis of the cranial sutures, low-set, dysplastic ears, micrognathia, and a short neck. Additional features include intestinal, cardiac, skeletal, and renal malformations. Band 16q21 is believed to be responsible for the distinctive aspects of the syndrome. Ophthalmolgic features include narrow and up- and downward slanting of the palpebral fissures, hypertelorism, strabismus, and epicanthus.[105,115,225,292]

Deletion 17p

An interstitial deletion of the short arm of chromosome 17 in the p11 band causes mental retardation with hypotonia, seizures, and craniofacial anomalies consisting of micro- and brachycephaly, prominent forehead, a broad face with a flattened midfacial region, broad nasal bridge, malformed and malpositioned ears, prominent jaw, and delayed dentition. Additional features include digital anomalies such as broad short hands, hearing loss, deep voice, and cardiac and genital anomalies. Ophthalmic features include up- or downward slanting of the palpebral fissures, strabismus, Brushfield spots of the iris, synophrys, and colobomatous microphthalmia.[207,260,328,339]

A deletion of the p13 region of the short arm of chromosome 17, Miller–Dieker syndrome, is associated with lissencephaly (smooth brain) and agyri or pachygyria. Additional malformations of the brain may be evident. Affected individuals have severe mental retardation with seizures and hypotonia. Ophthalmic manifestations include hypertelorism, upslanting and/or narrowing of the palpebral fissures, and epicanthus.[140]

Ring 17

Ring 17 is associated with mental retardation, microcephaly, and short stature. Features of neurofibromatosis I may be evident. Flecked retina with subretinal drusen-like deposits has been reported.[49]

Deletion 18p

The physical findings associated with the deletion (total or partial) of the short arm of chromosome 18 are broad. In the mildest form, affected individuals have microcephaly, mild mental retardation, short stature, webbed neck, and immunoglobulin abnormalities.[138] In the most severe form, median facial dysplasia with cebocephaly and/or incomplete morphogenesis of the brain may occur, with digital anomalies such as short fingers, high-set thumb(s), and syndactyly. Cardiac, renal, and gastrointestinal malformations are uncommon but may be evident. The ophthalmic features consistently include hypertelorism, epicanthus, blepharoptosis, and strabismus. Cataracts, retinal dysplasia, colobomatous microphthalmia, and synophthalmia/cyclopia have been reported.[113,156,188,208,311,395]

Deletion 18q

Partial deletion of the long arm of chromosome 18 produces a syndrome marked by mental and growth retardation with hypotonia. The facies is striking with microcephaly, midface hypoplasia, a carplike mouth with downward slanting margins, and a prominent antihelix and/or antitragus of the ears with a narrow or atretic canal and hearing loss. Cardiac and genitourinary malformations are common. The fingers taper markedly with a high frequency of whorl patterns, and simian creases may be evident. Toes have abnormal placement with the third toe placed above the second and fourth. Dimples may be evident on knuckles, knees, elbows, and shoulders. Ophthalmic abnormalities include epicanthus, hypertelorism, downward slanting of the palpebral fissures, nystagmus, strabismus, corneal abnormalities, cataracts, blue sclerae, dysplastic or atrophic optic nerve heads, and colobomatous microphthalmia.[60,70,92,208,239,309,354,390]

Ring 18

The physical findings of ring formation of chromosome 18 overlaps both the short arm and long arm deletion syndromes, although the manifestations are usually less severe than the monosomy 18 syndromes (see earlier). Ophthalmic features include epicanthus, hypertelorism, strabismus, nystagmus, blepharoptosis, colobomatous microphthalmia, and cyclopia.[78,156,190,208] Yanoff et al. histopathologically studied the eyes in the case of cebocephaly with a ring 18, and bilateral microphthalmia with cyst, intrascleral cartilage, intrachoroidal smooth muscle, and other anomalies were evident; however, no recognizable components of the optic system could be identified.[400]

Deletion 19p

Deletion of the short arm of chromosome 19 is associated with significant mental retardation and microcephaly. Facial features include low-set ears, flat nose, micrognathia, high-arched palate, and downturned corners of the mouth. Ophthalmic features hypertelorism and persistent hyperplastic primary vitreous.[162]

Deletion 20p

Deletion of the short arm of chromosome 20 causes growth delay and characteristisc facial features including a low and flat nasal bridge, maxillary hypoplasia, long philtrum, thin upper lip, small mandible, low-set ears, and a high-arched palate. Additional manifestations include upper airway obstruction, digital anomalies, and cardiac malformations. Ophthalmic features include epicanthus, hypertelorism, downward slanting of the palpebral fissures, strabismus, colobomata of the irides, and the anterior segment features of the Rieger or Alagille syndromes.[10,325]

Ring 21

The clinical features of ring 21 are similar to monosomy 21. Visceral anomalies are relatively consistent features. Reported ophthalmic manifestations include up- or downward slanting of the palpebral fissures and dysgenesis of the anterior segment similar to that of Peters' anomaly.[65,94,128,151,155,229]

Deletion 22q

The velo-cardio-facial (DiGeorge) syndrome has been associated with a deletion of the long arm of chromosome 22 in the region of band 11. The DiGeorge syndrome is characterized by aplasia of the thymus and parathyroids; the disorder may be referred to as the third and fourth pharyngeal pouch syndrome. Reported ophthalmic features include hypertelorism and up- or down-slanting of the palpebral fissures.[41,71,175,317]

Ring 22

Ring 22 causes mental retardation with microcephaly and craniofacial features including bulbous nose, high-arched palate, and large ears. Additional manifestations include renal anomalies such as polycystic kidneys and cardiac malformations. Ophthalmic features include epicanthus downslanting of the palpebral fissures, strabismus, synophrys, and proptosis.[117,125,161,204]

DUPLICATION SYNDROMES

Duplication 1q

Partial trisomy of the long arm of chromosome 1 is characterized by facial dysmorphism with deep-set eyes, a broad nasal bridge, retrognathia, and posteriorly rotated ears; mental retardation and seizures may be evident. Ophthalmic features include narrow horizontal palpebral fissures, synophrys, and colobomatous microphthalmia.[49,256,257,269,346]

Duplication 2p

Partial trisomy of the short arm of chromosome 2 is characterized by craniofacial features including microcephaly, a prominent forehead and/or glabella, short nose with a broad bridge and prominent tip, high-arched palate, micrognathia, pointed chin, and low-set and dysplastic ears; cardiac and genitourinary malformations and skeletal or digital anomalies may be present. Ophthalmic features include hypertelorism, epicanthus, strabismus, narrow palpebral fissures, blepharoptosis and blepharophimosis, nasolacrimal duct obstruction, cataract, retinal detachment and dysplasia, tortuosity of the retinal vessels, optic atrophy, persistent hyperplastic primary vitreous, and microphthalmia.[147,219,274,409]

Duplication 2q

Partial trisomy of the long arm of chromosome 2 is rare and characterized by growth retardation, microcephaly, a square facies, prominent glabella, micrognathia, cleft palate, cardiac malformations, and genitourinary malformations. Ophthalmic features include epicanthus, hypertelorism, up- or downward slanting of the palpebral fissures, strabismus, blepharitis, microcornea, anomalies of the anterior chamber angle, congenital glaucoma, dislocated lenses, macular hypoplasia with nystagmus, optic atrophy or optic nerve dysplasia, and colobomatous microphthalmia.[61,219,234,341,406]

Duplication 3p

Partial trisomy of the short arm of chromosome 3 is characterized by multiple anomalies including an unusual facial appearance with micro- and brachycephaly, frontal bossing with temporal indentations, a square-shaped face, a protruding upper lip with a long philtrum, and micrognathia. Skeletal anomalies including a short neck and syndactyly, hirsutism, and cardiac malformations may be evident. Ophthalmic features include hypertelorism, epicanthus, microphthalmia, and cyclopia.[129,179,368]

Duplication 3q

Partial trisomy of the long arm of chromosome 3, which is rare, is characterized by acro- and brachycephaly, hirsutism, facial features similar to the de Lange syndrome, synophrys, long eyelashes, hypogenitalism in both males and females, and cardiac malformations. Ophthalmic manifestations are common and include hypertelorism, epicanthus, up- or downward slanting of the palpebral fissures, synophrys, strabismus, nasolacrimal duct obstruction, cataract, corneal opacities, congenital glaucoma, nystagmus, and colobomatous microphthalmia.[4,53,90,118,183,301,316,337,368,386,411]

Duplication 4p

Partial trisomy of the short arm of chromosome 4 is a rare abnormality associated with dysmorphic facial features, malformed ears, depressed nasal bridge, short neck, prominent glabella and chin, abnormal genitalia in males, and skeletal anomalies; growth and mental retardation are consistent features. Ophthalmic features include hypertelorism, epicanthus, downslanting of the palpebral fissures, deeply set eyes, strabismus, blepharophimosis, bushy eyelashes, synophrys, nystagmus, and microphthalmia.[64,136,145,163]

Duplication 4q

Partial trisomy of the long arm of chromosome 4 is associated with microcephaly, micrognathia, a short neck, and syndactyly. Ophthalmic features include up- and downward slanting of the palpebral fissures, hypotelorism, epicanthus, strabismus, blepharoptosis and blepharophimosis, corneal clouding, and microphthalmia.[29,82,242,281,389,407]

Duplication 5p

Partial trisomy of the short arm of chromosome 5 is rare and the general features are relatively nonspecific; ophthalmic manifestations are common. Affected individuals have macro-dolicho-scaphocaphaly, low-set ears, depressed nasal bridge, macroglossia, micrognathia, cardiac malformations, long fingers, clubfeet, and seizures. Ophthalmic features include hypertelorism, upward slanting and/or narrowing of the palpebral fissures, epicanthus, strabismus, cataracts, nystagmus, and colobomatous microphthalmia.[44,176,196]

Duplication 5q

Duplication of the long arm of chromosome 5 is characterized by microcephaly, craniofacial dysmorphism with a short and receding forehead, prominent nasal bridge, low-set and/or dysplastic ears, a long or short philtrum, and a carp-shaped mouth or macrostomia. Additional features include digital anomalies and cardiac disease. Ophthalmic features include epicanthus, hypertelorism, and strabismus.[189]

Duplication 6p

Trisomy of the short arm of chromosome 6 is characterized by pre- and postnatal growth retardation. Affected individuals have a characteristic craniofacial dysmorphism with dolichocephaly, a high forehead with a high and broad nasal bridge, bulbous nose with hyperplastic nares, short philtrum, small mouth with thin lips, and micrognathia; choanal atresia, camptodactyly, syndactyly, and genitourinary malformations may be evident. Ophthalmic features include hypertelorism, strabismus, long lashes, blepharophimosis, blepharoptosis, optic atrophy, and microphthalmia.[112,329]

Duplication 6q

Trisomy of the long arm of chromosome 6 is characterized by minor dysmorphic features in infancy with development of turricephaly and a prominent forehead with or without microcephaly in childhood. The neck is broad, short, and webbed. The nipples are wide spaced with deformities of the chest and spine; joint contractures are common. Hypospadius and cryptorchidism may also be evident. Ophthalmic features include downward slanting of the palpebral fissures, epicanthus, hypertelorism, blepharoptosis, strabismus, hypoplastic supraorbital ridges, and thin, arched eyebrows.[50,55,350,355]

Duplication 7p

Duplication of the short arm of chromosome 7 causes dolichocephaly or microbrachycephaly, gaping fontanels, and wide sagittal and metopic sutures, large and low-set ears, and small mouth with downturned corners, micrognathia; other features include choanal atresia/stenosis, skeletal anomalies including hyperextensible joints, camptodactyly and rocker-bottom feet, joint contractures, and cardiac, central nervous system, and genitourinary malformations. Ophthalmic features include hypertelorism, epicanthus, up- or downward slanting of the palpebral fissures, and microphthalmia.[24,231]

Duplication 7q

Partial trisomy of the long arm of chromosome 7 in bands 2 to 3 causes pre- and postnatal growth retardation, delayed skeletal maturation including closure of the fontanelles, hypotonia, seizures, central nervous system malformations including hydrocephalus, hypoplasia of the corpus callosum, cerebral and cerebellar atrophy, and hypoplasia of the cerebellar vermis. Facial features include frontal bossing, depression of the nasal bridge, upturned nares, long philtrum, cleft palate, small mandible, dysplastic ears, and short neck and skeletal anomalies include scoliosis, hemivertebrae, absent ribs, joint laxity or stiffness, hip dislocation, camptodactyly, short midhands with a single transverse palmar crease, and long fingers and toes. Ophthalmologic features include hypertelorism, downward slanting and/or narrow palpebral fissures, epicanthus, strabismus, absent lateral rectus muscles, "prominent eyes," long lashes, optic nerve hypoplasia, and colobomatous microphthalmia/anophthalmia.[95,139,169,174,295,321,370,371]

Duplication 8p

Trisomy of the short arm of chromosome 8 is characterized by a high, prominent forehead, an everted lower lip, a poorly defined philtrum, macrostomia with gingival hypertrophy, a low nasal bridge and anteverted nostrils, and large, soft ears with excess folds. Hypotonia is common. Other features include flexion contractures and clubfeet; cardiac, central nervous system, and renal malformations; and spina bifida. Ophthalmic features include hypertelorism and upward slanting of the palpebral fissures.[56,111,217]

Duplication 8q

Duplication of the long arm of chromosome 8 causes growth retardation and craniofacial features including a prominent and short forehead, a broad and flat nose with a short septum, dysplastic ears, and a short upper lip. Additional manifestations include a funnel chest, hypertrichosis, and skeletal anomalies including coxa valga and brachy- and clinodactyly. Ophthalmic features include hypertelorism, upward slanting of the palpebral fissures, and colobomatous microphthalmia.[122,302,307]

Duplication 9p

Trisomy of the short arm of chromosome 9 is characterized by relatively consistent facial features including brachycephaly, bulbous nose, low-set and/or dysplastic ears, short philtrum, downturned corners of the mouth, cleft lip/palate, and a "worried appearance." Mental retardation and microcephaly occur in all cases. Delayed bone maturation, skeletal anomalies such as brachy- and clinodactyly and nail hypoplasia, and cardiac anomalies may be evident. Ophthalmic features include hypertelorism, downward slanting of the palpebral fissures, entropion, strabismus, cataracts, optic atrophy, and enophthalmia.[230,282,327,342,363,388,403]

Tetrasomy 9p

Tetrasomy of the short arm of chromosome 9 causes low birth weight, mental retardation, microcephaly, open sutures and fontanelles, and hydrocephalus; facial features include a bulbous, beaked nose, downward slanting mouth, micro- and retrognathia, protruding and malformed ears, and a short neck. Cardiac malformations and skeletal anomalies may be present. Ophthalmic features include hypertelorism, epicanthus, strabismus, and enophthalmia.[16,127,264]

Duplication 9q

Features of partial trisomy of chromosome 9, particularly including band 34 through the terminal region, include pre- and postnatal growth retardation, dolichocephaly, beaked nose, microstomia, retrognathia, and arachnodactyly. Ophthalmic features include epicanthus, hypotelorism, narrow palpebral fissures, strabismus, blepharoptosis, microphthalmia, and deep-set eyes.[6,281,331,359]

Duplication 10p

Duplication of the short arm of chromosome 10 causes mental and growth retardation. Craniofacial features include dolichocephaly, a narrow face, broad cheeks, high forehead, nose with a broad root and bulbous tip, thin lips, cleft lip or palate, fissured tongue, micrognathia, and small chin. Additional manifestations include cardiac and renal anomalies, hypoplastic or cystic lungs, and skeletal anomalies such as camptodactyly, scoliosis, and flexion deformities. Ophthalmic features include hypertelorism, upward slanting of the palpebral fissures, long, curled eyelashes, and colobomatous microphthalmia.[42,135,251,410]

Duplication 10q

Duplication of the long arm of chromosome 10 is characterized by severe growth retardation. Craniofacial features include microcephaly, high forehead, midfacial hypoplasia with a broad nasal bridge, an upturned nose, microstomia, micrognathia, cleft lip/palate, and a short neck. Additional features include skeletal anomalies such as generalized laxity, scoliosis, and camptodactyly, and cardiac and renal malformations. Ophthalmic manifestations include hypertelorism, epicanthus, downward slanting and/or narrow palpebral fissures, strabismus, enophthalmia, blepharoptosis and blepharophimosis, cataract, and microphthalmia.[20,96,114,180,186,273,410]

Duplication 11p

Individuals with duplication of the short arm of chromosome 11 have growth retardation and facial features including frontal bossing, a broad and flat nasal bridge, cleft lip/palate, and macroglossia; additional manifestations include hernia formation, cryptorchidism, hypospadias, and renal and cardiac malformations. Ophthalmic features include hypertelorism, epicanthus, downward slanting of the palpebral fissures, strabismus, blepharoptosis, conjunctival telangiectasia, Brushfield spots of the iris, nystagmus, and a retinal degeneration with abnormal rod responses on electroretinography.[87,170,340,358,377]

Duplication 11q

Individuals with duplication of the long arm of chromosome 11 have growth retardation, microcephaly with hypoplasia or aplasia of the corpus callosum, and facial dysmorphism including a short nose, long philtrum, micrognathia, low-set ears, and a high-arched palate or cleft palate. Some individuals have an unusual malformation of the clavicle; other features include cardiac or urinary malformations, cutis laxa, and neural tube defects. Ophthalmic features include hypo- or hypertelorism, epicanthus, downward slanting of the palpebral fissures, strabismus, conical corneal shape, and eccentric pupils.[68,144,270]

Duplication 12p

Partial trisomy of the short arm of chromosome 12 causes severe mental retardation, with characteristic facial features including midfacial hypoplasia, long philtrum, puffy cheeks with a thick, everted lower lip, a large tongue, and small ears; turribrachycephaly may be evident. Additional features include broad, short hands with clinodactyly, micrognathia, diastasis recti, and malformations of the heart and urinary tract. Ophthalmic features include hypertelorism, epicanthus, and downward slanting of the palpebral fissures.[14,152,277,281,289]

Duplication 12q

Trisomy of the long arm of chromosome 12 is associated with multiple craniofacial features including asymmetry with dolico- or brachycephaly, a narrow nasal bridge with anteverted nares, short upper lip, macrostomia, downturned corners of the mouth, scrotal tongue, and low-set and/or dysplastic ears. Skeletal anomalies may include proximal thumbs, brachymetatary and brachycarpy, and hip dislocations. Ophthalmic features include epicanthus, hypertelorism, upward slanting and/or narrow palpebral fissures, and heavy eyebrows.[73,220]

Duplication 13q

Partial duplication of the long arm of chromosome 13 causes mental and growth retardation with microcephaly; facial features include frontal bossing, long philtrum, dysplastic ears, stubby nose, and high arched palate; additional features include polydactyly, and genital abnormalities in males. Ophthalmic manifestations include hypo- or hypertelorism, epicanthus, up- or downward slanting of the palpebral fissures, strabismus, blepharoptosis, long lashes, synophrys, spherophakia, and colobomatous microphthalmia. The frequency of the specific anomalies is a function of the trisomic region.[30,85,132,233,244,261,310,349,397]

Duplication 14q

Duplication of the long arm of chromosome 14 is associated with growth retardation, microcephaly, and seizures. Features include a low anterior hairline, low-set and dysplastic ears, a prominent tip of the nose with a broad base, a large mouth with a thin upper lip, and micrognathia; the palate may be highly arched or clefted. Cardiac and genital malformations may be evident. Ophthalmic features include hypo- or hypertelorism, downward slanting of the palpebral fissures, blepharoptosis or blepharophimosis, strabismus, congenital glaucoma, microcornea, and microphthalmia.[15,89,268,276]

Duplication 15q

Duplication of long arm of chromosome 15 results in mental and postnatal growth retardation with microcephaly associated with craniofacial features including microdolichocephaly, prominent occiput, sloping forehead, large, low-set ears, prominent bulbous nose, long philtrum and a midline crease in the upper lip, high-arched palate, and micrognathia. Ophthalmic manifestations include downward slanting of the palpebral fissures, narrow palpebral fissures, epicanthus, strabismus, blepharoptosis, cataract, retinal detachment, and microphthalmia.[58,121,143,315,397]

Duplication of band 1 of the long arm of chromosome 15 causes severe mental retardation with the craniofacial features of an oval face with prominent supraorbital and zygomatic regions, full cheeks, a large nose, low-set ears, and a high-arched or cleft palate; microcephaly may be evident. Additional features include limb anomalies such as short, thick digits and rocker-bottom feet, cardiac malformations, and seizures. Signs and symptoms of the Prader–Willi syndrome may be evident. Ophthalmic manifestations include deep-set eyes, stabismus, and microphthalmia.[154,265]

Duplication 16p

Duplication of the short arm of chromosome 16 causes mental and prenatal growth retardation with seizures and craniofacial anomalies including a round head and face, sparse hair, cleft lip, and micrognathia. Additional manifestations include skeletal anomalies including joint contractures, long tapering fingers, absent, hypoplastic, or malpositioned thumbs; cardiac malformations; and inguinal hernia in males. Ophthalmic features include hypertelorism, sparse lashes, blepharoptosis, and up- or downward slanting of the palpebral fissures, narrowing of the palpebral fissures, and nystagmus.[134,198,223,293]

Duplication 16q

Duplication of the long arm of chromosome 16 causes postnatal growth retardation with hypotonia and characteristic craniofacial features including asymmetry with bitemporal narrowing, a high forehead, large metopic suture, prominent nose with a broad tip, thin upper lip, cleft palate, micrognathia, low-set, dysplastic ears, and a short neck. Other features include an imperforate or abnormally positioned anus; skeletal, gastrointestinal, and cardiac malformations; and dermatological abnormalities. Ophthalmic features include hypertelorism, epicanthus, up- and downward slanting and/or narrowing of the palpebral fissures, strabismus, decreased or long lashes, lid entropion, periorbital edema, deep-set globes, and strabismus.[17,39,146,313,338,406]

Duplication 17p

Duplication of the short arm of chromosome 17 is extremely rare. Features include pre- and postnatal growth retardation with severe developmental delay. Facial features include frontal bossing, a round face with midface hypoplasia, low-set ears, micrognathia, and cleft lip/palate. Cardiac malformations may occur. Ophthalmic features include hypertelorism, up- or downward slanting and/or narrowing of the palpebral fissures, blepharoptosis, and microphthalmia.[19,93,216]

Duplication 17q2

Duplication of the short arm of chromosome 17 in band 2 causes holoprosencephaly, polymicrogyria, a broad forehead and midface with a widow's peak, cleft palate, and a short neck. Additional features include skeletal anomalies such as scoliosis, shortening of the proximal limbs, brachy-, syn-, or polydactyly, and cardiac and genitourinary malformations. Ophthalmic features include hypertelorism and narrow palpebral fissures.[140,197,237]

Duplication 18p and q11

Duplication of the short arm of chromosome 18 with or without duplication of band 11 of the long arm causes prenatal growth retardation; craniofacial characteristics include microcephaly, a thin nose with a depressed bridge, narrow palate, malformed ears, micrognathia, and a short neck with redundant skin folds. Additional features include narrow shoulders, short sternum, widely spaced nipples, joint contractures, and digital anomalies; cardiac malformations may occur. Ophthalmic features include hypotelorism, downward slanting of the palpebral fissures, and strabismus.[101,150,354]

Duplication 18q

Duplication of the long arm of chromosome 18 causes distinctive craniofacial features including a broad, high forehead; prominent nasal bridge with absent frontonasal angle; bulbous nasal tip; and a large mouth with full lips. Epicanthus, blepharoptosis, synophrys, and enophthalmia occur in duplication of band 1.[108,119] Epicanthus, hypertelorism, and upward slanting of the palpebral fissures may be evident in duplication of band 2.[73,356]

Duplication 19q (de Grouchy Syndrome)

Duplication of the long arm of chromosome 19 causes severe pre- and postnatal growth retardation with microbrachycephaly and seizures; craniofacial features include open fontanelles, a flat facies, small nose with a flat bridge, low-set ears, short and prominent philtrum, downturned corners of the mouth, and short neck. Additional features include deformities of the chest, hands, and feet; cardiac, renal, bronchial, and vertebral anomalies; and genital malformations in males. Ophthalmic features include hypertelorism, downward slanting of the palpebral fissures, and blepharoptosis.[191,287]

Duplication 20p

Duplication of the short arm of chromosome 20 causes growth retardation with distinctive craniofacial features including wide cranial sutures, a round face with prominent cheeks, short nose with a broad upturned tip and large nares, long philtrum, large ears, and small chin. Additional features include skeletal, cardiac, and renal anomalies, hypogonadism, and macroorchidism. Ophthalmic manifestations include epicanthus, hypertelorism, up- or downward slanting of the palpebral fissures, strabismus, anterior segment abnormalities of the Rieger syndrome, colobomata, and enophthalmia.[18,31,100]

Duplication 22q

The "cat-eye" syndrome is a combination of two features, coloboma of the uveal tract (iris and/or choroid) and imperforate anus or anal atresia with retrovesical or rectovaginal fistula. The facies are unusual, with preauricular fistulas with skin tags, and a small chin may be evident. Most children have psychomotor retardation. Each of the three patients initially described had an extra acrocentric chromosome, smaller than either chromosome 21 or 22.[305] In those families in which more than one member has the extra chromosome, there has not been a correlation of the full syndrome with the presence of the extra chromosome. The origin of the extra chromosome was identified using DNA probes and is from within the long arm of chromosome 22 (q11 band); there are three or four copies of this region in affected individuals.[80,81,221] Ophthalmic features include hypertelorism, epicanthus, downward slanting of the palpebral fissures, strabismus, and colobomatous microphthalmia which is a consistent feature.[152,160,164]

Duplication of bands 12 and 13 of the long arm of chromosome 22 causes growth retardation with microcephaly and/or hydrocephalus, central nervous system malformations, short and broad nose, cleft lip and/or palate, and short neck; additional features include cardiac and genitourinary malformations and clubfoot. Ophthalmic features include hypertelorism, narrow palpebral fissures, corneal opacities, sclerocornea, and microphthalmia with orbital cyst.[3,288]

OTHER ANEUPLOIDY SYNDROMES

Triploidy

Triploidy causes multiple congenital anomalies and severe intrauterine growth retardation; the condition is lethal. Affected fetuses and infants have central nervous system malformations including hydrocephalus and hypoplasia of the cortex and/or cerebellum and anomalies of internal organs including the genitourinary, cardiac, intestinal, and endocrine systems. Hydatidiform mole may develop. Ophthalmic features include hypertelorism, cataracts, glaucoma, and colobomatous microphthalmia.[26,137,324,366]

Tetraploidy

The physical features of tetraploidy are similar to triploidy. Death occurs by or within the perinatal period. Reported ophthalmic features include hypertelorism, hypoplasia/aplasia of the optic tract, and microphthalmia.[137,304,391]

SEX-DETERMINING CHROMOSOMES

The syndromes caused by aneuploidy of the sex-determining chromosomes were described before the development of modern cytogenetic techniques.

Turner's Syndrome

Turner[365] described several females with sexual infantilism, webbed neck, and cubitus valgus, establishing as a clinical syndrome a previously described endocrinological disorder. The absence of "sex chromatin" in most Turner's syndrome patients was reported independently by three groups in 1954.[67,272,384] The first published 45,X karyotype[97] was confirmed by many laboratories within the same year. Approximately 80% of girls with Turner's syndrome have 45 chromosomes, a single X, and no sex chromatin (Barr bodies); the remaining 20% have other chromosomal variants. The unifying cytogenetic characteristic is the presence of a cell line that does not have two normal X chromosomes; it may lack the second X chromosome completely or have an abnormal second X chromosome (ring, fragment, deletion). Some patients are mosaic (45,X/46,XX) or have a long arm isochromosome (46,X,i(Xq)); an isochromosome is an abnormal chromosome with duplication of one arm forming two arms of equal length.

The typical findings in Turner's syndrome are sexual infantilism, short stature, webbed neck, broad shield chest with widely spaced nipples, increased carrying angle, small uterus, and multiple pigmented nevi. Recurrent ear infections are common. The ovaries consist of fibrous streaks with few or no follicles, and failure to feminize may be the presenting problem in the older girl with few of the physical stigmata. Coarctation of the aorta is common and may account for early childhood death. Autoimmune diseases, particularly Hashimoto thyroiditis and diabetes, have been associated with the syndrome. Turner's syndrome in some newborn infants is characterized by lymphedema of the hands and feet, which may persist into adulthood.

Blepharoptosis and strabismus are the most common ocular abnormalities. Cataracts may occur, particularly in association with diabetes. Refractive errors, corneal scars, blue sclera, and a variety of other anomalies have been reported.[13] The incidence of color blindness in females with 45,X Turner's syndrome equals that seen in normal males because only one X chromosome is present. In informative families, this defect may identify the origin of the single X.

Klinefelter's Syndrome

Klinefelter et al. described a syndrome of gynecomastia, small testes with hyalinization of seminiferous tubules, absent spermatogenesis but normal Leydig cell complement, and elevated urinary gonadotropins.[181] Patients with this clinical syndrome were shown to be chromatin positive by Plunkett and Barr[271] and to have 47,XXY chromosomal complement.[165] Males with more severe forms of Klinefelter's syndrome may have XXXY sex chromosomes and two Barr bodies, or XXXXY and three Barr bodies. Increasing numbers of X chromosomes cause greater physical and mental impairment. Males with XXXY are mentally retarded and may have radial-ulnar synostosis, scoliosis, microcephaly, cardiac malformations, and prognathism. The ophthalmic findings include epicanthal folds, hypertelorism, upward slant of palpebral fissures, strabismus, Brushfield spots, myopia, choroidal atrophy, and colobomatous microphthalmia.[59,98,137,394]

Eye anomalies are not usually seen in the XYY syndrome, although myopia, dislocation of the lens, retinal detachment, and colobomatous microphthalmia have been reported.[137,319]

References

1. Al-Awadi SA, Farag TI, Usha R, El-Khalifa MY, Sundareshan TS, Al-Othman SA. Brief clinical report: the long arm of chromosome 1 [del(1)(q32q42)]. Am J Med Genet 1986;23:931–933.

2. Alfi O, Donnell GN, Crandall BF, Derencsenyi A, Menon R. Deletion of the short arm of chromosome #9 (46,9p−): a new deletion syndrome. Ann Genet 1973;16:17–22.

3. Al-Gazali LI, Mueller RF, Caine A, et al. Two 46,XX,t(X;Y) females with linear skin defects and congenital microphthalmia: a new syndrome at Xp22.3. J Med Genet 1990;27:59–63.

4. Allderdice PW, Browne N, Murphy DP. Chromosome 3 duplication q21 → qter deletion p25 → pter syndrome in children of carriers of a pericentric inversion inv(3)(p25q21). Am J Hum Genet 1975;27: 699–718.

5. Allderdice PW, Davis JG, Miller OJ, et al. The 13q− deletion syndrome. Am J Hum Genet 1969;21:499–512.

6. Allderdice PW, Eales B, Onyett H, et al. Duplication 9q34 syndrome. Am J Hum Genet 1983;35:1005–1019.

7. Allen JC, Venecia G, Opitz JM. Eye findings in the 13 trisomy syndrome. Eur J Pediatr 1977;124:179–183.

8. Alvarado M, Bocian M, Walker AP. Interstitial deletion of the long arm of chromosome 3: case report, review, and definition of a phenotype. Am J Med Genet 1987;27:781–786.

9. Alvarez-Arratia MC, Rivera H, Moller M, Valdivia A, Vigueras A. De nove del(3)(q2800). Ann Genet 1984;27:109–111.

10. Anad F, Burn J, Matthews D, et al. Alagille syndrome and deletion of 20p. J Med Genet 1990;27:729–737.

11. Anneren G, Frodis E, Jorulf H. Trisomy 8 syndrome. Helv Paediatr Acta 1981;36:465–472.

12. Antle CM, Pantzar JT, White VA. The ocular pathology of trisomy 22: report of two cases and review. J Pediatr Ophthalmol Strabismus 1990;27:310–314.

13. Antonakou G, Levine R, Chrousos GP, et al. Ocular findings in Turner syndrome. A prospective study. Ophthalmology 1984;91: 926–928.

14. Armendares S, Salamanca F, Nava S, Ramirez S, Cantu J-M. The 12p trisomy syndrome. Ann Genet 1975;18:89–94.

15. Atkin JF, Patil S. Duplication of the distal segment of 14q. Am J Med Genet 1983;16:357–366.

16. Balestrazzi P, Croci G, Frassi C, Franchi F, Giovannelli G. Tetrasomy 9p confirmed by GALT. J Med Genet 1983;20:396–399.

17. Balestrazzi P, Giovannelli G, Landucci R, Dallapiccola B. Partial trisomy 16q resulting from maternal translocation. Hum Genet 1979;49:229–235.

18. Balestrazzi P, Virdis R, Frassi C, Negri V, Rigoli E, Bernasconi S. De novo trisomy 20p with macroorchidism in a prepuberal boy. Ann Genet 1984;27:58–59.

19. Bartsch-Sandoff M, Hieronimi G. Partial duplication of 17p. A new chromosomal syndrome. Hum Genet 1979;49:123–127.

20. Bass HN, Sparkes RS, Crandall F, Tannenbaum SM. Familial partial trisomy 10q(q23-qter) syndrome and paracentric inversion 3 (q13 q26) in the same patient. Ann Genet 1978;21:74–77.

21. Bateman JB, Maumenee IH, Sparkes RS. Peters' anomaly associated with partial deletion of the long arm of chromosome 11. Am J Ophthalmol 1984;97:11–15.

22. Beall MH, Falk RE, Ying K-L. A patient with an interstitial deletion of the proximal portion of the long arm of chromosome 4. Am J Med Genet 1988;31:553–557.

23. Benedict WF, Murphree AL, Banerjee A, Spina CA, Sparkes MC, Sparkes RS. Patient with 13 chromosome deletion: evidence that the retinoblastoma gene is a recessive cancer gene. Science. 1983; 219:973–975.

24. Berry AC, Honeycombe J, Macoun SJR. Two children with partial trisomy for 7p. Am Med Genet 1979;16:320–321.

25. Bialasiewicz AA, Mayer UM, Meythaler FH. Ophthalmologische befunde bei 11 q–deletionssyndrom. Klin Monatsbl Augenheilkd 1987;190:524–526.

26. Blackburn W, Miller R, Peyton W, et al. Comparative studies of infants with mosaic and complete triploidy: an analysis of 55 cases of birth defects. Birth Defects: Original Article Series. New York: March of Dimes Birth Defects Foundation, 1982;18(3B):251–274.

27. Blennow E, Brondum Nielsen K. Partial monosomy 8p with minimal dysmorphic signs. J Med Genet 1990;27:327–329.

28. Boilly-Dartigalongue B, Riviere D, Junien C, et al. Etude dun nouveau cas de monosomie partielle du chromosome 12, del(12)(p11.01–p12.109) confirmant la localisation du gene de la lactico-deshydrogenase B. Ann Genet 1985;28:55–57.

29. Bonfante A, Stella M, Rossi G. Partial trisomy 4q: two cases resulting from a familial translocation t(4;18) (q27;p11). Hum Genet 1979;52:85–90.

30. Bonioli E, Crisalli M, Monteverde R, Vianello MG. Karyotype–phenotype correlation in partial trisomy 13. Am J Dis Child 1981; 135:1115–1117.

31. Bown N, Cross I, Davison EV, Burn J. Partial trisomy 20p resulting from a recombination of a familial pericentric inversion. Hum Genet 1986;74:417–419.

32. Bowser Riley S, Buckton KE, Ratcliffe SG, Syme J. Inheritance of a ring 14 chromosome. J Med Genet 1981;18:209–213.

33. Breg WR, Steele MW, Miller OJ, Warburton D, deCapoa A, Allderdice PW. The cri du chat syndrome in adolescents and adults: clinical finding in 13 older patients with partial deletion of the short arm of chromosome no. 5(5p–). J Pediatr 1970;77:782–791.

34. Brocker-Vriends AHJT, Mooij PD, Van Bel F, Beverstock GC, Van De Kamp JJ. Monosomy 8p: an easily overlooked syndrome. J Med Genet 1986;23:153–154.

35. Brondum Nielsen K, Egede NF, Mouridsen I, Mohr J. Familial partial 7q monosomy resulting from segregation of an insertional chromosome rearrangement. J Med Genet 1979;16:461–466.

36. Bunin GR, Emanuel BS, Meadows AT, Buckley JD, Woods WG, Hammond GD. Frequency of 13q abnormalities among 203 patients with retinoblastoma. J Natl Cancer Inst 1989;81:370–374.

37. Burd L, Kerbeshian J, Fisher W, Martsolf JT. A case of autism and mosaic of trisomy 8. J Autism Dev Disord 1985;15:351–352.

38. Butler MG, Fogo AB, Fuchs DA, Collins FS, Dev VG, Phillips JA III. Brief clinical report and review: two patients with ring chromosome 15 syndrome. Am J Med Genet 1988;29:149–154.

39. Calva P, Frias S, Carnevale A, Reyes P. Partial trisomy 16q resulting from maternal translocation 11p/16q. Ann Genet 1984;27:122–125.

40. Cannizzaro LA, Emanuel BS. In situ hybridization and translocation breakpoint mapping. III. DiGeorge syndrome with partial monosomy of chromosome 22. Cytogenet Cell Genet 1985;39:179–183.

41. Cantu JM, Salamanca F, Buentello L, Carnevale A, Armendares S. Memoires et articles originaux. Trisomy 10p. A report of two cases due to a familial translocation rcp(10;21)(p11;p11). Ann Genet 1975;18:5–11.

42. Caputo AR, Wagner RS, Reynolds DR, Guo SQ, Goel AK. Down syndrome. Clinical review of ocular features. Clin Pediatr 1989;28:355–358.

43. Carnevale A, Hernandez M, Limon-Toledo I, Frias S, Castillo J, del Castillo V. A clinical syndrome associated with dup(5p). Am J Med Genet 1982;13:277–283.

44. Carter R, Baker E, Hayman D. Congenital malformations associated with a ring 4 chromosome. J Med Genet 1969;6:224–227.

45. Caspersson T, Zech L, Johansson C. Differential binding of alkylating fluorochromes in human chromosomes. Exp Cell Res 1970;60:315–319.

46. Catalano RA. Down syndrome. Surv Ophthalmol 1990;34:385–398.

47. Cavenee WK, Murphree AL, Shull MM, et al. Prediction of familial predispositional to retinoblastoma. N Engl J Med 1986;314:1201–1207.

48. Charles SJ, Moore AT, Davison BCC, Dyson HM, Willatt L. Flecked retina associated with ring 17 chromosome. Br J Ophthalmol 1991;75:125–127.

49. Chen H, Gershanik JJ, Mailhes JB, Sanusi ID. Omphalocele and partial trisomy 1q syndrome. Hum Genet 1979;53:1–4.

50. Chen H, Tyrkus M, Cohen F, et al. Familial partial trisomy 6q syndromes resulting from inherited ins (5:6) (q33;q15q27). Clin Genet 1976;9:631–637.

51. Chieri P, Iolster N. Monosomy 10qtr due to a balanced maternal translocation: t(10;8)(q23;p23). Clin Genet 1983;24:147–150.

52. Chitayat D, Hahm SYE, Iqbal MA, Nitowsky HM. Ring chromosome 6: report of a patient and literature review. Am J Med Genet 1987;26:145–151.

53. Chrousos GA, O'Neill JF, Traboulsi EI, Richmond A, Rosenbaum KN. Ocular findings in partial trisomy 3q. A case report and review of the literature. Ophthalmic Paediatr Genet 1988;9:127–130.

54. Chudley AE, Verma MR, Ray M, Riordan D. Letter to the Editor. Interstitial deletion of the long arm of chromosome 4. Am J Med Genet 1988;31:549–551.

55. Clark CE, Cowell HR, Telfer MA, Casey PA. Trisomy 6q25–6qter in two sisters resulting from maternal 6;11 translocation. Am J Med Genet 1980a;5:171–178.

56. Clark CE, Telfer MA, Cowell HR. A case of partial trisomy 8p resulting from a maternal balanced translocation. Am J Med Genet 1980;7:21–25.

57. Cogan DG, Kuwabara T. Ocular pathology of the 13–15 trisomy syndrome. Arch Ophthalmol 1964;72:246–253.

58. Cohen MM, Ornoy A, Rosenmann A, Kohn G. An inherited translocation t(4;15) (p16;q22) leading to two cases of partial trisomy 15. Ann Genet 1975;18:99–103.

59. Collier M, Chami M. Les manifestations of Klinefelter's syndrome. Bull Soc Ophtalmol Fr 1969;69:1073–1089.

60. Corney MJ, Smith S. Early development of an infant with 18q− syndrome. J Ment Defic Res 1984;28:303–307.

61. Cotlier E, Reinglass H, Rosenthal I. The eye in the partial trisomy 2q syndrome. Am J Ophthalmol 1977;84:251–258.

62. Cousineau AJ, Higgins JV, Scott-Emuakpor AB, Mody G. Brief clinical report: ring-11 chromosome: phenotype-karyotype correlation with deletions of 11q. Am J Med Genet 1983;14:29–35.

63. Cowell JK, Thompson E, Rutland P. The need to screen all retinoblastoma patients for esterase D activity: detection of submicroscopic chromosome deletions. Arch Dis Child 1987;62:8–11.

64. Crane J, Sujansky E, Smith A. 4p trisomy syndrome: report of 4 additional cases and segregation analysis of 21 families with different translocations. Am J Med Genet 1979;4:219–229.

65. Dallapiccola B, De Filippis V, Notarangelo A, Perla G, Zelante L. Ring chromosome 21 in healthy persons: different consequences in females and in males. Hum Genet 1986;73:218–220.

66. Daniele S, Pecorelli F, Tiepolo L, Armellini R, Liotti FS. Congenital ocular and other systemic abnormalities associated with ring-11 chromosome. Graefes Arch Clin Exp Ophthalmol 1986;224:317–320.

67. Decourt L, De Silva Sasso W, Chiorboli E, Fernandes JM. Sobre o sexo genetico nas pacientes dom sindrome de Turner. Rev Assoc Med Bras 1954;1:203–206.

68. de France HF, Beemer FA, Senders RCH, Gerards LJ, Cats BP. Partial trisomy 11q due to paternal t(11q;18p): further delineation of the clinical picture. Clin Genet 1984;25:295–299.

69. de France HF, Beemer FA, Senders RC, Schaminerr-Main SC. Trisomy 10 mosaicism in a newborn boy; delineation of the syndrome. Clin Genet 1985;27:92–96.

70. de Grouchy J, Royer P, Salmon C, Lamy M. Deletion partielle des bras longs du chromosome 18. Pathol Biol 1964;12:579–582.

71. de la Chapelle A, Herva R, Koivisto M, Aula P. A deletion in chromosome 22 can cause DiGeorge syndrome. Hum Genet 1981;57: 253–256.

72. Delicado A, Iniguez L, Lopez Pajares I, Omenaca F. Complete trisomy 9: two additional cases. Ann Genet 1985;28:63–66.

73. de Muelenaere A, Fryns JP, van den Berghe H. Familial partial distal 18q(18q22–18q23) trisomy. Clin Genet 1981;24:184–186.

74. de Muelenaere A, Fryns JP, van den Berghe H. Partial distal 12q trisomy. Ann Genet 1980;23:251–253.

75. Deroover J, Fryns JP, Parloir C, Haegeman J, Van Den Berghe H. Partial monosomy of the short arm of chromosome 9. Hum Genet 1978;44:195–200.

76. Dickinson AJ, Fielder AR, Young ID, Duckett DP. Ocular findings in Angelman's (happy puppet) syndrome. Ophthalmic Paediatr Genet 1990;11:1–6.

77. DiLiberti JH, McKean R, Webb MJ, Williams G. Trisomy 5p: delineation of clinical features. Birth Defects: Original Article Series. New York: March of Dimes Birth Defects Foundation, 1977;8(3C): 185–194.

78. Donlan MA, Donlan CR. Ring chromosome 18 in a mother and son. Am J Med Genet 1986;24:171–174.

79. Down JLH. Observations on an ethnic classification of idiots. Clin Lect Rep Lond Hosp 1866;3:259–262.

80. Duncan AMV, Hough CA, White BN, McDermid HE. Brief communication: breakpoint localization of the marker chromosome associated with the cat eye syndrome. Am J Hum Genet 1986;38:978–980.

81. Duncan AMV, Rosenfeld W, Verma RS. Letter to the editor: reevaluation of the supernumerary chromosome in an individual with cat eye syndrome. Am J Med Genet 1987;27:225–227.

82. Dutrillaux B, Laurent C, Forabosco A, et al. La trisome 4q partielle. a propos de trois observatrions. Ann Genet 1975;18:21–27.

83. Edwards JH, Harnden DG, Cameron AH, Crosse VM, Wolff OH. A new trisomic syndrome. Lancet 1960;1:787–789.

84. Elstner CL, Carey JC, Livingston G, Moeschler J, Lubinsky M. Further delineation of the 10p deletion syndrome. Pediatrics 1984; 73:670–675.

85. Escobar JI, Yunis JJ. Trisomy for the proximal segment of the long arm of chromosome 13. Am J Dis Child 1974;128:221–222.

86. Evans-Jones G, Howard PJ. A further case of monosomy 10qtr. Clin Genet 1983;24:216–219.

87. Falk RE, Carrel RE, Valente M, Creandall BF, Sparkes RS. Partial trisomy of chromosome 11: a case report. Am J Med Ment Defic 1977;77:383–388.

88. Farrell JW, Morgan KS, Black S. Lensectomy in an infant with cri du chat syndrome and cataracts. J Pediatr Ophthalmol Strabismus 1988;25:131–134.

89. Fawcett WA, McCord WK, Francke U. Trisomy 14q–. In: Bergsma D (ed) New chromosomal and malformation syndromes. Birth

Defects: Original Article Series. Miami: Symposium Specialists for National Foundation—March of Dimes, 1975;11(5):223–228.

90. Fear C, Briggs A. Familial partial trisomy of the long arm of chromosome 3 (3q). Arch Dis Child 1979;54:135–138.

91. Feingold M, Atkins L. A case of trisomy 9. Am J Med Genet 1973; 10:184–187.

92. Felding I, Kirstoffersson U, Sjostrom H, Noren O. Contribution to the 18q−syndrome. A patient with del(18)(q22.3qter). Clin Genet 1987;31:206–210.

93. Feldman GM, Baumer JG, Sparkes RS. Brief clinical report: the dup(17p) syndrome. Am J Med Genet 1982;11:299–304.

94. Ferrante E, Vignetti P, Antonelli M, Bruni L, Bertasi S, Chessa L. Partial monosomy for a 21 chromosome. Helv Paediatr Acta 1983; 38:73–80.

94a. Ferry AP, Marchevsky A, Strauss L. Ocular abnormalities in deletion of the long arm of chromosome II. Ann Ophthalmol 1981;13: 1373–1377.

95. Forabosco A, Baroncini A, Dalpra L, et al. The phenotype of partial dup(7q) reconsidered: a report of five new cases. Clin Genet 1988; 34:48–59.

96. Forabosco A, Bernasconi S, Giovannelli G, Dutrillaux B. Trisomy of the distal third of the long arm of chromosome 10. Report of a new case due to a familial translocation t(10;18)(q24;p11). Helv Paediatr Acta 1975;30:289–295.

97. Ford EC, Jones KW, Polani PE, de Almeida JC, Briggs JH. A sex-chromosome anomaly in a case of gonadal dysgenesis (Turner's syndrome). Lancet 1959;1:711–713.

98. Francois J, Leuven MT, Gombault P. Uveal coloboma and true Klinefelter syndrome. J Med Genet 1970;7:213–223.

99. Frangoulis M, Taylor C. Corneal opacities—a diagnostic feature of the trisomy 8 mosaic syndrome. Br J Ophthalmol 1983;67:619–622.

100. Franke U. Abnormalities of chromosomes 11 and 20. In: Yunis JJ (ed) New chromosomal syndromes. New York: Academic Press, 1977.

101. Fried K, Bar-Yockai A, Rosenblatt M, Mundel G. Partial 18 trisomy (with 47 chromosomes) resulting from a familial maternal translocation. Am J Med Genet 1978;15:76–78.

102. Friedrich U, Osterballe O, Stenbjerg S, Jorgensen J. A girl with karyotype 46,XX,del(7)(pter → q32:). Hum Genet 1979;51:231–235.

103. Friend SH, Bernards R, Rogelj S, et al. A human DNA segment with properties of the gene that predisposes to retinoblastoma and osteosarcoma. Nature (Lond) 1986;323:643–646.

104. Frydman M, Steinberger J, Shabtai F, Katznelson MBM, Varsano I. Interstitial deletion 2q14q21. Am J Med Genet 1989;34:476–479.

105. Fryns JP, Bande-Knops J, van den Berghe H. Partial monosomy of the long arm of chromosome 16: a distinct clinical entity? Hum Genet 1979;46:115–120.

106. Fryns JP, Bettens W, van den Berghe H. Distal deletion of the long arm of chromosome 6: a specific phenotype? Am J Med Genet 1986; 24:175–178.

107. Fryns JP, D'hondt F, Goddeeris P, van den Berghe. Full monosomy 21: a clinically recognizable syndrome? Hum Genet 1977;37:155–259.

108. Fryns JP, Detavernier F, van Fleteren A, van den Berghe H. Partial trisomy 18q in a newborn with typical 18 trisomy phenotype. Hum Genet 1978;44:201–205.

109. Fryns JP, Kleczkowska A, Buttiens M, Jonckheere P, Brouckmans-Buttiens K, van den Berghe H. Ring chromosome 15 syndrome. Ann Genet 1986;29:47–48.

110. Fryns JP, Kleczkowska A, Buttiens M, Marien P, van den Berghe H. Distal 11q monosomy. The typical 11q monosomy syndrome is due to deletion of subband 11q24.1. Clin Genet 1986;30:255–260.

111. Fryns JP, Kleczkowska A, Dereymaker AM, et al. Partial 8p trisomy due to interstitial duplication: karyotype: 46,XX,inv dup(8)(p21.1 → p22). Clin Genet 1985;28:546–549.

112. Fryns JP, Kleczkowska A, Moerman F, van den Berghe K, van den Berghe H. Partial distal 6p trisomy in a malformed fetus. Ann Genet 1986;29:53–54.

113. Fryns JP, Kleczkowska A, Vinken L, Geutjens J, Smeets E, Van Den Berghe H. Acrocentric/18p translocation in two mentally retarded males. Ann Genet 1986;29:107–111.

114. Fryns JP, Logghe N, van Eygen M, van den Berghe H. New chromosomal syndromes: partial trisomy of the distal portion of the long arm of chromosome number 10 (10q24 → 10qter): a clinical entity. Acta Paediatr Belg 1979;32:141–143.

115. Fryns JP, Proesmans W, Van Hoey G, van den Berghe H. Interstitial 16q deletion with typical dysmorphic syndrome. Ann Genet 1981;24:124–125.

116. Fryns JP, van Bosstraeten B, Malbrain H, van den Berghe H. Interstitial deletion of the long arm of chromosome 2 in a polymalformed newborn—karyotype: 46,XX,del(2)(q21;q24). Hum Genet 1977;39:233–238.

117. Fryns JP, van den Berghe H. Ring chromosome 22 in a mentally retarded child and mosaic 45,XX,−15,−22,+t(15;22) (p11;q11)/46,XX,r(22)/46,XX karyotype in the mother. Hum Genet 1979;47:213–216.

118. Fryns JP, van Eygen M, Logghe N, van den Berghe H. Partial trisomy for the long arm of chromosome 3 (3(q21 → qter)+) in a newborn with minor physical stigmata. Hum Genet 1978;40:333–339.

119. Fryns JP, Vinken L, Marien J, van den Berghe H. Partial trisomy 18q12, due to intrachromosomal duplication, is not associated with typical 18 trisomy phenotype. Hum Genet 1979;46:341–344.

120. Fujimoto A, Lin MS, Korula SR, Wilson MG. Trisomy 14 mosaicism with t(14;15)(q11;p11) in offspring of a balanced translocation carrier mother. Am J Med Genet 1985;22:333–342.

121. Fujimoto A, Towner JW, Ebbin AJ, Kahlstrom EJ, Wilson MG. Inherited partial duplication of chromosome no. 15. Am J Med Genet 1974;11:287–291.

122. Fujimoto A, Wilson MG, Towner JW. Familial inversion of chromosome no. 8. Humangenetik 1975;27:67–73.

123. Fujita H, Meng J, Kawamura M, Tozuka N, Ishii F, Tanaka N. Boy with a chromosome del (3)(q12q23) and blepharophimosis syndrome. Am J Med Genet 1992;44:434–436.

124. Funderburk SJ, Sparkes RS, Klisak I. Phenotypic variation in two patients with a ring chromosome 22. Clin Genet 1979;16:305–310.

125. Funderburk SJ, Sparkes RS, Klisak I. The 9p–syndrome. Am J Med Genet 1979;16:75–79.

126. Fung YK, Murphree AL, Tang A, Qian J, Hinrickhs SH. Structural evidence for the authenticity of the human retinoblastoma gene. Science 1987;236:1657–1661.

127. Garcia-Cruz D, Vaca G, Ibarra B, et al. Tetrasomy 9p: clinical aspects and enzymatic gene dosage expression. Ann Genet 1982;25:237–242.

128. Gardner RJM, Monk NA, Clarkson JE, Allen GJ. Ring 21 chromosome: the mild end of the phenotypic spectrum. Clin Genet 1986; 30:466–470.

129. Gimelli G, Cuoco C, Lituania M, et al. Dup(3)(p2–pter) in two families, including one infant with cyclopia. Am J Med Genet 1985;20: 341–348.

130. Ginsberg J, Ballard ET, Buchino JJ, Kinkler AK. Further observations of ocular pathology in Down's syndrome. J Pediatr Ophthalmol Strabismus 1980;17:166–171.

131. Ginsberg J, Bofinger MK, Roush JR. Pathologic features of the eye in Down's syndrome with relationship to other chromosomal anomalies. Am J Ophthalmol 1977;83:874–880.

132. Ginsberg J, Dignam PS, Buchino JJ, Kinkler AK. Ocular abnormality associated with partial duplication of chromosome 13. Ann Ophthalmol 1981;13:189–94.

133. Ginsburg J, Perrin EV, Sueoka WT. Ocular manifestations of trisomy 18. Am J Ophthalmol 1968;66:59–67.

134. Golden NL, Bilenker R, Johnson WE, Tischfield JA. Abnormality of chromosome 16 and its phenotypic expression. Clin Genet 1981;19:41–45.

135. Gonzalez CH, Billerbeck AEC, Wajntal A. Duplication 10p in a girl due to a maternal translocation t(10;14) (p11;p12). Am J Med Genet 1983;14:159–167.

136. Gonzalez CH, Sommer A, Meisner LF, Elejalde BR, Opitz JM. The trisomy 4p syndrome: case report and review. Am J Hum Genet 1977;1:137–156.

137. Gorlin RJ. Classical chromsome disorders. In: Yunis JJ (ed) New chromosomal syndromes. New York: Academic Press, 1977:59–117.

138. Gorlin RJ, Yunis J, Anderson VE. Short arm deletion of chromosome 18 in cebocephaly. Am J Dis Child 1968;115:473–476.

139. Grace E, Sutherland GD, Bain S, Bain AD. Partial trisomy of 7q resulting from a familial translocation. Ann Genet 1973;16:52–53.

140. Greenberg F, Stratton RF, Lockhart LH, Elder FFB, Dobyns WB, Ledbetter DH. Familial Miller–Dieker syndrome associated with pericentric inversion of chromosome 17. Am J Med Genet 1986; 23:853–859.

141. Greenberg F, Valdes C, Rosenblatt HM, Kirkland JL, Ledbetter DH. Hypoparathyroidism and T cell immune defect in a patient with 10p deletion synrome. J Pediatr 1986;109:489–492.

142. Greger V, Kerst S, Messmer E, Hopping W, Passarge E, Horsthemke B. Application of linkage analysis to genetic counseling in families with hereditary retinoblastoma. J Med Genet 1988;25:217–221.

143. Gregoire MJ, Boue J, Junien C, Pernot C, Gilgenkrantz S, Zergollern L. Duplication 15q22qter and its phenotypic expression. Hum Genet 1981;59:429–433.

144. Greig F, Rosenfeld W, Verma RS, Babu KA, David K. Duplication 11 (q22 → qter) in an infant. Ann Genet 1985;28:185–188.

145. Gustavson KH, Finley SC, Finley WH, Jalling B. A 4–5/21–22 chromosomal translocation associated with multiple congenital anomalies. Acta Paediatr 1964;53:172–181.

146. Hatanaka K, Ozaki M, Suzuki M, Murata R, Fujita H. Trisomy 16q13 → qter in a infant from a t(11;16)(q25;q13) translocation-carrier father. Hum Genet 1984;65:311–315.

147. Heathcote JG, Sholdice J, Walton JC, Willis NR, Sergovich FR. Anterior segment mesenchymal associated with partial duplication of the short arm of chromosome 2. Can J Ophthalmol 1991;26:35–43.

148. Heimonen OP, Slone D, Shapiro S. Birth defects and drugs in pregnancy. Littleton, MA: Publishing Sciences, 1977.

149. Helmuth RA, Weaver DD, Wills ER. Holoprosencephaly, ear abnormalities, congenital heart defect, and microphallus in a patient with 11q−mosaicism. Am J Med Genet 1989;32:178–181.

150. Hernandez A, Corona-Rivera E, Plascencia L, Nazara Z, Ibarra B, Cantu JM. De novo partial trisomy of chromosome 18(pter → q11:). Some observations on the phenotype mapping of chromosome 18 imbalances. Ann Genet 1979;22:165–167.

151. Hertz JM. Familial transmission of a ring chromosome 21. Clin Genet 1987;32:35–39.

152. Hoo JJ. 12p trisomy: a syndrome? Ann Genet 1976;19:261–263.

153. Hoo JJ, Robertson A, Fowlow SB, Bowen P, Lin CC. Letter to the editor: inverted duplication of 22pter → q11.21 in cat-eye syndrome. Am J Med Genet 1986;24:543–545.

154. Hood OJ, Rouse BM, Lockhart LH, Bodensteiner JB. Proximal duplications of chromosome 15: clinical dilemmas. Clin Genet 1986;29:234–240.

155. Houston CS, Chudley AE. Separating monosomy-21 from the "arthrogryposis basket." J Assoc Can Radiol 1981;32:220–223.

156. Howard RO. Chromosomal abnormalities associated with cyclopia and synophthalmia. Trans Am Ophthalmol Soc 1977;75:505–538.

157. Howard RO. Ocular abnormalities in the cri du chat syndrome. Am J Ophthalmol 1972;73:949–954.

158. Howard PJ, Clark D, Dearlove J. Retinal/macular pigmentation in conjunction with ring 14 chromosome. Hum Genet 1988;80:140–142.

159. Hreidarsson SJ, Stamberg J. Distal monosomy 14 not associated with ring formation. J Med Genet 1983;20:147–149.

160. Hsu LYF, Hirschhorn K. The trisomy 22 syndrome and the cat eye syndrome. In: Yunis JJ (ed) New chromosomal syndromes. New York: Academic Press, 1977:339–368.

161. Hunter AGW, Ray M, Wang HS, Thompson DR. Phenotypic correlations in patients with ring chromosome 22. Clin Genet 1977; 12:239–249.

162. Hurgoiu V, Suciu S. Occurrence of 19− in an infant with multiple dysmorphic features. Ann Genet 1984;27:56–57.

163. Hustinx TWJ, Gabreels FJM, Kirkels VGHJ, et al. Trisomy 4p in a family with a t(4;15). Ann Genet 1975;18:13–19.

164. Ioan D, Dumitriu L, Fabritius K, Simescu M, Maximilian C. The "cat eye" syndrome—reports of a case with hypothyroidism. Endocrinologie 1986;24:129–131.

165. Jacobs PA, Strong JA. A case of human intersexuality having a possible XXY sex determining mechanism. Nature (Lond) 1959;183: 302–303.

166. Jefferson RD, Burn J, Gaunt KL, Hunter S, Davison EV. A terminal deletion of the long arm of chromosome 4 [46,xx,del(4)(q33)] in an infant with phenotypic features of Williams syndrome. J Med Genet 1986;23:474–480.

167. Jenkins MB, Stang HJ, Davis E, Boyd L. Deletion of the proximal long arm of chromosome 3 in an infant with features of Turner syndrome. Ann Genet 1985;28:42–44.

168. Johnson VP, Aceto A, Likness C. Trisomy 14 mosaicism: case report and review. Am J Med Genet 1979;3:331–339.

169. Johnson DD, Michels VV, Aas MA, Dewald GW. Duplication of 7q31.2 → 7qter and deficiency of 18qter: report of two patients and literature review. Am J Med Genet 1986;25:477–488.

170. Journel H, Lucas J, Allaire C, et al. Trisomy 11p15 and Beckwith–Wiedemann syndrome: report of two new cases. Ann Genet 1985; 28:97–101.

171. Juberg RC, Haney NR, Stallard R. New deletion syndrome 1q43. Am J Hum Genet 1981;33:455–463.

172. Junien C, Turleau C, de Grouchy J, et al. Regional assignment of catalase (CAT) gene to band 11p13. association with the aniridia–Wilms' tumor–gonadoblastoma (WAGR) complex. Ann Genet 1980;23:165–168.

173. Kaminker CP, Dain L, Lamas MA, Sanchez JM. Brief clinical report: mosaic trisomy 9 syndrome with unusual phenotype. Am J Med Genet 1985;22:237–241.

174. Keith CG, Webb GC, Rogers JG. Absence of a lateral rectus muscle associated with duplication of the chromosome segment 7q32 → q34. J Med Genet 1988;25:122–125.

175. Kelley RI, Zackai EH, Emanuel BS, Kistenmacher M, Greenberg F, Punnett HH. The association of the DiGeorge anomalad monosomy of chromosome 22. J Pediatr 1982;101:197–200.

176. Khodr GS, Cadena G, Le KL, Kagan-Hallet KS. Duplication (5p14 → pter): prenatal diagnosis and review of the literature. Am J Med Genet 1982;12:43–49.

177. Kini KR, van Dyke DL, Weiss L, Logan MS. Ring chromosome 6: case report and review of literature. Hum Genet 1979;50:145–149.

178. Kivlin JD, Fineman RM, Williams MS. Phenotypic variation in the del(12p) syndrome. Am J Med Genet 1985;22:769–779.

179. Kleczkowska A, Fryns JP, van den Berghe H. Partial trisomy of chromosome 3(p14–p22) due to maternal insertional translocation. Ann Genet 1984;27:180–183.

180. Klep-de Pater JM, Bijlsma JB, de France HF, Leschot NJ, Duijndam-van den Berge M, van Hemel JO. Partial trisomy 10q. Hum Genet 1979;46:29–40.

181. Klinefelter HF Jr, Reifenstein EC Jr, Albright F. Syndrome characterized by gynecmastia, aspermatogenesis without A-Leydigism, and increased excretion of follicle-stimulating hormone. J Clin Endocrinol 1942;2:615–627.

182. Koenig R, Kessel E, Schoenberger W. Partial monosomy 10p syndrome. Ann Genet 1985;28:173–176.

183. Kondo I, Hirano T, Hamaguchi H, et al. A case of trisomy 3q21 → qter syndrome. Hum Genet 1979;46:141–147.

184. Koole FD, Velzeboer CMJ, van der Harten JJ. Ocular abnormalities in Patau syndrome. Ophthalmic Paediatr Genet 1990;11:15–21.

185. Kozma C, Hunt M, Meck J, Traboulsi E, Scribanu N. Familial Wolf–Hirschhorn syndrome associated with Rieger anomaly of the eye. Ophthalmic Paediatr Genet 1990;11:23–30.

186. Kroyer S, Niebuhr E. Partial trisomy 10q occurring in a family with a reciprocal translocation t(10;18) (q25;q23). Ann Genet 1975;18:50–55.

187. Kuchle HJ, Normann J, Lubbering I. Ein beitrag zum kongenitalen zystenauge. Klin Monatsbl Augenheilkd 1986;188:239–241.

188. Kuchle M, Kraus J, Rummelt C, Naumann GOH. Synophthalmia and holoprosencephaly in chromosome 18p deletion defect. Arch Ophthalmol 1991;109:136–137.

189. Kumar D, Heath PR, Blank CE. Clinical manifestations of trisomy 5q. J Med Genet 1987;24:180–183.

190. Kunze J, Stephan E, Tolksdorf M. Ring-chromosome 18. Human-genetik 1972;15:289–318.

191. Lange M, Alfi OS. Trisomy 19q. Ann Genet 1976;19:17–21.

192. Ledbetter DAL, Riccardi VM, Au WW, Wilson DP, Holmquist GP. Ring chromosome 15: phenotype, Ag-NOR analysis, secondary

aneuploidy, and associated chromosome instability. Cytogenet Cell Genet 1980;27:111–122.

193. Lee WH, Bookstein R, Hong F, Young LJ, Shew JY. Human retinoblastoma susceptibility gene cloning, identification, and sequence. Science 1987;235:1394–1399.

194. Lejeune J, Gautier M, Turpin R. Les chromosomes humains en cultur de tissues. C R Acad Sci (Paris) 1959;248:602–603.

195. Lejeune J, Lafourcade J, Berger R, et al. Trois cas de deletion partielle du bras court d'un chromosome 5. C R Acad Sci (Paris) 1963; 257:3098–3102.

196. Leschot NJ, Lim KS. Complete trisomy 5p: de novo translocation t(2;5)(q36;p11) with isochromosome 5p. Hum Genet 1979;46:271–278.

197. Lenzini E, Leszl A, Artifone L, Casellato R, Tenconi R, Baccichetti C. Partial duplication of 17 long arm. Ann Genet 1988;31:175–180.

198. Leschot NJ, de Nef JJ, Geraedts JPM, et al. Five familial cases with a trisomy 16p syndrome due to translocation. Clin Genet 1979;16: 205–214.

199. Levin H, Ritch R, Barathur R, Dunn MW, Teekhasaenee C, Margolis S. Brief clinical report: aniridia, congenital glaucoma, and hydrocephalus in a male infant with ring chromosome 6. Am J Med Genet 1986;25:281–287.

200. Levy I, Levy Y, Mammon A, Nitzan M, Steinherz R. Gastrointestinal abnormalities in the syndrome of mosaic trisomy 9. J Med Genet 1989;26:280–281.

201. Lewandowski RC Jr, Kukolich MK, Sears JW, Mankinen CB. Partial deletion 10q. Hum Genet 1978;42:339–343.

202. Lewandowski RC Jr, Yunis JJ. Trisomy 9 mosaicism. Clin Genet 1977;11:306–310.

203. Ligutic I, Brecevic L, Petkovic I, Kalogjera T, Rajic Z. Interstitial deletion 4q and Rieger syndrome. Clin Genet 1981;20:323–327.

204. Lindenbaum RH, Bobrow M, Barber L. Monozygotic twins with ring chromosome 22. J Med Genet 1973;10:85–89.

205. Lippe BM, Sparkes RS. Ring 14 chromosome: association with seizures. Am J Med Genet 1981;9:301–305.

206. Lipson MH. Brief clinical report: trisomy 14 mosaicism syndrome. Am J Med Genet 1987;26:541–543.

207. Lockwood D, Hecht F, Dowman C, et al. Chromosome subband 17p11-2 deletion: a minute deletion syndrome. J Med Genet 1988; 25:732–737.

208. Lurie IW, Lazjuk GI. Partial monosomies 18. Humangenetik 1972; 15:203–222.

209. Magenis RE, Toth-Fejel S, Allen LJ, et al. Comparison of the 15q deletions in Prader–Willi and Angelman syndrome: specific regions, extent of deletions, parental origin, and clinical consequences. Am J Med Genet 1990;35:333–349.

210. Mankinen CB, Sears JW, Alvarez VR. Terminal (1)(q43) long-arm deletion of chromosome no. 1 in a three-year-old female. Birth

244. Niebuhr E. Partial trisomies and deletions of chromsome 13. In Yunis JJ (ed) New chromosomal syndromes. New York: Academic Press, 1977:273–299.

245. Niebuhr E. The cri du chat syndrome. Hum Genet 1978;44:227–275.

246. Nielsen J, Homma A, Christiansen F, Rasmussen K, Saldana-Garcia P. The deletion 9p syndrome. A 61-year-old man with deletion of short arm 9. Clin Genet 1977;12:80–84.

247. Nielsen J, Homma A, Rasmussen K, Ried E, Sorensen K, Saldana-Garcia P. Deletion 14q and pericentric inversion 14. J Med Genet 1978;15:236–238.

248. Niikawa N, Jinno Y, Tomiyasu T, Fukushima Y, Kudo K. Ring chromosome 11 [46,XX,r(11)(p15q25)] associated with clinical features of the 11q− syndrome. Ann Genet 1981;24:172–175.

249. Nistrup Madsen H, Lundsteen C, Steinrud J. A case of partial deletion of the long arm of chromosome 7(7q34 → 7qter). Dan Med Bull 1983;30:14–16.

249a. O'Grady RB, Rothstein TB, Romano PE. D-group deletion syndromes and retinoblastoma. Am J Ophthalmol 1974;77:40–45.

250. O'Hare AE, Grace E, Edmunds AT. Deletion of the long arm of chromosome 11 [46,XX,del(11)(q24.1-qter)]. Clin Genet 1983;25:373–377.

251. Ohba KI, Ohdo S, Sonoda T. Trisomy 10p syndrome owing to maternal pericentric inversion. J Med Genet 1990;27:264–266.

252. Onufer CN, Stephan MJ, Thuline HC, Char F. Chromosome 13 long arm interstitial deletion associated with features of noonan phenotype. Ann Genet 1987;30:236–239.

253. Orye E, Craen M. A new chromosome deletion syndrome. Report of a patient with a 46,XY,8p-chromosome constitution. Clin Genet 1976;9:289–301.

254. Palka G, Verrotti A, Peca S, et al. Ring chromosome 11: a case report and review of the literature. Ann Genet 1986;29:55–58.

255. Palmer CG, Bader P, Slovak MI, Comings DE, Pettenati MJ. Partial deletion of chromosome 6p: delineation of the syndrome. Am J Med Genet 1991;39:155–160.

256. Palmer CG, Christian JC, Merritt AD. Partial trisomy 1 due to a "shift" and probable location of the duffy (fy) locus. Am J Hum Genet 1977;29:371–377.

257. Pan SF, Fatora SR, Sorg R, Garver KL, Steele MW. Meiotic consequences of an intrachromosomal insertion of chromosome no. 1: a family pedigree. Clin Genet 1977;12:303–313.

258. Park JP, Graham JM, Andrews PA, Wurster-hill DH. Ring chromosome 12. Am J Med Genet 1988;29:437–440.

259. Patau K, Smith DW, Therman E, Inhorn SL, Wagner HP. Multiple congenital anomaly caused by an extra autosome. Lancet 1960;1:790–793.

260. Patil SR, Bartley JA. Interstitial deletion of the short arm of chromosome 17. Hum Genet 1984;67:237–238.

261. Patil SR, Zellweger H. Partial trisomy 13. The myth of nonmongoloid trisomy G. Clin Pediatr 1981;20:534–536.

262. Peter J, Braun JT. Ocular pathology in trisomy 18 (Edward's syndrome). Ophthalmologica 1986;192:176–178.

262a. Peeden JN, Scarbrough P, Taysi K, et al. Ring chromosome 6: variability in phenotypic expression. Am J Med Genet 1983;16: 563–573.

263. Pellissier MC, Philip N, Voelckel-Baeteman MA, Mattei MG, Mattei JF. Monosomy 21: a new case confirmed by in situ hybridization. Hum Genet 1987;75:95–96.

264. Peters J, Pehl C, Miller K, Sandlin CJ. Case report of mosaic partial tetrasomy 9 mimicking Klinefelter syndrome. Birth Defects: Original Article Series. New York: March of Dimes Birth Defects Foundation, 1982;18(3B):287–293.

265. Pettigrew AL, Gollin SM, Greenberg F, Riccardi VM, Ledbetter DH. Duplication of proximal 15q as a cause of Prader–Willi syndrome. Am J Med Genet 1987;28:791–802.

266. Pfeiffer RA. Trisomy 8. In: Yunis JJ (ed) New chromosomal syndromes. New York: Academic Press, 1977:197–217.

267. Pfeiffer RA. Interstitial deletion of a chromosome 7 (q11.2q22.1) in a child with splithand/splitfoot malformation. Ann Genet 1984;27: 45–48.

268. Pfeiffer RA, Buttinghaus K, Struck H. Partial trisomy 14. Following a balanced reciprocal translocation t(14q–;21q+). Humangenetik 1973;20:187–189.

269. Pfeiffer RA, Englisch W. Partielle trisomie 1 (1q31–41) infolge intrachromosomaler insertion in 1p31.3 bei einem neugeborenen und der schwester der mutter. Monatsschr Kinderheilkd 1987;135:851–856.

270. Pihko H, Therman E, Uchida IA. Partial 11q trisomy syndrome. Hum Genet 1981;58:129–134.

271. Plunkett ER, Barr ML. Testicular dysgenesis affecting the seminiferous tubules principally with chromatin-positive nuclei. Lancet 1956;2:853–857.

272. Polani PE, Hunter WF, Lennox B. Chromosomal sex in Turner's syndrome with coarctation of the aorta. Lancet 1954;2:120–121.

273. Prieur M, Forabosco A, Dutrillaux B, Laurent C, Bernasconi S, Lejeune J. La trisome 10q24 → 10qter. Ann Genet 1975;18:218–221.

274. Pueschel SM, Scola PS, Mendoza T. Partial trisomy 2p. J Ment Defic Res 1987;31:293–298.

275. Ramer JC, Ladda RL, Frankel CA, Beckford A. A review of phenotype-karyotype correlations in individuals with interstitial deletions of the long arm of chromosome 2. Am J Med Genet 1989;32:359–363.

276. Raoul O, Rethore M-O, Dutrillaux B, Michon L, Lejeune J. Trisomie 14q partielle I.—Trisomie 14q partielle par translocation maternelle t(10;14)(p15.2;q22). Ann Genet 1975;18:35–39.

277. Ray M, Chuddley AE, Christie N, Seargeant L. A case of de novo trisomy 12p syndrome. Ann Genet 1985;28:235–238.

278. Reid CS, Stamberg J, Phillips JA. Monosomy for distal segment 6p: clinical description and use in localizing a region important for expression of Hageman factor. Pediatr Res 1983;17:217A.

279. Reiss JA, Brenes PM, Chamberlin J, Magenis RE, Lovrien EW. The 8p syndrome. Hum Genet 1979;47:135–140.

280. Reiss JA, Lovrien EW, Hecht F. A mother with Down's syndrome and her chromosomally normal infant. Ann Genet 1971;14:225–227.

281. Rethore M-O. Syndromes involving chromsomes 4, 9, and 12. In: Yunis JJ (ed) New chromosomal syndromes. New York: Academic Press, 1977:119–183.

282. Rethore M-O, Aurias A, Couturier J, Dutrillaux B, Prieur M, Lejeune J. Chromosome 8: trisome complete et trisomies segmentaires. Ann Genet 1977;20:5–11.

283. Reynolds JD, Golden WL, Zhang Y, Hiles DA. Ocular abnormalities in terminal deletion of the long arm of chromosome seven. J Pediatr Ophthalmol Strabismus 1984;21:28–32.

284. Riccardi VM. Trisomy 8: an international study of 70 patients. Birth Defects: Original Article Series. New York: March of Dimes Birth Defects Foundation, 1977;13(3C):171–184.

285. Riccardi VM, Hittner HM, Strong LC, Fernbach DJ, Lego R, Ferrel RE. Wilms tumor with aniridia/iris dysplasia and apparently normal chromosomes. J Pediatr 1982;100:574–577.

286. Riccardi VM, Sujansky E, Smith AC, Francke U. Chromosomal imbalance in the aniridia–Wilms' tumor association: 11p interstitial deletion. Pediatrics 1978;61:604–610.

287. Rivas F, Garcia-Cruz D, Rivera H, Plascencia L, Gonzalez RM, Cantu JM. 19q distal trisomy due to a de novo (19;22)(q13.2;p11) translocation. Ann Genet 1985;28:113–115.

288. Rivera H, Garcia-Esquivel L, Guadalupe M, Perez-Garcia RG, Martinez RMY. The 22q distal trisomy syndrome in a recombinant child. Ann Genet 1988;31:47–49.

289. Rivera H, Garcia-Esquivel L, Jimenez-Sainz M, Vaca G, Ibarra B, Cantu JM. Centric fission, centromere-telomere fusion and isochromosome formation: a possible origin of a de novo 12p trisomy. Clin Genet 1987;31:393–398.

290. Rivera H, Gonzalez-Flores SA, Rivas F, Sanchez-Corona J, Moller M, Cantu JM. Monosomy 13q32.3 → qtr: report of two cases. J Med Genet 1985;22:142–145.

291. Rivera H, Rivas F, Plascencia L, Cantu JM. Pure monosomy 21pter-q21 in a girl born to a couple 46,XX,t(14;21)(p12;q22) and 46,XY,t(5;18)(q32;q22). Ann Genet 1983;26:234–237.

292. Rivera H, Vargas-Moyeda E, Moller M, Torres-Lamas A, Cantu JM. Monosomy 16q: a distinct syndrome. Clin Genet 1985;28:84–86.

293. Roberts SH, Duckett DP. Trisomy 16p in a liveborn infant and a review of partial and full trisomy 16. J Med Genet 1978;15:375–381.

294. Rodrigues MM, Punnett HH, Valdes-Dapena M, Martyn LJ. Retinal pigment epithelium in a case of 18 trisomy. Am J Ophthalmol 1973;76:265–268.

295. Romain DR, Cairney H, Stewart D, et al. Three cases of partial trisomy 7q owing to rare rearrangements of chromosome 7. J Med Genet 1990;27:109–113.

296. Romain DR, Goldsmith J, Columbano-Green LM, Chapman CJ, Smythe RH, Parfitt RG. Partial monosomy 12p13.1–13.3. J Med Genet 1987;24:434–436.

297. Rutten FJ, Hustinx TWJ, Dunk-Tillemans AAW, Scheres JMJC, Tjon YST. A case of partial 9p monosomy with some unusual clinical features. Ann Genet 1978;21:51–55.

298. Rutzler L, Briner J, Sauer F, Schnid W. Mosaik-trisomie-8. Helv Paediatr Acta 1974;29:541–553.

299. Sachs ES, Hoogeboom AJM, Niermeijer MF, Schreuder GMT. Clinical evidence for localisation of HLA proximal of chromosome 6p22. Lancet 1983;1:659.

300. Salamanca-Gomez F, Nava S, Armendares S. Ring chromosome 6 in a malformed boy. Clin Genet 1975;8:370–375.

301. Salazar D, Rosenfeld W, Verma RS, Jhaveri RC, Dosik H. Partial trisomy of chromosome 3 (3q12 → qter) owing to 3q/18p translocation. Am J Dis Child 1979;133:1006–1008.

302. Sanchez O, Yunis JJ. Partial trisomy 8 (8q24) and the trisomy-8 syndrome. Humangenetik 1974;23:297–303.

303. Sandoval R, Sepulveda W, Gutierrez J, Be C, Altieri E. Prenatal diagnosis of nonmosaic trisomy 9 in a fetus with severe renal disease. Gynecol Obstet Investig 1999;48:69–72.

304. Scarbrough PR, Hersh J, Kukolich MK, et al. Tetraploidy: a report of three live-born infants. Am J Med Genet 1984;19:29–37.

305. Schachenmann G, Schmid W, Fraccaro M, et al. Chromosomes in coloboma and anal atresia. Lancet 1965;2:290.

306. Schinzel A. Incomplete trisomy 22. Hum Genet 1981;56:269–273.

307. Schinzel A. Partial trisomy 8q in half-sisters with distinct dysmorphic patterns not similar to the trisomy 8 mosaicism syndrome. Hum Genet 1977;37:17–26.

308. Schinzel A, Auf Der Maur P, Moser H. Partial deletion of long arm of chromosome 11[del(11)(q23)]: Jacobsen syndrome. J Med Genet 1977;14:438–444.

309. Schinzel A, Hayashi K, Schmid W. Structural aberrations of chromosome 18. II. The 18q−syndrome. Report of three cases. Humangenetik 1975;26:123–132.

310. Schinzel A, Hayaski K, Schmid W. Further delineation of the clinical picture of trisomy for the distal segment of chromosome 13. Hum Genet 1976;32:1–12.

311. Schinzel A, Schmid W, Luscher U, Nater M, Brook C, Steinmann B. Structural aberrations of chromosome 18. I, the 18p−syndrome. Archiv Genet 1974;47:1–15.

312. Schlessel JS, Brown WT, Lysikiewicz A, Schiff R, Zaslav AL. Monozygotic twins with trisomy 18: a report of discordant phenotype. J Med Genet 1990;27:640–642.

313. Schmickel R, Poznanski A, Himebaugh J. 16q trisomy in a family with a balanced 15/16 translocation. In: Bergsma D (ed) New chromosomal and malformation syndromes. Birth Defects: Origi-

nal Article Series. Miami: Symposium Specialists for National Foundation—March of Dimes. 1975;11(5):229–236.

314. Schmidt R, Eviatar L, Nitowsky HM, Wong M, Miranda S. Ring chromosome 14: a distinct clinical entity. J Med Genet 1981;18: 304–307.

315. Schnatterly P, Bono KL, Robinow M, Wyandt HE, Kardon N, Kelly TE. Distal 15q trisomy: phenotypic comparison of nine cases in an extended family. Am J Hum Genet 1984;36:444–451.

316. Schwanitz G, Schmid R-D, Grosse G, Grahn-Liebe E. Translocation familiale 3/22 mat avec trisomie partielle 3q. J Genet Hum 1977;25:141–150.

317. Schwanitz G, Zerres K. Partial monosomy 22 as result of an X/22 translocation in a newborn with DiGeorge syndrome. Ann Genet 1987;30:80–84.

318. Schwartz J, Chinitz J, Kushnick T. "Cri du chat" syndrome with additional findings of trisomy 17–18. Lancet 1968;88:303–305.

319. Schwinger E, Wiebusch D. Iris-und aderhautkolobom bein XYY-syndrom. Klin Monatsbl Augenheilkd 1970;156:873–877.

320. Seabright M. Rapid banding technique for human chromosomes. Lancet 1971;2:971–972.

321. Serville F, Broustet A, Sandler B, Bourdeau MJ, Leloup M. Trisomie 7q partielle. Ann Genet 1975;18:67–70.

322. Shapiro MB, France TD. The ocular features of Down's syndrome. Am J Ophthalmol 1985;99:659–663.

323. Shapiro SD, Hansen KL, Pasztor LM, et al. Deletions of the long arm of chromosome 10. Am J Med Genet 1985;20:181–196.

324. Sherard J, Bean C, Bove B, et al. Long survival in a 69,XXY triploid male. Am J Med Genet 1986;25:307–312.

325. Shohat M, Herman V, Melmed S, et al. Deletion of 20p 11.23-pter with normal growth hormone-releasing hormone genes. Am J Med Genet 1991;39:56–63.

326. Shokeir MHK. Complete trisomy 22. Clin Genet 1978;14:139–146.

327. Smart RD, Viljoen DL, Fraser B. Partial trisomy 9—further delineation of the phenotype. Am J Med Genet 1988;31:947–951.

328. Smith ACM, McGavran L, Robinson J, et al. Interstitial deletion of (17)(p11.2p11.2) in nine patients. Am J Med Genet 1986;24:393–414.

329. Smith BS, Petterson JC. An anatomical study of a duplication 6p based on two sibs. Am J Med Genet 1985;20:649–663.

330. Smith ACM, Sujansky E, Riccardi VM. Aniridia, mental retardation and genital abnormality in two patients with 46, XY, 11p−. Birth Defects 1977;13:3B.

331. Soltan HC, Jung JH, Pyatt Z, Singh RP. Partial trisomy 9q resulting from a familial translocation t(9;16)(q32;q24). Clin Genet 1984; 25:449–454.

332. Sparkes RS, Muller H, Klisak I, Abram JA. Retinoblastoma with 13q−chromosomal deletion associated with maternal paracsentric inversion of 13q. Science 1979;203:1027–1029.

333. Sparkes RS, Murphree AL, Lingua RW, et al. Gene for hereditary retinoblastoma assigned to human chromosome 13 by linkage to esterase D. Science 1983;219:971–973.

334. Sparkes RS, Sparkes MC, Wilson MG, et al. Regional assignment of genes for human esterase D and retinoblastoma to chromosome band 13q14. Science 1980;208:1042–1044.

335. Stallard R, Juberg RC. Partial monosomy 7q syndrome due to distal interstital deletion. Hum Genet 1981;57:210–213.

336. Stathacopoulos RA, Bateman JB, Sparkes RS, Hepler RS. The Rieger syndrome and a chromosome 13 deletion. J Pediatr Ophthalmol Strabismus 1987;24:198–203.

337. Steinbach P, Adkins WN, Caspar H, et al. The dup(3q) syndrome: report of eight cases and review of the literature. Am J Med Genet 1981;10:159–177.

338. Stratakis CA, Lafferty A, Taymans SE, Gafni RI, Meck JM, Blancato J. Anisomastia associated with interstitial duplication of chromosome 16, mental retardation, obesity, dysmorphic facies, and digital anomalies: molecular mapping of a new syndrome by fluorescent in situ hybridization and microsatellites to 16q13 (D16S419–D16S503). J Clin Endocrin Metab 2000;85:3396–401.

339. Stratton RF, Dobyns WB, Greenberg F, et al. Interstitial deletion of (17)(p11.2p11.2): report of six additional patients with a new chromosome deletion syndrome. Am J Med Genet 1986;24:421–432.

340. Strobel RJ, Riccardi VM, Ledbetter DH, Hittner HM. Duplication 11p11.3 → 14.1 to meiotic crossing-over. Am J Med Genet 1980;7:15–20.

341. Stromland K. Eye findings in partial trisomy 2q. Ophthalmic Paediatr Genet 1985;5:145–150.

342. Subrt I, Blehova B, Pallova B. Trisomy 9p resulting from maternal 9/21 translocation. Hum Genet 1976;32:217–220.

343. Suciu S, Nanulescu M. A case of 10p−syndrome. Ann Genet 1983; 26:109–111.

344. Sutherland GR, Carter RF, Morris LL. Partial and compelete trisomy 9: delineation of a trisomy 9 syndrome. Hum Genet 1976; 32:133–140.

345. Taillemite JL, Baheux-Morlier G, Roux C. Deletion interstitielle du bras long d'un chromosome II. Ann Genet 1975;18:61–63.

346. Taysi K, Singh Sekhon G. Partial trisomy of chromosome no. 1 in two adult brothers due to maternal translocation (1q−;6p+). Hum Genet 1978;44:277–285.

347. Taysi K, Strauss AW, Yang V, Padmalatha C, Marshall RE. Terminal deletion of the long arm of chromosome 10:q26 → qter: case report and review of the literature. Ann Genet 1982;25:141–144.

347a. Taysi K, Burel RM, Rohrbaugh JR. Terminal long arm deletion of chromosome 7 and retino-choroidal coloboma. Ann Genet 1982;25:159–161.

348. Telfer MA, Clark CE, Casey PA, Cowell HR, Stroud HH. Long arm deletion of chromosome 13 with exclusion of esterase D from 13q32–13qter. Clin Genet 1980;17:428–432.

349. Tharapel SA, Lewandowski RC, Tharapel AT, Wilroy RS Jr. Phenotype-karyotype correlation in patients trisomic for various segments of chromosome 13. J Med Genet 1986;23:310–315.

350. Tipton RE, Berns JS, Johnson WE, Wilroy RS, Summitt RL. Duplication 6q syndrome. Am J Med Genet 1979;3:325–330.

351. Tjio JH, Levan A. The chromosome number of man. Hereditas. 1956;42:1–6.

352. Townes PL, White M, Di Marzo SV. 4q−syndrome. Am J Dis Child 1979;33:383–385.

353. Traboulsi EI, Levine E, Mets M, Parelhoff ES, O'Neill JF, Gaasterland DE. Infantile glaucoma in Down's syndrome (trisomy 21). Am J Ophthalmol 1988;105:389–394.

354. Turleau C, Chavin-Colin F, Narbouton R, Asensi D, De Grouchy J. Trisomy 18q−. Trisomy mapping of chromosome 18 revisited. Clin Genet 1980;18:20–26.

355. Turleau C, de Grouchy J. Trisomy 6qter. Clin Genet 1981;19:202–206.

356. Turleau C, de Grouchy J. Trisomy 18qter and trisomy mapping of chromosome 18. Clin Genet 1977;12:361–371.

357. Turleau C, de Grouchy J, Chavin-Colin F, et al. Two patients with interstitial del (14q), one with features of Holt–Oram syndrome. Exclusion mapping of PI (alpha-10 antitrypsin). Ann Genet 1984;27:237–240.

358. Turleau C, de Grouchy J, Chavin-Colin F, Martelli H, Voyer M, Charlas R. Trisomy 11p15 and Beckwith–Wiedemann syndrome. A report of two cases. Hum Genet 1984;67:219–221.

359. Turleau C, de Grouchy J, Chavin-Colin F, et al. Partial trisomy 9q: a new syndrome. Humangenetik 1975;29:233–241.

360. Turleau C, de Grouchy J, Cornu A, Turquet M, Millet G. Trisomie 14 en mosaique par isochromosome dicentrique. Ann Genet 1980;23:238–240.

361. Turleau C, de Grouchy J, Perignon F, Lenoir G. Monosomie 7qter. Ann Genet 1979;22:242–244.

362. Turleau C, de Grouchy J, Ponsot G, Bouygues D. Monosomy 10qter. Hum Genet 1979;47:233–237.

363. Turleau C, de Grouchy J, Roubin M, Chavin-Colin F, Cachin O. Trisomie 9p pure 47,XX,+del(9)(q11) chez le pere. Ann Genet 1975;18:125–129.

364. Turleau C, Demay G, Cabanis M-O, Lenoir G, de Grouchy J. 6q1 monosomy: a distinctive syndrome. Clin Genet 1988;34:38–42.

365. Turner HH. A syndrome of infantilism, congenital webbed neck and cuitus valgus. Endocrinology 1938;23:566–574.

366. Uchida I, Freeman VCP. Triploidy and chromosomes. Am J Obstet Gynecol 1985;151:65–69.

367. Vachvanichsanong P, Jinorose U, Sangnuachua P. Trisomy 14 mosaeicism in a 5-year-old boy. Am J Med Genet 1991;40:80–83.

368. van Essen AJ, Kok K, van den Berg A, de Jong B, Stellink F. Partial 3q duplication syndrome and assignment of D385 to 3q25–3q28. Hum Genet 1991;87:151–154.

369. Verbraak FD, Pogany K, Pilon JW, et al. Congenital glaucoma in a child with partial 1q duplication and 9p deletion. Ophthalmic Paediatr Genet 1992;13:165–170.

370. Vogel W. Partial duplication 7q. In: Yunis JJ (ed) New chromosomal syndromes. New York: Academic Press, 1977:185–195.

371. Vogel W, Siebers J-W, Reinwein H. Partial trisomy 7q. Ann Genet 1973;16:277–280.

372. Voiculescu I, Back E, Duncan AMV, Schwaibold H, Schempp W. Trisomy 22 in a newborn with multiple malformations. Hum Genet 1987;76:298–301.

372a. Walknowska J, Peakman D, Weleber RG. Cytogenetic investigation of the cat-eye syndrome. Am J Ophthalmol 1977;84:477–486.

373. Walravens PA, Greensher A, Sparks JW, Wesenberg RL. Trisomy 8 mosaicism. Am J Dis Child 1974;128:564–566.

374. Warburg M, Mikkelsen M, Andersen SR, et al. Aniridia and interstitial deletion of the short arm of chromosome 11. Metab Pediatr Ophthalmol 1980;4:97–102.

375. Watson MS, Gargus JJ, Blakemore KJ, Katz SN, Breg WR. Chromosome deletion 1q42–43. Am J Med Genet 1986;24:1–6.

376. Watt JL, Olson IA, Johnston AW, Ross HS, Couzin DA, Stephen GS. A familial pericentric inversion of chromosome 22 with a recombinant subject illustrating a "Pure" partial monosomy syndrome. J Med Genet 1985;22:283–287.

377. Waziri M, Patil SR, Hanson JW, Bartley JA. Abnormality of chromosome 11 in patients with features of Beckwith–Wiedemann syndrome. J Pediatr 1983;102:873–876.

378. Wegner RD, Kunze J, Paust H. Monosomy 10qtr due to a balanced familial translocation: t(10;16)(q25.2;q24). Clin Genet 1981;19:130–131.

379. Weiss A, Margo CE. Bilateral microphthalmos with cyst and 13q deletion syndrome. Case report. Arch Ophthalmol 1987;105:29.

380. Wertelecki W, Breg WR, Graham JM, Ilinuma K, Puck SM, Sergovich FR. Trisomy 22 mosaicism syndrome and Ullrich–Turner stigmata. Am J Med Genet 1986;23:739–749.

381. Wiggs JL, Dryja TP. Predicting the risk of hereditary retinoblastoma. Am J Ophthalmol 1988;106:346–351.

382. Wilcox LM, Bercovitch L, Howard RO. Ophthalmic features of chromosome deletion 4p– (Wolf–Hirchhorn syndrome). Am J Ophthalmol 1978;86:834–839.

383. Wilkins LE, Brown JA, Nance WE, Wolf B. Clinical heterogeneity in 80 home-reared children with cri du chat syndrome. J Pediatr 1983;102:528–533.

384. Wilkins L, Grumbach MM, van Wyk JJ. Chromosomal sex in "ovarian agenesis." J Clin Endocrinol 1954;14:1270–1271.

385. Williams T, Zardawi I, Quaife R, Young ID. Complex cardiac malformation in a case of trisomy 9. J Med Genet 1985;22:230–233.

386. Wilson GN, Dasouki M, Barr M. Further delineation of the dup(3q) syndrome. Am J Med Genet 1985;22:117–123.

387. Wilson L, Hodes BL, Martin AO, Elias S, Ogata E, Simpson JL. Cytogenetic analysis of a case of "13q–syndrome." J Pediatr Ophthalmol Strabismus 1980;17:63–67.

388. Wilson GN, Raj A, Baker D. The phenotypic and cytogenetic spectrum of partial trisomy 9. Am J Med Genet 1985;20:277–282.

389. Wilson MG, Towner JW, Coffin GS, Forsman I. Inherited pericentric inversion of chromosome no. 4. Am J Hum Genet 1970;22:679–690.

390. Wilson MG, Towner JW, Forsman I, Siris E. Syndromes associated with the deletion of the long arm of chromosome 18[del(18q)]. Am J Med Genet 1979;3:155–174.

391. Wilson GN, Vekemans MJJ, Kaplan P. MCA/MR syndrome in a female infant with tetraploidy mosaicism: review of the human polyploid phenotype. Am J Med Genet 1988;30:953–961.

392. Wisniewski K, Dambska M, Jenkins EC, Sklower S, Brown WT. Monosomy 21 syndrome: further delineation including clinical, neuropathological, cyogenetic and biochemical studies. Clin Genet 1983;23:102–110.

393. Wolf U, Reinwein H, Porsch R, Schroter R, Baitsch H. Defizienz an den hurzen Armen eines Chromosoms nr. 4. Humangenetik 1965;1:397–413.

394. Wolkstein MA, Atkin AK, Willner JP, Mindel JS. Diffuse choroidal atrophy and Klinefelter syndrome. Acta Ophthalmol 1983;61:313–321.

395. Wulfsberg EA, Sparks RS, Klisak IJ, Teng A. Trisomy 18 phenotype in a patient with an isopseudodicentric 18 chromosome. J Med Genet 1984;21:151–153.

396. Wulfsberg EA, Weaver RP, Cunniff CM, Jones MC, Lyons K. Chromosome 10qter deletion syndrome: a review and report of three new cases. Am J Med Genet 1989;32:364–367.

397. Wyandt HE, Magenis RE, Hecht F. Abnormal chromsomes 14 and 15 in abortions, syndromes, and malignancy. In: Yunis JJ (ed) New chromosomal syndromes. New York: Academic Press, 1977:301–338.

398. Yamamoto Y, Okamoto N, Shiraiski H, Yanagisawa M, Kamoshita S. Deletion of proximal 6q: a clinical report and review of the literature. Am J Med Genet 1986a;25:467–471.

399. Yamamoto Y, Sawa R, Okamoato N, Matsui A, Yanagisawa M, Ikemoto S. Deletion 14q(q24.3 to q32.1) syndrome: significance of peculiar facial appearance in its diagnosis, and deletion mapping of Pi(a1-antitrypsin). Hum Genet 1986;74:190–192.

400. Yanoff M, Rorke LB, Niederer BS. Ocular and cerebral abnormalities in chromosome 18 deletion defect. Am J Ophthalmol 1970;70:391–402.

401. Yen FS, Podruch PE, Weisskopf B. A terminal deletion (14)(q31.1) in a child with microcephaly, narrow palate, gingival hypertrophy, protuberant ears, and mild mental retardation. J Med Genet 1989; 26:130–133.

402. Young RS, Bader P, Palmer CG, Kaler SG, Hodes ME. Brief clinical report: two children with de novo del(9p). Am J Med Genet 1983;14: 751–757.

403. Young RS, Reed T, Hodes ME, Palmer CG. The dermatoglyphic and clinical features of the 9p trisomy and partial 9p monosomy syndromes. Hum Genet 1982;62:31–39.

404. Young RS, Shapiro SD, Hansen KL, Hine LK, Rainosek DE, Guerra FA. Deletion 2q: two new cases with karyotypes 46,XY,del(2) (q31q33) and 46,XX,del(2)(q36). J Med Genet 1983;20:199–202.

405. Young RS, Weaver DD, Kukolich MK, et al. Terminal and interstitial deletions of the long arm of chromosome 7: a review with five new cases. Am J Med Genet 1984;17:437–450.

406. Yu CW, Chen H. De novo inverted tandem duplication of the long arm of chromosome 2(q34 → q37). Birth Defects: Original Article Series. New York: March of Dimes Birth Defects Foundation, 1982; 18(3B):311–320.

407. Yunis E, Giraldo A, Zuniga R, Egel H, Ramirez E. Partial trisomy 4q. Ann Genet 1977;20:243–248.

408. Yunis E, Gonzalez T, Torres de Caballero OM. Partial trisomy 16q. Hum Genet 1977;38:347–350.

409. Yunis E, Gonzalez J, Zuniga R, Torres de Caballero OM, Mondragon A. Direct duplication 2p14 → 2p23. Hum Genet 1979; 48:241–244.

410. Yunis JJ, Lewandowski RC Jr. Partial duplication 10q and duplication 10p syndromes. In: Yunis JJ (ed) New chromosomal syndromes. New York: Academic Press, 1977:219–244.

411. Yunis JJ, Quintero L, Castaneda A, Ramirez E, Leibovici M. Partial trisomy 3q. Hum Genet 1979;48:315–320.

412. Yunis JJ, Ramsay N. Retinoblastoma and subband deletion of chromosome 13. Am J Dis Child 1978;132:161–163.

413. Zatterale A, Pagnao L, Fioretti G, et al. Clinical features of monosomy 10qtr. Ann Genet 1983;26:106–108.

414. Zurcher VL, Golden WL, Zinn AB. Distal deletion of the short arm of chromosome 6. Am J Med Genet 1990;35:261–265.

4

Craniofacial Syndromes and Malformations

Marilyn T. Miller and Anna Newlin

The explosion of knowledge in the area of genetics, and a greater desire by patients and their families to know the cause and risk of recurrence of genetic malformations, have resulted in greater attention to errors of morphogenesis. For physicians who do not confront these problems regularly, the vocabulary often is confusing and unclear. Increasing effort has been made to clarify definitions for better communication of ideas. Improved classification of malformations and clusters of associated anomalies will assist in better diagnosis and treatment and more accurate risk counseling. Spranger et al.[219] Cohen,[38–40] Herrmann and Opitz,[100] and others have attempted to define more precisely commonly used terms.

TERMINOLOGY

Malformation: a morphological defect of an organ, part of an organ, or larger region resulting from an intrinsically abnormal developmental process. The risk of recurrence depends on the etiology of the malformation (e.g., genetic, teratogenic).

Congenital anomalies: all forms of developmental defects present at birth, whether caused by genetic, chromosomal, or environmental factors.

Dysmorphology: the study of congenital anomalies. The term *dysmorphic* describes an individual with obvious multiple and severe malformations.

Sequence: pattern of multiple anomalies derived from a single structural defect or mechanical factor (e.g., Möbius sequence).

Developmental field: a group of cells or a region that responds as a coordinated unit to embryonic interaction; defects in developmental fields result in multiple malformations (e.g., formation of the lens depends on interaction with the optic cup). Many malformations are field defects.[177]

Syndrome: pattern of anomalies thought to be pathologically related. The term implies a single cause, not a field defect.

Disruption: a morphological defect resulting from the extrinsic breakdown of, or an interference with, an originally normal developmental process (e.g., amniotic bands). As these are usually nonrecurring events, counseling will indicate low risk for future family members.

Deformation: abnormal form, shape, or position of a part of the body caused by a mechanical process (e.g., intrauterine compression).

Association: statistically related association of anomalies not identified as a sequence or syndrome (e.g., CHARGE association).

A disturbance to a group of cells in a single developmental *field* may result in multiple malformations. A single structural defect or factor causing a cascade of secondary anomalies is referred to as a *sequence*, with a domino-type effect. A sequence implies heterogeneous causative factors. Pierre Robin syndrome (cleft palate, glossoptosis, micrognathia, and respiratory problems) may represent a sequence caused by abnormal descent of the tongue due to mandibular hypoplasia. This sequence has been reported in many syndromes, including Stickler, fetal alcohol, and chromosomal syndromes. In contrast, a syndrome implies a single cause, even if the etiological agent is not yet identified.

The term *syndrome* is used in many ways, often utilizing a variety of definitions. It may be attached to an assortment of signs and symptoms for which the etiology is known (e.g., Down's syndrome, Marfan syndrome, trisomy 13), or it may be used to describe a group of findings for which the cause is poorly understood. The term *disease* is more frequently used with a group of signs and symptoms associated with progression or deterioration (e.g., diabetes). This separation is not always precise, and there are many examples of overlapping in which the term disease is used in a way that is more consistent with the definition of syndrome and vice versa. Although the etiology is known in some syndromes, the basic defect in many malformation syndromes remains unknown, with the name of the syndrome based on a wide variety of things, such as the physician's or patient's name, the striking feature, and mythical designation. The number and types of abnormalities ascribed to many syndromes vary not only in the frequency with which the syndrome has been observed and reported in the literature but also in the underlying pleiotropic characteristics of the syndrome. The term *phenotypic spectrum* was used by Opitz et al.[178] to describe the number of abnormalities reported for a given syndrome and their frequency in a controlled population. This approach helps to separate findings that are specific to the syndrome from those that are just a chance occurrence. A given anomaly may be clearly or questionably related to the syndrome or may be a chance occurrence; rarely, it may occur at a significantly lower frequency than would occur in a controlled population. This latter situation would suggest that the syndrome in some way protects the organism from a given abnormality. Various malignancies show increased correlations with a syndrome, whereas a few have the opposite relationship. For example, the association of Wilm's tumor with aniridia is well appreciated, but patients with osteogenesis imperfecta may be more resistant to cancer.[143]

A weak recurring pattern is described as an *association*. This term implies that the defects occur with more frequency than would be expected by chance but do not show a pattern that can be clearly defined as a syndrome. The *CHARGE association* (ocular Coloboma, Heart defects, choanal Atresia, developmental or mental Retardation, and Genitourinary and Ear anomalies) is an example that may represent a variety of yet unidentified etiologies.[180] If a definite etiology is established (e.g., a chromosomal abnormality) then, more precisely, that individual has a syndrome.

Cohen[38–40] reported that new syndromes are described at a rate of approximately one or more per week. In a typical scenario, an infant with multiple anomalies is examined. An attempt is made to arrive at a specific diagnosis from classic textbooks.[85,113,151,237]   computer-based   CD-ROM   programs,[9] London dysmorphology,[142] online databases,[149,176] and consultations with geneticists. If these investigations do not delineate a specific syndrome, the patient is presumed to represent an *unknown genesis syndrome*, in which the causes are unknown but the findings are thought to represent a unique pattern. The patient is then described in the literature, and the reaction of the scientific community is awaited.

At times, investigators have failed to recognize a previously described syndrome, and future correspondence will clarify the existing syndrome that the patient exhibits. Another possibility is that on seeing this constellation of findings, other physicians report additional cases, and this group of patients is classified into a category referred to as a *recurring pattern syndrome*. As more examples are observed, the validity of this new syndrome and the description of the spectrum of clinical manifestations increase. The etiology of the syndrome may not be appreciated at the time or even in the future, but if the specific cause is later described, these patients represent a *known genesis syndrome* and are subcategorized into such groups as (1) chromosomal defect, (2) enzyme deficiency, (3) environmental factor, (4) single gene syndrome, or (5) diseases or familial syndromes. The appreciation of developmental genes (e.g., Hox genes) has expanded the spectrum of possible genetic causation.

The study of many cases is required to establish whether any group of patients with similar but not identical findings represent different etiologies (heterogeneity) or the same cause with variable manifestations (pleiotropism).

One problem confronting less experienced physicians is that textbook descriptions frequently characterize and illustrate only the classic cases or severely affected patients, and more minimally affected individuals may not be recognized. Figure 4-1 shows examples of mildly, moderately, and severely affected children with mandibulofacial dysostosis, a dominantly inherited condition with high penetrance but variable expressivity. Frequently, other family members with the syndrome are not identified until a diagnosis is made in a severely affected child.

Children with congenital malformations and syndromes involving craniofacial structures are at a significant risk for ocular anomalies. The number of syndromes and isolated malformations is great, and the spectrum of eye problems is vast. Therefore, the development of an approach to the dysmorphic child is more productive than an attempt to memorize all ocular pathological changes reported in the literature. It is useful to consider these ocular findings in two general categories.

1. *Ocular complications secondary to abnormal size, shape, or position of bony and soft tissue changes in orbital structures.* These complications may occur during development (disruption or deformation) or may be acquired after birth. These derived changes can be anticipated from the malformations present in the

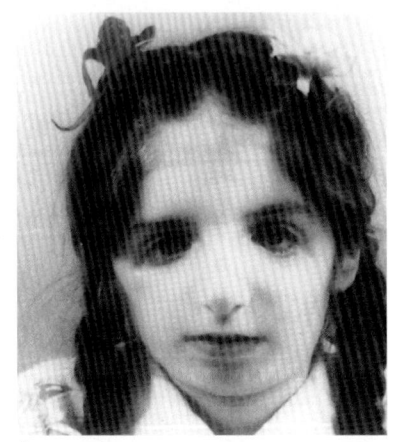

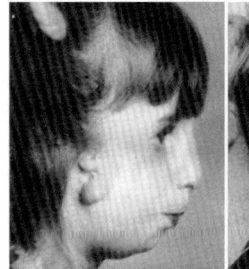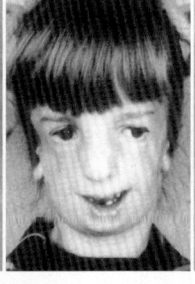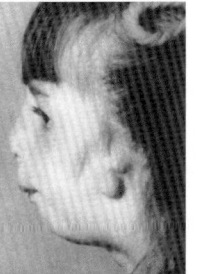

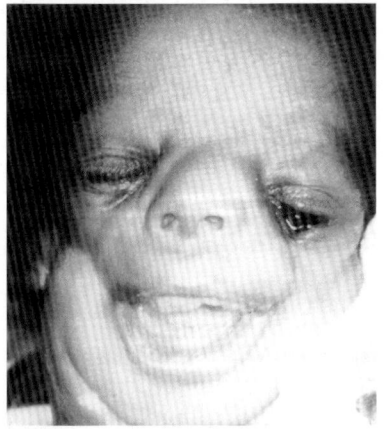

surrounding tissues. They are not necessarily specific to a syndrome but are the result of a type of deformity or mechanical factors. The same anomaly may occur in separate syndromes.

There are numerous common examples of secondary complications. Abnormalities in orbital size or position may result in many commonly listed and often severe ocular findings. For example, in craniosynostosis the resultant shallow orbits may result in corneal exposure or ulceration and motility disturbances. If the craniosynostosis causes extensive cranial suture closure, increased intracranial pressure may ensue with papilledema and optic atrophy.

2. *Intrinsic ocular pathology.* Examples include primary malformations associated with craniofacial syndromes, such as myopia and retinal pathological changes in Stickler syndrome, anterior segment developmental anomalies seen in fetal alcohol syndrome and many chromosomal anomalies, and Duane's syndrome, associated with many craniofacial malformation syndromes.

OPHTHALMOLOGIC EXAMINATION

Most ophthalmic findings are detected during the routine complete eye examination. The modifications of the examination consist of a more detailed search for milder forms of the "anticipated pathology," the recording of negative findings, and baseline measurements of anatomic relationships. These additions aid in a retrospective review of ocular manifestations in a particular syndrome, studies of the natural history with and without surgical intervention, and in devising coordinated treatment plans for a patient who is frequently being cared for by practitioners in multiple specialties of medicine.

Cycloplegic refraction and careful examination of the lids, palpebral fissures, anterior segment, pupils, and fundus, as well as special study of the optic disc, are routine and mandatory.

FIGURE 4-1A–C. Mandibulofacial dysostosis (Treacher Collins syndrome) in three children with different degrees of severity of the syndrome: **(A)** lid colobomas; **(B)** lower lid notching with absent cilia nasally, severe microtia with hearing deficit; **(C)** severe midface hypoplasia, facial clefts, lower lid coloboma, severe external ear malformations, and hearing loss.

Motility evaluation should include measurements in the primary position and all fields of gaze, with particular attention to the presence or absence of A- or V-pattern deviations and limitations of versions and ductions. Intraocular pressure measurements, visual field examination, exophthalmometry, corneal sensitivity tests, color vision tests, and tests of binocular vision should be performed when possible and desirable. When visual or structural abnormalities are noted, less routine tests, such as fluorescein angiography, visualization of the lacrimal system by radiologic techniques and electrophysiology, visual field analysis, and other tests may be appropriate. When abnormalities are numerous or serious ophthalmic disease is strongly suspected, examination under anesthesia may be necessary if the patient cannot co-operate. Before such a procedure is undertaken, however, consultation with other medical personnel should be conducted to anticipate anesthesia or sedation complications or to combine procedures that are scheduled to be completed. Patients with multiple craniofacial malformations are frequently at increased risk for complications and must be monitored more closely.

Some evaluations should be performed in patients with craniofacial anomalies that are not usually part of a routine eye examination, including measurements and documentation of certain anatomic relationships: (1) inner and outer canthal distances, (2) interpupillary distance, (3) palpebral fissure size, (4) position of the lacrimal puncta, (5) obliquity of the palpebral fissure, and (6) asymmetry of orbits and orbital structures. These measurements serve two purposes. First, they prevent errors of recording false impressions such as pseudohypertelorism caused by soft tissue changes in the canthal area such as telecanthus. In addition, they provide useful data for the study of the syndrome characteristics and serve as a baseline if reconstructive surgery is performed. With greater success in surgical correction of severe craniofacial anomalies, there has been renewed interest in the study of growth patterns of abnormal facial structures, necessitating detailed documentation of normal and abnormal findings. Accurate normal values are necessary for these comparisons (Fig. 4-2).[85,95,107,113]

If proptosis or exophthalmos is observed, careful measurements should be obtained. The instrument used to measure proptosis either reflects the personal preference of the examiner or is the one most readily available but should be standard for each examination. Because many patients are children, a simple type may be the most useful.

Interpupillary distance is an important observation in this group of patients. Most published values represent the interpupillary distance obtained while the patient is fixating on a distant target, which may be difficult to accomplish in a child. If the measurement can be made only at the near position, this fact should be recorded, and the distance measurement can be estimated by adding approximately 3 mm. If an ocular deviation is present, the left eye is covered so that the right eye fixes and the distance from the midpupil of the right eye to the midpoint over the nasal bridge is recorded. The right eye is then covered, and a similar measurement is made on the left side. The addition of the two values represents the interpupillary distance (usually for near). A more accurate and reproducible method of measuring orbital separation is the radiologic measurement of the bony intraorbital distance. It is appropriate to calculate separately the anatomic distance for each half of the face, not only for interpupillary values but also for intercanthal values, as asymmetry is present in many craniofacial syndrome entities. The difference between the values obtained for each half of the face is an indication of the degree of asymmetry in the orbital region.

To obtain more accurate values for the degree of orbital separation, Pryor[190] proposed the use of canthal measurement, believing that the sum of the inner and outer canthal distances divided by two is an accurate estimate of the interpupillary measurement. This may not be true if there are anomalies of the soft tissue structures, such as in individuals with primary telecanthus, which is discussed later in the section on hypertelorism.

PROTOTYPES OF CRANIOFACIAL SYNDROMES

It is beyond the scope of this chapter to list all the craniofacial syndromes and their ocular findings. Detailed information on rare syndromes must be obtained from standard texts of syndromes, from computerized databases, or from the specific literature. Many ocular findings are not syndrome specific but are the result of a particular anatomic derangement that may occur in multiple syndromes. The syndromes described here were selected for further description either because they were char

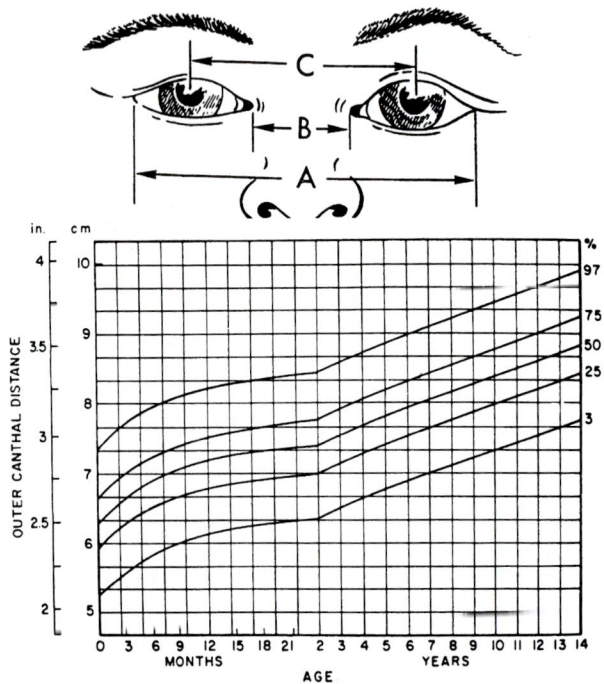

A

FIGURE 4-2. Facial measurements at different ages: *A*, outer canthal distance; *B*, inner canthal distance; *C*, interpupillary distance. (From Feingold M, Bossert WH. Birth Defects 1974;10:13, with permission.)

acteristic of a common group of craniofacial syndromes or because they had unusual or severe ocular malformations.

CRANIOSYNOSTOSIS

Cohen,[38–40] in his comprehensive book on craniosynostosis, described the historical interest and intrigue shown for patients with craniosynostosis, who are characterized by an unusual-shaped skull because of cranial and suture abnormalities. Descriptions appeared in mythical writings, religious treatises, and the literature of a broad scope of medical disciplines.

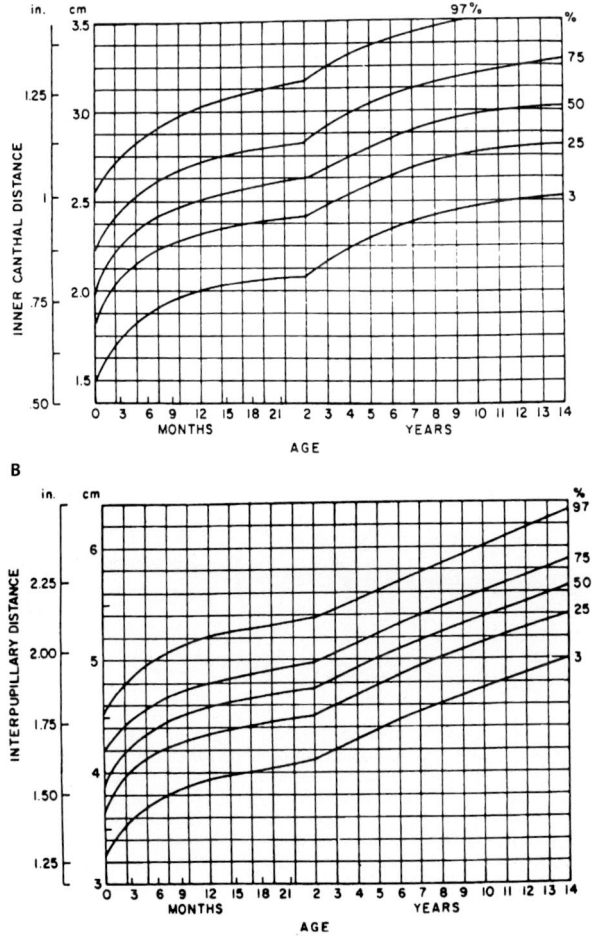

FIGURE 4-2. (continued).

Virchow[243] advanced the principle that closure of one or more cranial sutures resulted in compensatory growth in the other areas of the skull. An illustration of different ways in which compensatory growth could be manifested is shown in

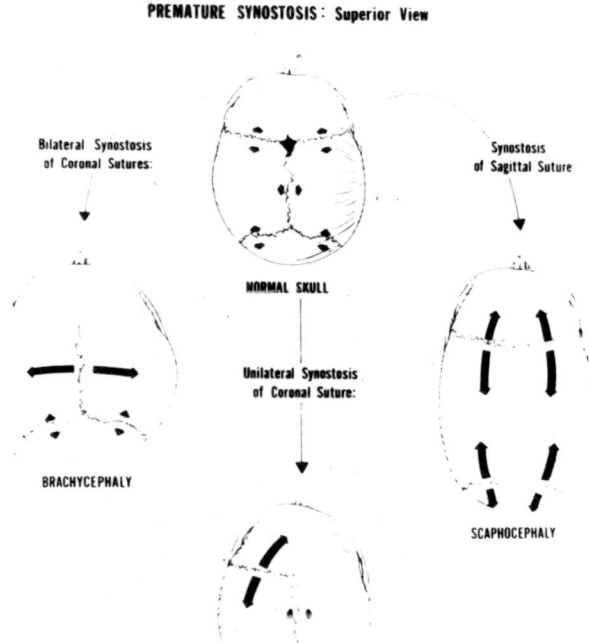

FIGURE 4-3. Effect of premature closure of various sutures on cranial morphology. Note that growth is inhibited perpendicularly to synostotic suture and expansion of skull occurs in area of open suture. Brachycephaly results from premature closure of the coronal suture, causing a short but laterally expanded head. Plagiocephaly (*lower*) results from asymmetrical closure of one coronal suture, causing anterior posterior elongation of the anterior aspect of the skull. A long narrow skull results from premature closure of the sagittal, causing anterior posterior elongation of the skull.

Figure 4-3. This boat-shaped head deformity is caused by fusion of the sagittal suture, which causes a decrease in the lateral growth and an increased anteroposterior growth, resulting in a skull shape that resembles the keel of a boat. Another cranial synostosis, *oxycephaly* (tower head deformity), results from early fusion of the coronal sutures plus part of the sagittal suture producing increased vertical diversion to the skull. The overall incidence for all forms of craniosynostosis is 1 in 2,000 to 1 in 2,500 live births.[130,131] *Sagittal synostosis* is the most common, with an incidence of 1 in 5,250.[131] *Coronal synostosis* is the second most common form, with an overall incidence of 1 in 16,000 in males and 1 in 8,000 in females.[130,131]

In many craniosynostosis syndromes, the particular suture showing premature closure is not necessarily characteristic of that syndrome, and patients with the same syndrome may manifest different combinations of suture closure. However, in some cases there does seem to be a characteristic cranial shape and facial appearance. Facial sutures are also involved, resulting in the midface hypoplasia and orbital dystopia. The ophthalmologist is more frequently consulted in cases of patients with monogenic syndromes, such as Crouzon and Apert syndromes, but the principles outlined and the types of problems and malformations may be applied to other causes of craniosynostosis. Craniosynostosis, whether isolated or part of a syndrome, is a major concern because of the potentially serious secondary, and in some cases primary, disturbances to ocular structures. The diagnosis of craniosynostosis and determination of the suture(s) involved are usually initiated by clinical findings, which include assessment of craniofacial shape, movement or lack of movement of the calvarial bones during infancy, and the presence or absence of sutural ridging, and can be confirmed by an X-ray of the skull or head CT examination.[89] In some instances, particularly with sagittal or coronal involvement, plain X-rays may suffice. If radiographic interpretation is equivocal, CT imaging is mandatory.

OCULAR FINDINGS

The ocular findings associated with craniosynostosis are potentially a serious threat to vision. Fortunately, the most serious ocular complications are often preventable if recognized early and treated promptly.[64] Other findings, such as strabismus and rarer anomalies, can be treated with appropriate surgery or other therapeutic modalities in a prioritized manner determined by the ophthalmologist and the craniofacial team.

Routine ocular examination, with special attention to positional relationships of the ocular adnexa, reveals most abnormalities. In addition to the standard history, more detailed questions about symptoms that suggest corneal exposure or changes in vision should be included. Because incomitant motility problems are common, a detailed evaluation of limitation of movement in all fields of gaze is indicated. Intraocular pressure, visual fields, and corneal sensitivity should be determined, and exophthalmometry should be performed when appropriate and possible. Special precaution should be exercised if a sedated examination is planned because of the frequent associated respiratory problems. Special imaging procedures, such as MRI and CT, are often routinely done in these patients. Small cuts (1.5–3 mm) through the orbit should be taken to provide more detailed information on the position and size of the ocular muscles. This information will be particularly useful if strabismus surgery is contemplated.

Visual loss is the most serious ophthalmologic complication seen in patients with craniosynostosis. It may be present at birth and can progress; it may also be a complication of reconstructive surgery. Therefore, many patients require ophthalmologic surveillance from infancy through adulthood or until their condition is stable. Visual loss may result from acquired ocular pathology, such as papilledema, optic atrophy, corneal exposure, or amblyopia secondary to strabismus or anisometropia. Several low-frequency ocular malformations may cause poor visual acuity and are generally noted during infancy in the course of a standard examination.

Optic nerve findings may reflect elevated intracranial pressure or possibly be secondary to local anatomic changes in the optic canal. Because the presence of craniosynostosis is currently recognized earlier than in years past, there seems to be a decreased incidence of papilledema and optic atrophy; however, these findings are still possible, and any routine ophthalmologic evaluation must include the status of the optic nerve.[124,125] Ophthalmologic evidence of increased intracranial pressure frequently necessitates earlier neurosurgical intervention. Some authors have recommended the use of visual evoked potential (VEP) and fluorescein angiography in some cases to aid in evaluation of optic nerve status.[91]

Increased tortuosity and a blurred optic disc border suggest the presence of increased intracranial pressure but also can exist without evidence of abnormal intracranial pressure. The causes of the pseudopapilledema and vessel changes are not always clear. Optic atrophy may also be noted without documented papilledema, thus raising the question whether some cases are caused by local compression of the optic nerve.

Proptosis (sometimes called exorbitism) seen in many craniosynostosis syndromes is caused by the shallow orbits and midface hyperplasia. This finding is quantitatively different from exophthalmos secondary to tumors and pseudotumors in patients with normal orbits and may show a different rate of progression. However, the ophthalmic symptoms and problems are similar. The degree of proptosis may vary greatly in patients with the same syndrome, ranging from minimal changes to severe corneal exposure mandating surgical intervention to prevent cornea ulceration and blindness. Figures 4-4 and 4-5 show the variations present in two patients with Crouzon syndrome. The patient shown in Figure 4-4 required immediate intervention and ultimately had fairly good visual function without long-term effects of the severe proptosis noted in infancy. The patient shown in Figure 4-5 had no corneal complications and required no special therapy for the proptosis.

Occasionally, during the examination of patients with marked exorbitism, slight retraction of the lid may cause luxation of the globe. Luxation may occur spontaneously or with manipulation of the lids. This dramatic finding may be frightening to the examining ophthalmologist, especially if it occurs when the exophthalmos is measured with an instrument placed on the lateral orbit. Fortunately, the patients or their families usually know how to gently push the eye back by pulling the lid over it. If luxation is not reduced promptly, secondary conjunctival edema may ensue, making it more difficult to reduce the luxated globe. If the globe remains unprotected, severe corneal exposure will follow, necessitating aggressive therapeutic intervention to prevent serious complications.

Severe proptosis from the reduced orbital volume may necessitate a different surgical treatment different from other causes of proptosis. If conservative management is insufficient to prevent corneal damage, a tarsorrhaphy (usually lateral) may be indicated as a temporary or permanent measure, depending on the long-term management plan for the facial deformity in the patient. Eyelid surgery should be deferred if extensive reconstructive surgery is anticipated in the near future, unless the corneal integrity is severely threatened. Tarsorrhaphy may protect the cornea and diminish the proptotic appearance by narrowing the abnormally wide palpebral fissure, but the improvement may be short lived and recurrence may result from constant mechanical force on the sutured lids. The definitive

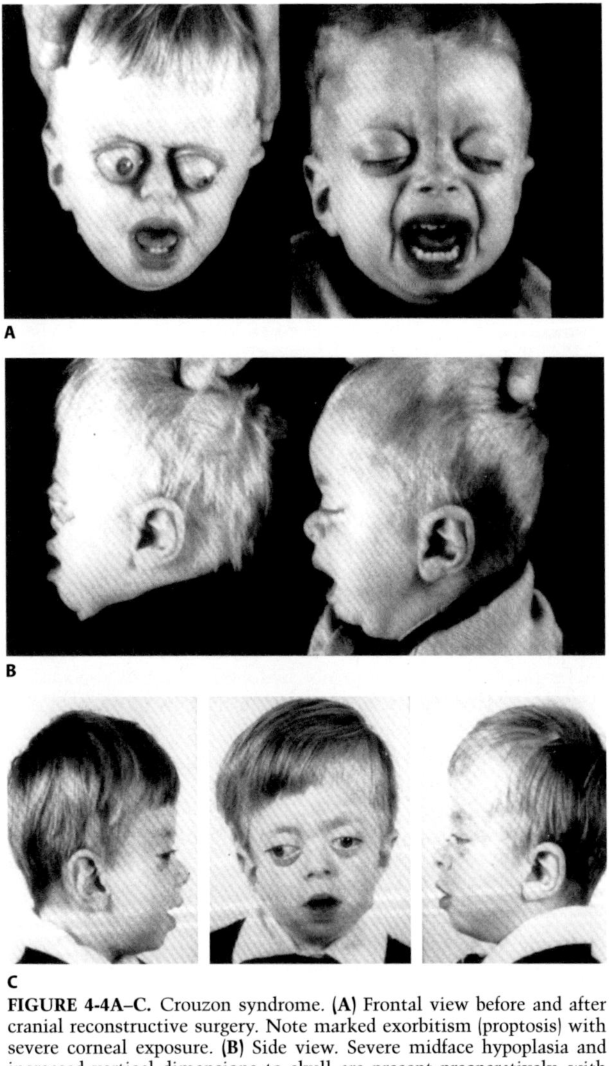

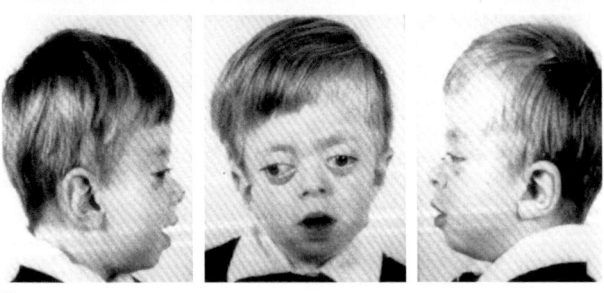

A

B

C

FIGURE 4-4A–C. Crouzon syndrome. **(A)** Frontal view before and after cranial reconstructive surgery. Note marked exorbitism (proptosis) with severe corneal exposure. **(B)** Side view. Severe midface hypoplasia and increased vertical dimensions to skull are present preoperatively, with improvement postoperatively. **(C)** At age 5 years, the patient had no signs of serious corneal exposure, but large exotropia exists that will require future ocular muscle surgery.

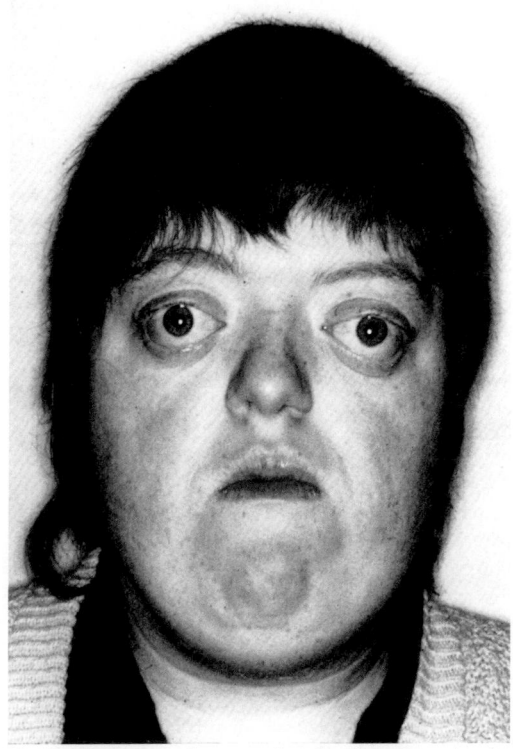

FIGURE 4-5. Crouzon syndrome: patient has less severe involvement and has never had evidence of corneal exposure.

solution is reconstructive surgery that creates a larger orbit. Standard decompression techniques that are useful for tumors or hyperthyroidism are not suitable.

Other causes of visual impairment include unusual refractive error and amblyopia due to anisometropia or strabismus. The treatment of refractive error and amblyopia is standard but may be hindered by difficulty in fitting glasses that are comfortable for patients with nose, eye, ear, and orbital malformations.

In the early literature, authors attributed all cases of strabismus to poor visual acuity, but this was proved to be incorrect. Although decreased visual acuity may be an important factor in some patients, strabismus is often the result of related anatomic and mechanical factors. The ocular deviation in the primary position is most frequently exotropia (Fig. 4-4) but also can be esotropia or straight eyes. A more consistent finding is the presence of an exotropia in the upgaze position with straight eyes or esotropia in downgaze, producing the V configuration.[126,158,160] Many patients also have associated overaction of the inferior oblique muscles. A subgroup of patients shows limitations in various fields of gaze. Although some of these findings may be attributed to mechanical effects of abnormally shaped and positioned orbits, there is good evidence that a number of patients have an abnormal insertion, structure, or orientation of the extraocular muscles.[52,59,146,252] It is unclear whether this represents a pleiotropic effect of the gene or secondary changes in the position of the muscles of the globe caused by local mechanical factors that occur during embryogenesis.

Most information about strabismus relates to patients with Crouzon and Apert syndromes, and there is some disagreement as to the ideal timing of surgical intervention for strabismus. Some physicians recommend early surgery, but many prefer to defer surgery until after the facial reconstructive surgery.[27,160] Reconstructive surgery of the midface in craniosynostosis may not affect the degree or pattern of ocular motility, but in some cases a substantial effect does occur (in contrast to patients with hypertelorism and median facial cleft in whom reconstructive surgery has been observed to significantly affect the ocular motility).[31] Attainable goals of therapy in most patients are good vision in both eyes and a cosmetically acceptable position of the eyes in the primary position of gaze. Because of the potential anatomic abnormalities of ocular muscle and the orbits, it is often impossible to align the eyes in all fields of gaze, and so the surgery is more directed to a straight primary position.[27,147,160]

Intrinsic ocular pathology is less frequent than secondary pathology, but it may include a few rare anomalies, such as iris colobomas, cataract, vitreous opacity, and medullated nerve fibers, along with the ocular muscle abnormalities. Keratoconus has occasionally been observed, as have changes in iris illumination and fundus pigmentary changes.[21,145] There is frequently a disturbance in the lacrimal outflow system with recurrent dacryocystitis.

PATHOGENESIS

The causes of craniosynostosis are known to be heterogeneous. The premature closure of the suture may result from a number of pathogenic mechanisms and has been reported in chromosomal, monogenetic, and teratogenic syndromes; in nutritional deficiency; and in other syndromes of unknown genesis.[39]

Most cranial and facial sutures do not close until adulthood, but a few synostose spontaneously early in development (premaxial, maxiofacial, axillary, and metopic). The reason for this predictably age-related synostosis is unknown, but it has been proposed to be related to the functional environment of a particular suture and the need for adaptive skeletal change in the craniofacial area.[137,138,140,211]

RECURRENCE RISK

Simple cases of craniosynostosis are often sporadic occurrences. Syndromic types frequently show autosomal dominant inheritance (Crouzon or Apert, Pfeiffer, and Saethre–Chotzen syndromes), although a few show autosomal recessive (Carpenter's syndrome) or other forms of inheritance.

ROLE OF THE OPHTHALMOLOGIST

The ophthalmologist is an indispensable member of the craniofacial team for this group of patients. Initially, examination of the optic nerve status as an indicator of intracranial pressure is most crucial. This evaluation, along with determination of whether there is vision-threatening corneal exposure, will determine whether emergency surgical intervention by the craniofacial team is necessary. Subsequently, the identification and treatment of strabismus, amblyopia, refractive errors, dacryocystitis, and mild corneal exposure may require frequent ophthalmologic visits. An ophthalmologist's consultation will be a factor in determining the time and extent of reconstructive craniofacial surgery. Major strides forward in the field of reconstructive surgery for the craniosynostosis group of patients has led to functional and cosmetic improvement for many and has resulted in increased knowledge of the pathophysiology of craniofacial structures.[21,232]

Ocular complications after major reconstructive surgery are potentially serious. Direct or indirect damage to the neurological pathways to the eye can result in permanent visual loss. Fortunately, blindness has been a rare complication. In a combined report of 793 cases,[253] 2 patients sustained permanent visual loss; in another study of 75 cases,[54] only 2 patients had severe visual complications. Choy et al.[30] reported their complications in reconstructive surgery, and Diamond et al.,[60] Morax,[168] and Choy et al.[31] reported ocular alignment changes after surgery. The cause of serious complications was not uniform in the few reported cases, although postoperative hematoma and nerve decompression was reported in some cases.

Changes in lid position may occur after midface surgery, requiring secondary ptosis surgery. Because the levator muscle is often normal from a neuromuscular standpoint, resection may have a greater effect than one would predict if the ptosis were congenital. Because lacrimal system dysfunction is common postoperatively and is related to an increased incidence of lacrimal excretory system anatomic anomalies or damage due to reconstructive surgery, the timing of lacrimal surgery depends on the severity of symptoms (particularly recurrent infection) and the potential effect of future surgery on the anatomy. Preoperative tearing is best treated after reconstructive surgery unless recurrent severe dacryocystitis exists that cannot be medically treated. This issue must be discussed with the craniofacial team to arrive at an appropriate decision.[54,253]

Apert Syndrome

Apert syndrome is characterized by craniosynostosis midface hypoplasia and syndactyly of extremities (Fig. 4-6). Its transmission is believed to be autosomal dominant, but most cases are sporadic and caused by high neonatal mortality and reduced fitness of affected individuals.[42]

Blank[23] estimated a frequency of 1 in 160,000 population, but Cohen[45] believed the prevalence may be higher. Prenatal diagnosis is possible.[135]

SYSTEMIC FINDINGS

Craniosynostosis of the coronal suture is characteristic with associated findings of midface deficiency, high-arched palate, syndactyly of the hands and feet involving digits two through four,[45] and central nervous system anomalies. The cranial base is malformed, and frequently there is bulging of the bregma. A trilobulated shaped skull (cloverleaf) has also been reported. The nasal bridge is depressed, and the nose is humped. Fused cervical ver-

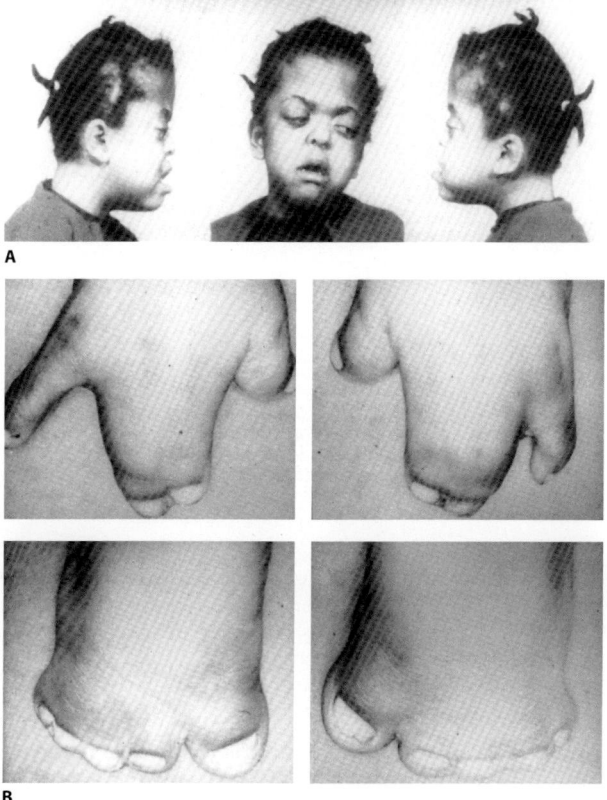

FIGURE 4-6A,B. Apert syndrome: (**A**) facial view; (**B**) syndactyly of hands and feet.

tebrae, usually involving C5–C6, have been reported in two-thirds of patients by Cohen and Kreiborg.[35] Mental deficiency appears more commonly than in Crouzon syndrome, even when no abnormalities of intracranial pressure are documented, and may be dependent on time of craniofacial surgery.[197]

OCULAR FINDINGS

Ocular findings are frequent.[27] Mild hypertelorism, downward slanting of palpebral fissures, and proptosis are commonly seen,

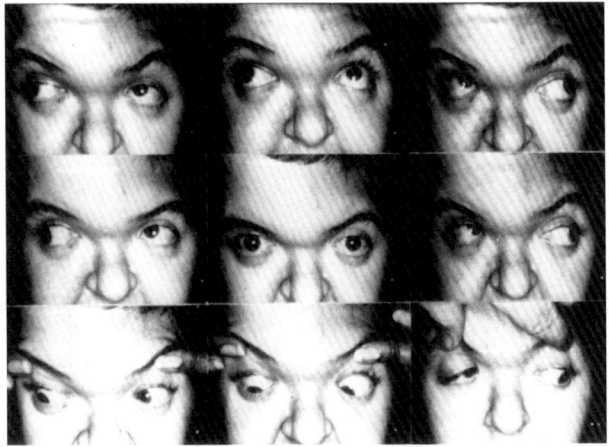

FIGURE 4-7. Apert syndrome. Ocular motility showing a small exotropia in primary position with a large exotropia looking up and esotropia looking down. Both inferior oblique muscles are overacting.

along with a characteristic V-pattern strabismus (Fig. 4-7). Abnormal origins, size, or insertion of ocular muscles may be present.[52,143] Infrequent findings include an albinotic appearance of the fundus, congenital glaucoma, and keratoconus.[85,145]

GENETICS

Two very specific changes in adjacent amino acids in the fibroblast growth factor receptor 2 (FGFR2) gene: Pro250Arg and Ser252Trp account for 97% of all mutations in Apert syndrome. The Ser252Trp mutation is more common, seen in 71% of Apert syndrome patients compared to the Pro253Arg mutation, which is seen in 26%. Cleft palate is more common in patients with Ser252Trp, whereas the degree of syndactyly is more prominent in the patients with Pro253Arg.[183,184,215] In Apert syndrome, the clinical manifestations within a family usually show little variability. Apert syndrome shows full penetrance, meaning that all individuals carrying a mutation for Apert syndrome will exhibit some phenotypic manifestation, even if fairly subtle. Affected individuals have a 50% chance of passing the disease-causing mutation to each one of their children. An advanced paternal age effect in new mutations has been conclusively demonstrated at the molecular level in Apert syndrome.[167] Germline mosaicism (where the mutation is confined to a percentage of the gonadal cells) has been observed. The limited number of different mutations in Apert syndrome (Ser252Trp, Pro253Arg) greatly facilitate diagnostic confirmation in addition to rendering feasible prenatal diagnosis via amniocentesis or chorionic villi sampling (CVS) in an at-risk pregnancy.

Pfeiffer's Syndrome

SYSTEMIC

Pfeiffer's syndrome is similar to Apert syndrome (see page 714), but also is characterized by very shallow orbits (already part of Apert) and short broad thumbs and toes. Corneal exposure is an important problem in these children.

Pfeiffer's syndrome is both clinically and molecularly heterogeneous. Cohen[35,47] has proposed three clinical subtypes with varying degrees of severity. This separation is often not clinically distinct in any patient but does allow a way of determining general prognosis.

Pfeiffer's syndrome types 2 and 3 are more common than type 1. Patients with Pfeiffer's syndrome type 1 can exhibit a spectrum of craniofacial involvement ranging from moderate to severe midfacial hypoplasia. Skeletal features encompass broad and medially deviated thumbs and great toes; variable degrees of brachydactyly can occur as well. Associated findings may include hearing loss or hydrocephalus. Intellect is usually normal. Overall, Pfeiffer's syndrome type 1 has a more favorable prognosis than types 2 and 3.

Craniofacial involvement in Pfeiffer's syndrome type 2 is more severe that in type 1, with cloverleaf skull and extreme proptosis (often to the point of inability to close eyelids). Not surprisingly, developmental delay and mental retardation are common. Skeletal findings are similar to type 1 with broad and medially deviated thumbs and great toes and a variable degree of brachydactyly. Additionally, ankylosis of the elbows and knees can occur. Associated findings have included choanal stenosis or atresia, laryngotracheal abnormalities, hydrocephalus, seizures, and increased risk for early death.

Pfeiffer's type 3 is almost identical to type 2; however, the skull shape is turribrachycephalic. The cognitive, skeletal features, and associated findings are those of type 9.

GENETICS

Inheritance is autosomal dominant with complete penetrance and variable expressivity. Mutations causing Pfeiffer's syndrome have been found on FGFR1 and FGFR2. A single common missense mutation, Pro250Arg, has been associated in five unrelated families with a relatively mild form of Pfeiffer's syndrome type 1.[170,199] Multiple mutations are known in FGFR2 and have been associated with a variety of phenotypes including Pfeiffer's. Rutland et al.[208] and Schell et al.[211] suggested that genotype–phenotype correlations can be drawn between the mutation in FGFR1 and those on FGFR2. Severe craniosynostosis and midfacial hypoplasia, more pronounced proptosis, and perhaps broader thumbs are more likely to be associated with mutations on FGFR2 than with the single mutation in FGFR1. In about 45% of Pfeiffer's syndrome patients, no mutation has been identified. With familial Pfeiffer's syndrome, when a specific mutation is known in advance, prenatal diagnosis is possible by CVS or amniocentesis. Ultrasonographic examination may show cloverleaf skull in type 2.

Table 4-1 compares the clinical features of FGFR craniosynostosis syndromes, and Table 4-2 summarizes the molecular basis.

Carpenter's Syndrome

Carpenter's syndrome, also known as acrocephalo-polysyndactyly type II, is a variation of Apert syndrome characterized by preaxial polydactyly on the side of the thumb or big toe, syndactyly, brachycephaly, synostosis, obesity, hypogonadism, mental retardation, shallow orbits, proptosis, and laterally placed intercanthi.[43,201]

TABLE 4-1. Distinguishing Clinical Features in the FGFR-Related Craniosynostosis Syndromes.

Thumbs:	Great toes:
Normal	Normal
Occasionally fused to fingers	Occasionally fused to toes
Broad, deviated	Broad, deviated
Hands:	Feet:
Normal	Normal
Bone syndactyly	Bone syndactyly
Variable brachydactyly	Variable brachydactyly

TABLE 4-2. Prevalence and Molecular Basis of FGFR-related Craniosynostosis Syndromes.

Syndrome	Incidence	Proportion of FGFR1 mutations	Proportion of FGFR2 mutations	Proportion of FGFR3 mutations
Isolated coronal synostosis	?Common			5%
Crouzon	1.6/100,000		95%	5%
Apert	1/100,000		100%	
Pfeiffer type 1	1/100,000	5%	95%	
Pfeiffer type 2	1/100,000	100%		
Pfeiffer type 3	1/100,000	100%		

GENETICS

Inheritance is autosomal recessive and the molecular basis is unknown to date. In all cases, examination of the parents has been normal.

Crouzon Syndrome

Crouzon syndrome occurs in approximately 1 in 25,000 births.[46] The coronal suture is most frequently involved, but different combinations of sutures have been reported in 75% of cases.[125,126] Craniofacial findings in Crouzon syndrome are similar to those for Apert syndrome and other types of craniosynostosis, but the prevalence of various malformations and the family history are different, and there are no anomalies of the hands or feet (although a radiographic metacarpal-phalangeal profile may reveal shortening.[171] About 5% of individuals have acanthosis nigricans, which can appear after the neonatal period. This finding is associated with a specific mutation in the FGFR3 gene. Progressive hydrocephalus occurs in approximately 30% of affected individuals, often with tonsillar herniation.

OCULAR FINDINGS

Proptosis occurs in most patients and may be severe, with vision-threatening corneal exposure necessitating reconstructive surgery earlier than usual. Optic atrophy and blindness are also more frequent than in other types of craniosynostosis syndromes. Low-frequency anomalies reported include keratoconus, iris and corneal malformations, glaucoma, and ectopia lentis.[85]

Abnormal location and position of ocular muscles have been reported frequently in both Crouzon and Apert syndromes. These findings may be due to a bias of the type of patients more frequently referred to an ophthalmologist, or they may represent a true increased prevalence in these particular forms of craniosynostosis.

GENETICS

Crouzon syndrome has a clear autosomal dominant mode of inheritance, with about 67% of cases being familial.[44] Variability of expression characterizes Crouzon syndrome. Most of the mutations associated with Crouzon syndrome are located in FGFR2. With the milder phenotype that can be seen in Crouzon syndrome, inheritance of the mutant gene from an affected parent is common. To date, about a half dozen mutations found in patients and families with Crouzon are identical to those that cause Pfeiffer's syndrome, and one 9-bp deletion overlaps with an 18-bp deletion in Pfeiffer's syndrome (see Table 4-2). When a specific mutation is known in advance, prenatal diagnosis is possible by CVS or amniocentesis.

PLAGIOCEPHALY

Plagiocephaly is defined as asymmetry of the skull caused by unilateral or asymmetrical involvement of the cranial sutures or a deformation defect from compression on the head.[26,33] Female preponderance is noted in both types of plagiocephaly.[26] Figure 4-8A shows a patient with plagiocephaly. Frequently, the asymmetry is best observed by looking down on a patient's head (Fig. 4-8B).

SYSTEMIC FINDINGS

Plagiocephaly is sometimes divided into a frontal type involving a corneal suture or an occipital type involving the lambdoidal suture. Unilateral coronal synostosis is estimated to occur in 1 per 10,000 births, 10 times more frequently than lambdoidal synostosis.[26] Deformational plagiocephaly is more frequent, but many of these infants are not referred to craniofacial centers because of the natural history of improvement of this form of plagiocephaly. The following discussion concerns

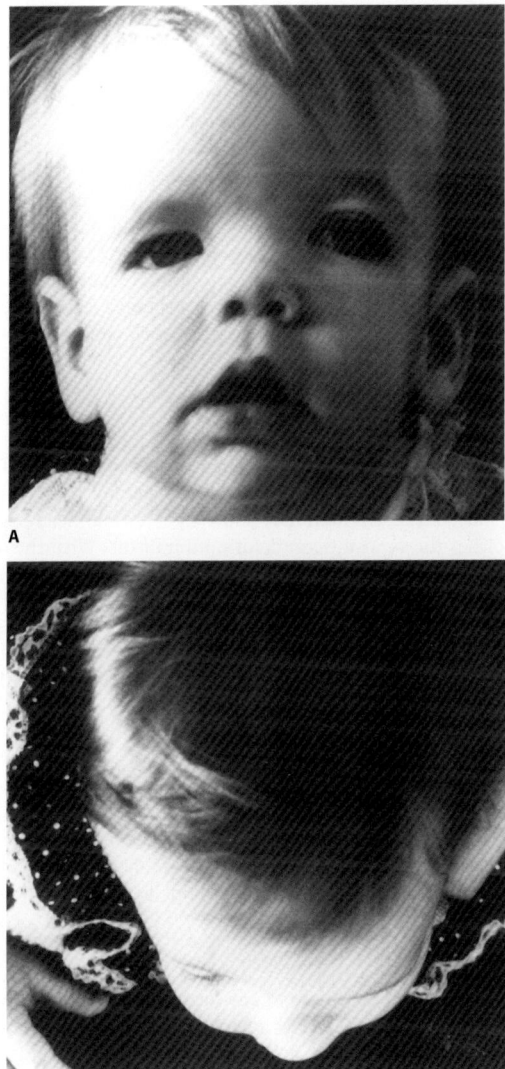

FIGURE 4-8A,B. Synostotic plagiocephaly in child (**A**). (**B**) As viewed from above.

the frontal type of plagiocephaly, which is the most common and of greatest concern to the ophthalmologist.

In the synostotic form, the orbit is elevated on the affected side and the nasal root is also deviated on that side. Usually the ear is supraplaced, the forehead flattened, and the palpebral fissure more flattened on the involved side. Craniofacial growth will be altered. The most reliable diagnostic tests are standard radiographs or CT scans. Primary radiographic findings may be unreliable in the first few months of life[26] and may need to be repeated if deformity remains or progresses, even when the initial early radiographic evaluation did not disclose any abnormality. Three-dimensional CT scans, although expensive, give more information on the degree of deformity or orbital dysmorphology.[148,241]

OCULAR FINDINGS

Affected patients have a high incidence of vertical strabismus. The strabismus pattern depends on the type and degree of plagiocephaly. These children may show an abnormal head position with either the synostotic or deformation forms. With the deformation type, the head tilt is often more to the affected side, whereas with the synostosed form the tilt is to the opposite side, often with a hypertropia secondary to a superior oblique muscle palsy[187] on the side of the abnormal orbit as well as a classic upslanted overacting inferior oblique muscle. Surgery similar to that for a routine superior oblique palsy may be indicated. These patients should be examined carefully because they may exhibit other types of patterns or motility disturbances.

It is possible that other ocular symptoms or signs ascribed to craniosynostosis may exist that are limited to the affected side. However, because an adequate number of sutures are opened in most cases, there usually is no optic nerve damage or increased intraocular pressure. There are exceptions to this rule, however.

ROLE OF THE OPHTHALMOLOGIST

The diagnosis and treatment of any form of strabismus is usually the most important task in synostotic plagiocephaly. Torticollis with deformation plagiocephaly is treated with physical therapy and head helmets. Although the differentiation between these forms appears clear in some cases, the relationship of the head position to the observed strabismus is not clear.

GENETICS

Gripp et al.[90] found a pro250-to-arg (P250R) amino acid substitution in FGFR3 in 4 of 37 patients with synostotic anterior plagiocephaly. This same mutation was identified in patients with Muenke nonsyndromic coronal synostosis as well as in individuals with Saethre–Chotzen syndrome. In 3 mutation-positive patients with full parental studies, a parent with an extremely mild phenotype was found to carry the same mutation. None of the 6 patients with nonsynostotic plagiocephaly and none of the 4 patients with additional suture synostosis had the FGFR3 mutation.

HYPERTELORISM

Hypertelorism is an anatomic description that indicates an increased distance between the orbits (greater than 2 standard deviations from normal values). Hypertelorism is thought to be the consequence of arrest in development of the greater wings of the sphenoid, making them smaller than the lesser wings and thus fixing the orbits in the widely separated fetal position. The most accurate diagnoses involve radiologic methods. The exact location for measuring the intraorbital distance may vary among different investigators, but there are appropriate established norms for the various locations.[17] A less accurate clinical determination is to measure the interpupillary distance (previously described in the introduction of the chapter).

Soft tissue variations may result in a false diagnosis of hypertelorism. The most common cause of pseudohypertelorism is an increased distance between the medial canthi (i.e., telecanthus). If the abnormality is confined to the soft tissue, the term primary telecanthus is sometimes used. Patients with increased intraorbital distance and proportional increased intercanthal distances are at times referred to as having secondary telecanthus. Therefore, secondary telecanthus is not "pseudo"-hypertelorism, as there is a true increase in the orbital distance. A combination of telecanthus and lateral displacement of the lacrimal puncta occurs in some patients (Fig. 4-9); this is seen most commonly in Waardenburg syndrome but also is seen in a few other syndromes, such as blepharonasofacial syndrome.[192]

Hypertelorism, a nonspecific finding in many dysmorphic individuals, is associated with a large, heterogeneous group of

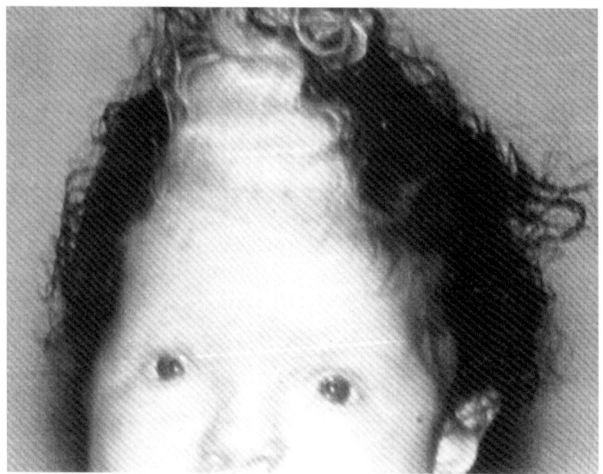

FIGURE 4-9. Waardenburg syndrome with forelock and primary telecanthus.

etiologies, such as craniofacial syndromes, teratogenic deformities, and disruptions.[41] Hypertelorism is a characteristic finding of a variety of chromosomal aberrations.[85] No single specific ocular abnormality is associated with the various types of hypertelorism, but dysfunction of the lacrimal excretory system caused by disturbed midline anatomy exists in many patients without regard to etiology of the hypertelorism. Lacrimal duct probings are not always successful because of these anatomic changes, and more complex diagnostic evaluations of the lacrimal system are needed.

Strabismus, usually exotropia, is frequently present if the hypertelorism is severe. If the bony orbits are abnormal in more respects than in their horizontal position (e.g., craniosynostosis), other motility disturbances also may be present.

GENETICS

The recurrence risk is determined by the etiology of the hypertelorism. For example, if the cause is associated with Crouzon syndrome, the recurrence risk would be 50%, whereas frontonasal dysplasia usually occurs sporadically and thus has a low recurrence risk.

Frontonasal Dysplasia (Median Face Cleft Syndrome; Frontonasal Malformation)

In frontonasal dysplasia, hypertelorism is the sine qua non. Other characteristic findings are bifidum occultum anterior cranium; midline clefting of nose, upper lip, premaxilla, and palate; and widow's peak (Fig. 4-10). There may also be notching of alae nasi. Intellectual development is usually normal. Midbrain anomalies, including septo-optic dysplasia, have been reported in addition to interhemispheric lipomas.[73] Sphenoethmoid encephalocele may be associated with frontonasal dysplasia and optic disc anomalies[133] and may represent a separate entity within the spectrum of anomalies. Primary telecanthus superimposed on secondary telecanthus has been reported in some patients.

Frontonasal dysplasia is a developmental field defect of midfacial development. Clinical features include a broad nose, hypertelorism, low anterior hairline, and sometimes bony defects of

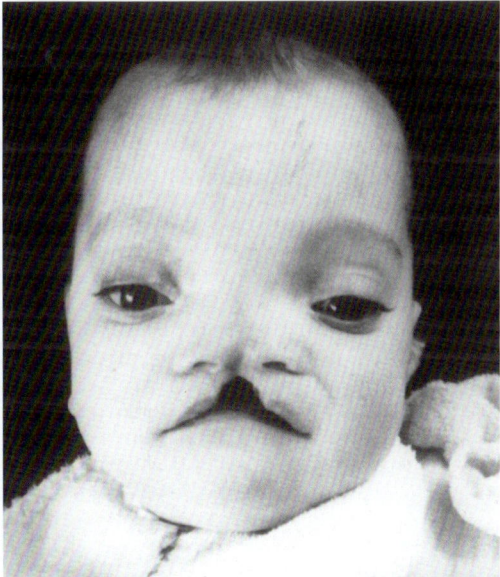

FIGURE 4-10. Median facial cleft syndrome: patient has hypertelorism, cleft lip, bifid nose, and exotropia.

the forehead.[57] There are reports of this malformation occurring with central nervous system anomalies, in particular frontal encephaloceles and agenesis of the corpus callosum. A few patients show some of the characteristics of Goldenhar's syndrome (oculosyndrome auriculovertebral) with lid colobomas, epibulbar dermoids or lipodermoids, and vertebral anomalies.[172]

Computed tomography and MRI are useful in the evaluation of patients with hypertelorism. The facial structures are better delineated by CT, but cerebral and ocular anomalies are more detailed on magnetic resonance images.

OCULAR FINDINGS

Ocular findings are common and varied, with strabismus being the most common.[118] Exotropia occurs in many patients and seems related to the degree of hypertelorism. An overacting inferior oblique muscle may also be present. Duane's syndrome has been reported. Uveal coloboma, and microphthalmia have been noted in a few cases.[11,181] Optic atrophy is much rarer than in patients with craniosynostosis.

ROLE OF THE OPHTHALMOLOGIST

Routine ophthalmologic examination will reveal any low-incidence anomalies but in most patients the strabismus, usually exotropia, becomes the ophthalmologist's main concern in addition to any ocular complications that may ensue after reconstructive surgery.

The exotropia appears to have a mechanical etiology due to the large separation of the orbits. Tessier[253] noted that the intraorbital distance is much greater anteriorly than posteriorly. There may be a relative normal relationship horizontally between the optic canals. This related difference results in an increased angulation of the orbits. When the intraorbital distance is reduced in reconstructive surgery, the degree of the exotropia frequently decreases or is eliminated.[141] In a few patients esotropia with diplopia may actually occur postoperatively, which suggests that delaying strabismus surgery until after reconstructive surgery may give better results.

GENETICS

The disorder is thought most often to be sporadic and is known to occur with a high frequency in twins. Both autosomal dominant and autosomal recessive modes of inheritance have been suggested, without completely convincing evidence in either case. Autosomal recessive inheritance was suggested by the inbred kindred reported by Moreno,[169] who reviewed the conflicting literature on the genetics of this anomaly. An X-linked dominant form has also been suggested as a possibility.[76]

Hypotelorism

Hypotelorism, like hypertelorism, is an anatomic description and not a syndrome diagnosis. The intrapupillary distance must be considered in relationship to the head size so that relative hypotelorism in a microcephalic head would have a different implication than true hypotelorism in a head with normal circumference. Hypotelorism may occur with isolated median cleft lip and a few other craniofacial anomalies with a normal brain,[85] but many times it is an indication of abnormal brain development such as holoprosencephaly.

ROLE OF THE OPHTHALMOLOGIST

In the examination of a child with hypotelorism, it is most important for the ophthalmologists to be aware of possible central nervous system anomalies and to refer the patient for further medical evaluation. If there are any ocular developmental anomalies, the child should be treated in the standard way.

GENETICS

Hypotelorism is an etiologically heterogeneous entity. The recurrence risk of hypotelorism with or without holoprosencephaly depends on the etiology. Many cases are sporadic, but there are a few conditions that have some recurrence risk. Relatives should be examined for mild forms of hypotelorism, bifid nose, pituitary deficiency, and dental anomalies.

HOLOPROSENCEPHALY

Holoprosencephaly, which occurs with a frequency of 1 in 16,000 live births and about 1 in 200 spontaneous abortions, is a spectrum of central nervous system malformations involving midline structures. It is an etiologically heterogeneous entity, including teratogenic causes such as maternal diabetes.

DeMeyer et al.[58] outlined the facial dysmorphism that they proposed predicted different types of holoprosencephaly. At one extreme is cyclopia with a single median eye sometimes associated with a proboscis. There may be varying degree of doubling of the ocular structures in this severe developmental anomaly. Less severe malformations of the face and brain may be associated with iris coloboma.[36,37] Occasionally, holoprosencephaly is not accompanied by characteristic facial features, but significant hypotelorism implies central nervous system malformations and usually mental retardation, and the child should be worked up with that possibility in mind. In *Aicardi's syndrome*, hypotelorism, costovertebral defects, mental deficiency, arrhinencephaly, agenesis/dysgenesis of the corpus callosum, seizures, and other central nervous systems anomalies are associated with choroidoretinal lacunae.[63] Flexion spasms in the infant represent the usual mode of clinical presentation in the Aicardi syndrome. This group of findings is confined almost exclusively to girls, suggesting X-linked dominant inheritance with lethality in hemizygous males. All cases would, on this hypothesis, be new mutations. There are many recognized syndromes and chromosomal anomalies with holoprosencephaly.[36,37,119,163]

PATHOGENESIS

Holoprosencephaly indicates a midline cleavage anomaly of the embryonic forebrain. As it is seen in cases of known chromosomal, genetic, and teratogenic factors, this seems to best fit into the category of a developmental field defect.

Sulik and Johnston[226] suggested that these complex facial and central nervous system anomalies can be traced to a defect in development that occurs near the third week of gestation. They were able to produce this defect by administering alcohol in a mouse model.

GENETICS

The recurrence risk of holoprosencephaly depends on the etiology. Relatives should be examined for mild forms of hypotelorism, bifid nose, pituitary deficiency, and dental anomalies. Holoprosencephaly can be chromosomal, multifactorial, or monogenic in origin and may be associated with other midline malformations. Autosomal dominant holoprosencephaly is a rare but well-documented entity. The transmitting parent may be normal or have a single central maxillary incisor as the only manifestation of a midline abnormality. At least 12 genetic loci have been associated with holoprosencephaly, including the sonic hedgehog gene (SHH) at 7q36.[246] Sporadic cases account for two-thirds of cases, and the recurrence risk after an isolated case is predicted to be 13% to 14%.[175]

MANDIBULOFACIAL DYSOSTOSIS (TREACHER COLLINS, FRANCESCHETTI–ZWAHLEN–KLEIN SYNDROMES)

Mandibulofacial dysostosis (MFD) has many names depending on the medical specialty or the country of origin in which it is reported. Although this syndrome was first described in the literature in the 1800s by Berry,[20] detailed descriptions of the major manifestations were later published.[71,239] It occurs in 1 in 25,000 to 1 in 50,000 births with more than 50% new mutations and some relationship incidence related to paternal age.[115]

SYSTEMIC FINDINGS

The disorder shows an unusually wide range of expressivity and involves structures primarily derived from the first branchial arch, groove, and pouch. The complete form is characterized by (1) coloboma or notching of the outer part of the lower eyelid; (2) lack of development of the malar bone and mandible; (3) antimongoloid slant of the palpebral fissures; (4) large mouth (macrostomia), abnormal (highly arched) palate, and anomalies of dentition; (5) malformations of the external and middle ear; (6) atypical hairline with projections toward the check; and (7) blind fistulas between the ears and angles of the mouth (see Fig. 4-1). The condition is almost always bilateral. Incomplete and abortive cases are common. The abnormalities are bilateral and usually quite symmetrical contrasted with hemifacial microsomia. Intelligence is usually normal.

A cleft palate exists in about 35% of patients, with an additional 30% to 40% of patients showing more minor palatal anomalies.[85] The temporal orbital wall is affected with secondary hypoplasia and malposition of soft tissues. Consistent bony abnormalities include absence or severe hypoplasia of the zygomatic process of the temporal bone and deformities of the orbital rim, zygoma, mandible, and of the medial pterygoid plates with hypoplasia of the pterygoid muscles. There is micrognathia, macrostomia, and downward displacement of the external ear. In many patients, the external auditory meatus is absent. In addition to the external ear anomalies, middle ear dysplasia with fusion of absence of the ossicles may result in hearing deficits. Preauricular ear tags and fistulas may be present as abnormal anterior hairline patterns.

OCULAR FINDINGS

Although a variety of ocular abnormalities have been reported, vision is usually normal, and most of the ophthalmic defects are confined to the soft and hard tissues surrounding the globe. In the more severe cases there is a complete coloboma of the lower lid, which gives the lid a triangular shape. All structures of the lid may be affected at, and medial to, the site of the coloboma. In less-severe cases, only a notch of an S-shaped configuration of the lower lid exists, often with a decrease in the cilia of the lid medially. Significant astigmatism has been observed in a number of patients with off-axis cylinders, suggesting a possible relationship between the refraction and the defects in the surrounding soft and hard tissue.[158]

The lacrimal puncta may also be involved or absent.[13] Wang et al.[747] examined 14 patients with mandibulofacial dysostosis and described in detail the changes observed in fissure length (decreased), shortening of the eyelid on forced closure, and the previously described punctal and lower lid anomalies.

Low-incidence anomalies include upper eyelid colobomas, corneal guttata, and ptosis.[174,247]

PATHOGENESIS

Teratogenic doses of isotretinoin and vitamin A have produced malformations resembling those seen in mandibulofacial dysostosis abnormalities in neural crest development.[189,228] Possible mechanisms suggested were disturbance of migration of neural crest cells or increased programmed cell death due to selective cytotoxicity.

GENETICS

The inheritance is clearly autosomal dominant in most cases, with markedly variable expressivity. It is not unusual to encounter a classical case and then find other family members with mild previously unrecognized manifestations. The risk of recurrence for future children and offspring is 50%. The paternal age was noted to be older in the estimated 50% to 60% of new mutations.[115] There seems to be no sex or racial predilection.[203]

There is variable expression within families; some patients are mildly affected, and others are so severely affected that they die shortly after birth.[203] The gene locus for the Treacher Collins syndrome was finally mapped to chromosome 5Q32–q33.3 by Jabs and coworkers,[111] and Dixon and coworkers[62]; and the Treacher Collins Syndrome Collaborative Group[238] isolated the locus for the TCOF1 gene in 1996. Although TREACLE was the initial designation for the gene for Treacher Collins syndrome, it is now used to designate the protein product. Dixon[61] reviewed the clinical and molecular features of Treacher Collins syndrome. A total of 51 mutations in the TCOF1 gene had been identified to date, all of which result in introduction of premature termination codons into the reading frame, suggesting haploinsufficiency as the molecular mechanism underlying the disorder. Splendore et al.[218] screened 28 families with a clinical diagnosis of Treacher Collins syndrome for mutations in the 25 coding exons of TCOF1 and their adjacent splice junctions through SSCP and direct sequencing. Pathogenic mutations were detected in 26 patients, yielding the highest detection rate reported so far for this disease (93%).

When a specific mutation is known in advance, prenatal diagnosis is possible by CVS or amniocentesis. Otherwise, ultrasound imaging in the second trimester can be used to view the fetal profile for micrognathia and maxillary hypoplasia, features suggestive of the disorder. Additionally, presence of polyhydramnios with no visible stomach bubble can be an indicator of reduced fetal swallowing due to marked micrognathia.

ROLE OF THE OPHTHALMOLOGIST

Most of these patients require no ophthalmologic treatment other than routine management of strabismus, if it exists, and correction of the refractive error (although it may be somewhat difficult to fit eyeglasses because of the ear deformity). A few patients have tearing secondary to malformed positions of the palpebral fissures and other lacrimal anomalies that require treatment.[13] The primary treatment for severe cases consists of reconstruction of the hypoplastic facial bones and surgical correction of the ear deformities.

The management of mandibulofacial dysostosis also includes early recognition of hearing deficits and cosmetic correction of any major facial defects. Patients are usually of normal intelligence. Because some patients have narrow airways, extreme care is recommended during endotracheal intubation.

NAGER SYNDROME (PREAXIAL ACROFACIAL DYSOSTOSIS)

Patients with Nager syndrome resemble those with mandibulofacial dysostosis with the additional finding of limb deformities. The mandibulofacial dysostosis is characterized mainly by severe micrognathia and malar hypoplasia. The limb deformities consist of absence of the radius, radioulnar synostosis, and hypoplasia or absence of the thumbs. This syndrome is usually sporadic, and there are reported systemic findings of small stature, malformation of the thumbs, radial deformities, and kidney malformations.[85] McDonald and Gorski[150] presented a summary of 76 previously reported cases and added 2 new cases. They favored inheritance as a pleiotropic disorder with markedly variable penetrance and expressivity, but granted that the occurrence of affected sibs with normal parents suggested genetic heterogeneity with the existence of an autosomal recessive form. They found 5 families with normal parents and 2 affected siblings. Zori et al[262] suggested that the gene for this disorder may reside on chromosome 9, at q32.

OCULO-AURICULO-VERTEBRAL SPECTRUM (HEMIFACIAL MICROSOMIA, GOLDENHAR'S SYNDROME, FACIAL MICROSOMIA)

Hemifacial microsomia encompasses a heterogeneous spectrum of conditions characterized by malformations involving the ear, oral, and mandibular structures. There are no absolute minimum criteria for diagnosis, and the incidence of this syndrome complex is unknown. Goldenhar's syndrome is considered by many to be a variant in the group and is estimated to represent 10% of the total group.[205] The frequency of the total group is estimated about 1 in 5600 population with a 3:2 male-to-female ratio.[85,86]

SYSTEMIC FINDINGS

The phenotypic spectrum is large and extremely variable. Unilateral facial involvement (usually the right side) or marked asymmetry is present in about 70% of cases.[85] The mandibular ramus and condyle are frequently severely involved.

Ear malformations range from anotia to only ear tags, with intermediate malformations involving size, position, or configuration (Fig. 4-11). Hearing loss may be caused by inner, middle, and external ear lesions. Preauricular tags are present in 40% cases and may be bilateral even in patients in whom the condition appears to be unilateral. Supranumerary tags usually follow an imaginary line extending from the tragus of the ear to the corner of the mouth. Preauricular pits may be present.

Central nervous system anomalies occur in 5% to 15% of cases,[5,48,213] and cranial nerve involvement of the trigeminal and facial nerves occurs in 10% to 20% of cases.[85] Autism has been reported.[132]

Cervical spine anomalies also vary widely and include fusional defects, spina bifida, Klippel–Feil anomalies, and scoliosis. The combined presence of this group of malformations occurs in about 55% of cases.[85]

Macrostomia is common, especially in patients with mandibular malformations and, to a lesser extent, epibulbar dermoids.[85] Cleft palate and occasionally cleft lip and dental anomalies are also seen.

Heart, lung, and kidney malformations are reported in 5% to 50% of cases[48] but less frequently than in the craniofacial anomalies.

OCULAR FINDINGS

The designation of Goldenhar's syndrome implies epibulbar or conjunctival lipodermoids with vertebral anomalies in addition to other characteristic findings. Ocular findings are thus more prevalent in this variant.

Ocular and adnexal findings were reported by Hertle et al.[102] in 67% of cases in a facial microsomia series, with ptosis or a narrow palpebral fissure on the affected side in 10% of cases. Epibulbar dermoid and conjunctival lipodermoids occur fre-

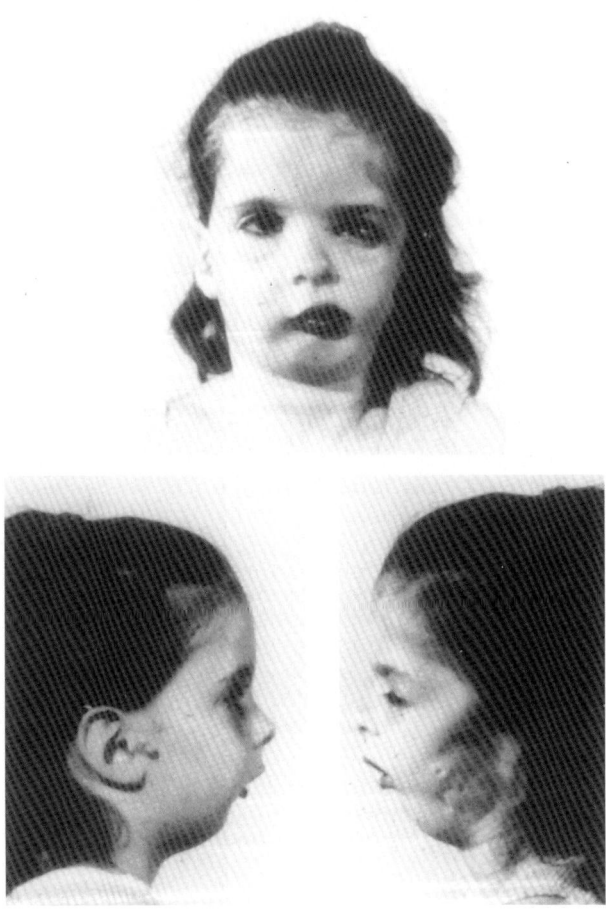

A
FIGURE 4-11A,B. Hemifacial microsomia: Goldenhar variant, at **(A)** 5 years and **(B)** 10 years. Patient shows bilateral involvement (ear tags) but with marked asymmetrical effects of ear structures. She also had conjunctival lipodermoids, Duane's syndrome, mild microphthalmia, and anisometropia with amblyopia.

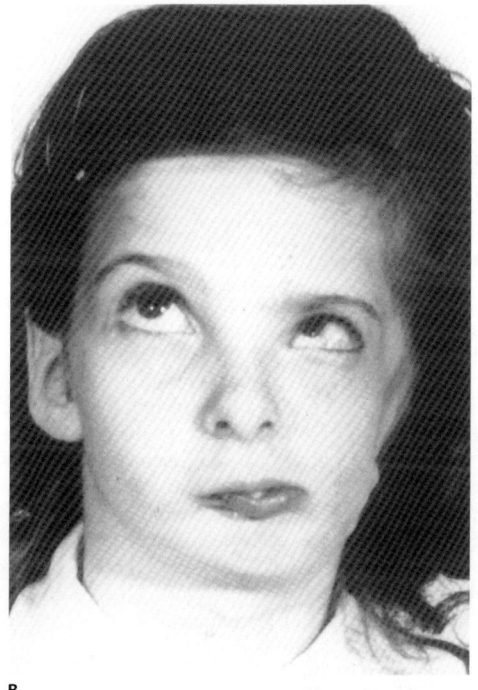

FIGURE 4-11B. (continued).

quently[15] and most often inferotemporally. Conjunctival lipodermoids may be inconspicuous. Upper lid colobomas are noted in about 20% of cases.[15] There appears to be a higher incidence of associated anophthalmia in cases with severe central nervous system anomalies.[85] Hertle et al.[102] reviewed 49 cases of facial microsomia (5 bilateral, 44 unilateral); visual loss was noted in 8% of cases, amblyopia in 16%, refractive errors in 27%, and strabismus in 22%.

Strabismus is usually comitant, but there is an increased occurrence of Duane's syndrome[15,154,155,185] and other incomitant types of strabismus.[4] Low-incidence anomalies include uveal colobomas,[15] corneal anesthesia and corneal ulcers,[166,217,244,250] iris coloboma,[68] optic nerve hypoplasia, and retinal abnormalities.[144]

PATHOGENESIS

Branchial arch anomalies are believed to represent a nonspecific syndrome complex due to multiple etiologies and are pathogenetically heterogeneous.[85] Poswillo[188] believed that vascular disruption in the region of the developing ear and jaw was the initiating cause. Such disruption may cause a local disturbance or may affect migrating neural crest cells.

GENETICS

Most cases are sporadic, with rare concordance in monozygotic twins and a few reported families with characteristics of this heterogeneous complex.[205] A similar phenotype has been observed in a few children with chromosomal anomalies, teratogenic causes, and amniotic band syndrome. Genetic counselors estimate a 2% to 3% empirical recurrence risk for future siblings in families with apparently isolated cases.[205] Kaye et al.[117] analyzed the families of 74 probands by examining relatives to identify ear malformations, mandibular anomalies, and other craniofacial abnormalities. They concluded that the hypothesis of no genetic transmission could be rejected; the evidence favored autosomal dominant inheritance, whereas recessive and polygenic models were not distinguishable.

ROLE OF THE OPHTHALMOLOGIST

Cosmetic and functional ocular malformations are common but extremely variable. In a few patients, the most important challenge may be cosmetic, with anophthalmia or microphthalmia. Many patients require routine treatment of refractive errors, amblyopia, and strabismus. If corneal sensation is decreased, artificial tears may be indicated.

Epibulbar dermoids may result in astigmatism in the affected eye, and treatment should address amblyopia and cosmetic appearance. Small, epibulbar dermoids and many conjunctival lipodermoids require only observation unless they increase in size. If surgical removal is necessary, care should be taken, as symblepharon formation may occur; removal is usually best limited to a readily visible section.[152] After removal, the astigmatism often changes only slightly. If the posterior aspect of a large lipodermoid is not visible, radiographic imaging may determine the extent of the lesion.

FETAL ALCOHOL SYNDROME

A pattern of malformations has been observed in children born to women who have a history of alcohol abuse during pregnancy. These dysmorphic features, along with other symptoms and signs, have been designated the fetal alcohol syndrome (FAS).[114,116] Recognition of the spectrum of features of this syndrome and insight into the probable prevalence in the general population have emerged during the past two decades, but the observation that the ingestion of large amounts of alcohol by women during pregnancy may result in harm to the fetus has been known for centuries.[240,249]

This pattern of anomalies in children with typical FAS results in a recognizable gestalt (Fig. 4-12). At the other end of

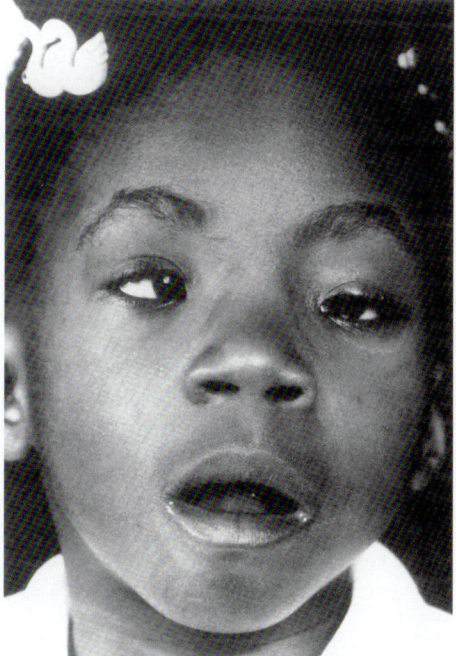

FIGURE 4-12. Fetal alcohol syndrome: note telecanthus, asymmetrical ptosis, and strabismus.

the spectrum are mildly affected children with fetal alcohol effects (FAE) who may manifest an assortment of malformations. Alcohol-related birth defects (ARBD) is a term used to describe these varied effects.

It is difficult to determine the exact incidence of FAS, FAE, or ARBD, but estimates range from 1 or 2 live births in 1000 to partial expression in up to 3 to 5 in 1000.[32] If the 2 in 1000 statistic is accurate, then FAS ranks among the top three causes of mental retardation and is the most preventable. Other studies have suggested that 1 in 30 women abuse alcohol during pregnancy and that 6% of their offspring show noticeable effects. If true, this would make FAS one of the leading causes of mental retardation worldwide.[32]

The critical amount of alcohol required to produce FAS or any malformation in the fetus or functional effects has not been established, but a definite risk of developing the syndrome is believed to exist with an intake of 89 ml per day of absolute alcohol (average of six drinks).[32] Intake of lesser amounts of alcohol (e.g., two drinks per day) carries no established risks but is believed to cause an increased incidence of fetal anomalies. For some malformations, there may be no safe level of alcohol consumption, and binge drinking may result in a malformation even if the average number of drinks consumed per week is low.[88,97,222]

CLINICAL MANIFESTATIONS

The typical clinical findings of FAS include (1) facial abnormalities consisting of palpebral fissure changes, thin vermilion border of the upper lip, flat philtrum, and epicanthal folds; (2) mental retardation, varying from mild to severe; (3) low weight and decreased body length at birth and persisting into childhood; and (4) abnormalities of the cardiovascular and skeletal systems (see Fig. 4-12).

Numerous abnormalities of the central nervous system have been described, including abnormal corpus callosum and polymicrogyria.[81] Some anomalies implicate abnormal neural migration.[85] Holoprosencephaly has also been reported as a possible result of in utero alcohol exposure in both human and mouse studies.[227]

Alcohol is a well-established behavioral teratogen.[222] Children with FAS are frequently hyperactive, show poor motor function, and have difficulty learning.[222] Mental retardation is usually mild to moderate. A wide variety of cardiac, skeletal, vertebral, pulmonary, and renal malformations have been described.

OCULAR FINDINGS

The ocular manifestations initially described were soft-tissue changes of small palpebral fissure, telecanthus, ptosis, epicanthus, and some low-incidence anomalies (Figs. 4-12, 4-13). As the number of ophthalmologic reports increased, more serious manifestations that significantly decrease visual acuity were noted.[157,159,224,225]

Telecanthus (increased distance between medial canthi) is a characteristic finding in the typical FAS gestalt and seems to be more prominent than decreased distance between the lateral canthi. Although blepharophimosis (decrease in all fissure measurements) has been mentioned in the literature, telecanthus is probably a more accurate description in most patients. Ptosis,

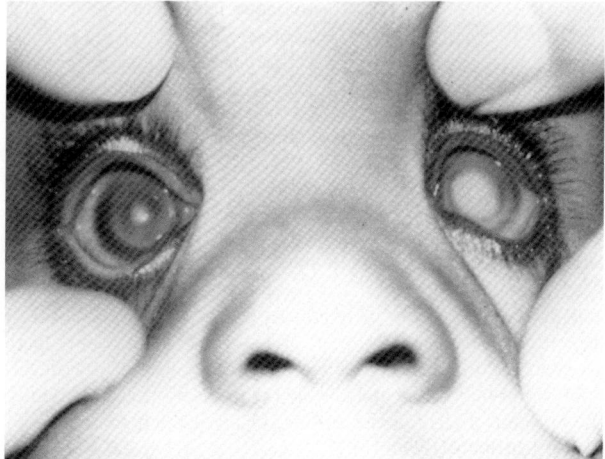

FIGURE 4-13. Fetal alcohol syndrome (FAS): patient has developmental anomaly of anterior segment characteristic of Peters' anomaly. There was a typical history of heavy alcohol intake during mother's pregnancy, and child had the characteristic findings of FAS.

often asymmetrical or unilateral, is also a common finding along with epicanthus.

Strabismus is common and usually comitant.[159,224] Although anisometropia or structural eye defects may predispose to ocular deviations in some patients, the strabismus in most cases appears to be primary.

Hypoplastic or abnormal-appearing optic discs have been noted in many cases of FAS.[159,224] Strömland[225] reported this finding in 40% of cases in her series. The hypoplasia seems to be less severe than that described in septo-optic dysplasia, and there may not be associated nystagmus. Tortuosity of the retinal vessels is also very common. Its significance is unknown but may be related to the length of vessels versus the size of the eye.

Developmental anomalies of the anterior segment, ranging from a posterior embryotoxon to a severely ectatic opaque cornea, have been described[157,225] (Fig. 4-13). One report in the literature suggests that unilateral or asymmetrical anterior segment anomalies are associated with significant myopia in the less-involved or uninvolved eye, suggesting that high myopia may be a forme fruste of anterior segment developmental anomalies.[157] Steep corneal curvatures have been observed in cases of FAS,[78] implicating the cornea as the significant factor in cases of high myopia.

Refraction in FAS may range from high hyperopia to high myopia, but the distribution is abnormal, with more cases in the two tails of the distribution curve of refractive errors.[224]

PATHOGENESIS

The teratogenic effect of alcohol may be mediated through multiple mechanisms. The development of the central nervous system may be adversely affected at different times of gestation and by different mechanisms and may extend beyond organogenesis to histogenesis.[193] Decreased blood flow to the uterus and placenta resulting in hypoxia, fetal acidosis, alteration in migration of neural crest cells, and shortage of nutrients have all been postulated as possible effects of alcohol on the developing embryo.[193] There may be factors in the mother that modify the amount of alcohol the embryo receives, such as the rate of detoxification of alcohol.

RECURRENCE RISK

As with most teratogenic agents, the susceptibility of the embryo or fetus varies greatly due to maternal and genetic variables and dosage and timing of intake variables.[2] If the mother does not change her drinking habits, subsequent pregnancies will also have an increased risk of FAS or fetal alcohol effects, but no absolute number can be applied because of the many variables.

ROLE OF THE OPHTHALMOLOGIST

Every child suspected of having FAS or fetal alcohol effects should undergo a complete eye examination to detect the ocular manifestations that could result in severely reduced visual acuity. Treatment of the most common problems, such as refractive errors, strabismus, and amblyopia, should follow standard practices. If the child is in an undesirable socioeconomic environment, compliance with treatment may be poor. The visual potential of the child should be conveyed to the educational authorities for appropriate school placement. Severe ocular malformations, such as Peters' anomaly, may require extensive and prolonged therapy, and the ophthalmologist becomes an indispensable member of the team to assist in establishing treatment priorities.

HALLERMANN–STREIFF SYNDROME (FRANÇOIS DYSCEPHALIC SYNDROME, OCULOMANDIBULODYSCEPHALY)

Although Hallerman–Streiff syndrome (HSS) had been described previously in the literature, in 1960 François[74] published a detailed review and delineation of the characteristic features of this syndrome. Ophthalmologic findings are present in most cases[6,28,67,72,221,229] and frequently require surgical and medical treatment. The risks of anesthesia are increased because of obstruction of the upper airways, and this must be considered if early surgery is necessary to remove the congenital cataracts.

SYSTEMIC FINDINGS

Dyscephaly, small stature, dental anomalies, and hypotrichosis occur in 80% to 100% of affected individuals. Final adult height is usually 2 to 5 standard deviations below the mean.[85] Prematurity is noted in about one-third of affected individuals, with normal birth weight in two thirds of cases.[22] The face is small, with a pointed, thin, pinched nose. The mandible is hypoplas-

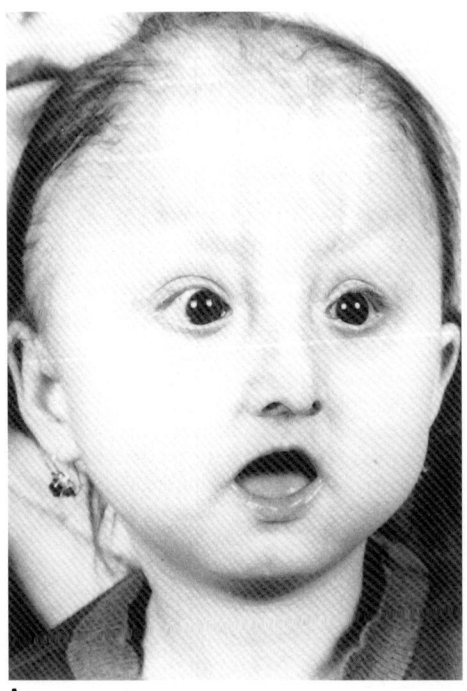

A

FIGURE 4-14A,B. Hallermann–Streiff syndrome: characteristic findings of alopecia, small pinched nose, small stature, hypoplastic mandible. **(A)** Frontal view. **(B)** Side view.

tic, with displacement of the temporomandibular joint (Fig. 4-14). A double chin with a central cleft and high-arched palate is noted in all cases, and absent teeth and malocclusion are common. Mental retardation has been reported in about 15% to 33% of cases.[22,85]

The typical finding of alopecia may be missed if the patient is wearing a wig. Occasionally, the thickness of the hair is normal but the hair structure is abnormal.[82] Cutaneous atrophy is present in most cases. Cohen[34] warned of the potential complications related to the narrow upper airway for anesthesia and sedation.[209] Snoring and/or daytime hypersomnolence are indications for sleep studies. Robinow[200] also emphasized the risks

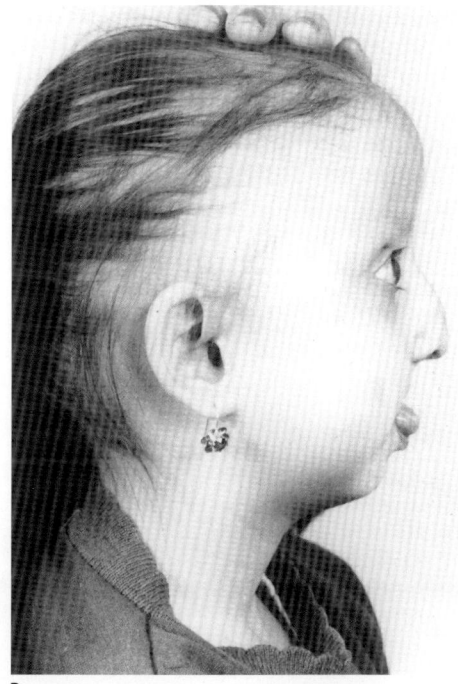

B

FIGURE 4-14B. (continued).

of problems with upper airway obstruction in HSS, particularly in the neonatal period and in infancy. Obstruction may result from small nares and glossoptosis secondary to micrognathia and these may lead to cor pulmonale. Other low-incidence anomalies have also been reported.

OCULAR FINDINGS

Although Hallermann–Streiff syndrome is rare, most affected individuals require ophthalmologic care throughout their lives because of the severity and frequency of ocular findings, the most common of which is congenital cataracts, occurring in 80% to 90% of cases.[22] One unusual characteristic of these cataracts is that they often spontaneously resorb.[14,187,259] Microphthalmia is also a common finding (78%–83%). Nystagmus and strabismus are frequently seen as would be expected, many times secondary to ocular defects. Visual acuity is frequently reduced because of the ocular malformation, but glaucoma may be primary or secondary.[108] Other ocular conditions reported in more than 10% of cases are uveitis, blue sclera, sparse eyebrows and eyelashes, fundus anomalies, downslanted palpebral fissures, iris atrophy, and congenital and corneal anomalies.[12] Many other anomalies have been noted with low frequency.[210]

PATHOGENESIS

The pathophysiology of Hallermann–Streiff syndrome is unknown. François[74] demonstrated connective tissue changes in elastin and postulated a primary disturbance in the metabolism of glycoproteins.

GENETICS

Almost all cases are sporadic, making the risk of recurrence very low. There are a few exceptions in the literature, such as occasional reports of an associated chromosomal anomaly[28] and a few atypical cases with familial involvement.[123] Some authors argue for autosomal dominant transmission with de novo mutation.[22] Cohen[34] gave a long review in which he pointed out that all cases have been sporadic; that the disorder has been both concordant and discordant in monozygotic twins; and that an affected female with two normal children was reported by Ponte.[187] Cohen stated: "I cannot accept any of the familial cases recorded to date."

ROLE OF THE OPHTHALMOLOGIST

Ophthalmologic consultation should be obtained immediately after diagnosis, and these patients should be monitored for the rest of their lives.[206] If the cataracts are advanced, early surgery may be indicated, followed by appropriate optical correction and amblyopia therapy, if indicated. Because the eyes are microphthalmic and surgery is frequently performed when patients are young, early insertion of intraocular lenses would be very risky. The frequency of secondary or primary glaucoma necessitates close monitoring of intraocular pressure. Other ocular findings (e.g., strabismus, uveitis, and nystagmus) should be treated as usual.

MÖBIUS SEQUENCE

Möbius syndrome/sequence is known to ophthalmologists because of the apparent combination of facial palsy (seventh nerve) and abducens palsy (sixth nerve) with or without limb or other systemic anomalies. This description, although frequently found in textbooks, oversimplifies the ocular motility findings and implies a well-defined syndrome, which is not the case.

The association of cranial nerve palsies with craniofacial and limb malformations is well recognized in the literature, occurring in a number of syndromes, although the differentiation between many of these syndromes is not distinct. Recognizing the overlapping of these entities, Hall[96] grouped them under the collective heading of "oromandibular limb hypogenesis syndromes" (OMLH), and included Möbius syndrome and other conditions Observed limb anomalies range from mild changes, such as syndactyly of digits, to amputation defects of the limb.[85,204] Because the proximal limb structures are characteristically normal or near normal, Temtamy and McKusick[231] referred to this group of syndromes as "terminal transverse defects with orofacial malformations" (TTV-OFM). The term sequence is preferred because multiple etiologies appear to cause the embryologic developmental error.

SYSTEMIC ANOMALIES

The severity of limb deformities, especially involving the feet, are believed by some[231] to be somewhat specific. The craniofacial anomalies vary greatly and include micrognathia, tongue malformations, facial and oral clefts, oligodontia, and paresis of other cranial nerves. Cranial nerve palsies may occur in any of these entities but become the distinguishing criteria for Möbius sequence (Fig. 4-15). Although the associations of restricted horizontal movements of the eye and facial nerve palsy had been noted in the late 1800s, Möbius[164,165] created a separate diagnostic entity, which ultimately bore his name.

Facial nerve paresis and abduction deficiency are usually bilateral, but unilateral involvement has also been reported. Asymmetry, especially of the facial nerve paresis, is often noted. Systemic findings are common, and it is the patients with severe systemic findings and cranial nerve palsies in whom syndrome delineation is confusing and frequently somewhat arbitrary. Deficiency of the sternal head of the pectoralis major muscle

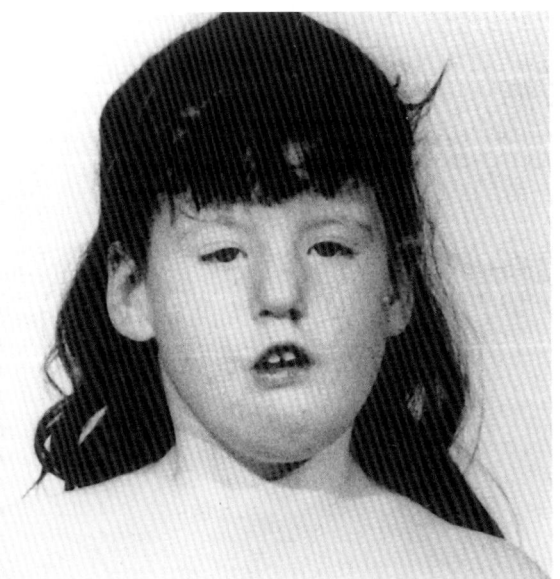

FIGURE 4-15. Möbius syndrome: note masklike facies. Patient also has marked limitation of abduction and Poland syndrome (deficiency in sternal head of pectoralis major plus ipsilateral hand anomaly).

(Poland anomaly), at times associated with an ipsilateral hand deformity (Poland syndrome), is another interesting malformation that has been reported in a number of cases but most frequently occurs in patients with Möbius-like syndromes.

Autosomal spectrum disorder (ASD) was reported previously by Gillberg and Steffenburg[79] and has been reaffirmed in a multidiscipline study.[112,162].

OCULAR FINDINGS

Sixth nerve paresis is the classic description of the major strabismus finding in Möbius sequence, but a closer look at the motility description in many patients shows variable horizontal limitations of movement with occasional vertical involvement.

Miller et al.[161] and Miller and Strömland[162] described various patterns of strabismus. (1) Bilateral limitation of abduction with no observable fissure change or significant limitation of adduction. This type represents the patients with classic Möbius syndrome described in the literature. Esotropia may be present in the primary position. (2) Bilateral marked limitation of both abduction and adduction. These patients appear to have a horizontal gaze paresis, and a subset of patients will demonstrate greater adduction on convergence than on horizontal versions.[104,162,220] There may be no ocular motility deviation in the primary position. Changes in fissures are difficult to assess due to limited horizontal movement. A number of patients described in the literature as having a sixth nerve palsy and partial third nerve palsy with normal vertical movements seem to fit better in this group of apparent gaze palsy patterns, because a partial third nerve palsy involving only the medial recti seems improbable. (3) Bilateral limitation of abduction, limitation of adduction, and retraction on adduction (Duane type). The clinical ocular motility pattern of a few patients clearly resembled that of a typical patient designated as having Duane's syndrome. (4) Asymmetrical or unilateral ocular motility disturbances. This pattern was noted in a very small number of cases in the literature. (5) Both horizontal and significant vertical limitation of movement. This finding was also uncommon. The motility disturbances were frequently bizarre and asymmetrical, resembling more of a congenital fibrosis pattern than cranial nerve palsies, although some cases in the literature are mentioned as demonstrating involvement of both third and sixth cranial nerves.[220,258] A few patients have been described in the literature as showing complete ophthalmoplegia, and they may be similar to our group number 5.[134] Other ocular malformations are rare, although coloboma, heterochromia cyclitis, and nystagmus have been reported.[49,77,110,231]

PATHOGENESIS

Most cases of Möbius sequence have no known cause, although two known teratogens (misoprostol, thalidomide) have been associated with some cases. One concept[101,231] is that these conditions fall into a formal genesis syndrome, "i.e., syndromes that have similar mechanisms of production of anomalies but are etiologically heterogeneous."[178]

Vascular disruption has been proposed as another mechanism for the production of the constellation of malformations seen in the Möbius sequence.[16,55,139] The cause of these vascular interruptions may be multiple: environmental, genetic, or local accidents in development, but the final result is ischemia, edema, and hypoxia to the embryonic tissues or cranial nerve nuclei supplied by that vessel. Hyperthermia has been implicated in a few cases.[81] The vascular disruption theory has been strengthened by some of the pathological findings at autopsy[234,257] and on imaging studies.[129,260] There is some evidence that there is a zone of vulnerability in the developing brainstem.[136]

Abbott et al.[1] reported eight cases of Möbius syndrome with a marked decrease of horizontal saccades with limited abduction and adduction. Abnormal innervation has occasionally been suggested as a possible etiology for this set of clinical findings.[103,161]

The use of the abortifacient drug misoprostol in early pregnancy has been associated with children having characteristics of Möbius sequence when abortion attempt has been unsuccessful after an attempted self-induced abortion.[70,83,84]

GENETICS

Although instances of occasional families showing autosomal recessive or dominant inheritance have been described, many of these families may represent other entities. Most cases of Möbius syndrome appear to occur sporadically.[85] Unless a positive family history exists, the recurrence risk has been estimated by Baraitser[10] to be about 2%. To date, three Möbius syndrome loci have been mapped: MSB1 to 13q12.2–q13, MSB2 to 3q21–q22, and MSB3 to 10q21.3–q22.1. Therefore, in familial cases, linkage studies are possible.[127,216,242,261]

ROLE OF THE OPHTHALMOLOGIST

The ophthalmologic symptoms are primarily related to strabismus and occasionally to corneal exposure due to the seventh nerve paresis. Because these patients have multiple systemic problems, they should not be on the same therapeutic timetable as the child with typical comitant congenital esotropia without other malformations. Epicanthus and facial configuration may accentuate a relatively small-angle squint. The esotropia may improve with age. Patients with marked limitation of abduction and adduction frequently have little deviation in the primary position of gaze, thus requiring no surgical intervention for strabismus. Further weakening of the medial recti (if there is associated limitation of adduction) should be approached with caution. If a large esotropia exists in the primary position, medial rectus recessions and recess-resect surgeries have reportedly improved the cosmetic appearance in the primary position in some patients.[1,202]

WILDERVANCK SYNDROME (CERVICO-OCULO-ACOUSTIC SYNDROME)

Wildervanck[255] noted the combination of hearing loss, Klippel–Feil deformity, and an eye motility disturbance (Duane's retraction syndrome) in a case report. He further described the triad in 1960 in a group of 21 patients and called this combination of findings the *cervico-oculo-acoustic syndrome*.[254]

SYSTEMIC FINDINGS

The first characteristic of the triad noted in Wildervanck syndrome is hearing loss, usually secondary to a congenital inner ear anomaly, although mixed forms have been described.[50] Regular and computed tomography of otologic structures have demonstrated frequent abnormalities of the middle ear structures and semicircular canals.[66,212,256] The hearing loss is primarily bilateral, but unilateral cases occur.[66]

The secondary characteristic of the triad is Klippel–Feil anomaly of the spine consisting of fusion of one or more cervical (occasionally thoracic) vertebrae, resulting in a short webbed neck (Fig. 4-16). Movement is restricted in all directions. Other spinal anomalies have also been described.[56,75] There may be asymmetry of the face and other low-incidence anomalies.[75] This syndrome (at least profound childhood deafness and Klippel–Feil malformation) may be responsible for at least 1% of deafness among females.

OCULAR FINDINGS

The third characteristic of the triad is Duane's syndrome, either bilateral or unilateral, with a spectrum of horizontal limitation patterns.[154,196]

Epibulbar dermoids have been noted in a number of cases[121] and low-incidence anomalies such as subluxation of lens[223] and pseudopapilledema[120] have been reported. Paradoxical lacrimation, Klippel–Feil anomaly, and Duane's syndrome have been reported together.[25]

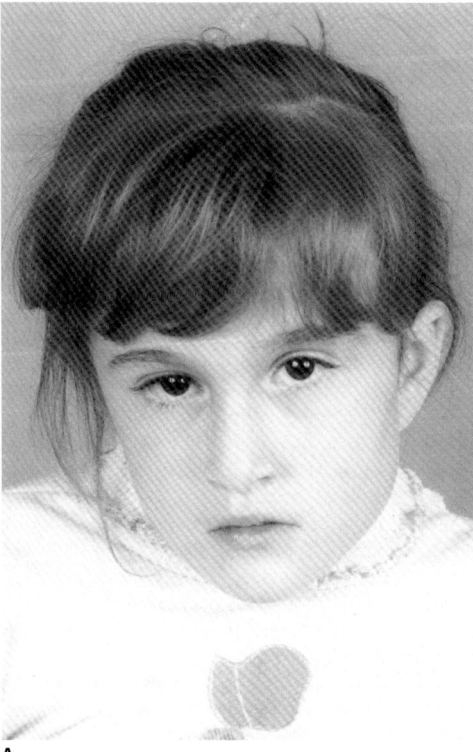

A

FIGURE 4-16A,B. Wildervanck syndrome: patient has short, webbed neck due to Klippel–Feil anomaly of spine. Additionally, she has a bilateral neurosensory deafness and unilateral Duane syndrome. **(A)** Frontal view. **(B)** Side view.

PATHOGENESIS

The developmental defect causing Wildervanck syndrome is unknown. Although this syndrome has certain distinct characteristics (female preponderance, familial pattern), there is considerable overlap with other conditions. In the Fraser and MacGillivray[75] review of the literature, dermoids were noted in four cases. The authors concluded that intermediate forms exist between cervico-oculo-acoustic syndrome and other first-arch

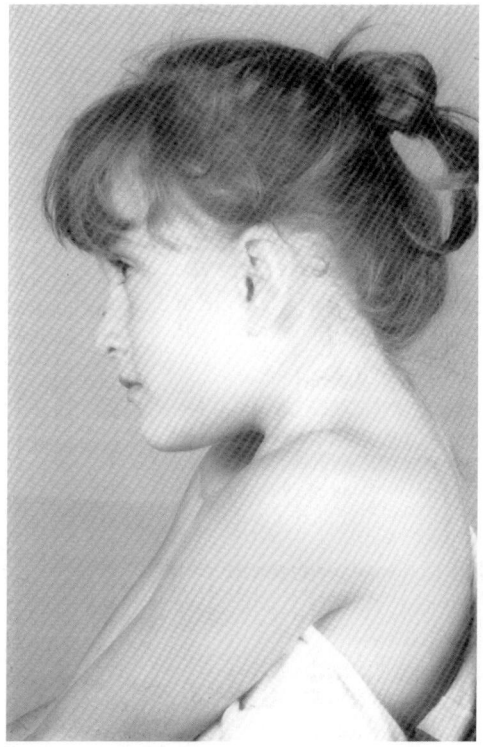

B

FIGURE 4-16B. (continued).

conditions such as Goldenhar's syndrome. However, the familial pattern and strong preponderance of females in Wildervanck syndrome are significantly different findings from those of hemifacial microsomia.

The early effects of *thalidomide* intake (days 21 to 25 of gestation) produce a high incidence of Duane's syndrome with external or internal ear anomalies, paradoxical lacrimation, facial nerve palsy, and a few lipodermoids; all findings are reported also in Wildervanck syndrome, which suggests that the timing of the developmental insult is an important factor in producing this group of malformations.[155] In thalidomide embryopathy, spinal anomalies are not as prominent as in Wildervanck and Goldenhar syndromes.

GENETICS

Genetic counseling is difficult because of the confusion about the inheritance pattern. Although the frequency of the isolated forms of Duane's syndrome is higher in females (60%–70%), there is an almost complete predominance of females in Wildervanck syndrome, leading some authors to suggest an X-linked dominant inheritance with lethality in males. Often patients manifest only part of the syndrome, and Kirkham[122] postulated autosomal dominant inheritance with incomplete penetrance and variable expressivity with partial sex limitation. He reviewed 112 cases of Duane syndrome and noted 12 cases with perceptive deafness, 5 with Klippel–Feil anomaly, and only 2 with the complete triad. Wildervanck[255] also observed variable expressivity of this syndrome and suggested that only two characteristics of the triad are needed to make the diagnosis. Interestingly, 1 patient in his original report had epibulbar dermoids. Wildervanck, in an extensive 1978 review of the subject, concluded that polygenic inheritance with limitation to females is most likely.[254]

WAARDENBURG SYNDROME (KLEIN–WAARDENBURG SYNDROME)

A detailed description was given by Waardenburg[245] of a previously described syndrome characterized by developmental anomalies of the eyelids, nasal root, and eyebrows, along with other findings of heterochromia iridis, white forelock, and sensorineural deafness. On the basis of clinical and genetic criteria, four types of Waardenburg syndrome are recognized. The primary differentiating aspect is the presence (type I) or absence (type II) of the lateral displacement of the medial canthus and lacrimal puncta.[7] Waardenburg syndrome type III (Klein–Waardenburg) is similar to type I, but is also characterized by musculoskelatal anomalies (an ortho-osteomyomo dysplasia of the upper limbs, or with abnormalities of the arms). Waardenburg type IV (Shah–Waardenburg syndrome) is the association of Waardenburg syndrome with congenital aganglionic megacolon (Hirschsprung disease).[65]

SYSTEMIC FINDINGS

The white forelock is present in 30% to 40% of patients[85] but may disappear with age or affect only a few hairs (see Fig. 4-9). It may be evident at birth, or soon afterward, or develop later. Young patients frequently dye the white hair, so a specific question must be asked. Premature graying in less than 10% or other pigmentation and changes of hair, lashes, or eyebrows have been noted. The nasal root is broad and may be associated with hypoplastic alar cartilage.[85]

An important characteristic is the sensorineural deafness, reported to occur more frequently in type II (75% of cases),[93] which has been shown to manifest malformations of the organ of Corti and other inner ear structures.[92,194] There are different combinations of hearing loss: unilateral or bilateral, severe or moderate, and total or partial.

OCULAR FINDINGS

Telecanthus (increased distance between medial canthi), usually with further displacement of lacrimal puncta, is the most striking adnexal finding in type I. Although the illusion of hypertelorism occurs in many patients, a true increase between the orbits exist in about 10%.[182] Synophrys is frequent in both types but more so in type I.

Partial or complete heterochromia of one or both irides is seen in both types. The fundi may be albinotic.[56,80] Strabismus has been noted in 10% of cases.[56] Low-incidence anomalies include cataract, microphthalmia, and ptosis.[80,85] Other ocular anomalies (e.g., cataracts, microphthalmia) have been reported occasionally.

GENETICS

Waardenburg syndrome is both a clinically and genetically heterogeneous disorder.[85,195] It follows autosomal dominant inheritance for most, if not all, cases of type I, II and III, and is autosomal recessive for type IV, with variable penetrance and phenotypic expression of different clinical features. All four types show marked variability, even within families.[195] Waardenburg syndrome type I is caused by "loss of function" mutations in the PAX3 gene on chromosome 2q37. PAX3 is a transcription factor expressed during embryonic development. Recently, 11 mutational changes in the PAX3 gene were identified in patients with Waardenburg syndrome type I. Waardenburg syndrome type II is a genetically heterogeneous disorder, with about 15% of cases heterozygous for mutations in the microphthalmia-associated transcription factor (MITF) gene on 3p12, the human homologue of the mouse microphthalmia (mi) gene.[173] Mutations in the PAX3 gene are associated not only with Waardenburg syndrome type I but also with type III.[109] However, in type III, some but not all patients are homozygotes, whereas in type II they are heterozygotes. Type IV is caused by mutations in the genes for endothelin-3 (EDN3)[65] or one of its receptors, endothelin beta-receptor (EDNRB) on chromosome 13.[65,191] EDNRB mutations are dosage sensitive; heterozygosity predisposes to isolated Hirschprung disease with incomplete penetrance, whereas homozygosity results in more complex neurocristopathies associating with congenital aganglionic megalocolon and Waardenburg syndrome features.

Families with type IV have been found to have mutations in SOX10 that are likely to result in haploinsufficiency of the SOX10 product.[128,186] MITF transactivates the gene for tyrosinase, a key enzyme for melanogenesis, and is critically involved in melanocyte differentiation. Absence of melanocytes affects pigmentation in the skin, hair, and eyes and hearing function in the cochlea. Therefore, hypopigmentation and hearing loss in Waardenburg syndrome type II are likely to be the results of an anomaly of melanocyte differentiation caused by MITF mutations. The molecular mechanism by which PAX3 mutations cause the auditory-pigmentary symptoms in type I and type III awaited explanation until Watanabe provided evidence that PAX3 directly regulates MITF. He suggested that the failure of this regulation due to PAX3 mutations causes the auditory-pigmentary symptoms in at least some individuals with type I.[250] Because all these forms show marked variability even within families, at present it is not possible to predict severity, even when a mutation is detected. Clinical molecular testing, which entails direct DNA testing of PAX3, is available for Waardenburg type I, whereas only research studies are available for type II. Prenatal diagnosis by CVS or amniocentesis is possible when a specific mutation is known in advance. In the absence of molecular investigations, careful canthal and punctal measurements will help in the diagnosis. Family members may show different manifestations of the syndrome.

ROLE OF THE OPHTHALMOLOGIST

The management of Waardenburg syndrome consists of early detection and treatment of deafness and significant ocular anomalies. Intelligence of patients is normal, and lifespan is unaffected except possibly for type IV. At present there are diagnostic molecular tests for type I and research tests for type II; therefore, the diagnosis remains, for the most part, a clinical one in which careful canthal and punctal measurements will help in the diagnosis. Family members may show different manifestations of the syndrome.

CHARGE ASSOCIATION

An association is a nonrandom collection of malformations that are not recognized as a clearly defined syndrome but that occur together more frequently than would be expected by chance. A number of chromosomal anomalies have been reported in patients manifesting many of the characteristic findings of CHARGE association; this makes the terminology confusing, and perhaps these cases should be referred to as CHARGE syndrome. Hall[94] and Hittner et al.[106] had noted certain malformations that seemed to occur together. In 1981, Pagon et al.[180] suggested the mnemonic CHARGE to designate a certain heterogeneous group of anomalies (coloboma; heart defects; choanal atresia; retarded growth; development or central nervous anomalies; genital hypoplasia; and ear malformations or deafness) that may result from abnormal migration or interaction of cephalic neural crest cells.[214,248]

Ascertainment bias will affect the percentage of each anomaly in any series, but colobomas is one of the more common findings, perhaps because it is often one of the most conspicuous malformations and is noted early in infancy. Colobomas has been reported to occur in a high percentage (75%–95%) of cases in many series. The presence of three or four characteristics (CHARGE) in a patient with no other recognizable syndrome suggests the CHARGE association. Consideration of this diagnosis will remind the physician to carefully evaluate other systems.

SYSTEMIC FINDINGS

The most common systemic findings are heart defects (85%) (septal and other types), choanal atresia (79%) (unilateral or bilateral), retarded development or central nervous system anomalies (100%) (e.g., mental retardation, encephaly, microcephaly, and other structural abnormalities), genital hypoplasia (34%) (usually in boys), and ear anomalies (91%) (small or malformed external ears or sensorineural deafness) (62%). Many other systemic anomalies have also been reported, including microphthalmia, cleft palate, facial palsy, and swallowing difficulties.[85,180] Autism has been noted in a few cases[69] (Miller and Strömland, personal observation).

OCULAR FINDINGS

The typical colobomas may involve the iris, choroid, or optic nerve, and may be asymmetrical or unilateral, and associated with varying degrees of microphthalmia.[29,106,207] High myopia or hyperopic refractive errors and nerve palsies have been noted.[106] Strabismus, nystagmus, and amblyopia may be associated findings, possibly often secondary to asymmetry of involvement, although it is possible in cases of strabismus and nystagmus that the etiology may be central nervous system pathological changes.

GENETICS

Most cases are sporadic, but affected families have been described with suggested autosomal dominant or recessive modes of inheritance.[53,85,106,180] Chromosomal anomalies have also been described multiple times, but no consistent locus has emerged. Recurrence risk is low. In a review of 47 cases, Tellier et al.[230] noted a significantly higher mean paternal age at conception, which, together with concordance in monozygotic twins and the existence of rare familial cases, supported the role of genetic factors such as de novo dominant mutation or subtle submicroscopic deletion or chromosome rearrangement.

DEFORMATION SYNDROMES

Congenital deformations resulting from intrauterine restraint are common, usually disappear, and rarely have long-term consequences. They occur in about 2% of infants and may involve craniofacial structures. Congenital torticollis is one of the possible resultant deformations with an ophthalmologic implication, as it may suggest congenital superior oblique muscle palsy.

Torticollis may result from plagiocephaly with mechanical effects on ocular motility (described earlier). Occasionally, fetal head constraint may cause craniosynostosis, particularly of sagittal, corneal, or metopic sutures.[85]

Deformations due to an abnormal uterine environment (e.g., breech or restricted area with a twin) may not cause significant increase in subsequent pregnancies unless the underlying problem continues. Deformational plagiocephaly is frequently a late gestational or postnatal deformity, but the important differential diagnosis is craniosynostosis because the treatment of these different etiologies is important.

DISRUPTION SYNDROMES

Disruptions are breakdowns or interference in an originally normal development. One cause of disruption anomalies could be disturbance of the vascular supply of the embryo in an area destined to form craniofacial sutures. Another cause is aberrant bands from premature amniotic rupture (see following).

RECURRENCE RISK

The recurrence risk for disruption-type anomalies is low because most are chance occurrences.

AMNIOTIC BAND SYNDROME (AMNIOTIC RUPTURE SEQUENCE, ADAM COMPLEX, STREETER BANDS)

Premature amniotic rupture of the sac, resulting in amniotic bands, may produce deformities, disruptions (breakdown in normal development), and malformations.[81,153,179,235] These aberrant bands can produce severely malformed structures.

The collection of fetal malformations resulting from the entanglement or attachment of amniotic remnants following rupture of the amniotic sac is referred to as the amniotic band syndrome (ABS), among other names (listed in heading). The diagnosis is frequently difficult to make because of the wide spectrum of potential deformities that might be produced depending on the number and location of the bands and the timing of their formation.

Amniotic bands have been noted in 2% of malformed infants, and are estimated to occur at a frequency of 1 in 10,000 live births,[8] but may be more common in abortuses.[85] With few exceptions of possible familial occurrence and relation to amniocentesis, most cases appear to be sporadic and thus recurrence risk is very low. The sex distribution is usually equal, although male predominance has been reported. Amniotic bands have been proposed to be an occasional cause of isolated lid and ocular defects, but this relationship is difficult to establish unless other characteristic systemic anomalies are also present or if actual bands are visible at the time of birth (a rare occurrence).

Modern techniques in ultrasonography and the subsequent utilization of this procedure in many pregnancies have resulted in reports of intraamniotic membranes in a number of patients, even though the procedure was performed for routine indications in cases with no identifiable risk factors. Some infants were found to have malformations consistent with amniotic band syndrome at the time of birth, but other infants with these unusual sonographic findings were found to be normal at birth, which has raised the question of occurrence of "innocent" amniotic bands. Herbert et al.[99] reported one case in which intraamniotic strandlike structures were observed on ultrasonography that were later found on the placenta at time of delivery.

SYSTEMIC FINDINGS

The anomalies are rarely alike in affected individuals, but there is often a pattern of malformations that include one or more of the following: (1) facial clefts that do not conform to normal embryologic patterns; (2) skull defects, including asymmetrical encephaloceles; (3) constrictive anomalies of limbs, which in their most severe forms may cause amputations; (4) umbilical cord abnormalities; (5) compression-related defects; and (6) visceral malformations. A variety of infrequent findings have also been reported in the literature.[105,153,155,179,235]

OCULAR FINDINGS

Observed ocular anomalies include lid colobomas (frequently with adjacent corneal opacities) and contiguous facial clefts, hypertelorism, palpebral fissure changes, microphthalmia or

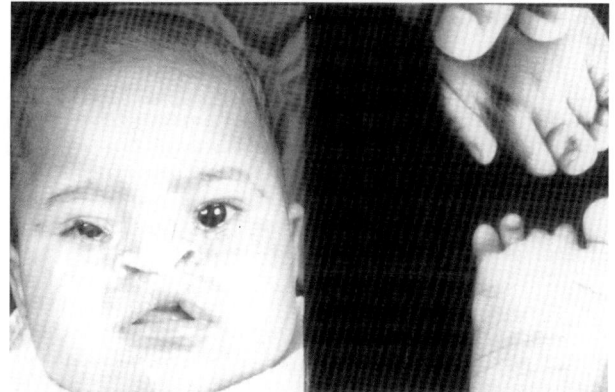

FIGURE 4-17. Amniotic band syndrome: note facial clefts and skin indentation (secondary to intrauterine bands) involving face and lids, causing secondary corneal opacity. Child has typical ring constriction and amputation anomalies of hands and feet caused by bands.

anophthalmia, and strabismus[19,24,153] (Fig. 4-17). A unilateral coloboma of the globe, perhaps the most interesting finding, has been reported occasionally.[18,156,236] A lacuna-type defect of the retina has been reported in patients with ABS.[98]

PATHOGENESIS

Malformations may result from distortion and cleavage of formed structures or interference of normal embryologic development. The cause of the eye malformation often appears to be consistent with the proposed mechanism of action of the bands. Corneal leukomas are usually located adjacent to lid defects and facial clefts. In some cases, a fissure in the skin, similar to the constriction defects in the extremities, was noted next to lid or corneal defects. When distortion is severe in the involved orbital area, microphthalmos or anophthalmia may result.

GENETICS

Some cases are possibly autosomal recessive, but for the majority the cause for amnion disruption remains unknown.

PSYCHOSOCIAL CONSIDERATIONS

Craniofacial malformations may occur alone, coupled with facial malformations, or part of a broader pattern of malformations. In any of these instances, the psychosocial impact for the family can be considerable. The birth of a dysmorphic or malformed infant often precipitates a major family crisis that can disrupt the usual pathways for parent–infant bonding. Parental reaction and adjustment depend on many factors including cultural background, social factors, attitudes, and established coping patterns.

Generally parents with malformed infants go through an identifiable sequence of complex emotional reactions, although the amount of time required to work through the problems of each stage varies. The initial period is usually one of overwhelming shock. Some parents do not react with shock, but tend to intellectualize the problem and focus on the facts relating to their infant's condition. A second stage of disbelief follows, in which most parents practice denial, the intensity of which varies considerably. Feelings of sadness and anger follow the stage of disbelief. A gradual lessening of sadness, anger, and anxiety gives way to a new stage of equilibrium in which the parents become increasingly comfortable with their situation and develop confidence in their ability to care for their infant. This new equilibrium takes a variable amount of time to reach. During the period leading up to it, parents deal with the responsibility for their child's problems and achieve an adequate adaptation. Some parents may remain in a state of chronic sorrow for a protracted period of time.

Parents attach great importance to the approach and the general attitude of family, friends, and the medical and nursing staff. Kindness, sensitivity, and empathy make deep and lasting impressions. Parents often have little or no experience with their child's diagnosis, and may feel extremely isolated, as if they are the only ones to have a child with this particular condition. It can be extremely helpful to provide the family with resources through which they can network with other families. This assistance is helpful in "demystifying" the condition, and talking to other parents helps provide emotional support in addition to offering a venue for exchange of practical information. A parent who has had to grapple with a similar circumstance can provide critical validation of another parent's feelings. Following is a list of national and international resources that typically provide networking services; disorder-specific information written for families; newsletters which address a myriad of topics including medical management issues and recent advances in medical research; and listings of local and national meetings and educational conferences, to name a few. It can be useful for families to contact one or several organizations to be placed on their mailing list, as this is an easy way for families to stay informed of any research advances or relevant studies.

- AboutFace International
  123 Edward Street, Suite 1003
  Toronto, Ontario
  M5G 1E2 Canada
  Phone: 800-665-FACE
  Email: info@aboutfaceinternational.org
  Web: *www.aboutfaceinternational.org*
- American Cleft Palate-Craniofacial Association
  104 South Estes Drive, Suite 204
  Chapel Hill, NC 27514
  Phone: 919-933-9044
  Fax: 919-933-9604
  Email: cleftline@aol.com
  Web: *www.cleftline.org*
- Australian Cranio-Facial Unit
  Women's and Children's Hospital
  72 King William Road
  North Adelaide, SA 5006
  Australia
  Phone: 61-8-82047235
  Fax: 61-8-82047080
  Email: dstone@wch.sa.gov.au
  Web: *www.wch.sa.gov.au/acfu*
- Children's Craniofacial Association
  P.O. Box 280297
  Dallas, TX 75243-4522
  Phone: 800-535-3643; 972-994-9902
  Fax: 972-240-7607
  Email: DNKM90A@prodigy.com
  Web: *www.masterlink.com/children*
- Crouzon Support Network
  P.O. Box 1272
  Edmonds, WA 98020
  Email: penny@crouzon.org
  Web: *www.crouzon.org*

- Let's Face It
  P.O. Box 29972
  Bellingham, WA 98228-1972
  Phone: 360-676-7325
  Email: letsfaceit@faceit.org
  Web: *www.faceit.org*

CONCLUSIONS

With identification of more human genes involved with various malformations or malformation syndromes, more information about DNA and protein interactions will emerge from genetic and biochemical experimentation. Additional extracellular components, such as hormones, growth factors, and cytokines that modulate skull development, will also undoubtedly be discovered, yielding a wealth of contributing factors to study.

Acknowledgments. This work was supported in part by core grant EY 1792 from the National Eye Institute, Bethesda, Maryland, by an unrestricted research grant from Research to Prevent Blindness, Inc., New York, New York, and by the Lions of Illinois Foundation, Maywood, Illinois.

References

1. Abbott RL, Metz HS, Weber AA. Saccadic velocity studies in Möbius syndrome. Ann Ophthalmol 1978;10:619–623.
2. Abel EL. Fetal alcohol syndrome in families. Neurotoxol Teratol 1988;10:1–2.
3. Abel EL, Sokol RJ. Incidence of fetal alcohol syndrome and economic impact of FAS-related anomalies. Drug Alcohol Depend 1987;19:51–70.
4. Aleksic S, Budzilovich G, Choy A, et al. Congenital ophthalmoplegia in oculoauriculovertebral dysplasia: hemifacial microsomia (Goldenhar–Gorlin syndrome). Neurology 1979;26:638–644.
5. Aleksic S, Budzilovich G, Greco MA, et al. Intracranial lipomas, hydrocephalus and other CNS anomalies in oculoauriculo-vertebral dysplasia (Goldenhar–Gorlin syndrome). Child's Brain 1984;11:285–297.
6. Aracena T, Sangueza P. Hallermann–Streiff–François syndrome. J Pediatr Ophthalmol 1977;14:373–378.
7. Arias S. Waardenburg syndrome: two distinct types. Am J Med Genet 1980;6:99–100.

8. Baker CJ, Rudolph AJ. Congenital ring constrictions and intrauterine amputations. Am J Dis Child 1971;121:393.

9. Bankier A. POSSUM (Pictures of Standard Syndromes and Undiagnosed Malformations), Murdoch Institute, Royal Children's Hospital, Melbourne, Victoria. World Wide Web: http://www.possum.net.au.

10. Baraitser M. Genetics of Möbius syndrome. J Med Genet 1977; 14:415–417.

11. Baraitser M, Winter RM. Iris coloboma, ptosis, hypertelorism and mental retardation. J Med Genet 1988;25:41–43.

12. Barrucand D, Benradi C, Schmitt J. Syndrome de François: a propos de deux cas. Rev Otoneuroophtalmol 1978;50:305–326.

13. Bartley GB. Lacrimal drainage anomalies in mandibulofacial dysostosis. Am J Ophthalmol 1990;109:571–574.

14. Basiakos H, Miller MT, Tessler H. Anterior uveitis in Hallermann–Streiff syndrome. In: Proceedings of International Ophthalmologic Congress, Amsterdam, The Netherlands. Kugler/Ghedini, 1986.

15. Baum JL, Feingold M. Ocular aspects of Goldenhar's syndrome. Am J Ophthalmol 1973;250–257.

16. Bavinck JN, Weaver DD. Subclavian artery supply disruption sequence: hypothesis of a vascular etiology for Poland, Klippel–Feil, and Möbius anomalies. Am J Med Genet 1986;23:903–918.

17. Becker MH, McCarthy JG, Chase N, et al. Computerized axial tomography of craniofacial malformations. Am J Dis Child 1976; 130:17.

18. BenEzra D, Frucht Y. Uveal coloboma associated with amniotic band syndrome. Can J Ophthalmol 1983;18:136.

19. BenEzra D, Frucht Y, Paez JH, et al. Amniotic band syndrome and strabismus. J Pediatr Ophthalmol Strabismus 1982;19:33.

20. Berry GA. Note on a congenital defect (coloboma?) of the lower lid. Ophthalmol Hosp Rep Lond 1889;12:255–257.

21. Bertelsen TI. The etiology of the premature synostosis of the cranial sutures. Acta Ophthalmol (Copenh) 1958;36(suppl 51):1–176.

22. Bitoun P, Timsit J-C, Trang H, et al. A new look at the management of the oculo-mandibulo-facial syndrome. Ophthalmic Paediatr Genet 1992;13:19–26.

23. Blank CE. Apert's syndrome, a type of acrocephalosyndactyly: observations on a British series of 39 cases. Ann Hum Genet 1960;24: 151–164.

24. Braude L, Miller MT, Cuttone J. Ocular abnormalities in the amniogenic band syndrome. Br J Ophthalmol 1981;65:299.

25. Brik M, Athayde A. Bilateral Duane's syndrome, paroxysmal lacrimation and Klippel–Feil anomaly. Ophthalmologica 1973;167:1–8.

26. Bruneteau RJ, Mulliken JB. Frontal plagiocephaly: synostotic, compensational, or deformational. Plast Reconstr Surg 1992;89:21–31.

27. Bunsic JR. The ocular aspects of Apert syndrome. Clin Plast Surg 1991;18:315–319.

28. Caspersen I, Warburg M. Hallermann–Streiff syndrome. Acta Ophthalmol (Copenh) 1968;46:385–390.

29. Chestler RJ, France TD. Ocular findings in CHARGE syndrome: six case reports and a review. Ophthalmology 1988;95:1613–1619.

30. Choy A, Margolis S, Breinin G. Ophthalmologic complications of craniofacial surgery. In: Converse JM, McCarthy JG, Wood-Smith D (eds) Symposium on diagnosis and treatment of craniofacial anomalies. St. Louis: Mosby, 1979:519.

31. Choy A, Margolis S, Breinin G, et al. Analysis of preoperative and postoperative extraocular muscle function in surgical translocation of bony orbits: a preliminary report. In: Converse JM, McCarthy JG, Wood-Smith D (eds) Symposium on diagnosis and treatment of craniofacial anomalies. St. Louis: Mosby, 1979:128–136.

32. Clarren SK, Smith DW. The fetal alcohol syndrome. N Engl J Med 1978;298:1063.

33. Clarren SK. Plagiocephaly and torticollis: etiology, natural history, and helmet treatment. J Pediatr 1981;98:92.

34. Cohen MM. Hallermann–Streiff syndrome: a review. Am J Med Genet 1991;41:488–499.

35. Cohen MM, Kreiborg S. Visceral anomalies in the Apert syndrome. Am J Med Genet 1993;45:758–760.

36. Cohen MM Jr. Holoprosencephaly and cytogenetic findings: further information. Am J Med Genet 1989;34:265.

37. Cohen MM Jr. Perspectives on holoprosencephaly. Part III. Spectra, distinctions, continuities, and discontinuities. Am J Med Genet 1989;34:271–288.

38. Cohen MM Jr. Syndromology: an updated conceptual overview. I. Syndrome concepts, designations, and population characteristic. Int J Oral Maxillofac Surg 1989;18:216–222.

39. Cohen MM Jr. Syndromology: an updated conceptual over-view. II. Syndrome classifications. Int J Oral Maxillofac Surg 1989;18:223–228.

40. Cohen MM Jr. Syndromology: an updated conceptual overview. III. Syndrome delineation. Int J Oral Maxillofac Surg 1989;18:281–285.

41. Cohen MM Jr, Richieri-Costa A, Guion-Almeida ML, et al. Hypertelorism: interorbital growth, measurements, and pathogenetic considerations. Intl J Oral Maxillofacial Surg 1995;24(6):387–395.

42. Cohen MM Jr. Apert syndrome. In: Cohen MM Jr (ed) Craniosynostosis: diagnosis, evaluation and management. Part VIII, 2nd edn. New York: Oxford Press, 2000:316.

43. Cohen MM Jr. Carpenter syndrome. In: Cohen MM Jr (ed) Craniosynostosis: diagnosis, evaluation and management. Part VIII, 2nd edn. New York: Oxford Press, 2000:377–379.

44. Cohen MM Jr. Crouzon syndrome. In: Cohen MM Jr (ed) Craniosynostosis: diagnosis, evaluation and management. Part VIII, 2nd edn. New York: Oxford Press, 2000:361–365.

45. Cohen MM Jr. Epidemiology of craniosynostosis. In: Cohen MM Jr (ed) Craniosynostosis: diagnosis, evaluation and management. Part III, 2nd edn. New York: Oxford Press, 2000:112–118.

46. Cohen MM Jr. History, terminology, and classification of craniosynostosis. In: Cohen MM Jr (ed) Craniosynostosis: diagnosis, evaluation and management. Part III, 2nd edn. New York: Oxford Press, 2000: 103–111.

47. Cohen MM Jr. Pfeiffer syndrome. In: Cohen MM Jr (ed) Craniosynostosis: diagnosis, evaluation and management. Part VIII, 2nd edn. New York: Oxford Press, 2000:354.

48. Cohen MM Jr, Rollnick BR, Kaye CI. Oculoauriculovertebral spectrum: an updated critique. Cleft Palate J 1989;26:276–286.

49. Cohen SC, Thompson JW. Varients of Möbius syndrome and central neurologic impairment. Ann Otol Rhinol Laryngol 1987;96:93–100.

50. Cremers CWRJ, Hoogland GA, Kuypers W. Hearing loss in the cervico-oculo-acoustic (Wildervanck) syndrome. Arch Otolaryngol 1984;110:54–57.

51. Cross HE, Pfaffenback DD. Duane's retraction syndrome and associated congenital malformations. Am J Ophthalmol 1972;73:442–449.

52. Cuttone JM, Brazis PT, Miller MT, et al. Absence of the superior rectus muscle in Apert's syndrome. J Pediatr Ophthalmol Strabismus 1979;16:349–354.

53. Davenport SLH, et al. The spectrum of clinical features in CHARGE syndrome. Clin Genet 1986;29:298–310.

54. David D, Poswillo D, Simpson D. The craniosynostoses: causes, natural history and management. New York: Springer-Verlag, 1982.

55. D'Cruz OF, Swisher CN, Jaradeh S, et al. Möbius syndrome: evidence for a vascular etiology. J Child Neurol 1993;8:260–265.

56. Delleman JW, Hageman MJ. Ophthalmological findings in 34 patients with Waardenburg syndrome. J Pediatr Ophthalmol 1978;15: 341–345.

57. DeMeyer W. The median cleft face syndrome: differential diagnosis of cranium bifidum occultum, hypertelorism, and median cleft nose, lip and palate. Neurology 1967;17:961–971.

58. DeMeyer WE, et al. The face predicts the brain: diagnostic significance of median facial anomalies for holoprosencephaly (arhinencephaly). Pediatrics 1964;34:256–263.

59. Diamond GR, Katowitz JA, Whitacker LA, et al. Variations in extraocular muscle number and structure in craniofacial dysostosis. Am J Ophthalmol 1980;90:415–418.

60. Diamond GR, Katowitz JA, Whitaker LH, et al. Ocular alignment after craniofacial reconstruction. Am J Ophthalmol 1980;90:248–250.

61. Dixon MJ. Treacher Collins syndrome. Hum Mol Genet 1996;XX: 1391–1396.

62. Dixon MJ, Read AP, Donnai D, et al. The gene for Treacher Collins syndrome maps to the long arm of chromosome 5. Am J Hum Genet 1991;49:17–22.

63. Donnenfeld AE, Packer RJ, Zackai EH, et al. Clinical, cytogenetic, and pedigree findings in 18 cases of Aicardi syndrome. Am J Med Genet 1989;32:461–467.

64. Dufier JL, Vinurel MC, Renier D, et al. Les complications ophthalmologiques des craniofaciostenoses. A propos de 244 observations. J Fr Ophtalmol 1986;9:273–280.

65. Edery P, Attie T, Amiel J, et al. Mutation of the endothelin-3 gene in the Waardenburg–Hirschsprung disease (Shah–Waardenburg syndrome). Nat Genet 1996;12:442–444.

66. Evenberg G, Ratjen MD, Serenson H. Wildervanck's syndrome. Klippel–Feil's syndrome associated with deafness and retraction of the eyeball. Br J Radiol 1963;36:562–567.

67. Falls HF, Schull WJ. Hallermann–Streiff syndrome: a dyscephaly with congenital cataracts and hypotrichosis. Arch Ophthalmol 1960;63: 409–420.

68. Feingold M, Gellis SS. Ocular abnormalities associated with the first and second arch syndromes. Surv Ophthalmol 1969;14:30–42.

69. Fernell E, Olsson VA, Karlgren-Leitner C, et al. Autistic disorders in children with CHARGE association. Dev Med Child Neurol 1999; 41(4):270–272.

70. Fonseca W, Alencar AJC, Mota FSB, et al. Misoprostol and congenital malformations. Lancet 1991;338:56.

71. Franceschetti A, Klein D. Mandibulo-facial dysostosis: new hereditary syndrome. Acta Ophthalmol (Kbh) 1949;27:143–224.

72. François J. François' dyscephalic syndrome. Birth Defects Orig Artic Ser 1982;18(6):595–619.

73. François J, Eggermont E, Evens L, et al. Agenesis of the corpus callosum in the median facial cleft syndrome and associated ocular malformations. Am J Ophthalmol 1973;76:241–245.

74. François MJ. A new syndrome: dyscephalia with bird face and dental anomalies, nanism, hypotrichosis, cutaneous atrophy, microphthalmia and congenital cataract. Arch Ophthalmol 1960;60:842–862.

75. Fraser WI, MacGillivray RC. Cervico-oculo-acoustic dysplasia (the "syndrome of Wildervanck"). J Ment Defic Res 1968;12:322–329.

76. Fryburg JS, Persing JA, Lin KY. Frontonasal dysplasia in two successive generations. Am J Med Genet 1993;46:712–714.

77. Gadoth N, Beidner B, Torok G. Möbius syndrome and Poland anomaly: case report and review of the literature. J Pediatr Ophthalmol Strabismus 1979;16:374–376.

78. Garber JM. Steep corneal curvature: a fetal alcohol syndrome landmark. J Am Optom Assoc 1984;55:595–598.

79. Gillberg C, Steffenburg S. Autistic behaviour in Moebius syndrome. Acta Paediatr 1989;79:314–26.

80. Goldberg MJ. Waardenburg's syndrome with fundus and other anomalies. Arch Ophthalmol 1966;76:797–810.

81. Goldstein F, Arulananthan K. Neural tube defects and renal anomalies in a child with fetal alcohol syndrome. J Pediatr 1978;93:636–637.

82. Golomb RS, Porter PS. A distinct hair shaft abnormality in the Hallermann–Streiff syndrome. Cutis 1975;16:122–128.
83. Gonzalez CH, Marques-Dias MJ, Kim CA, et al. Congenital abnormalities in Brazilian children associated with misoprostol misuse in first trimester of pregnancy. Lancet 1998;351(9116):1624–1627.
84. Gonzalez CH, Vargas FR, Perez AB, et al. Limb deficiency with or without Möbius sequence in seven Brazilian children associated with misoprostol use in the first trimester of pregnancy. Am J Med Genet 1993;47(1):59–64.
85. Gorlin RG, Cohen MM, Hennekam RCM (eds). Syndromes of the head and neck, 4th edn. New York: Oxford University Press, 2001.
86. Grabb WC. The first and second branchial arch syndrome. Plast Reconstr Surg 1965;36:485–508.
87. Graham JM, Edwards MJ, Lipson AH, et al. Gestational hyperthermia as a cause for Möbius syndrome. Teratology 1988;37:461.
88. Graham JM, Hanson JW, Dabry BL, et al. Independent dysmorphology evaluations at birth and 4 years of age for children exposed to varying amounts of alcohol in utero. Pediatrics 1988;81(6):772–778.
89. Greenwood Genetics Center. Growth references from conception to adulthood. Proc Green Genet Ctr 1988;1.
90. Gripp W, McDonald-McGinn DM, Gaudenz K, et al. Identification of a genetic cause for isolated unilateral coronal synostosis: a unique mutation in the fibroblast growth factor receptor 3. J Pediatr 132(4):714–716.
91. Gupta S, Supriyo G, Mridula R, et al. The optic nerve in children with craniosynostosis. Doc Ophthalmol 1993;(83):271–278.
92. Hageman MJ. Audiometric findings in 34 patients with Waardenburg syndrome. J Laryngol Otolaryngol 1977;91:575–584.
93. Hageman MJ, Delleman JW. Heterogeneity in Waardenburg syndrome. Am J Hum Genet 1977;29:468–485.
94. Hall B. Choanal atresia and associated multiple anomalies. J Pediatr 1979;95:395–398.
95. Hall JG, Foster-Iskenius UG, Allanson JE (eds). Handbook of normal physical measurements. New York: Oxford, 1989.
96. Hall BD. Aglossia-adactylia. Birth Defects 1971;7:233–236.
97. Hanson JW, Streissguth AP, Smith DW. The effects of moderate alcohol consumption during pregnancy on fetal growth and morphogenesis. J Pediatr 1978;92:457–460.
98. Hashemi K, Traboulsi EI, Chavis R, et al. Chorioretinal lacuna in the amniotic band syndrome. J Pediatr Ophthalmol Strabismus 1991;28:238–239.
99. Herbert WNP, Seeds JW, Cefalo RC, et al. Prenatal detection of intraamniotic bands: implications and management. Obstet Gynecol 1985;65(suppl 3):36S.
100. Herrmann J, Opitz JM. Naming and nomenclature of syndrome. Birth Defects 1974;10:69–86.

101. Herrmann J, Pallister PD, Gilbert EF, et al. Studies of malformation syndromes of man, XXXXIB: nosologic studies in the Hanhart and Möbius syndrome. Eur J Pediatr 1976;122:19–55.

102. Hertle RW, Quinn GE, Katowitz JA. Ocular and adnexal findings in patients with facial microsomias. Ophthalmology 1992;99:114–119.

103. Hickey WF, Wagner MD. Bilateral congenital absence of abducens nerve. Virchows Arch 1983;402:91–98.

104. Hicks AM. Congenital paralysis of lateral rotators of eyes with paralysis of muscles of face. Arch Ophthalmol 1943;30:38–42.

105. Higginbottom MD, Jones KL, Hall BD, et al. The amnion band disruption complex: timing of amnion rupture and variable spectra of consequent defects. J Pediatr 1979;95:544.

106. Hittner HM, Hirsch NJ, Kreh GM, et al. Colobomatous microphthalmus, heart disease, hearing loss and mental retardation. J Pediatr Ophthalmol Strabismus 1979;16:122–128.

107. Hoffman WY, McCarthy JG, Cutting CB, et al. Computerized tomographic analysis of orbital hypertelorism repair: spatial relationship of the globe and the bony orbit. Ann Plast Surg 1990;25(2):124–131.

108. Hopkins DJ, Horan EC. Glaucoma in the Hallermann–Streiff syndrome. Br J Ophthalmol 1970;54:416–422.

109. Hoth CF, Milunsky A, Lipsky N, et al. Mutations in the paired domain of the human PAX3 gene cause Klein–Waardenburg syndrome (WS-III) as well as Waardenburg syndrome type I (WS-I). Am J Hum Genet 1993;52:455–462.

110. Huber A, Kraus-Mackiw E. Heterochromiezyklitis Fuchs bei Möbius-syndrome. Klin Monatsbl Augenheilkd 1981;178:182–185.

111. Jabs EW, Li X, Coss CA, et al. Mapping the Treacher Collins syndrome locus to 5Q31.35–q33.3. Genomics 1991;11:193–198.

112. Johansson M, Wentz E, Fernell E, et al. Autism spectrum disorders in Möbius sequence: a comprehensive study of 25 individuals. Dev Med Child Neurol 2001;43:338–345.

113. Jones KL. Smith's recognizable pattern of human malformations, 4th edn. Philadelphia: Saunders, 1997.

114. Jones KL, Smith DW. Recognition of the fetal alcohol syndrome in early infancy. Lancet 1973;1:999.

115. Jones KL, Smith DW, Harvey MAS, et al. Older paternal age and fresh gene mutations: data on additional disorders. J Pediatr 1976;86:84–88.

116. Jones KL, Smith DW, Ullehand CN, et al. Pattern of malformation in offspring of chronic alcoholic mothers. Lancet 1973;1:1267.

117. Kaye CI, Martin AO, Rollnick BR, et al. Oculoauriculovertebral anomaly: segregation analysis. Am J Med Genet 1992;43:913–917.

118. Kinsey JA, Streeten BW. Ocular abnormalities in the median cleft face syndrome. Am J Ophthalmol 1977;83:261–266.

119. Kinsman SL, Plawner LL, Hahn JS. Holoprosencephaly: recent advances and new insights. Curr Opin Neurol 2000;13(2):127–132.

120. Kirkham TH. Cervico-oculo-acousticus syndrome with pseudopapilloedema. Arch Dis Child 1969;44:504–508.

121. Kirkham TH. Duane's syndrome and familial perceptive deafness. Br J Ophthalmol 1969;53:335–339.

122. Kirkham TH. Inheritance of Duane's syndrome. Br J Ophthalmol 1970;54:323–329.

123. Koliopoulos J, Palimeris G. Atypical Hallermann–Streiff–François syndrome in three successive generations. J Pediatr Ophthalmol 1975;12:235–239.

124. Kreiborg S. Craniofacial growth in plagiocephaly and Crouzon syndrome. Scand J Plast Reconstr Surg 1981;5:187–197.

125. Kreiborg S. Craniofacial growth in premature craniofacial synostosis. Scand J Plast Reconstr Surg 1981;15:171–184.

126. Kreiborg S. Crouzon syndrome. Scand J Plast Reconstr Surg Suppl 1981;18:1–198.

127. Kremer H, Kuyt L P, van den Helm B, et al. Localization of a gene for Moebius syndrome to chromosome 3q by linkage analysis in a Dutch family. Hum Mol Genet 1996;5:1367–1371.

128. Kuhlbrodt K, Schmidt C, Sock E, et al. Functional analysis of SOX10 mutations found in human Waardenburg–Hirschsprung patients. J Biol Chem 1998;273:23033–23038.

129. Kuhn MJ, Clark HB, Morales A, et al. Group III Möbius syndrome: CT and MR findings. AJNR 1990;11:903–904.

130. Lajeunie E, Le Merrer M, Bonaïti-Pel\u0003lie C, et al. Genetic study of nonsyndromic coronal craniosynostosis. Am J Med Genet 1995;55:500–504.

131. Lajeunie E, Le Merrer M, Bonaiti-Pelie C, et al. Genetic study of scaphocephaly. Am J Med Genet 1996;62(3):282–285.

132. Landgren M, Gillberg C, Strömland K. Goldenhar syndrome and autistic behavior. Dev Med Child Neurol 1992;34:999–1005.

133. Lees MM, Hodgkins P, Reardon W, et al. Frontonasal dysplasia with optic disc anomalies and other midline craniofacial defects: a report of six cases. Clin Dysmorphol 1998;7(3):157–162.

134. Legum C, Godel V, Nemet P. Heterogeneity and pleiotropism in the Möbius syndrome. Clin Genet 1981;20:254–259.

135. Leonard CO, Daikoku NH, Winn K. Prenatal fetoscopic diagnosis of the Apert syndrome. Am J Med Genet 1982;1:5–9.

136. Leong S, Ashwell KW. Is there a zone of vascular vulnerability in the fetal brain stem? Neurotoxicol Teratol 1997;19:265–275.

137. Lewanda AF, Meyers GA, Jabs EW. Craniosynostosis and skeletal dysplasias: fibroblast growth factor receptor defects. Proc Assoc Am Physicians 1996;1:19–24.

138. Lewanda AF, Traboulsi EI, Jabs EW. Syndromes with craniofacial anomalies. In: Traboulsi E (ed) Genetic disease of the eye. New York: Oxford University Press, 1998:777–796.

139. Lipson AH, Gillerot Y, Tannenberg AE, et al. Two cases of maternal antenatal splenic rupture and hypotension associated with Moebius syndrome and cerebral palsy in offspring. Further evidence for a utero placental vascular aetiology for the Moebius syndrome and some cases of cerebral palsy. Eur J Pediatr 1996;55(9):800–804.

140. Li X, Park W-J, Pyeritz RE, et al. Effect on splicing of a silent FGFR2 mutation in Crouzon syndrome (letter). Nat Genet 1995;9:232–233.

141. Lloyd L. Craniofacial reconstruction: ocular management of orbital hypertelorism. Trans Am Ophthalmol Soc 1975;73:123.

142. London Dysmorphology Data Base version 2.2, Oxford Medical Databases. London, Oxford University Press.

143. Lynch HT, Lemon HM, Krush AJ. A note on "cancer-susceptible" and "cancer-resistant: genotypes." Nebr State Med J 1966;51:209–211.

144. Margolis S, Aleksic J, Charles N, et al. Retinal and optic nerve findings in Goldenhar-Gorlin syndrome. Ophthalmology 1984;91:1327–1333.

145. Margolis S, Choy AE, Breinin GM. Retinal findings in Apert's syndrome and Crouzon's disease. In: Converse JM, Wood-Smith D (eds) Symposium on diagnosis and treatment of craniofacial anomalies. St. Louis: Mosby, 1979:263–268.

146. Margolis S, Packter BR, Brenin GM. Structural alterations of extraocular muscle associated with Apert's syndrome. Br J Ophthalmol 1977;61:683–689.

147. Marsh JL, Galic M, Vannier MW. The surgical correction of surgical of craniofacial dysmorphology in Apert syndrome. Clin Plast Surg 1991;18:251–275.

148. Marsh JL, Vannier MA. Three-dimensional surface imaging from CT scans for the study of craniofacial dysmorphology. J Craniofac Genet Dev Biol 1989;6:61.

149. Maxwell Online, Inc. Birth Defects Encyclopedia Online (BDEO). McLean, VI: Maxwell.

150. McDonald MT, Gorski JL. Nager acrofacial dysostosis. J Med Genet 1993;30:779–782.

151. McKusick VA. Mendelian inheritance in man. Catalogs of human genes and genetic disorders, 12th edn. Baltimore: Johns Hopkins University Press, 1998.

152. McNab AA, Wright JE, Caswell AG. Clinical features and surgical management of dermolipomas. Aust NZJ Ophthalmol 1990;18:159–162.

153. Miller ME, Graham JM, Higginbottom MC, et al. Compression-related defects from early amnion rupture: evidence of mechanical teratogenesis. J Pediatr 1981;98:292.

154. Miller MT. Association of Duane retraction syndrome with craniofacial malformations. J Craniofac Genet Dev Biol Suppl 1985;1:273–282.

155. Miller MT. Thalidomide embryopathy: a model for the study of congenital incomitant horizontal strabismus. Trans Am Ophthalmol Soc 1991;89:623–674.

156. Miller MT, Deutsch TA, Cronin C, et al. Amniotic bands as a cause of ocular anomalies. Am J Ophthalmol 1987;104:270–279.

157. Miller MT, Epstein RJ, Sugar J, et al. Anterior segment anomalies associated with the fetal alcohol syndrome. J Pediatr Ophthalmol Strabismus 1984;21:8–18.

158. Miller MT, Folk ER. Strabismus associated with craniofacial anomalies. Am Orthopt J 1975;25:27–36.

159. Miller MT, Israel J, Cuttone J. Fetal alcohol syndrome. J Pediatr Ophthalmol Strabismus 1981;18:6–15.

160. Miller MT, Pruzansky S. Craniofacial anomalies. In: Peyman GA, Sanders DR, Goldberg MF (eds) Principles and practice of ophthalmology, vol 3. Philadelphia: Saunders, 1980:2354.

161. Miller MT, Ray V, Owens P, et al. Möbius and Möbius-like syndromes (TTV-OFM, OMLH). J Pediatr Ophthalmol Strabismus 1989; 26:176–188.

162. Miller MT, Strömland K. The Möbius sequence: a relook. J Am Assoc Pediatr Ophthalmol Strabismus 1999;3:199–208.

163. Ming JE, Muenke M. Holoprosencephaly: from Homer to Hedgehog. Clin Genet 1998;53(3):155–163.

164. Möbius PJ. Uber angeborene doppelseitige Abducens-Facialis-Lahmung. MMW 1888;35:91–94.

165. Möbius PJ. Uber infantile Keinschwund. MMW 1892;39:41–55.

166. Mohandessan MM, Romano PE. Neuroparalytic keratitis in Goldenhar–Gorlin syndrome. Am J Ophthalmol 1978;85:111–113.

167. Moloney DM, Slaney SF, Oldridge M, et al. Exclusive paternal origin of new mutations in Apert syndrome. Nat Genet 1996;13(1):48–53.

168. Morax S. Changing of the eye position after craniofacial surgery. In: Caronni EP (ed) Craniofacial surgery. Boston: Little, Brown, 1985: 200–210.

169. Moreno FH. The spectrum of frontonasal dysplasia in an inbred pedigree. Clin Genet 1980;7(2):137–142.

170. Muenke M, Schell U, Hehr A, et al. A common mutation in the fibroblast growth factor reception 1 gene in Pfeiffer shndrome. Nat Genet 1994;269–274.

171. Murdoch-Kinch CA, Ward RE. Metacarpophalangeal analysis in acrocephalosyndactyly syndromes. Am J Med Genet 1997;73:61–66.

172. Naidich TP, Osborn RE, Bauer B, et al. Median cleft face syndrome: MR and CT data from 11 children. J Comput Assist Tomogr 1988;12: 57–64.

173. Nobukuni Y, Watanabe A, Takeda K, et al. Analyses of loss-of-function mutations of the MITF gene suggest that haploinsufficiency is a cause of Waardenburg syndrome type 2A. Am J Hum Genet 1996;59:76–83.

174. Nucci P, Brancato R, Carones F, et al. Mandibulofacial dysostosis and cornea guttata. Am J Ophthalmol 1989;109:204.

175. Odent S, Le Marec B, Munnich A, et al. Segregation analysis in nonsyndromic holoprosencephaly. Am J Med Genet 1998;77:139–143.

176. Online Mendelian Inheritance in Man, OMIM (TM). McKusick–Nathans Institute for Genetic Medicine, Johns Hopkins University (Baltimore, MD) and National Center for Biotechnology Information, National Library of Medicine (Bethesda, MD), 2000. World Wide Web URL: http://www.ncbi.nlm.nih.gov/omim/.

177. Opitz JM. The developmental field concept. Am J Med Genet 1985; 21:1–11.

178. Opitz JM, Herrmann J, Dieker H. The study of malformation syndromes in man. In: Harris H, Hirschern K (eds) Birth defects, vol 5. New York: Plenum, 1969:1–10.

179. Ossipoff V, Hall B. Etiologic factors in the amniotic band syndrome: a study of 24 patients. Birth Defects 1978;12:177.

180. Pagon RA, Graham JM, Zonana J, et al. Coloboma, congenital heart disease and choanal atresia with multiple anomalies: CHARGE association. J Pediatr 1981;99:223–227.

181. Pallotta R. Iris coloboma, ptosis, hypertelorism, and mental retardation: a new syndrome possibly localised on chromosome 2. J Med Genet 1991;28:342–344.

182. Pantke OA, Cohen MM Jr. The Waardenburg syndrome. Birth Defects 1971;7:147–152.

183. Park W-J, Meyers GA, Li X, et al. Novel FGFR2 mutations in Crouzon and Jackson–Weiss syndromes show allelic heterogeneity and phenotypic variability. Hum Mol Genet 1995;4:1229–1233.

184. Park WJ, Theda C, Maestri NE, et al. Analysis of phenotypic features and FGFR2 mutations in Apert syndrome. Am J Hum Genet 1995;57(2):321–328.

185. Pieroni D. Goldenhar's syndrome associated with bilateral Duane's retraction synrrome. J Pediatr Ophthalmol 1969;6:16–18.

186. Pingault V, Bondurand N, Kuhlbrodt K, et al. SOX10 mutations in patients with Waardenburg–Hirschsprung disease. Nat Genet 1998; 18:171–173.

187. Ponte F. Further contribution to the study of the syndrome of Hallermann–Streiff. Ophthalmologica 1962;143:399–408.

188. Poswillo D. The pathogenesis of the first and second branchial arch syndrome. Oral Surg 1973;35:302–309.

189. Poswillo D. The pathogenesis of Treacher Collins syndrome (mandibulofacial dysostosis). Br J Oral Surg 1975;13:1–26.

190. Pryor HB. Objective measurement of interpupillary distance. Pediatrics 1969;44:973.

191. Puffenberger EG, Hosoda K, Washington SS, et al. A missense mutation of the endothelin-B receptor gene in multigenic Hirschsprung's disease. Cell 1994;79:1257–1266.

192. Putterman AM, Pashayan H, Pruzansky S. Eye findings in the blepharo-naso-facial malformation syndrome. Am J Ophthalmol 1973; 76:825.

193. Randall CL, Ulla E, Anton RF. Perspectives on the pathophysiology of fetal alcohol syndrome. Alcohol Clin Exp Res 1990;14:807–812.

194. Rarey KE, Davis LE. Inner ear anomalies in Waardenburg's syndrome with Hirschsprung's disease. Int J Pediatr Otorhinolaryngol 1984;8: 181–189.

195. Read AP, Newton VE. Waardenburg syndrome. J Med Genet 1997;34: 656–665.

196. Regenbogen L, Godel V. Cervico-oculo-acoustic syndrome. Ophthalmic Paediatr Genet 1985;6:183–187.
197. Renier D, Arnaud E, Cinalli G, et al. Prognosis for mental function in Apert syndrome. J Neurosurg 1996;85:66–72.
198. Robb RM, Boger WP III. Vertical strabismus associated with plagiocephaly. J Pediatr Ophthalmol Strabismus 1983;20(2):58–63.
199. Robin NH, Feldman GJ, Mitchell HF, et al. Linkage of Pfeiffer syndrome to chromosome 8 centromere and evidence for genetic heterogeneity. Hum Mol Genet 1994;3:2153–2158.
200. Robinow M. Respiratory obstruction and cor pulmonale in the Hallermann–Streiff syndrome. Am J Med Genet 1991;41:515–516.
201. Robinson LK, James HI, Mubarak SJ, et al. Carpenter syndrome: natural history and clinical spectrum. Am J Med Genet 1985;20:461–469.
202. Rodrigues-Alves CA, Caldeira JAF. Möbius syndrome: a case report with multiple congenital anomalies. J Pediatr Ophthalmol 1975;12:103.
203. Rogers BO. Berry–Treacher Collins syndrome: a review of 200 cases. Br J Plast Surg 1964;17:109–137.
204. Rogers GL, Hatch GF, Gray I. Möbius syndrome and limb abnormalities. J Pediatr Ophthalmol Strabismus 1977;14:134–138.
205. Rollnick BR, Kaye CI. Hemifacial microsomia and variants: pedigree data. Am J Med Genet 1983;15:233–253.
206. Ronen S, Rozenmann Y, Isaacson M, et al. The early management of a baby with Hallermann–Streiff–François syndrome. J Pediatr Ophthalmol Strabismus 1979;6:119–121.
207. Russell-Eggitt HI, Blake K, Taylor D, et al. The eye in the CHARGE association. Br J Ophthalmol 1990;74:421–426.
208. Rutland P, Pulleyn LJ, Reardon W, et al. Identical mutations in the FGFR2 gene cause both Pfeiffer and Crouzon phenotypes. Nat Genet 1995;9:173–176.
209. Sataloff RT, Roberts BR. Airway management in Hallermann–Streiff syndrome. Am J Otolaryngol 1984;5:64–67.
210. Schanzlin DJ, Goldberg DB, Brown SI. Hallermann–Streiff syndrome associated with sclero-cornea, aniridia, and a chromosomal abnormality. Am J Ophthalmol 1980;90(3):411–415.
211. Schell U, Hehr A, Feldman GJ, et al. Mutations in FGFR1 and FGFR2 cause familial and sporadic Pfeiffer syndrome. Hum Mol Genet 1995;4(3):323–328.
212. Schild JA, Mafee MF, Miller MT. Wildervanck syndrome: the external appearance and radiologic findings. Int J Pediatr Otorhinolaryngol 1984;7:305–310.
213. Shokeir MHK. The Goldenhar syndrome: a natural history. Birth Defects Orig Artic Ser 1977;13:67–83.
214. Siebert JR, Graham JM Jr., MacDonald C, et al. Pathologic features of the CHARGE association: support for involvement of the neural crest. Teratology 1985;31:333–336.

215. Slaney SF, Oldridge M, Hurst JA, et al. Differential effects of FGFR2 mutations on syndactyly and cleft palate in Apert syndrome. Am J Hum Genet 1996;58:923–932.

216. Slee JJ, Smart RD, Viljoen DL. Deletion of chromosome 13 in Moebius syndrome. J Med Genet 1991;28:413–414.

217. Snyder DA, Swartz M, Goldberg MF. Corneal ulcers associated with Goldenhar syndrome. J Pediatr Ophthalmol 1977;14:286–290.

218. Splendore A, Silva EO, Alonso LG, et al. High mutation detection rate in TCOF1 among Treacher Collins syndrome patients reveals clustering of mutations and 16 novel pathogenic changes. Hum Mutat 2000;16:315–322.

219. Spranger J, Benirschke K, Hall JG, et al. Errors of morphogenesis: concepts and terms. J Pediatr 1982;100:160–165.

220. Sprofkin BE, Hillman IW. Möbius syndrome: congenital oculofacial paralysis. Neurology 1956;6:50–54.

221. Steele RW, Bass JW. Hallermann–Streiff syndrome: clinical and prognostic considerations. Am J Dis Child 1970;120:462–465.

222. Streissguth AP. The behavioral teratology of alcohol: performance behavioral, and intellectual deficits in prenatally exposed children. In: West J (ed) Alcohol and brain development. New York: Oxford University Press, 1986:3–44.

223. Strisciuglio P, Raia V, Di Meo A, et al. Wildervanck's syndrome with bilateral subluxation of lens and facial paralysis. J Med Genet 1983; 20:72–73.

224. Strömland K. Ocular abnormalities in the fetal alcohol syndrome. Acta Ophthalmol Graphic Systems, Goteborg, Sweden, 1985;63: suppl 171.

225. Strömland K. Ocular involvement in the fetal alcohol syndrome. Surv Ophthalmol 1987;31:277–284.

226. Sulik KK, Johnston MC. Embryonic origin of holoprosencephaly: interrelationshps of the developing brain and face. Scanning Electron Microsc 1982;1:309–322.

227. Sulik KK, Johnston MC. Sequence of developmental alterations following acute ethanol expsoure in mice: craniofacial features of the fetal alcohol syndrome. Am J Anat 1983;166:257–269.

228. Sulik KK, Smiley SJ, Turvey TA, et al. Pathogenesis of cleft palate in Treacher Collins, Nager, and Miller syndromes. Cleft Palate J 1989;26:209–216.

229. Sugar A, et al. Hallermann–Streiff–François syndrome. J Pediatr Ophthalmol 1971;8:234–238.

230. Tellier AL, Cormier-Daire V, Abadie V, et al. CHARGE syndrome: report of 47 cases and review. Am J Med Genet 1998;76(5):402–409.

231. Temtamy SA, McKusick VA. The genetics of hand malformations. Birth Defects 1978;14:73–91.

232. Tessier P. The definitive plastic surgical treatment of the severe facial deformities of craniofacial dysostosis. Crouzon's and Apert's diseases. Plast Reconstr Surg 1971;48:419–422.

233. Tessier P. Orbital hypertelorism. Scand J Plast Reconstr Surg 1972;6: 135.

234. Thakkar N, O'Neil W, Durally J, et al. Möbius syndrome due to brain stem tegmental necrosis. Arch Neurol 1977;34:124–126.

235. Torpin R. Amniochorionic mesoblastic fibrous strings and amnion bands: associated constricting fetal malformation or fetal death. Am J Obstet Gynecol 1965;91:65.

236. Tower P. Coloboma of lower lid and choroid, with facial defects and deformity of hand and forearm. Arch Ophthalmol 1953;50:333.

237. Traboulsi EL. Genetic diseases of the eye. New York: Oxford University Press, 1998.

238. Treacher Collins Syndrome Collaborative Group. Positional cloning of a gene involved in the pathogenesis of Treacher Collins syndrome. Nat Genet 1996;12(2):130–136.

239. Treacher Collins E. Case with symmetrical congenital notches in the outer part of each lower lid and defective development of the malar bone. Trans Ophthalmol Soc UK 1960;20:190–192.

240. Ullehand CN. The offspring of alcoholic mothers. Ann NY Acad Sci 1972;197:167–169.

241. Vannier MW. Radiologic evaluation of craniosynostosis. In: Craniosynostosis: diagnosis, evaluation and management. Part IV, 2nd edn. New York: Oxford Press, 2000:1148–1157.

242. Verzijl HTFM, van den Helm B, Veldman B, et al. A second gene for autosomal dominant Moebius syndrome is localized to chromosome 10q, in a Dutch family. Am J Hum Genet 1999;65:752–756.

243. Virchow R. Uber den Cretinismus, namentlich in Franken, und uber pathologische Schadelformen. Verh Phys Med Gesellsch (Wurzburg) 1851;2:230–270.

244. von Bijsterveld OP. Unilateral corneal anesthesia in oculoauriculovertebral dysplasia. Arch Ophthalmol 1969;82:189–190.

245. Waardenburg PJ. A new syndrome combining developmental anomaly of the eyelids, eyebrows and nose root with congenital deafness. Am J Genet 1951;3:195–253.

246. Wallis D, Muenke M. Mutations in holoprosencephaly. Hum. Mutat 2000;16:99–108.

247. Wang FM, Millman AL, Sidoti PA, et al. Ocular findings in Treacher Collins syndrome. Am J Ophthalmol 1990;110:280–286.

248. Warburg M. Ocular coloboma and multiple congenital anomalies: the CHARGE association. Ophthalmic Paediatr Genet 1983;2:189–899.

249. Warner RH, Rossett HL. The effects of drinking on offspring. J Stud Alcohol 1975;36:1395–1419.

250. Watanabe A, Takeda K, Ploplis B, et al. Epistatic relationship between Waardenburg syndrome genes MITF and PAX3. Nat Genet 1998;18:283–286.

251. Weidle EG, Thiel HJ, Lisch W, et al. Corneal complications in Goldenhar–Gorlin syndrome. Klin Monatsbl Augenheilkd 1987;190: 436–438.

252. Weinstock FJS, Hardesty HH. Absence of superior recti in craniofacial dysostosis. Arch Ophthalmol 1965;74:152–153.

253. Whitacker LA, Munro IRF, Sayler KE, et al. Combined report and complications in 793 craniofacial operations. Plast Reconstr Surg 1979;64:198–203.

254. Wildervanck LS. The cervico-oculo-acusticus syndrome. In: Vinken PJ, Bruyn GW, Myrianthopoulos NC (eds) Handbook of clinical neurology, vol 32. Amsterdam: North-Holland, 1978:123–130.

255. Wildervanck LS. Een cervico-oculo-acusticussyndroom. Ned Tijdschr Geneeskd 1960;104:2600–2605.

256. Wildervanck LS, Hoeksema PE, Penning L, et al. Radiological examination of the inner ear of deaf mutes presenting the cervico-oculo-acousticus syndrome: with a summary of roentgenologic and pathologico-anatomical findings in other endogenous forms of deafness. Acta Otolaryngol 1966;61:445–453.

257. Wilson ER, Mirra SS, Schwartz JF. Congenital diencephalic and brain stem damage. Acta Neuropathol 1982;57:70–74.

258. Wishnick MD, Nelson L, Hupport L, et al. Möbius syndrome and limb abnormalities with dominant inheritance. Ophthalmic Paediatr Genet 1983;2:77–81.

259. Wolter JR, Jones DH. Spontaneous cataract absorption in Hallermann–Streiff syndrome. Ophthalmologica 1965;50:401–408.

260. Yoon K, Yoo SJ, Suh DC, et al. Möbius syndrome with brain stem calcification: prenatal and neonatal sonographic findings. Pediatr Radiol 1997;27:150–152.

261. Ziter FA, Wiser WC, Robinson A. Three-generation pedigree of a Möbius syndrome variant with chromosome translocation. Arch Neurol 1997;34:437–442.

262. Zori RT, Gray BA, Bent-Williams A, et al. Preaxial acrofacial dysostosis (Nager syndrome) associated with an inherited and apparently balanced X;9 translocation: prenatal and postnatal late replication studies. Am J Med Genet 1993;46:379–383.

Connective Tissue, Skin, and Bone Disorders

Elias I. Traboulsi

CONNECTIVE TISSUE DISORDERS

Pseudoxanthoma Elasticum

Pseudoxanthoma elasticum (Grönbald–Strandberg syndrome) (PXE) affects about 1 in 70,000 to 1 in 100,000 individuals. It is characterized by skin abnormalities in the neck, axilla, and other flexural areas, breaks in Bruch's membrane with formation of *angioid streaks*, and disruption of arterial walls producing gastrointestinal and other hemorrhages, calcification, and occlusive vascular changes. The vasculopathy is characterized by fragmentation and calcification of the elastic component of the media, leading to vascular fragility and atherosclerosis. The vasculopathy results in gastrointestinal hemorrhages, neurological abnormalities,[122] coronary atherosclerotic heart disease, renal failure and hypertension, and peripheral vascular disease.[36] The disease becomes manifest in the third decade, but gastrointestinal hemorrhage has been reported as early as 6 or 7 years of age. Mitral valve prolapse occurs in 70% of patients.[155] Cutaneous findings are characteristic and consist of yellowish, xanthomatous lesions that coalesce to form peau d'orange plaques in areas of skin folds such as the neck, axilla, and genital, popliteal, and periumbilical regions. Mucosal lesions can also be present on the lower lip, rectum, and vagina. Skin biopsy reveals fragmentation and clumping of elastic fibers in the dermis with scattered calcifications.

The gene causing both recessive and dominant varieties of PXE has been mapped to chromosome 16p13.1[272] and identified as the ABCC6 (MRP6) gene, a member of the ATP transporter family. Molecules presumably transported by ABCC6 may be essential for extracellular matrix deposition or turnover of connective tissue at specific sites in the body.[15] Given the high expression of ABCC6 in liver and kidney, ABCC6 substrates may be transported into the blood. A deficiency of specific ABCC6 substrates may affect a range of connective tissue sites throughout the body and specifically the elastic fiber assembly.

A number of mutations that support autosomal recessive inheritance have been found, and an R114X mutation was found in families segregating autosomal dominant and autosomal recessive PXE. Initial debates as to number of varieties and modes of inheritance were caused by the variability of disease expression within families and among patient groups; some have predominant ocular disease with mild cutaneous findings and vice versa. Based on a study of 180 cases, Pope[213-215] postulated the existence of two dominant and two recessive varieties with 47% of cases having recessive disease. Neldner[193] found that 97% of patients probably had recessive disease. An additional recessive variant with severe ocular findings and relatively mild cutaneous and vascular changes may exist in Afrikaners and Belgian patients.[61,293] The classic variety involving skin, blood vessels, and the eye corresponds to type I recessive in Pope's classification. Histopathological findings may allow preclinical diagnosis in familial instances.[100]

Angioid (blood vessel-like) streaks occur in 85% of patients with PXE, and 70% of these patients experience subsequent visual loss.[46,96] The streaks represent linear discontinuities in Bruch's membrane starting at the optic nerve head and radiating toward the equator of the globe. The elastic layer of Bruch's membrane is abnormal and calcific; this leads to cracks involving the full thickness of the membrane.[37] Fibrovascular proliferation from the choroid and through the crack may lead to serous or hemorrhagic detachment of the retinal pigment epithelium. Angioid streaks may remain stationary or may progress intermittently in number, length, or width. Visual symptoms result from retinal hemorrhages, extension of angioid streaks into the macula, choroidal atrophy or sclerosis, and retinal pigment epithelial atrophy. Angioid streaks are best visualized using fluorescein angiography.[119,236] Other ocular findings in PXE include a peau d'orange appearance to the fundus and scattered punched-out chorioretinal lesions in the fundus periphery (Fig. 5-1).[37,255] Secretan et al.[245] analyzed the retinal and choroidal vascular abnormalities in eyes with angioid streaks (AS) associated with

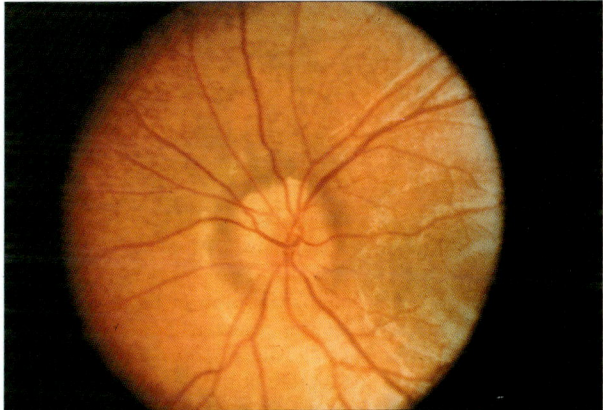

FIGURE 5-1. Fundus of patient with pseudoxanthoma elasticum. Note peau d'orange appearance and optic nerve head drusen.

PXE. Color photographs and fluorescein angiograms of 54 eyes of 27 consecutive patients with AS and PXE were examined retrospectively. Four (7%) of the 54 eyes had a major vascular abnormality at the level of the disc; this took the form of a large vascular loop corresponding to an arteriovenous communication between retina and choroid in 3 eyes (6%) and an anastomosis between two retinal arteries in 1 eye (2%).

The management of patients with PXE consists of treatment of vascular complications and cardiac valvular and myopathic lesions, and, when possible, photocoagulation of choroidal neovascularization that may complicate the AS. Because testing for the genetic mutation(s) responsible for PXE is not routine, genetic counseling must be done with caution. Sherer et al.[254] described four families in which one or more children were diagnosed with PXE. Detailed examination of the parents was carried out, including skin biopsy and ophthalmologic examination. In three of the four families, one parent had limited phenotypic expression, such as ocular findings without skin lesions or very mild skin lesions with no ocular findings. In the other family, one parent had very mild skin and ocular disease. All four affected parents had diagnostic skin biopsy findings. In none of the four families was the inheritance pattern clear cut. Although the inheritance pattern of PXE has been debated, clinically significant stigmata of PXE, which are not always readily apparent, can occur in successive generations. Therefore, all first-degree relatives of affected patients should undergo a full dermatological examination as well as a funduscopic examination. If even mild typical skin or eye findings are present, then skin biopsy should be performed.

Ehlers–Danlos Syndrome

There are several types of Ehlers–Danlos syndrome (Table 5-1). Characteristic joint hyperextensibility and skin laxity are demonstrated in Figure 5-2. Ehlers–Danlos syndrome type VI (lysyl hydroxylase deficiency) is the form of most interest to ophthalmologists because of the potential for rupture of the globe or retinal detachment following minor trauma. Judisch et al.[131] observed spontaneous rupture of the globe in the absence of lysyl hydroxylase deficiency. Their patient probably had the syndrome of macrocephaly–Ehlers–Danlos VI phenotype reported later by Cadle et al. in 1985.[29] Other similar patients have been reported since and have had normal levels of lysyl hydroxylase.[238,313] Zlotogora et al.[313] divided patients with the so-called brittle cornea syndrome into two groups. The first group comprises Tunisian Jewish patients with red hair and ocular fragility, and the second larger group is composed of patients of

TABLE 5-1. Clinical Features of Ehlers–Danlos Syndrome.

Type, inheritance, gene, and locus	Clinical features	Ocular features
I (gravis) OMIM #130000 Autosomal dominant COL5A1 gene defects 2q31, 17q21.31–q22, 9q34.2–q34.3	Most common; hyperextensible skin; easy bruisability; cigarette-paper scarring; difficult healing; six different errors of metabolism	Stretchable lids; retinal detachment has been reported
II (mitis) OMIM #130010 Autosomal dominant COL5A1 and COL5A2 gene defects 9q34.2–q34.3	Like type I but milder; may be most common form of EDS	None
III (benign hypermobility) OMIM #130020 Autosomal dominant COL3A1 gene defect 2q31	Severe hypermobility of all joints without musculoskeletal abnormalities; minimal skin changes; autosomal dominant	None

TABLE 5-1. (continued)

Type, inheritance, gene, and locus	Clinical features	Ocular features
IV (ecchymotic or Sack) OMIM #130050 Autosomal dominant COL3A1 gene defect 2q31	Abnormalities of medium and large arteries with spontaneous arterial rupture at a young age; bowel perforation; thin and transparent skin; minimal hyperextensibility of joints and skin laxity	None
V OMIM #305200 X-linked recessive	Minimal joint hypermobility; marked skin hyperextensibility; mitral valve prolapse	None
VI (ocular) OMIM #225400 Autosomal recessive Lysyl hydroxylase deficiency 1p36.3–p36.2	Hypotonia in infancy followed by severe scoliosis, recurrent joint dislocations and stretchable skin; high risk for catastrophic arterial rupture	Blue sclerae; spontaneous rupture of globe; glaucoma; keratoconus
VII (dermatosparaxis) OMIM #225410 Autosomal recessive ADAMTS2 gene defect 5q23	Short stature; extreme generalized joint hypermobility; moderate skin stretchability and bruisability	Hypertelorism; epicanthus
VIII OMIM #130080 Autosomal dominant	Accompanying periodontosis	None
IX OMIM #304150 X-linked Cu(2+)-transporting ATPase, alpha polypeptide defect Xq12–q13	Occipital bony horns; loose stools; obstructive uropathy; bladder diverticulae; joint laxity; hooked nose; short broad clavicles; fused carpal bones; mild mental retardation	None
X OMIM #225310 Autosomal dominant Possible fibronectin defect 2q34	Mild clinical findings	None
XI OMIM #147900 Autosomal dominant	Familial joint instability	None

Source: Based on information from Online Mendelian Inheritance in Man, OMIM (TM). McKusick–Nathans Institute for Genetic Medicine, Johns Hopkins University (Baltimore, MD) and National Center for Biotechnology Information, National Library of Medicine (Bethesda, MD), 2000. World Wide Web URL: http://www.ncbi.nlm.nih.gov/omim/

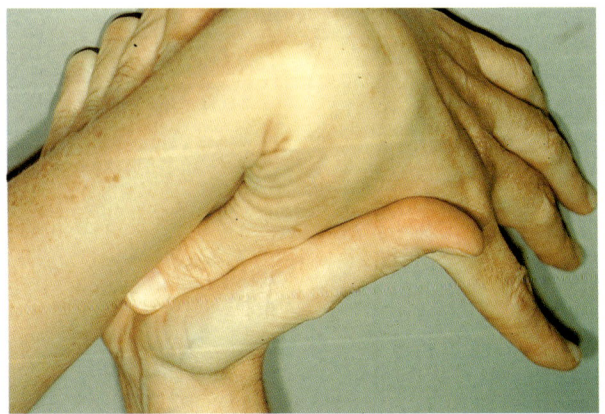

A

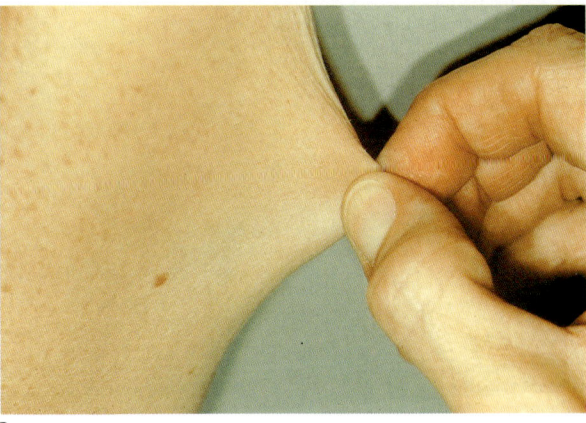

B

FIGURE 5-2A,B. Hyperextensible joint (**A**) and elastic skin (**B**) in a patient with Ehlers–Danlos syndrome.

different ethnic backgrounds who are not redheaded. The locus for this syndrome may be closely linked for the gene(s) responsible for hair color. Ocular findings that are occur in some patients with Ehlers–Danlos syndrome (EDS) include myopia, microcornea, keratoconus, and occasionally retinal detachment and glaucoma. Their prevalence, however appears to be low or the same as the general population.[177]

One of the most challenging problems facing ophthalmologists who care for patients with EDS type VI and ocular fragility is the repair of the ruptured globe. Macsai et al.[165] described an alternative to corneal transplantation and suturing in these patients. They performed a 360° conjunctival peritomy, removed the epithelium from the keratoglobus cornea, and sutured a ring of Descemet's membrane and endothelium from a fresh donor corneoscleral ring to the patient's sclera with 9-0 nylon suture. The conjunctiva was brought into position and tacked down over the edge of the donor graft. A full-thickness penetrating keratoplasty was performed 4 months later. This procedure was performed on both eyes with a final visual acuity OU of 20/100.

Marfan Syndrome

In its classical form, Marfan syndrome is characterized by the presence of abnormalities of the eye (ectopia lentis), aorta (dilatation of the aortic root and aneurysm of the ascending aorta and aortic aneurysm), and skeleton (dolichostenomelia, upper segment/lower segment ratio 2 SD below mean for age, pectus excavatum, and kyphoscoliosis).[11,220] In addition to these three major criteria, auxiliary signs may be present, such as myopia, mitral valve prolapse, *arachnodactyly*, joint laxity, tall stature, pes planus, striae distensae, pneumothorax, and dural ectasia. The clinical diagnosis may be difficult in mild cases, and the spectrum of patients with connective tissue abnormalities simulating the Marfan syndrome is wide. The identification of *fibrillin*, a major component of connective tissue,[242] as the defective gene in Marfan syndrome following the mapping of the disease to chromosome 15,[56,57,133,289] has stirred up interest in this glycoprotein and its role in connective tissue diseases.

About 35% of patients with the Marfan syndrome do not develop lens subluxation.[172] There have been reports of large families with Marfan syndrome without ectopia lentis in which the disease could not be linked to the fibrillin gene[18] but maps to chromosome 3p24.2–p25.[45] Marfan syndrome affects 1 in 20,000 persons.[220]

Ocular findings are present in at least 60% of patients with Marfan syndrome.[4,50,172] A number of ocular histopathological studies have been published.[60,67,223,296] The most characteristic and usually diagnostic ocular abnormality is *subluxation of the crystalline lens* (Fig. 5-3). The degree of subluxation varies from mild superior and posterior displacement, evident only on

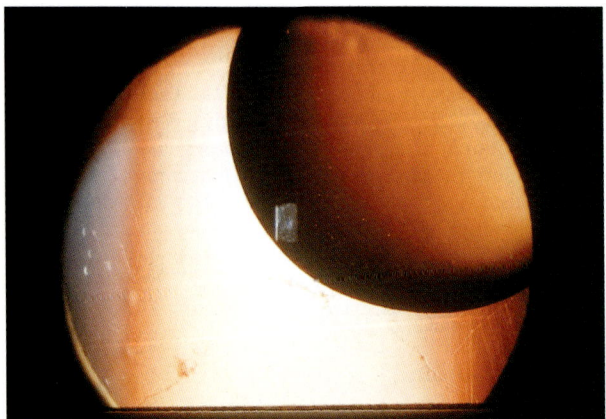

FIGURE 5-3. Subluxated lens of a patient with Marfan syndrome. Note stretched zonules inferonasally.

maximal pupillary dilation, to significant subluxation placing the equator of the lens in the pupillary axis. Although superior and temporal displacement of the lens is most common, inferior, nasal, or lateral subluxation also occurs. Subluxation of the lens is slowly progressive in some patients and most noticeable in the first few years of life or in the late teens and early twenties; in most patients, however, no progression of the displacement is noted over the years. Total dislocation in the vitreous cavity is unusual early in life, but has been documented in older patients where it may, rarely, be complicated by phacolytic glaucoma. Lens dislocation into the pupil or the anterior chamber is characteristic of untreated homocystinuria.

In the Marfan syndrome, stretched zonular fibers can be seen through the dilated pupil. In places where zonules have ruptured, a straightening of the lens contour is noted and has been falsely labeled as a coloboma of the lens. *Microspherophakia* is present in about 15% of patients and results in high myopia. The cornea is flat with keratometric readings in the high 40s in about 20% of patients. *Megalocornea* (corneal diameter measuring more than 13.5 mm) may be present in some patients. The iris has a thin velvety texture, and the pupil is difficult to dilate in the more severely affected patients where there is atrophy of the dilator muscle fibers. *Iridodonesis* results from lens subluxation.

Wheatley and coworkers studied the distribution of fibrillin in normal ocular tissues and found the glycoprotein to be ubiquitous in the cornea, sclera, anterior chamber angle, uvea, zonules, lens capsule, and optic nerve septae.[306] They concluded that ocular abnormalities in the Marfan syndrome could be correlated to the pattern of distribution of fibrillin in the eye. Further studies of sections and/or flat mounts of lens capsules from normal autopsy eyes, and surgical capsulotomy specimens from patients with senile cataracts and from patients with the Marfan syndrome, showed three distinct and adjacent zones in the equatorial and periequatorial regions of the normal lens capsule: zone I, a 0.75-mm-wide peripheral ring of the anterior capsule that contained radial bundles of fibrillin fibers which appeared to suspend the central part of the capsule; zone II, a 1-mm-wide meshwork of fibrillin-rich fibers that encircled the equator and served as an insertion platform for zonular fibers; and zone III, composed of radial, 0.1-mm-wide bands arranged in a periodic fashion in the most peripheral part of the posterior capsule. Fibrillin fibers were abnormal and disrupted in all three zones in patients with the Marfan syndrome.[185] From these observations and a later study by Traboulsi et al.,[287] it was concluded that fibrillin is a major constituent of the peripheral and equatorial areas of the lens capsule, that it may play a role in the ability of the lens to change its configuration during accommodation, and that the observed qualitative and quantitative abnormalities in fibrillin expression in the lens capsule of patients with the Marfan syndrome support a causal relationship to lens abnormalities in these patients.[185,287]

Strabismus is more common in the Marfan syndrome than in the general population of the United States.[124] Exotropia occurs in about 10% of patients and esotropia in 2%. Strabismic or anisometropic or ametropic amblyopia should be suspected in all patients with reduced visual acuity, especially if the reduction is asymmetrical. In many cases, amblyopia responds surprisingly well to treatment despite years of uncorrected high errors of refraction. Open-angle glaucoma is significantly more common in patients with the Marfan syndrome in all age groups as compared to the general population and becomes more prevalent in this disease with increasing patient age.[123] Pupillary block is unusual but has been documented. Phacolytic glaucoma has been noted in older patients with mature dislocated lenses and carries a guarded prognosis because of the complex vitreoretinal surgery needed to extract the hard cataractous lenses. Retinal detachment may occur spontaneously in eyes with axial myopia, or following cataract extraction, especially in longer eyes. Cataracts develop earlier than in the general population and, in most cases, are the indication for lens extraction. Occasionally poor vision from high astigmatic errors of refraction from lenses whose equator is in the middle of a small pupillary area leads to a surgical decision. Finally, recurrent dislocation into the anterior chamber, rare as it might be in the Marfan syndrome, may prompt lens extraction.

Infants and children with the Marfan syndrome can be severely affected and present major therapeutic challenges from the orthopedic and cardiovascular standpoints.[101,188,269] Recent advances in the medical and surgical management of these patients has allowed them to survive longer than into the third or fourth decade as was the case in the past.[100,170,192] Mitral valve disease in childhood and dissecting aortic aneurysm in adults remain the most frequent causes of death. The mainstay in the treatment of this disease relies on the prevention of cardiac complications using beta-blocking agents. Careful and repeated phakic or aphakic refractions are necessary to achieve the best possible vision. Patients should try both aphakic and phakic corrections and see which one they prefer. Extraction of subluxated lenses should only be performed after careful consideration of phakic and aphakic optical correction and of the level of visual acuity, its fluctuation with lens movement, and the age of the patient. This author still has not removed a lens in a patient with Marfan syndrome for optical reasons. The hesitance arises from concerns for retinal detachment, the rate of which may approach 25% in elongated globes. Visual prognosis is very good if amblyopia is treated and appropriate optical correction is instituted early. Retinal detachment remains the leading cause of severe visual loss. Early detection of glaucoma is essential. Prenatal diagnosis of the Marfan syndrome is possible using ultrasonography if the fetus is severely affected.[243] In families in which linkage to fibrillin is demonstrated or where a specific mutation in the fibrillin gene is present, linkage analysis or direct gene sequencing may allow prenatal diagnosis.

Osteogenesis Imperfecta

Four clinical types of osteogenesis imperfecta are recognized[11,26,27,258,259] (Table 5-2). The disease has a frequency of about 1 in 20,000 live births. The clinical manifestations involve the

TABLE 5-2. Clinical Features of the Four Types of Osteogenesis Imperfecta.

Type, OMIM #, inheritance, gene and locus	Clinical findings	Ocular findings
I (tarda) Autosomal dominant OMIM #166200 COL1A1, COL1A2 or others 17q21.31–q22; 7q22.1	Most common type; mild to moderate severity; multiple bone fractures from minor trauma; teeth are usually normal; age-dependent hearing loss in 50%; little or no deformity	Intensely blue sclerae that remain blue throughout life; low ocular rigidity reduced central corneal thickness
II (congenita) Autosomal dominant OMIM #166210 COL1A1 gene defect q22.1ts 17q21.31–q22; 7q22.1	Lethal perinatal form; severe bone deformities	Dark blue sclerae
III Autosomal dominant	Progressive deforming disease; variable severity of dental and hearing problems	None
IV (with normal sclerae) Autosomal dominant OMIM #166220 COL1A1 or COL1A2 17q21.31–q22	Least severe; resembles Ehlers–Danlos syndrome; mild bone deformity; short stature	Normal sclerae

skeleton, ears, eyes, teeth, skin, and joints.[160,228] Osteogenesis imperfecta is caused by abnormalities of the alpha$_1$ or alpha$_2$ chains of type I collagen. There is failure of type I collagen fibers to mature to their normal diameter. Mutations in the COL1A1 (chromosome 17) and COL1A2 genes (chromosome 7) account for most cases in all four types. The location of the mutation in the gene seems to determine the clinical phenotype.[27,305] The diagnosis of osteogenesis imperfecta is based on clinical, dental, and radiologic criteria. Individuals with OI type I have bright *blue sclerae* that remain intensely blue throughout life (Fig. 5-4). In types III and IV, the sclerae may be blue at birth, but the intensity of the color decreases such that by adolescence or early adulthood the sclera appear normal. The blue coloration results from the visualization of the underlying choroid through a thin sclera. Ocular rigidity was found to be reduced in a group of 16 patients with different types of OI.[134] The perilimbal region is often whiter than the remaining sclera, resulting in the so-called *Saturn's ring*. Electron microscopy reveals reduction in the

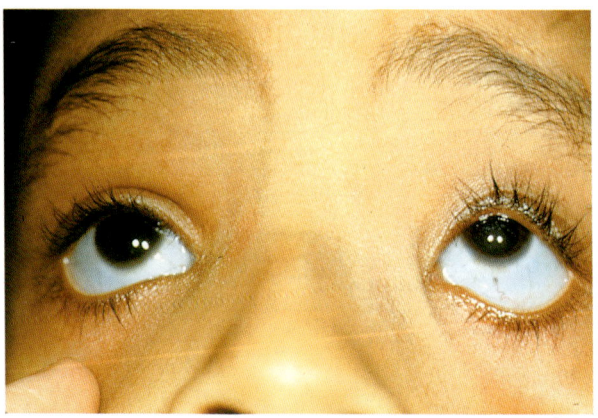

FIGURE 5-4. Blue sclerae in a child with osteogenesis imperfecta.

diameter of collagen fibers and change in their cross-striation pattern.[35] Blue sclerae are also present in type VI Ehlers–Danlos syndrome and in small children with hypophosphatasia. Optic nerve damage may result from deformities or fractures of calvarial bones. Posterior embryotoxon, keratoconus, and megalocornea have been observed. Rare ocular findings include congenital glaucoma, cataracts, choroidal sclerosis, and subhyaloid hemorrhage.[137] In a series of 53 patients, central corneal thickness was reduced to a mean 0.443 mm as compared to 0.522 in normal controls ($p < 0.001$).[211] Hyperopia is common. Spontaneous rupture of the globe is very rare.

The management of patients with osteogenesis imperfecta consists of aggressive orthopedic management of fractures to prevent extensive deformities of the extremities and spine. Patients with the severe congenital form rarely survive beyond the first few years of life. A better prognosis for life is found in the milder forms of the disease, especially types I and IV. Many patients become wheelchair bound because of extensive limb deformities.

Weill–Marchesani Syndrome

The Weill–Marchesani syndrome[168,301] is a rare autosomal recessive condition characterized by congenital short stature, brachycephaly, short stubby spadelike hands and feet, and ocular abnormalities in the form of *microspherophakia* and *ectopia lentis*.[226] The incidence of this disease is about 1 in 100,000 individuals. Patients are of normal intelligence. One parent is usually short with or without stubby hands and no ocular abnormalities, indicating that the gene for this disorder is not completely recessive. Family members in previous generations may also be identified as carriers based on stature.[98,143]

Ocular abnormalities are only present in homozygotes.[128] The microspherophakic lens tends to move into the pupillary area, leading to pupillary block and glaucoma.[309] Total dislocation into the anterior chamber may occur. Myopia is most often caused by the spherophakia, but may be axial, and ranges from 3 to more than 20 diopters. Lenticular diameter may be as small as 6.75 mm, and the sagittal diameter of the lens may be increased by 25%.[178] A peripheral iridectomy relieves pupillary block in most patients, but lens extraction may be necessary to control intraocular pressure elevation. Mydriatics are preferred over miotics for the relief of pupillary block; cycloplegics, however, have been reported to induce pupillary block in these patients.[311]

Cohen Syndrome

Cohen syndrome is characterized by congenital hypotonia, mid-childhood truncal obesity, narrow hands and feet, and a typical facial appearance with a high nasal bridge, open mouth with prominent central incisors, short philtrum, and micrognathia.[31,42,197,198] Some patients have delayed puberty but no documentable endocrinological abnormalities.[7,54] Granulocytopenia may be present, and Warburg and coworkers[299] postulated the existence of two types, type I (with granulocytopenia) and type II (without granulocytopenia). Cohen syndrome can be differentiated from Bardet–Biedl syndrome by the absence of polydactyly and hypogenitalism; both feature a progressive retinal dystrophy that is, however, much more severe in the Bardet–Biedl syndrome. Cohen syndrome is inherited in an autosomal recessive fashion,[70,82,145] and the gene has been mapped to 8q22–q23.[277]

Night blindness with poor vision and constricted visual fields are universal. Downslanting of the palpebral fissures occurs in all patients. A pigmentary retinopathy with progressive chorioretinal atrophy develops as early as the first decade of life. The electroretinogram is nonrecordable, and bony spicules are seen in the retinal periphery. Progressive myopia is one of the hallmarks of the disease and is present in the majority of patients.[299] Cataracts develop in some patients in the fourth and fifth decades of life.[196]

No specific treatment is available. Despite the granulocytopenia, patients with Cohen syndrome do not seem prone to infection.[299]

Stickler Syndrome (Hereditary Progressive Arthro-Ophthalmopathy)

This syndrome is a clinically heterogeneous group of dominantly inherited disorders of collagen.[109,173,204,270,280,294] Four genetic loci have been identified. The most common type, STL1 or membranous vitreous type, is caused by mutations in the COL2A1 gene on 12q14.[79,84] The other forms include STL2 or beaded vitreous type caused by mutations in COL11A1, STL3 or nonocular type caused by mutations in COL11A2, and an additional form whose locus has not be identified yet.[264]

The incidence of Stickler syndrome is estimated at 1:20,000. Optiz et al.[204] believe that Stickler syndrome is more common than Marfan syndrome. Some features are common to more than one clinical subtype; these include sensorineural hearing loss in about 25% of patients, cleft palate in about 25%, and a progressive arthropathy that is often subtle early in life but becomes most pronounced in the fourth or fifth decade. Although most patients have increasing stiffness, soreness, and arthritic changes, some have hyperextensible joints. Flattening of the epiphyseal centers on X-rays is present early in life, and, together with congenital myopia, constitute the minimal diagnostic criteria for the Stickler syndrome. Mitral valve prolapse is present in 45% of patients.[163]

The ocular findings include congenital and sometimes stable high myopia, presenile cataracts, and vitreoretinal degeneration; Retinal detachment is common.[144,266] In the most common STL1 type the vitreous is liquefied with midperipheral circumferential condensations or veils (Fig. 5-5). Radial perivascular patches of lattice degeneration are present in the posterior pole and midperiphery (Fig. 5-6). Glaucoma develops in about 5% of cases. Rarely, patients develop subluxation of the lens.

The management of patients with Stickler syndrome includes the prevention of retinal detachment through repeated careful ophthalmoscopic examinations and prophylactic treatment of retinal holes. Patients with cleft palate receive appro-

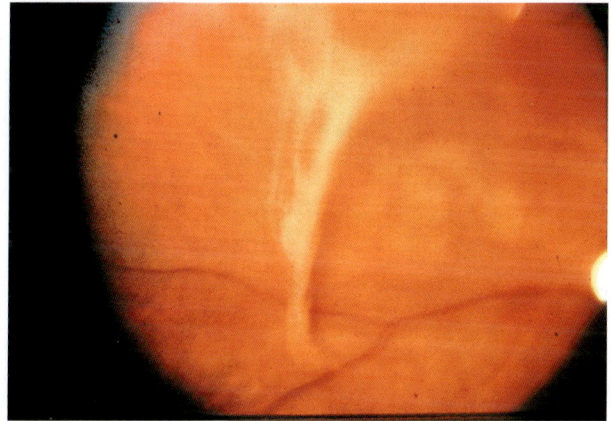

FIGURE 5-5. Vitreous veil in a patient with Stickler syndrome.

priate surgical treatment. Screening for hearing loss is mandatory in infants with Stickler syndrome. Newborns with the *Pierre Robin malformation complex* should be routinely screened for the presence of other anomalies suggestive of Stickler syndrome. Stickler syndrome should also be suspected

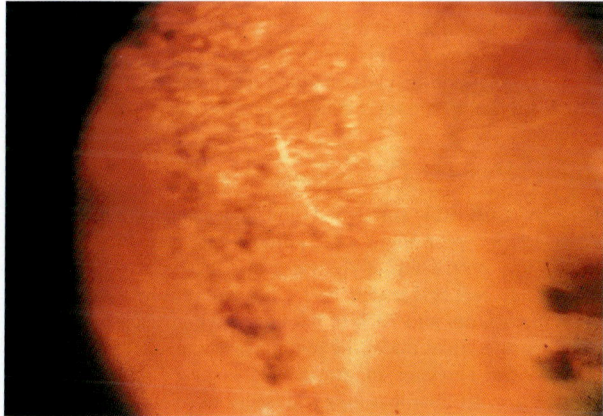

FIGURE 5-6. Peripheral area of circumferential lattice degeneratiom in a patient with Stickler syndrome.

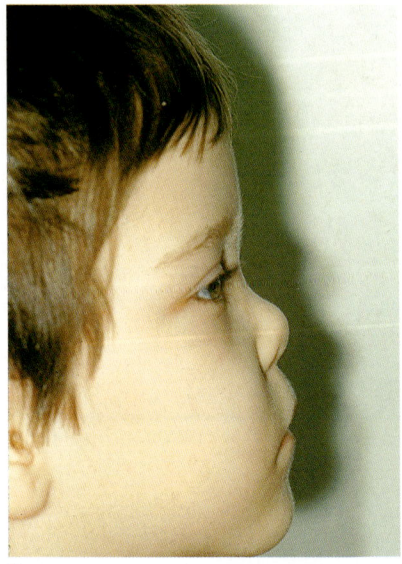

A

FIGURE 5-7A–C. Typical flat facial appearance of a patient with Kniest syndrome (**A**). Note enlarged interphalangeal joints (**B**) and knees (**C**).

in dominantly inherited myopia with or without retinal detachment and deafness. The diagnosis should also be suspected in dominantly inherited cleft palate, mild spondyloepiphyseal dysplasia, and in dominantly inherited mitral valve prolapse.

Kniest Dysplasia

Patients with this autosomal dominant bone dysplasia have short stature, prominent wide joints, short trunk with a broad thorax and protrusion of the sternum, and a flat midface with depressed nasal bridge (Fig. 5-7). Cleft palate is present in about 40% of patients and 75% of patients have hearing loss. X-rays demonstrate widening of the metaphyses and narrowing of joint spaces. The cartilage in growth plates has a "Swiss cheese" appearance on histopathological sections; this appearance is caused by the dilated endoplasmic reticulum complex in chondrocytes. The disorder results from mutations in COL2A1,[308] the

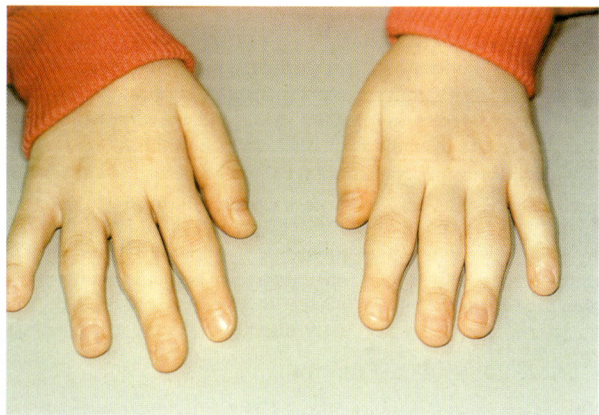

B

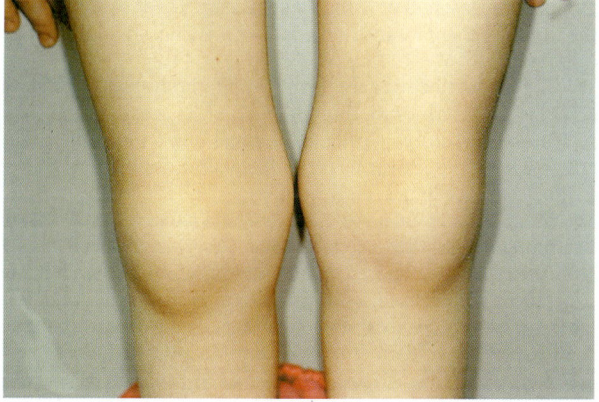

C

FIGURE 5-7B–C. (continued).

same gene that causes Stickler syndrome.[310] It appears that Kniest dysplasia results from shorter type II collagen monomers and that alteration of a specific domain of COL2A1 that may span from exons 12 to 24 results in the Kniest phenotype.

Patients with Kniest dysplasia have a severe vitreoretinal degeneration that resulted in retinal detachment in five eyes of seven patients in one series.[175] The retinal detachments frequently result from giant tears or retinal dialysis. All patients in one series had congenital severe myopia averaging −15.25 diopters and oblique astigmatism averaging +3.00 diopters. The myopia did not progress with increasing age. Some patients developed cataracts in the first or second decade of life. Subluxation of the lens and glaucoma are rare findings.

Careful retinal examination should be performed at regular intervals with prophylactic cryotherapy of retinal breaks or vitrectomy as required. Cataract surgery should be carefully weighed against the high incidence of aphakic retinal detachment in these patients. No specific treatment is available for the bone dysplasia.

Chondrodysplasia Punctata

There are several genetically and clinically distinct types of chondrodysplasia punctata. Some are autosomal recessive while others are autosomal or X-linked dominant. These diseases share the radiologic appearance of punctate calcific stippling of the epiphyses.

The X-linked dominant forms of chondrodysplasia punctata (CDPX2, *Conradi–Hunermann disease*) is characterized by typical facial features with a saddle nose and a flat, sometimes grooved nasal tip, linear ichthyosiform skin changes, cataracts, scoliosis and leg length discrepancies.[105,167,191,268] Skin lesions are present at birth in about 30% of cases and affect areas of flexion and moisture. Intelligence is normal. Progressive scoliosis is a prominent feature. Stippled epiphyses are characteristic, but the stippling may fade or disappear with age leaving areas of defective ossification. Sectoral or wedge-shaped cortical cataracts are usually present at birth or early in life. There is little or no progression, with good visual prognosis. The linear skin changes and the wedge-shaped lenticular changes are thought to be due to Lyonization.[16,52] The gene for CDPX2 maps to Xp11.23–p11.22 and codes for the delta(8)-delta(7) sterol isomerase emopamil-binding protein.[22] The X-linked recessive form, CDPX1, is due to mutations in the arylsulfatase E gene at Xp22.3 with significant variability of clinical manifestations in carrier males and females.[252]

In the autosomal dominant form of chondrodysplasia punctata (Conradi–Hunermann syndrome),[47,120] limb shortening is not asymmetrical.[251,265] The nose has a flattened tip with a short columella and a depressed nasal bridge. Although males and females are affected, there appears to be an excess of females in patients assigned to the autosomal dominant group by Spranger et al.,[268] suggesting that some of these females probably have the X-linked variety. Cataracts are rarely present.

In the rhizomelic, autosomal recessive form of chondrodysplasia punctata, there is marked proximal shortening of the (rhizomelic, at the root) arms and legs with splaying of the long bones and abnormal ossification of epiphyses of both the humerus and femur. A depressed midface with saddle nose deformity, frontal bossing, and high arched palate are constant findings. Patients may have low birth weight and fail to thrive. Flexion contractures, dislocation of the hips, and microcephaly are common (Fig. 5-8). *Rhizomelic chondrodysplasia punctata*

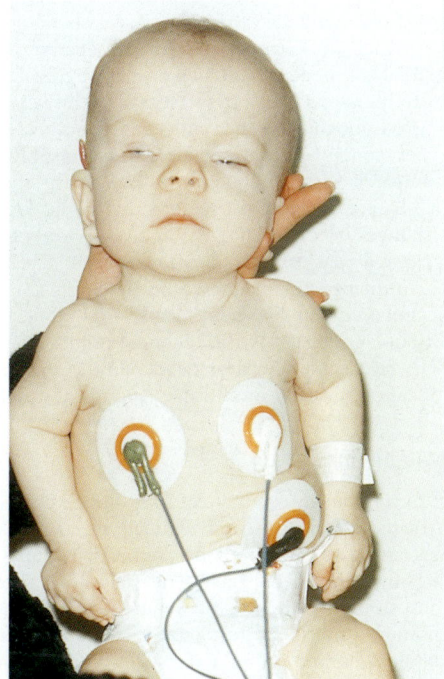

FIGURE 5-8. One-year-old boy with rhizomelic chondroplasia punctata. Note short humeri and atypical facial features.

is caused by an abnormality in peroxisomal function.[111,203,298] Cataracts occur in all patients.[65,284] The eyes are otherwise normal on histopathological examination (D. Wilson and R. Weleber, personal communications). The rhizomelic autosomal recessive form of chondrodysplasia punctata maps to 6q22–q24 and results from mutations in the PEX7 gene that encodes the peroxisomal type 2 targeting signal receptor PTS2.[21]

Cataract surgery is performed if lenticular opacities are visually significant in the dominant varieties of the disease. In the rhizomelic form, cataract surgery was withheld in the past because of poor prognosis for life, but with current survival of patients with this disease late into the first decade, we favor early surgery and visual rehabilitation. Life expectancy and mental development are normal in the dominant varieties. Orthopedic problems are frequent from the asymmetrical shortening of the limbs or scoliosis.

Spranger et al. concluded that the form of chondrodysplasia punctata to which the Conradi–Hunermann eponym is appropriately applied has predominantly epiphyseal, frequently asymmetrical calcifications and dysplastic skeletal changes, a relatively good prognosis, and autosomal dominant inheritance.[268] They concluded that cataracts occur in only 17% of cases as compared with a frequency of 72% in the rhizomelic form, which is recessive and is usually lethal in the first year of life. Skin changes occur in about 28% of cases of both forms. Happle suggested that cataracts are consistently absent in the autosomal dominant form and present in about two-thirds of the rhizomelic and X-linked dominant forms.[105]

Conditions confused with chondrodysplasia punctata include Zellweger cerebrohepatorenal syndrome and multicentric epiphyseal ossification in multiple epiphyseal dysplasia.

Homocystinuria

Homocystinuria is an autosomal recessive disease characterized in the untreated state by mental retardation, coarse fair hair, malar flush, and a thromboembolic diathesis. Patients have a marfanoid body habitus and have lens dislocation, hence the clinical confusion with the Marfan syndrome. Two main categories of homocystinuria are recognized.[190] The most common type or classical homocystinuria is caused by a deficiency of cystathionine β-synthase, which catalyzes the transsulfuration of homocysteine to cystathionine in the presence of pyridoxine.

Cystathionine β-synthase has been mapped to 21q22.3.[149] The second type of homocystinuria is caused by impaired activity of 5-methyltetrahydrofolate-homocysteine methyltransferase. About 50% of patients with classical homocystinuria clear the urine of homocystine after dietary supplementation with pyridoxine. There is an association between homocystinuria and a schizophrenia-like picture in some patients.[19] Vitamin B_6 nonresponders are usually mentally retarded; responders are of normal intelligence. Accumulation of homocystine proximal to the enzyme block may be responsible for the arteriosclerosis, abnormal platelet adhesiveness, and frequent cerebral thromboses. It has also been proposed that the accumulated homocystine interferes with collagen and elastin cross-linking, hence leading to the observed connective tissue defects.

Subluxation of the lenses is noted by age 5 years in 38% of untreated patients and in all patients by age 25 years. The direction of subluxation is usually inferior or inferonasal.[50] The lenses may dislocate into the anterior chamber, and patients present with a red eye and cloudy cornea. The lens is found in the pupillary area or in the anterior chamber (Fig. 5-9). Lens extraction is frequently complicated by retinal detachment, vitreous hemorrhage, and glaucoma. Cystic and pigmentary changes of unclear

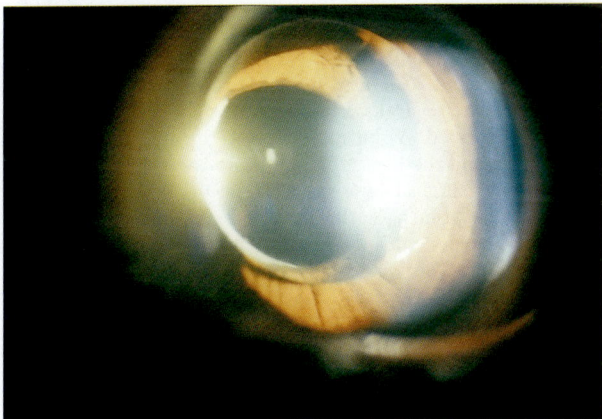

FIGURE 5-9. Lens totally dislocated into the anterior chamber of a 7-year-old girl with untreated homocystinuria.

significance have been noted in the retinal periphery of some patients with the disease.

Lens fringe or ragged zonules have been described in some patients with homocystinuria.[223,224] A characteristic thick periodic acid–Schiff- (PAS-) positive layer composed of short filaments of zonular origin is demonstrated histopathologically over the ciliary epithelium. The degree of zonular abnormality is related to the age of the patient.

All patients with dislocated lenses without a clear history of trauma should have quantification of serum amino acids to rule out homocystinuria. An episode of anterior dislocation of the crystalline lens in a patient with presumed Marfan syndrome should suggest the diagnosis of homocystinuria. Patients with homocystinuria are initially supplemented with 50 to 1000 mg/day of oral vitamin B_6; this leads to clinical and biochemical improvement in about 50% of patients. Nonresponders are started on a diet low in methionine and supplemented with cystine. Betaine facilitates the conversion of serum homocystine to methionine and significantly reduces the symptoms of homocystinuria. Recent studies have demonstrated that neonatal screening, detection of the disease at birth, and appropriate therapy prevent the development of mental retardation, myopia, and subluxation of the lens. Patients with homocystinuria are placed on platelet antiaggregation agents such as dipyridamole and acetylsalicylic acid to prevent vasoocclusive or thromboembolic events.

In patients who present with lens dislocation into the anterior chamber, dilation of the pupil and positional manipulation may be sufficient to return the lens to the posterior chamber. Patients are then placed on miotics and a peripheral laser iridotomy is performed. With time, however, the pupillary sphincter may infarct and the lens subluxates into the anterior chamber, necessitating surgical removal. Because of the risk of thromboembolic phenomena with general anesthesia and the complications of surgery, conservative management of the dislocated lens is preferred. Survival is good in vitamin B_6 responders, and a normal lifespan is expected. Patients with other types have shortened survival depending on the type of mutation, severity of the disease at diagnosis, and the time of institution of therapy. The need for any surgery should be carefully evaluated. Death from general anesthesia has been reported on several occasions. Good hydration and medications that inhibit platelet aggregation should be given before surgery.

SKIN DISORDERS

Albinism

Albinism refers to the absence or reduction in the amount of *melanin* in the skin, eye, or both. Diseases featuring albinism are genetically determined and involve defects of melanogenesis. In tyrosinase-negative oculocutaneous albinism, the defect involves the enzyme *tyrosinase*, which catalyzes the conversion of tyrosine to dihydroxyphenylalanine (DOPA) and of DOPA to DOPA quinone.[141] In type II or tyrosinase-positive albinism, as well as in autosomal recessive ocular albinism and in the Prader–Willi plus albinism syndrome, the defect lies in the P gene located on 15q11–q13.

Albinism has an overall prevalence of about 1 in 20,000 individuals. In the United States, the frequency of tyrosinase-negative albinism is 1 in 39,000 of the white population and 1 in 28,000 of the black population, with a gene frequency of 1%. The prevalence of X-linked ocular albinism is about 1 in 50,000.[142] There are nine forms of oculocutaneous albinism, at least two forms of ocular albinism and a number of disorders with dermal hypopigmentation without ocular albinism. Clinically, patients who have no skin, hair, or ocular pigment and do not tan at all have tyrosinase-negative oculocutaneous albinism. Patients who have any amount of pigment, and those who develop a suntan, are classified as having type II or tyrosinase-positive albinism. The hairbulb incubation test is the definitive way to assign patients into one of these two categories, but is of no practical value as the diagnosis can be made with relative certainty based on clinical findings.[138] Patients with the *Chediak–Higashi* syndrome have tyrosinase-positive oculocutaneous albinism and susceptibility to gram-positive infections and lymphoreticular malignancies. They have characteristic giant cytoplasmic inclusions in peripheral leukocytes.[307] In the *Hermanski–Pudlak syndrome*,[110] which is very common in Puerto Ricans, there is defective platelet aggregation and patients develop progressive restrictive lung disease and bowel disorders that may lead to death in the third and fourth decades of life (Fig. 5-10). The gene for tyrosinase has been mapped to 11q14–q22.[8]

Ocular albinism is X-linked recessive[78] and has been mapped to the short arm of the X chromosome.[14,210] Pedigree analysis and the presence of a mosaic pattern of retinal pigment epithelium

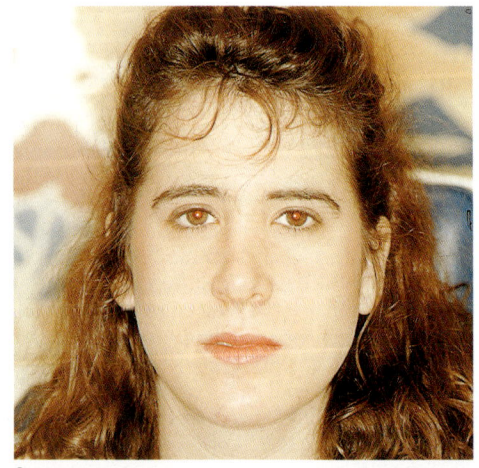

A

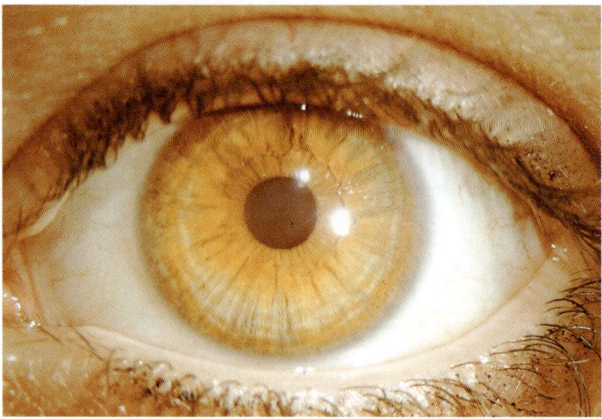

B

FIGURE 5-10A–C. Hermansky–Pudlak syndrome. Note the darkly pigmented hair (**A**) and brown iris (**B**). Transillumination (**C**) shows large defects in the pigmented iris epithelium.

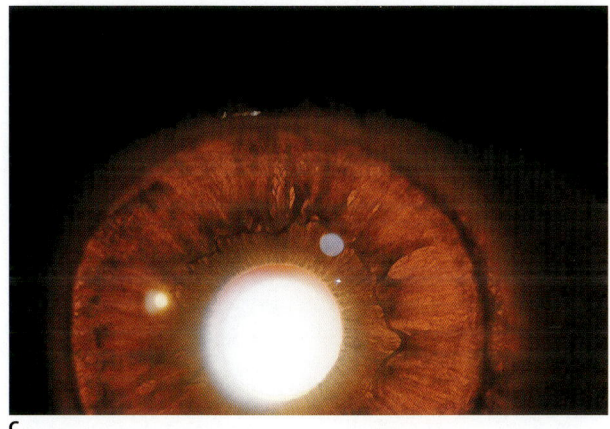

C

FIGURE 5-10C. (continued).

(RPE) and choroidal pigmentation in carrier females allow diagnosis. Skin biopsies reveal *macromelanosomes* in melanocytes,[200] a finding that indicates that the skin is involved as well. Black patients may retain a fair amount of uveal pigment, leading to the picture of ocular albinism cum pigmento.[199] Rarely, patients appear to have autosomal recessive ocular albinism.[188] Such patients have mutations in the P gene on chromosome 15q11–q13.[157] The P protein is a transmembrane polypeptide that may transport small molecules such as tyrosine, the precursor of melanin. Ocular albinism is a leading cause of nystagmus in male infants and children. Slit lamp examination for iris transillumination and examination of the ocular fundus of carrier mothers are essential to rule out this condition in the child with nystagmus.

The ocular features of albinism include nystagmus, strabismus, macular hypoplasia, and absence of pigment in the retinal pigment epithelium and uveal tract with iris transillumination, prominence of choroidal vessels, and high astigmatic refractive errors.[142] Although photophobia is generally believed to be a major symptom of albinos, this has not been a universal experience, and sunglasses may further compromise the reduced visual acuity of some patients. Abnormal decussation of temporal optic nerve fibers in the optic chiasm is present in most, if not all, forms of albinism.[62] Visual acuity in patients with albinism usually clusters around 20/100 to 20/200, although acuities as good as 20/40 have been observed in some patients with tyrosinase-positive oculocutaneous albinism. The association of oculocutaneous albinism and anterior chamber cleavage malformations may not be coincidental[292] (and personal observations).

Children with albinism should be carefully refracted and any error of refraction fully corrected to prevent anisometropic amblyopia. Strabismus is corrected surgically, although patients never achieve binocular vision. Referrals for special education and low-vision aids may be necessary, although most children attend regular school. Monocular telescopes may be prescribed at 5 or 6 years of age. Albino children, as are all children with low vision, are allowed to hold their reading material as close to their eyes as they wish; they should be seated in the front row in class.

Ochronosis

Ochronosis refers to the deposition of golden-yellowish-brownish pigment in the skin and eyes of patients with *alkaptonuria*. This autosomal recessive disorder affects 1 of 250,000 newborns and results from a deficiency of the enzyme homogentisic acid oxidase or homogenitsate 1,2-dioxygenase, whose gene maps to 3q21–q24.[69] The disease is most common in Slovakia and in the Dominican Republic. Homogentisic acid is an intermediate in the degradation pathway of tyrosine and phenylalanine. When it accumulates in the disease, it is excreted unchanged in the urine. It is then transformed into the ochronotic pigment benzoquinone acetic acid and its polymers in cartilage and connective tissue through the action of homogentisic acid polyphenol oxidase. In the urine homogentisic acid is oxidized to melanin-like products, especially in an alkaline pH, resulting in the dark urine of patients with alkaptonuria and the black diapers of babies with the disorder. The diagnosis of alcaptonuria relies on the demonstration of homogentisic acid in the urine because it is absent in normal individuals.[151]

Exogenous ochronosis may develop in persons who use carbolic acid (phenol) dressings chronically for the treatment of ulcers. Less commonly it may be seen in black women who use hydroquinone bleaching creams and in patients who have taken large doses of some antimalarial agents.[51]

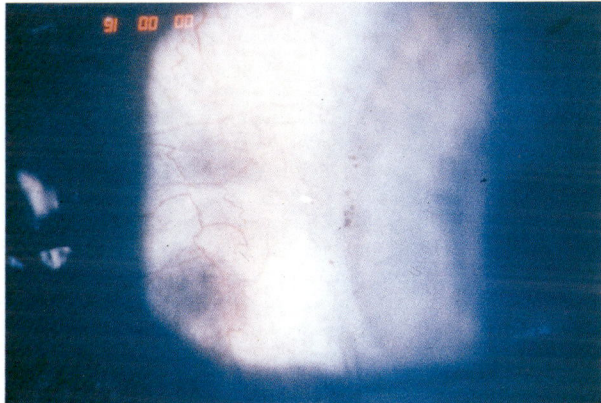

FIGURE 5-11. Episcleral, scleral and corneal deposits in a patient with ochronosis.

The deposition of ochronotic pigment in connective tissue leads to arthropathy, prostatic and renal stones, and cardiovascular changes. The disease, especially the spondyloarthropathy, may be disabling, but lifespan is not shortened. Skin pigmentation is most visible in areas of increased sweat follicles such as the axilla and the anogenital area and in thin skin, especially over cartilage such as that of the ears, nose, extensor tendons of the hand, and costochondral junctions.

Bilateral scleral pigmentation starts in the third decade of life and is variable. It is typically most pronounced near the insertion of the rectus muscles (Fig. 5-11). Less commonly, corneal globular areas of pigmentation are present in the peripheral cornea.[3]

Mayatepek et al.[176] suggested that supplementation of ascorbic acid in doses of 1 g/day represents a simple and rational treatment in patients with alkaptonuria. The arthropathy is treated with analgesics and physiotherapy. Joint replacement may be necessary in advanced cases.

Ichthyosis

Ichthyosis refers to the presence of cutaneous scales, hence the terminology (Greek *ichthys*, fish). Ichthyosis is a feature of a number of distinct genetic and nongenetic disorders.[126,303] Most patients, however, fall into one of the following categories. (1) *Ichthyosis vulgaris*, which is dominantly inherited, has its onset in childhood and occurs in 1 in 5300 live births.[304] The scales are fine and white and involve the trunk and limbs, sparing the flexor areas. Ocular findings are restricted to mild scaling of the lids. (2) *X-linked ichthyosis*, which is caused by a deficiency of the enzyme steroid sulfatase,[182,250] and affects 1 in 6,200 males.[304] The onset is in the first 6 months of life. The scales are large and yellow and involve the neck, trunk, and limbs including the flexor areas. The lids are affected, and there may be pre-Descemet's fine irregular gray punctate stromal deposits from limbus to limbus in affected males and carrier females; these deposits do not lead to any corneal dysfunction, and patients are asymptomatic. The absence of corneal deposits does not exclude the diagnosis of X-linked ichthyosis because in some authors' experience they are present in only 50% of cases.[126] (3) *Lamellar ichthyosis*, which is autosomal recessive and exceedingly rare, affects 1 in 300,000 individuals.[304] It is caused by mutations in the keratinocyte transglutaminase (TGM1) on14q11.2.[241] Genetic heterogeneity exists, and there is a second locus on 2q33–q35 as well as a third locus on 19p12–q12. Scales are present at birth; they are large and polygonal and involve all the skin of the body including palmar and plantar surfaces. The nails are thickened. Ocular findings include scaling of the lids with ectropion, lagophthalmos, and anterior segment exposure (Fig. 5-12). (4) *Epidermolytic hyperkeratosis*, which is also exceedingly rare, has an incidence of 1 in 300,000. It is autosomal dominant with scaling at birth. The scales are generalized, coarse, and verrucous and may be associated with bullae; they involve the eyelids. There is a nonbullous sporadic form of ichthyosiform erythroderma that also affects the eyelids.

Ichthyosis is also a feature of other genetic disorders such as the *Sjogren–Larsson syndrome*[261] and *Refsum disease* (phytanic acid storage disease), both autosomal recessive, and the dominant *KID (keratitis, ichthyosis, and deafness) syndrome*,[262] in which recurrent episodes of keratitis lead to corneal opacification and vascularization. Deafness is present early in life and is not progressive.

Jay and coworkers[126] found increased peripheral fundus pigmentation in 21 of 62 patients with different types of ichthyosis; this finding remains unexplained. The same authors observed the corneal deposits in all patients with X-linked ichthyosis

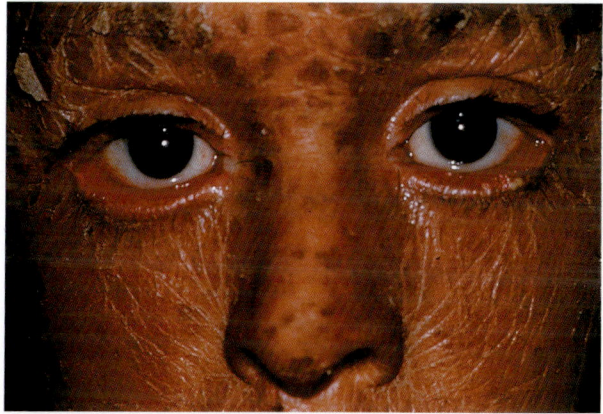

FIGURE 5-12. Bilateral ectropion in a patient with recessive lamellar ichthyosis.

older than 25 years but only in one-third of those under 25 and in 3 of 22 patients with dominant ichthyosis vulgaris.[126]

The management of ichthyosis consists of softening the skin using hydrating emollients such as petrolatum jelly. Keratolytic agents may be used to remove the scales, and retinoic acid reduces scale formation. The ocular surface in patients with lamellar ichthyosis and ectropion must be kept lubricated using ointments. Surgical correction of the ectropion is occasionally necessary. Prenatal diagnosis is possible in X-linked ichthyosis.[104]

Incontinentia Pigmenti (Bloch–Sulzberger Syndrome)

Incontinentia pigmenti was described by Bloch[17] and Sulzberger.[275] This genodermatosis is inherited in an X-linked dominant fashion that is usually lethal prenatally in males,[281] with rare exceptions.[77] In affected females, it causes highly variable abnormalities of the skin, hair, nails, teeth, eyes, and central nervous system. The prominent skin signs occur in four classic cutaneous stages: perinatal inflammatory vesicles, verrucous patches, a distinctive pattern of hyperpigmentation, and dermal scarring. The disease is caused by mutations in the *NEMO* gene and is referred to as IP2, or "classical" incontinentia pigmenti. Sporadic incontinentia pigmenti, so-called IP1, maps to Xp11 and is categorized as *hypomelanosis of Ito*. The evolution of lesions has been interpreted as representing death of cells that have the mutant-bearing X chromosome as the active one and their replacement by cells with a normal active X. The erythematous eruption with linear vesiculation in the newborn period is followed by a verrucous stage. After a few months, the verrucous growth is eliminated and is replaced by hyperpigmented areas that eventually disappear at about age 20 years.

In addition to the cutaneous abnormalities, 20% of patients have skeletal abnormalities including hemivertebrae, kyphoscoliosis, syndactyly, and leg length discrepancies. Hypodontia, delayed tooth eruption, and conical teeth are frequent.[33,187]

About 35% of patients have significant ocular abnormalities,[32] which are generally unilateral or markedly asymmetrical; 20% of patients have significant visual loss, mostly from retinal disease. The development of a retrolental mass of glial tissue may lead to confusion with retinoblastoma or retinopathy of prematurity. The eye with the mass is usually microphthalmic. Evidence of previous intraocular inflammation in some eyes with a retrolental mass has led to the presumption of an inflammatory etiology for the ocular process. An alternative pathogenetic mechanism is based on an ischemic etiology, such as may be the case in retinopathy of prematurity. Abnormal vascular anastomoses with peripheral zones of decreased perfusion and preretinal fibrosis were present in 17 of 19 patients reported by Watzke and coworkers.[300] Less common ocular findings include cataracts in 4% of patients, uveitis in 2%, and blue sclerae in 2%.[32] Other abnormalities include nystagmus, strabismus, microphthalmos, ptosis, pigmentation of the conjunctiva, corneal scarring, absence of the anterior chamber, optic atrophy, persistence of the hyaloid artery, and myopia.[77]

In a series of articles, Goldberg reported on the nature of the ocular complications of incontinentia pigmenti. He emphasizd that the ocular and cerebral abnormalities associated with this disease are far worse than the name would indicate. Although some patients have normal vision, total blindness or permanent visual deficiency may occur. Retinal vascular abnormalities, involving the periphery as well as the macula, appear to represent the primary disease process in the eye. Retinal detachment may then ensue, resulting from mechanisms that seem analogous to those of retinopathy of prematurity. Optic nerve atrophy and occipital lobe infarction are additional causes of severe visual dysfunction in some patients. He reported, for the first time, neonatal infarction of the macula in this disease.[92]

There is no specific therapy for the skin disorder. Cryotherapy[221] and laser photocoagulation have been used with some success in patients in whom the retinal disease was detected early.[34]

Cockayne Syndrome

The disease is named after Edward Alfred Cockayne (1880–1956), a London physician with particular interest in hereditary cutaneous diseases of children.

Cockayne syndrome is an autosomal recessive condition characterized by growth retardation, a progeroid facies with a small head, disproportionate long limbs, photodermatitis, and skeletal malformations with knee contractures resulting in a horse-riding stance.[40,41,207] In the classical form of Cockayne syndrome (type I), the symptoms are progressive and typically become apparent after the age of 1 year. An early onset or congenital form of Cockayne syndrome (type II) is apparent at birth.[164,189,208] Interestingly, unlike other DNA repair diseases, Cockayne syndrome is not linked to cancer.

Clinical features of type I become evident in the first 2 years of life. There is disproportionate dwarfism with cachexia, and patients develop progressive kyphoscoliosis, ankylosis and a horse-riding stance. The limbs are long and the hands and feet are large.[229,256] Patients are microcephalic and have a progeroid facies with lack of subcutaneous fat, prominence of the facial bones, and enophthalmos. Sensorineural deafness[253] and progressive neurodegeneration with mental deficiency, cerebellar ataxia, chorioathetosis, epilepsy, extrapyramidal tract signs, intracranial calcifications, and peripheral neuropathy become evident with time.[53] Photodermatitis of sun-exposed areas such as the cheeks is a prominent feature. Death ensues in the second to fourth decades. After exposure to UV radiation (found in sunlight), people with Cockayne syndrome can no longer perform a certain type of DNA repair, known as "transcription-coupled repair." This type of DNA repair occurs "on the fly," just as the DNA that codes for proteins is being replicated. Two genes defective in Cockayne syndrome, CSA and CSB, have been identified so far. The CSA gene is found on chromosme 5. Both genes code for proteins that interact with components of the transcriptional machinery and with DNA repair proteins. Cultured fibroblasts from patients with Cockayne syndrome are very sensitive to the lethal effects of ultraviolet-C (UVC) light. There is defective recovery of DNA and RNA replication, but no increase in chromosomal breakage or abnormalities in DNA repair as in *xeroderma pigmentosum* or Bloom syndrome.[113,153,222] Genetic heterogeneity has been demonstrated, and three complementation groups have been identified.[158,278] Patients with Cockayne syndrome are not at an increased risk for cancer.[249] Prenatal diagnosis is possible.[159] Patients may have hyperbetaglobulinemia, hyperinsulinemia, and hyperlipoproteinemia.

Enophthalmos is present in all patients with Cockayne syndrome and is caused by loss of subcutaneous and orbital fat. Visual acuity is surprisingly well preserved in most of patients in the face of advanced optic atrophy and retinal dystrophic changes.[286] Strabismus (exotropia or esotropia) is common. Nystagmus was present in 6 of 46 cases in one review.[209] A characteristic ocular finding in Cockayne syndrome is the poor pupillary response to dilating agents; this may result from atrophy of the dilator iris muscle fibers, as evidenced by peripheral iris transillumination defects in some patients. Pigment dispersion in the anterior and posterior chambers has been documented by histopathological studies by Levin and coworkers.[161] Raised inferior corneal lesions, band keratopathy and recurrent erosions have been described in some patients[23,43] and are probably caused by corneal exposure in neurologically impaired patients. Cataracts have been described in about 15% of patients with Cockayne syndrome[209] and were present in both of Cockayne's original patients.[40,41] Hyperopic errors of refraction as high as +10.00 diopters are present in the majority of patients.

Pigmentary retinopathy is one of the most consistent physical feature of the Cockayne syndrome. The fundus has a salt-and-pepper appearance with optic atrophy and arteriolar narrowing. Patients have been reported who lacked the typical salt-and-pepper appearance and exhibited denser black pigmentation in the posterior pole.[23] There is a variable degree of reduction of scotopic and photopic electroretinographic responses, most pronounced in older patients. Ocular histopathological studies in one case[161] revealed degeneration of all retinal layers; pigment migration into the photoreceptor layer; thinning of the choriocapillaris; and moderate atrophy of the optic nerve with gliosis. The retinal pigment epithelium was intact with excessive intracellular deposition of lipofuscin. Unusual pigmented cells were present in the retinal and subretinal space. There was widespread pigment dispersion in the anterior and posterior chambers and in the trabecular meshwork. The cornea was normal.

The management of patients with Cockayne syndrome consists of shielding the skin from ultraviolet light using sunscreen lotions. Errors of refraction and strabismus should be corrected early and cataracts extracted as in infants and children who are otherwise normal.

Focal Dermal Hypoplasia (Goltz–Gorlin Syndrome)

The major diagnostic criterion for the Goltz–Gorlin syndrome is the presence of focal areas of dermal thinning with protrusion of fat. The dermal hypoplasia forms reticular, vermiform, cribriform, and sometimes linear streaks.[93–95] The cutaneous streaks are reddish-brown, and telangiectasias and nodules of herniated fat may be covered by thin strands of connective tissue. The lesions are present at birth in the form of an erosive dermatosis. Papillomas of the lips, gums, anus, and vulva are frequent. The hair may be sparse, or there may be localized areas of scalp hypoplasia or poliosis. Nails may be dystrophic or absent, and there is marked hypoplasia of the teeth with late eruption and irregular placement. Patients are short and microcephalic, and there may be a variety of skeletal abnormalities involving the spine or digits. Radiologic findings are characteristic and show linear striations of long bones (osteopathia radiata), generalized osteoporosis, and widening of the symphysis pubis. Other systemic findings include joint hypermobility, congenital heart defects, asymmetry of the face, ear anomalies, deafness, genitourinary abnormalities, and defects of the abdominal wall. Patients may be severely retarded but some are remarkably intelligent.

Ocular abnormalities occur in about 60% of cases[114] and include widely spaced eyes, nasolacrimal duct obstruction, ptosis, ectropion, strabismus, nystagmus, microphthalmia, coloboma, aniridia, heterochromia, hypo- and hyperpigmentation of the retina, and optic atrophy. Furthermore, patients may have benign tumors of the lids and lid margins.

This disease is presumed to be X-linked dominant with lethality in males. The linear cutaneous and bony abnormalities are probably due to Lyonization (random inactivation of the X chromosome in different cell lines in the body). The management of patients with the Goltz–Gorlin syndrome is multidisciplinary, and individual abnormalities are approached as needed.

Linear Nevus Sebaceous

This condition consists of a triad of midline facial linear *nevus of Jadahsson*, neurological abnormalities such as seizures or mental retardation, and ocular abnormalities. A large number of cases have been reported since the original description by Feuerstein and Mims.[2,71]

The characteristic skin lesion may involve all the structures on one side of the face and consists of a smooth or verrucous yellow plaque and areas of alopecia. Histologically, there is papillomatous hyperplasia with hyperkeratosis of the epidermis and closely packed sebaceous glands. Malignant degeneration has been reported after puberty.[129] The majority of patients have seizures in the first year of life and are mentally retarded. Structural anomalies of the brain such as cerebral and cerebellar hypoplasia, cortical atrophy, and hydrocephalus may occur.

The nevus may involve the periocular and adnexal structures, resulting in ptosis, lid coloboma, and choristomatous lesions that may be epibulbar and lead to strabismus and amblyopia. Uveal coloboma and microphthalmia have been reported. One patient had a choroidal osseous choristoma with an overlying choroidal neovascular membrane.[152] One patient with linear nevus sebaceous and bilateral optic nerve hypoplasia has been reported by Katz and coworkers.[136] Traboulsi et al. highlighted the the association of posterior osseous and/or cartilaginous ocular choristomas with *epibulbar choristomas* in this condition.[282a] They reported four patients with epibulbar lesions and peripapillary lesions. Three patients had the triad of posterior osseous/cartilaginous ocular choristomas, anterior epibulbar choristomas, and *nevus sebaceus of Jadassohn*, and one patient had anterior epibulbar choristomas and posterior osseous/cartilaginous ocular choristomas. Ultrasonography and computed tomography were valuable in detecting scleral ossification or epibulbar cartilage or both. The ophthalmoscopic findings were similar to those of a choroidal osteoma. The authors concluded that the presence of posterior osseous/cartilaginous ocular choristomas in a patient with epilepsy or epibulbar lesions or both suggests the diagnosis of nevus sebaceus of Jadassohn or organoid nevus syndrome.

Oculodermal Melanocytosis

In the nevus of Ota[206] there is increased pigmentation of the episclera, uvea, and periocular skin, which may extend to involve the forehead or the nose, usually in the distribution of the first and second branches of the trigeminal nerve (Fig. 5-13). Ten percent of cases are bilateral. Oral and nasal mucosal involvement may occur, as can tympanic membrane, meningeal, orbital, and brain melanocytosis. In one-third of cases dermal involvement occurs without ocular melanocytosis; less commonly, the eye is affected without the skin. Isolated iridal melanosis may occur and, because of the nodular iris thickening, can be confused with neurofibromatosis. The lesions are not composed of nevus cells but rather of groups of dendritic or fusiform cells containing large melanin granules; these cells are located in the deep dermis and do not involve the basal epithelial layer that normally contains the dermal pigment. The

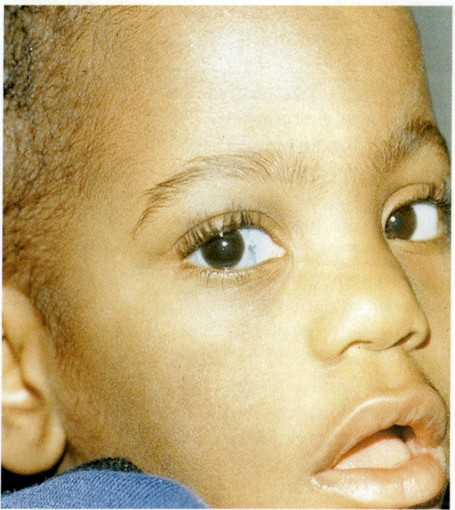

FIGURE 5-13. Young boy with nevus of Ota involving the upper face and episclera.

involved skin and episcleral areas take on a bluish-grayish appearance, and skin involvement may be difficult to detect in blacks in whom oculodermal melanocytosis (ODM) is more common than in whites. ODM is most commonly found in the Oriental race.[73] In a study of 194 Thailandese patients, Teekhasaenee and coworkers[279] found elevated intraocular pressures in the affected eyes of 10.3% of patients; 3 patients had infantile glaucoma, 14 had ocular hypertension or open-angle glaucoma, and 3 had acute angle-closure glaucoma. Additionally, 9.8% of patients had a cup-to-disc ratio greater by 0.2 or more in the ipsilateral eye in the absence of elevated intraocular pressure. ODM is associated with an increased incidence of uveal, cutaneous,[195] orbital, and intracranial melanoma.[59] Exact risk estimates are not available but are probably low. Patients with ODM should be examined frequently for the development of nodular cutaneous or uveal lesions and for the possible advent of glaucoma.

Xeroderma Pigmentosum

Xeroderma pigmentosum (XP) refers to a group of autosomal recessive conditions in which ultraviolet light-induced damage to nuclear DNA cannot be repaired through the normal endonuclease initiated multistep process. There is genetic heterogeneity, which can be demonstrated in vitro by cell complementation studies from different types of XP. At least nine different complementation groups (A through I) have been identified.[72] The discussion of these types and their molecular mechanisms are beyond the scope of this chapter. Defective DNA repair occurs in all nucleated cells including conjunctival cells.[194] The disease has a frequency of 1 in 250,000 in the United States and 1 in 40,000 in Japan, and is more frequent in countries where consanguinous marriages are common. Ultraviolet-induced damage is reflected clinically by sensitivity to sunlight, most noticeable in exposed areas. This sensitivity decreases with age. Freckling of the skin develops first, followed by dryness and scaling. Finally, hypopigmentation and telangiectasia develop along with actinic keratosis, keratoacanthomas, and verrucous papules.

Kraemer et al. examined reports of 132 patients with xeroderma pigmentosum.[147] Malignant skin neoplasms were present in 70% of the patients with XP at a median age of 8 years; 57% of the patients had basal cell or squamous cell carcinoma, and

22% had melanoma. The frequency of melanomas, resembling the frequency of nonmelanoma skin cancers, anterior eye cancers, and tongue cancers but not that of internal neoplasms, was increased 1000 fold or more in patients with XP who were younger than 20 years. The authors suggested that DNA repair plays a major role in the prevention of cutaneous cancers in the general population, and that sunlight exposure is responsible for the induction of melanoma as well as nonmelanoma skin cancers in patients with XP, although acting by different mechanisms for the two types of skin cancer.

About 20% of patients with XP have neurological abnormalities that may be more common in certain complementation subgroups of the disease. The neurological abnormalities include mental retardation in 80% of cases; microcephaly in 35%; progressive sensorineural deafness in 20%; spasticity and late onset of ataxia and choreoathetoid movements; abnormal electroencephalogram in 11%; and loss of neurons in the cerebral cortex or demyelination of the dorsal columns.

Ocular complications are limited to the anterior segment of the eye and occur in 40% to 80% of patients. The majority of patients have photophobia. Conjunctivitis, keratitis, and dryness of the ocular surface are common. Lid lesions with ectropion or entropion may occur. Squamous cell carcinoma develops in 13% of patients[64] and tends to involve the limbus and interpalpebral fissure area and to spread over the cornea. Conjunctival melanosis and melanoma have been described, as well as an angiosarcoma of the limbal area that developed in a granulomatous mass.[13]

Management of patients with xeroderma pigmentosum consists of protection from ultraviolet light and chemical carcinogens. Regular skin and ocular examination with photography are required with excision of suspicious tumors. More extensive surgical management such as dermabrasion, dermatome shaving, and skin transplantation may be required in advanced cases. Corneal complications of this disorder may require penetrating keratoplasty for visual rehabilitation. Surgery is rarely undertaken in these eyes because of multiple associated problems involving the ocular surface and the lids. Jalali et al.[125] reported three cases of successful penetrating keratoplasty in xeroderma pigmentosum and reviewed 9 cases reported earlier. Successful grafts were initially achieved in all 12 eyes. Graft failure occurred due to an untreated rejection episode in only 1 eye. Another eye was treated by exenteration for recurrent ocular malignancies. The authors recommended penetrating kerato-plasty in carefully selected patients.

Oral retinoids have been demonstrated to prevent new neoplasms but the dosage was toxic. Survival is reduced because of the development of malignant neoplasms. Early detection and prophylaxis from ultraviolet light has resulted in a reduction of malignant tumors and improvement of survival. There is a 70% chance of survival to age 40 years.

Ectodermal Dysplasia

The ectodermal dysplasias are characterized by abnormal hair, teeth, and nails and decreased or absent sweating. Ectodermal dysplasia occurs either as an isolated condition or in association with other systemic abnormalities. Freire-Maia[83] has catalogued more than 100 types of ectodermal dysplasias.

One condition of interest to the ophthalmologist is the association of ectodermal dysplasia with ectrodactyly and cleft lip/palate (EEC). Ectrodactyly refers to the absence of one or more digits derived from the central ray of the hand or foot, resulting in a cleft or lobster-claw deformity (Fig. 5-14).

The EEC syndrome was first described by Eckholdt and Martens in 1804 and was further delineated and named by Rudiger and coworkers.[240] Since then, numerous cases have been reported but the exact incidence of this disorder is unknown. The mode of inheritance is autosomal dominant with incomplete penetrance. Although frequent, ectrodactyly is not essential for the diagnosis, and patients without facial clefting have a characteristic facial appearance with maxillary hypoplasia, a short philtrum, and a broad nasal tip.[85] Genitourinary abnormalities are also a component of the *EEC syndrome*.[234] Tucker and Lipson[290] observed choanal atresia and vesicoureteric reflux in one patient. It seems that no sign is obligatory for the diagnosis.[85] Anneren and coworkers[5] suggested that low birth weight and polysyndactyly (without ectrodactyly) may be features of the EEC syndrome.

Patients with EEC are photophobic and have a chronic blepharitis. There is a reduction or absence of meibomian gland orifices at the lid margins, which results in decreased secretion of the oily component of tears and instability of the tear film. The lacrimal puncta, canaliculi, and lacrimal sacs are absent. Despite normal production of tears, the absence of oily secretion and instability of the tear film lead to a relative dry eye syndrome

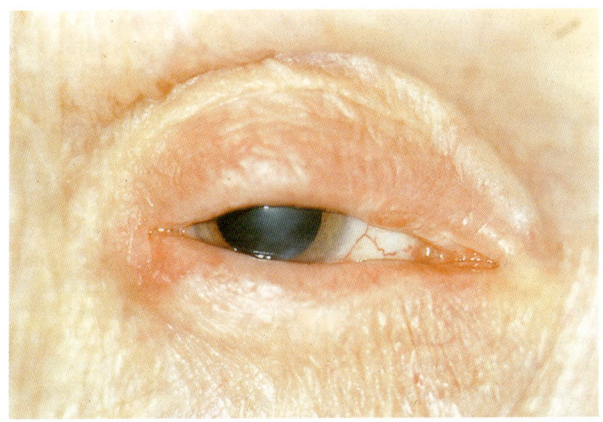

A

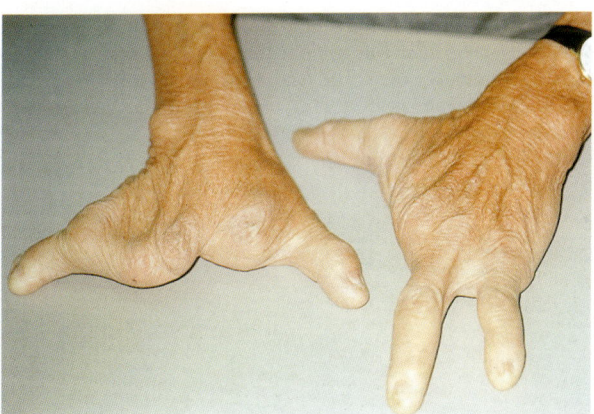

B

FIGURE 5-14A,B. Total madarosis (loss of lashes) in an adult with ectrodactyly–ectodermal dysplasia–clefting (EEC) syndrome (**A**). Note absent and fused fingers resulting in lobster-claw hand deformity (**B**).

with corneal vascularization and scarring. The corneal problems may, however, be due to the underlying ectodermal dysplasia. Treatment icludes surgical correction of the cleft and limb anomalies. Ocular lubricants are used to stabilize the tear film and reduce corneal scarring.

Another rare condition of interest to the ophthalmologist is the ectodermal dysplasia–ectrodactyly–macular dystrophy (EEM) syndrome. It is inherited in an autosomal recessive fashion and characterized by sparse hair, small and missing teeth, terminal transverse limb defects, and macular pigmentary changes.[1,202]

Juvenile Xanthogranuloma

Juvenile xanthogranuloma (JXG) is a benign histiocytic inflammatory condition affecting mostly infants and children in the first few years of life. JXG does not evolve into any of the histiocytosis-X group of conditions. Its etiology is unknown, although there is some evidence that it may represent a histioxanthomatous response to local tissue injury. JXG is present at birth in 30% of cases. Most cases, however, are detected in the first 2 years of life.

Cutaneous lesions may be as few as two or three in number (Fig. 5-15) or as many as several hundred. The lesions characteristically involve the scalp, face, neck, upper trunk, and proximal upper extremities. Varying in size from 1 to 20 mm, skin lesions may be relatively flat or may be elevated. Lesions thin with time and turn from orange-yellow to brown in color and then disappear, leaving a hypo- or hyperpigmented scar. Histo-

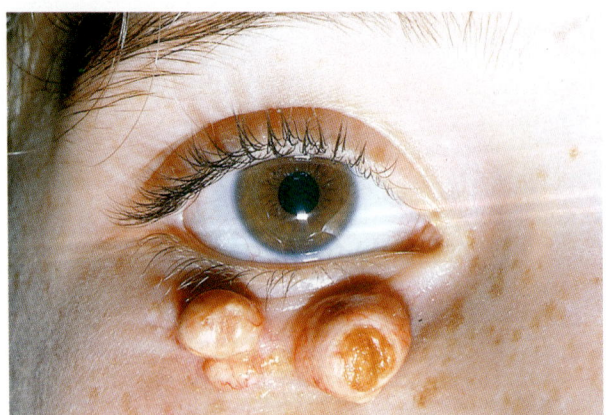

FIGURE 5-15. Multiple unusually large xanthogranulomas in a 10-year-old girl.

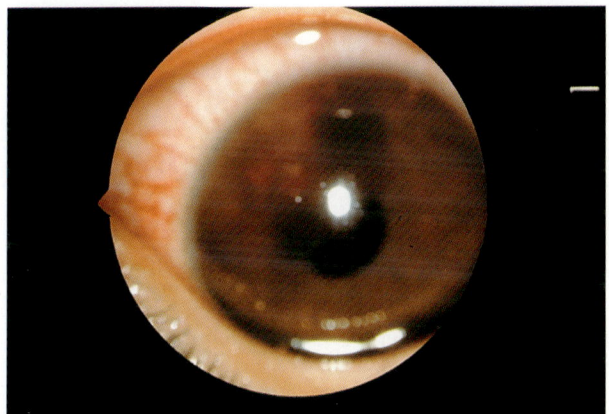

FIGURE 5-16. Hyphema in a 1-year-old girl with juvenile xanthogranu-loma. Tumor is partially masked by hemorrhage in superior aspect of the iris.

logically, skin lesions are composed of nodules of histiocytic pro-liferation with foam cell formation. Touton giant cells with cir-cularly arranged nuclei are characteristic.

Cutaneous and ocular lesions spontaneously regress over 3 to 6 years. Rarely, xanthomatous lesions have involved other tissues such as muscle, salivary glands, kidneys, testes, perios-teum, bone, colon, ovaries, pericardium, and myocardium. Metabolic and radiologic evaluations of patients with JXG have been consistently normal.

Ocular lesions may precede, follow, or occur simultaneously with the skin lesions. Occasional bilateral cases have been recorded. The iris and ciliary body are most commonly involved, but choroidal and retinal lesions have been reported. Other loca-tions include the lids, orbit, and extraocular muscles, and rarely the cornea, conjunctiva, and sclera. Iris lesions may be nodular or diffusely infiltrating. Because of their vascularity, iris lesions can spontaneously bleed, and JXG is a leading cause of sponta-neous hyphema in childhood (Fig. 5-16). This event may lead to glaucoma that may be relatively resistant to medical therapy. Infants with JXG may present with an irritated red eye or with corneal enlargement and clouding because of glaucoma. Rarely, patients may have an asymptomatic iris nodule or heterochro-mia irides.

Treatment of JXG is only indicated in the case of uveal involvement to prevent serious ocular complications. Topical steroids with or without systemic steroids are used. Radiation therapy may be of benefit in very selected cases if other therapeutic measures fail.

Erythema Multiforme and Stevens–Johnson Syndrome

Erythema multiforme is characterized by target-shaped skin lesions with or without erythematous macules, papules, wheals, bullae, and ulcerations of mucous membranes. The Stevens–Johnson syndrome refers to the severe form of erythema multiforme with extensive skin and mucous membrane involvement along with fever and affection of the kidneys, gastrointestinal tract, and central nervous system.[269] The mortality rate from the Stevens–Johnson syndrome ranges from 5% to 20%.[38] Both conditions affect primarily children and young adults, and while males and females are equally affected in erythema multiforme, more males are affected in Stevens–Johnson syndrome.

The disease is precipitated by infections or medications, most notoriously by herpetic infections, *Mycoplasma pneumoniae*, and sulfonamides. In many cases it is uncertain whether the medications or the infection for which they were given are the culprits. Histologically, there is a vasculitis that involves the superficial dermal vessels. Helper/inducer T lymphocytes and Langerhans' cells predominate in the dermis whereas cytotoxic/suppressor cells are found in the epidermis. In the conjunctiva there is an immune complex vasculitis with infiltration of the substantia propria by helper/inducer T cells.[6] The lesions of erythema multiforme typically involve the abdomen, the extensor surfaces of the legs and arms, and the dorsal aspects of the hands and feet. There usually is severe pruritus. The lesions, which usually appear in crops, subside within 2 to 6 weeks. Mucosal involvement occurs in about one-third of patients and affects the conjunctiva and buccal surfaces. The nose, genitalia, and anal region are rarely involved, but when they are stenosis may occur. Tracheal lesions occur in about 50% of patients with Stevens–Johnson syndrome and may result in constriction and asphyxiation; death, however, usually ensues from renal and central nervous system complications. Ten percent to 15% of patients with erythema multiforme have recurrences that are usually precipitated by herpetic infections. Episodic conjunctival inflammation may also follow the Stevens–Johnson syndrome.[74]

In the ocular surface, squamous metaplasia and conjunctival scarring lead to a dry eye state, trichiasis, corneal ulceration, scarring, and neovascularization.

The treatment of erythema multiforme and Stevens–Johnson syndrome consists of carrying patients over the period when the disease is most severe and managing the complications of systemic involvement. Antipruritic agents are helpful. Antibiotics are used to treat underlying or precipitating infections. High-dose systemic steroids may be used but their value is doubtful. Topical corticosteroid drops started early may prevent conjunctival scarring. Tear supplementation, lubricants, and bandage contact lenses are used to treat the ocular surface disorder. Topical retinoic acid may be of some value because of the squamous metaplasia. Oral acyclovir may be used in recurrent disease if a relation to recurrent herpetic infections is established.

SKELETAL DYSPLASIAS AND RELATED DISORDERS

Oculo-dento-osseous Dysplasia

Oculo-dento-osseous dysplasia (ODOD) is a malformation syndrome involving the hair, face, eyes, teeth, and bones.[97,183] The mode of inheritance generally autosomal dominant but a recessive variety probably exists.[90,282] Patients with ODOD have a characteristic facies with scarce eyebrows, narrow and short palpebral fissures, microcornea or microphthalmia, and a small nose with hypoplastic alae nasae and a prominent columella (Fig. 5-17A). The dental enamel is dysplastic, and microdontia or hypodontia may be present. Skeletal abnormalities are most prominent in the distal parts of the extremities with camptodactyly (position of permanent flexion) or syndactyly of the ulnar two or three digits; the toes are short and frequently lack second metatarsals (Fig. 5-17B). Other skeletal abnormalities include calvarial hyperostosis, a heavy mandible with an obtuse angle between the body and rami, plump clavicles, thickened ribs, and poorly tubulated long bones. Generalized hair abnormalities are manifested by hypotrichosis, trichorrhexis, and dry hair. Less common abnormalities include cleft lip/palate,

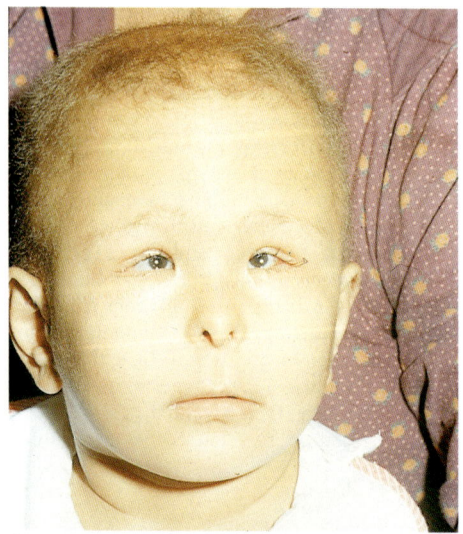

A

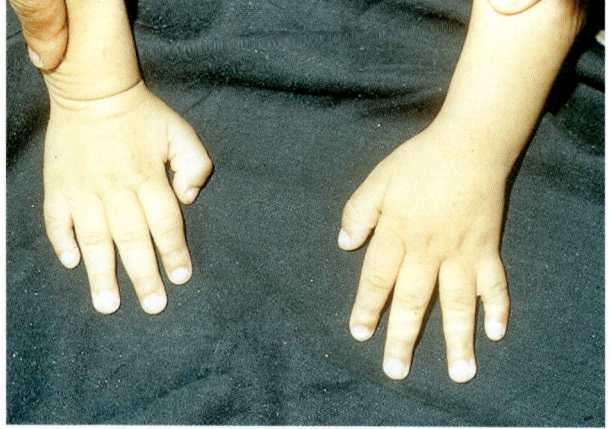

B

FIGURE 5-17A,B. One-year-old girl with oculo-dento-osseous dysplasia (**A**). Note syndactyly and camptodactyly of fourth and fifth fingers in both hands (**B**).

conductive hearing loss, hip dislocation, and osteopetrosis. Intellect is generally normal.

Lid abnormalities in ODOD include telecanthus and epicanthal folds in the majority of cases. Hypotelorism is present in 40% of cases.[66] Convergent strabismus is a frequent finding. There may be anterior segment dysgenesis, and the eye may be of low normal size or microphthalmic.[130] Anterior segment dysgenesis may be more severe in the rarer presumed recessive form of ODOD.[282] Remnants of the pupillary membrane are frequently present. Cataracts have been reported in two cases.[12,103] Posterior segment abnormalities have included remnants of the hyaloid system[103,282] and increased numbers of retinal vessels at the optic disc.[130]

Glaucoma has been reported in a total of 12 patients with ODOD.[285] Glaucoma can develop in ODOD at different ages and is caused by a variety of mechanisms, the most important of which is anterior segment dysgenesis. In infancy, it is probably due to trabeculodysgenesis. The onset of glaucoma in the patients reported by Meyer-Schwikerath,[183] Weintraub et al.,[302] and Dudgeon and Chisholm[58] was in childhood or early adulthood. An adult-onset open-angle type of glaucoma may occur, such as in one member of the family reported by Dudgeon and Chisholm.[58] Finally, angle-closure glaucoma has been reported by Sugar[273] in one eye of one patient who had infantile glaucoma in the other eye and in another patient he had previously reported[274]; the mechanism in this situation appears to be the presence of a lens of normal size in a small globe with a crowded anterior segment. Glaucoma is the most common cause of visual loss in patients with ODOD. Regular intraocular pressure measurements should be initiated as early as possible after diagnosis, especially in the presence of tearing, photophobia, and hazy or enlarged corneas. The management of glaucoma in ODOD patients is difficult, and multiple surgeries may be required.

Osteopetrosis (Albers–Schonberg Disease)

In osteopetrosis, failure of bone absorption occurs because of a defect in osteoclast function; this results in generalized bone sclerosis and the formation of bone that is more brittle than normal. There are characteristic radiologic findings, especially in the infantile form of the disease, with a sandwich appearance to the vertebral bodies and a masklike appearance to the skull. Two main categories are recognized: a more benign, autosomal dominant form, which is diagnosed in adulthood, and a severe, autosomal recessive, "malignant" infantile category that is probably heterogeneous. Patients with the adult form are diagnosed when X-rays are taken for other reasons or when they present with fractures from minimal trauma. In the infantile form of malignant osteopetrosis, which occurs in about 0.5 to 1 per 100,000 live births, there is extramedullary hematopoiesis when bone marrow spaces are obliterated; this leads to hepatosplenomegaly, frontal bossing, anemia, thrombocytopenia, and their complications. Another form of recessive infantile osteopetrosis that results from a deficiency of the enzyme carbonic anhydrase II features renal tubular acidosis and cerebral calcifications with milder skeletal affection than the lethal type.[150,263] A third and milder form of recessive osteopetrosis also exists with short stature, macrocephaly, disproportionate shortness of the limbs, recurrent fractures, and mild to moderate anemia.[132]

Deafness and optic atrophy occur secondary to a generalized thickening of calvarial bones that narrow the foramina transmitting cranial nerves, especially the third, fourth, and seventh nerves. Patients may have anosmia and facial palsy. A retinal dystrophy has also been reported in the recessive form of the disease, in addition to the compressive optic neuropathy may contribute to visual loss.[139,239] Decreased vision leads to nystagmus and strabismus. Because of the bony abnormalities in the skull, patients with the infantile type of osteopetrosis have widely spaced eyes and may develop exophthalmos.

High doses of calcitriol and a low-calcium diet may increase osteoclast activity.[140] Bone marrow transplantation has been used successfully in a few patients with the infantile form of the disease.[39]

Other Related Systemic and Craniofacial Disorders

See Chapter 5 for discussion of mandibulofacial dysostosis (Treacher Collins syndrome), oculoauriculo-vertebral dysplasia (Goldenhar's syndrome, hemifacial microsomia), Waardenburg syndrome, and Hallermann–Streiff–François syndrome (oculo-mandibulofacial syndrome, François' dyscephalic syndrome).

References

1. Albrectsen B, Svendsen IB. Hypotrichosis, syndactyly, and retinal degeneration in two siblings. Acta Dermato-Venereol 1956;1:96–101.

2. Alfonso I, Howard C, Lopez P, Palomino JA, Gonzalez CE. Linear nevus sebaceous syndrome. A review. J Clin Neuro-ophthalmol 1987;7:170–177.

3. Allen RA, O'Malley C, Straatsma BR. Ocular findings in hereditary ochronosis. Arch Ophthalmol 1961;65:657–668.

4. Allen RA, Straatsma BR, Apt L, Hall JF. Ocular manifestations of the Marfan syndrome. Trans Am Acad Ophthalmol Otolaryngol 1967;71:13–38.

5. Anneren G, Anderson T, Lindgren PG, Kjartansson S. Ectrodactyly-ectodermal dysplasia-clefting syndrome (EEC): the clinical variation and prenatal diagnosis. Clin Genet 1991;40:257–262.

6. Bahn AK, Fujikawa LS, Foster CS. T cell subsets and Langerhans cells in normal and diseased conjunctiva. Am J Ophthalmol 1982; 94:205–212.

7. Balestrazzi P, Corrini L, Villani G, Bolla MP, Casa F, Bernasconi S. The Cohen syndrome: clinical and endocrinological studies of two new cases. J Med Genet 1980;17:430–432.

8. Barton DE, Kwon BS, Francke U. Human tyrosinase gene, mapped to chromosome 11(q14–q21), defines second region of homology with mouse chromosome 7. Genomics 1988;3:17–24.

9. Beighton H. X-linked inheritance in the Ehlers-Danlos syndrome. Br Med J 1968;2:409–411.

10. Beighton P. Serious complications in the Ehlers–Danlos syndrome. Br J Ophthalmol 1970;54:263–268.

11. Beighton P, de Paepe A, Danks D, et al. International nosology of heritable disorders of connective tissue, Berlin 1986. Am J Med Genet 1988;29:581–594.

12. Beighton P, Hamersma H, Raad M. Oculodentoosseous dysplasia: heterogeneity or variable expression? Clin Genet 1979;16: 169.

13. Bellows RA, Lahav M, Lepreau FJ, Albert M. Ocular manifestations of xeroderma pigmentosum in a black family. Arch Ophthalmol 1974;92:113–117.

14. Bergen AAB, Sammans C, Schuurman EJM, et al. Multiplant linkage analysis in X-linked ocular albinism of the Nettleship–Falls type. Hum Genet 1991;88:162–166.

15. Bergen AA, Plomp AS, Schuurman EJ, et al. Mutations in ABCC6 cause pseudoxanthoma elasticum. Nat Genet 2000;25:228–231.

16. Bick D, Curry CJR, McGill JR, Schorderet DF, Bux, Moore CM. Male infant with ichthyosis, Kallmann syndrome, chondrodysplasia punctata, and an Xp chromosome deletion. Am J Med Genet 1989;33:100–107.

17. Bloch B. Eigentumliche, bisher nicht beschriebene Pigment-affektion (incontinentia pigmenti). Schweiz Med Wochenchr 1926;56:404.

18. Boileau C, Jondeau G, Babron M-C, et al. Autosomal dominant Marfan-like conneective tissue disorder with aortic dilation and skeletal anomalies not linked to the fibrillin gene. Am J Hum Genet 1993;53:46–54.

19. Bracken P, Coll P. Homocystinuria and schizophrenia. Literature review and case report. J Nerv Ment Dis 1985;173:51–55.

20. Brailey WA. Double microphthalmos with defective development of iris, teeth, and anus: glaucoma at an early age. Tr Ophthalmol Soc UK 1890;10:139.

21. Braverman N, Steel G, Obie C, et al. Human PEX7 encodes the peroxisomal PTS2 receptor and is responsible for rhizomelic chondrodysplasia punctata. Nat Genet 1997;15:369–376.

22. Braverman N, Lin P, Moebius FF, et al. Mutations in the gene encoding 3 beta-hydroxyseroid-delta(8), delta(7)-isomerase cause X-linked dominant Conradi–Hunermann syndrome. Nat Genet 1999; 22:291–294.

23. Brodrick JD, Dark AJ. Corneal dystrophy in Cockayne's syndrome. Br J Ophthalmol 1973;57:391.

24. Burgdorf WH, Dick GF, et al. Focal dermal hypoplasia in a father and daughter. J Am Acad Dermatol 1981;4:273–277.

25. Burian AM, Allen L. Histologic study of patients with Marfan's syndrome. Arch Ophthalmol 1961;65:323–333.

26. Byers PH, Wallis CA, Willing MC. Osteogenesis imperfecta: translation of mutation to phenotype. J Med Genet 1991;28:433–442.

27. Byers PH. Osteogenesis imperfecta. In: Riyce BM, Steinmann B (eds). Connective tissue and its heritable disorders: molecular, genetic and medical aspects. New York: Wiley-Liss, 1993:317–350.

28. Cadera W, Silver MM, Burt L. Juvenile xanthogranuloma. Can J Ophthalmol 1983;18:169–174.

29. Cadle RG, Hall BD, Waziri M. Phenotypic Ehlers–Danlos, type VI with normal lysyl hydroxylase activity and macrocephaly (Abstract). Am J Hum Genet 1985;37:A48.

30. Cameron JA, Cotter JB, Risco JM, Alvarez H. Epikeratoplasty for keratoglobus associated with blue sclera. Ophthalmology 1991;98: 446–452.

31. Carey JC, Hall BD. Confirmation of the Cohen syndrome. J Pediatr 1978;93:239–244.

32. Carney RG Jr. Incontinentia pigmenti. A world statistical analysis. Arch Dermatol 1976;112:535–542.

33. Carney RG. Incontinentia pigmenti. A report of five cases and review of the literature. Arch Dermatol Syphilol 1951;64:126–135.

34. Catalano RA. Incontinentia pigmenti. Am J Ophthalmol 1990;110: 696–700.

35. Catalano RA, Lopatynsky M, Tasman WS. Treatment of proliferative retinopathy associated with incontinentia pigmenti. Am J Ophthalmol 1990;110:701–702.

36. Chan CC, Green WR, de la Cruz ZC, et al. Ocular findings in osteogenesis imperfecta congenita. Arch Ophthalmol 1982;100: 1459–1463.

37. Clarkson JG, Altman RD. Angioid streaks. Surv Ophthalmol 1982; 26:235–246.

38. Claxton RC. Review of 31 cases of Stevens–Johnson syndrome. Med J Aust 1963;1:963.

39. Coccia PF, Krivit W, Cervenka J, et al. Successful bone-marrow transplantation for infantile malignant osteopetrosis. N Engl J Med 1980;302:701.

40. Cockayne EA. Dwarfism with retinal atrophy and deafness. Arch Dis Child 1936;11:1.

41. Cockayne EA. Dwarfism with retinal atrophy and deafness. Arch Dis Child 1946;21:52.

42. Cohen MM, Hall BD, Smith DW, Graham CB, Lampert KJ. A new syndrome with hypotonia, obesity, mental deficiency, and facial, oral, ocular and limb anomalies. J Pediatr 1973;83:280–284.

43. Coles R. Ocular manifestations of Cockayne's syndrome. Am J Ophthalmol 1969;67:762.

44. Collins TE. Cases with symmetrical congenital notch in the outer part of each lower lid and defective development of the malar bone. Tr Ophthalm Soc UK 1900;20:190–192.

45. Collod G, Babron M-C, Jondeau G, et al. A second locus for Marfan syndrome maps to chromosome 3p24.2–p25. Nat Genet 1994;8: 264–268.

46. Connor PJ, Juergens JL, Perry HO, et al. PXE and angioid streaks. A review of 106 cases. Am J Med 1961;30:53.

47. Conradi E. Vorzeitiges Auftreten von Knochenunjd eigenartigen Verkalkungskernen bei Chondrodystrophia foetalis hypoplastica. Jahrb Kinderheilkd 1914;80:86.

48. Cooper PH, Frierson HF, Kayne AL, et al. Association of juvenile xanthogranuloma with juvenile myeloid leukemia. Arch Dermatol 1984;120:371–375.

49. Crolla JA, Gilgenkrantz S, de Grouchy J, Kajii T, Bobrow M. Incontinentia pigmenti and X-autosome translocations: non-isotopic in situ hybridization with an X-centromere-specific probe (p SV2X5) reveals a possible X-centromeric breakpoint in one of five published cases. Hum Genet 1989;81:269–272.

50. Cross HE, Jensen AD. Ocular manifestations in the Marfan syndrome and homocystinuria. Am J Ophthalmol 1973;75:405–420.

51. Cullison D, Abele DC, O'Quinn JL. Localized exogenous ochronosis. J Am Acad Dermatol 1983;8:882–889.

52. Curry CJR, Magenis RE, Brown M, et al. Inherited chondrodysplasia punctata due to a deletion of the terminal short arm of an X chromosome. N Engl J Med 1984;311:1010–1015.

53. Dabbagh O, Swaimann KF. Cockayne syndrome. MRI correlates of demyelination. Pediatr Neurol 1988;3:113–116.

54. De Toni T, Cafiero V. Sexual development in a girl with Cohen syndrome. J Pediatr 1982;100:1001–1002.

55. DeWeerd-Kastelein EA, Keijzer W, Bootsma D. Genetic heterogeneity of xeroderma pigmentosum demonstrated by somatic cell hybridization. Nature (Lond) 1972;238:80–83.

56. Dietz HC, Cutting GR, Pyeritz RE, et al. Marfan syndrome caused by a recurrent de novo missense mutation in the fibrillin gene. Nature (Lond) 1991;352:337–339.

57. Dietz HC, Pyerritz RE, Hall BD, et al. The Marfan syndrome locus: confirmation of assignment to chromosome 15 and identification of tightly linked markers at 15q15–q21.3. Genomics 1991;9:355–361.

58. Dudgeon J, Chisholm IA. Oculo-dento-digital dysplasia. Trans Ophthalmol Soc UK 1974;94:203.

59. Dutton JJ, Anderson RL, Schelper RL, et al. Orbital malignant melanoma and oculodermal melanocytosis: report of two cases and review of the literature. Ophthalmology 1984;91:497–507.

60. Dvorak-Theobald G. Histologic eye findings in arachnodactyly. Am J Ophthalmol 1941;24:1132–1137.

61. De Paepe A, Viljoen D, Matton R, et al. Pseudoxanthoma elasticum: similar autosomal recessive subtye in Belgian and Afrikaner families. Am J Med Genet 1991;38:16–20.

62. Drager UC. Albinism and visual pathways. N Engl J Med 1986;314: 1636–1638.

63. Eddy DD, Farber EM. Pseudoxanthoma elasticum. Internal manifestations: a report of cases and a statistical review of the literature. Arch Dermatol 1962;86:729–740.

64. El-Hefnawi H, Mortada A. Ocular manifestations of xeroderma pigmentosum. Br J Dermatol 1965;77:261–276.

65. Eustis S. Rhizomelic chondrodysplasia punctata. J Pediatr Opthalmol Strabism.

66. Fara M, Gorlin RJ. The question of hypercurtosis in oculoden-toosseous dysplasia [Letter]. Am J Med Genet 1981;10:101.

67. Farnsworth PN, Burke P, Dotto ME, et al. Ultrastructural abnormalities in Marfan's syndrome lens. Arch Opthalmol 1977;95: 1601–1606.

68. Feinberg A, Menter MA. Focal dermal hypoplasia (Goltz syndrome) in a male: a case report. S Afr Med J 1976;50:554–555.

69. Fernandez-Canon JM, Granadino B, Beltran-Valero de Bernabe D, et al. The molecular basis of alkaptonuria. Nat Genet 1996;14:19–24.

70. Ferre P, Fournet JP, Courpotin C. Le syndrome de Cohen, une affection autosomique recessive? Arch Fr Pediatr 1982;39:159–180.

71. Feuerstein RC, Mims LC. Linear nevus sebaceus with convulsions and mental retardation. Am J Dis Child 1962;104:675–679.

72. Fischer E, Keijzer W, Thelmann HW, et al. A ninth complementation group in xeroderma pigmentosum, XP I. Mutat Res 1985;145: 217–225.

73. Fitzpatrick TB, Zeller R, Kukita A, Kitamura H. Ocular and dermal melanocytosis. Arch Ophthalmol 1956;56:830–832.

74. Foster CS, Fong LP, Azar D, et al. Episodic conjunctival inflammation after Stevens–Johnson syndrome. Ophthalmology 1988;95: 453–462.

75. Foster CS. Erythema multiforme. In: Gold DH, Weingeist TA (eds) The eye in systemic disease. Philadelphia: Lippincott, 1990:637–638.

76. Franceschetti A, Klein D. The mandibulo-facial dysostosis: a new hereditary syndrome. Acta Ophthalmol 1949;27:143–224.

77. François J. Incontinentia pigmenti (Block–Sulzberger syndrome) and retinal changes. Br J Ophthalmol 1984;68:19–25.

78. François J, Deweer JP. Albinisme oculaire lie au sexe et alterations caracteristiques du fond d'oeil chez les femmes heterozygotes. Ophthalmologica 1953;126:209–221.

79. Francomano CA, Liberfarb RM, Hirose T, et al. The Stickler syndrome is closely linked to COL 2A1, the structural gene for tye II collagen. Pathol Immunopathol Res 1988;7:104–106.

80. Francomano CA, Liberfarb RM, Hirose T, et al. The Stickler syndrome: evidence for close linkage to the structural gene for type II collagen. Genomics 1987;1:293–296.

81. Freedman J. Xeroderma pigmentosum and band-shpaed nodular corneal dystrophy. Br J Ophthalmol 1977;61:96–100.

82. Friedman E, Sack J. The Cohen syndrome: report of five new cases and a review of the literature. J Craniofacial Genet Dev Biol 1982;2:193–200.

83. Freire-Maia N, Pinheiro M. Ectodermal dysplasias: a clinical and genetic study. New York: Liss, 1984.

84. Fryer AE, Upadhyaya M, Littler M, et al. Exclusion of COL 2A1 as a candidate gene in a family with Wagner–Stickler syndrome. J Med Genet 1990;27:91–93.

85. Fryns JP, Legius E, Dereymaeker AM, Van Den Bergh H. EEC syndrome without ectrodactyly: report of two new families. J Med Genet 1990;27:165–168.

86. Gaasterland DE, Rodrigues MM, Moshell AN. Ocular involvement in xeroderma pigmentosum. Ophthalmology 1982;89:980–986.

87. Giebel LB, Tripathi RK, Strunk KM, et al. Tyrosinase gene mutations associated with type IB ("yellow") oculocutaneous albinism. Am J Hum Genet 1991;48:1159–1167.

88. Gilgenkrantz S, Mitchell G, Frezal J, et al. Linkage studies do not confirm the cytogenic location of incontinentia pigmenti on Xp11. Hum Genet 1988;80:282.

89. Giller H, Kaufmann WC. Ocular lesions in xeroderma pigmentosum. Am J Ophthalmol 1959;62:130–133.

90. Gillespie FD. A hereditary syndrome: "dysplasia oculodentodigitalis." Arch Ophthalmol 1964;71:187.

91. Glesby MJ, Pyeritz RE. Association of mitral valve prolapse and systemic abnormalities of connective tissue. A phenotypic continuum. JAMA 1989;262:523–528.

92. Goldberg MF. The blinding mechanisms of incontinentia pigmenti. Ophthalmic Genet 1994;15:69–76.

93. Goltz RW, Peterson WC, Gorlin RJ, Ravits HG. Focal dermal hypoplasia. Arch Dermatol 1962;86:708–717.

94. Goltz RW, et al. Focal dermal hypoplasia syndrome: a review of the literature and report of two cases. Arch Dermatol 1970;101:1–11.

95. Goltz RW. Focal dermal hypoplasia syndrome: an update [Editorial]. Arch Dermatol 1992;128:1108–1111.

96. Goodman RM, Smith EW, Paton D, et al. Pseudoxanthoma elasticum: a clinical study and histopathological study. Medicine (Baltim) 1963;42:297–334.

97. Gorlin RJ, Meskin LH, Geme JW. Oculodentodigital dysplasia. J Pediatr 1963;63:69.

98. Gorlin RJ, L'Heureux PR, Shapiro I. Weill–Marchesani syndrome in two generations: genetic heterogeneity or pseudodominance? J Pediatr Ophthalmol Strabismus 1974;11:139–144.

99. Gorski JL, Burright EN, Harnden CE, Stein CK, Glover TW, Reyner EL. Localization of DNA sequences to a region within xp11.21 between incontinentia pigmenti (IP1) X-chromosomal translocation breakpoints. Am J Hum Genet 1991;48:53–64.

100. Gott VL, Pyeritz RE, Magovern GJ Jr, et al. Surgical treatment of aneurysm of the ascending aorta in the Marfan syndrome: results of composite-graft repair in 50 patients. N Engl J Med 1986;314:1070–1074.

101. Gruber MA, Graham TP Jr, Engel E. Marfan syndrome with contractural arachnodactyly and severe mitral regurgitation in a premature infant. J Pediatr 1978;93:80–82.

102. Gutmann DH, Brooks ML, Emanuel BC, McDonald-McGinn DM, Zackai EH. Congenital nystagmus in a (46XX/45X) mosaic woman from a family with X-linked congenital nystagmus. Am J Hum Genet 1991;39:167–169.

103. Guttierez-Diaz A, Alonso MI, Borda M. Oculodentodigital dysplasia. Ophthalmic Paediatr Genet 1982;1:227.

104. Hahnel R, Hahnel E, Wysocki SJ, Wilkinson SP, Hockey A. Prenatal diagnosis of X-linked ichthyosis. Clin Chim Acta 1982;120:143–152.

105. Happle R. X-linked dominant chondrodysplasia punctata. Review of the literature and report of a case. Hum Genet 1979;53:65–73.

106. Happle R, Lenz W. Striation of bones in focal dermal hypoplasia: manifestation of mosaicism? Br J Dermatol 1977;96:133–138.

107. Harris A, Lankester S, Haan E, et al. The gene for incontinentia pigmenti: failure of linkage studies using DNA probes to confirm cytogenic localization. Clin Genet 1988;34:1.

108. Hausser I, Anton-Lamprecht I. Early preclinical diagnosis of dominant pseudoxanthoma elasticum by specific ultrastructural changes of dermal elastic and colagen tissue in a family at risk. Hum Genet 1991;87:693–700.

109. Hermann J, France T, Spranger JW, Opitz JM, Wiffler C. The Stickler syndrome (hereditary arthro-ophthalmopathy). BDOAS 1975;XI(2):76–103.

110. Hermansky F, Pudlak P. Albinism associated with hemorrhagic diathesis and unusual pigment reticular cells in the bone marrow: report of two cases with histochemical studies. Blood 1959;14:162.

111. Heymans HSA, Oorthuys JWE, Nelck G, Wanders RJA, Schutgens RBH. Rhizomelic chondrodysplasia punctata: another peroxisomal disorder. N Engl J Med 1985;313:187–188.

112. Heymans HSA, Oorthuys JWE, Nelck G, Wanders RJA, Dingemans KP, Schutgens RBH. Peroxisomal abnormalities in rhizomelic chondrodysplasia punctata. J Inherit Metab Dis Suppl 1986;2:329–331.

113. Hoar DI, Waghorne C. DNA repair in Cockayne syndrome. Am J Hum Genet 1978;30:590.

114. Holden JD, Akers WA. Goltz's syndrome: focal dermal hypoplasia, A combined mesoectodermal dysplasia. Am J Dis Child 1967;114: 292–300.

115. Hollister DW, Godfrey M, Sakai LY, Pyeritz RE. Immunohistologic abnormalities of the microfibrilllar fiber system in the Marfan syndrome. N Engl J Med 1990;323:152–159.

116. Holmes LB, Walton DS. Hereditary microcornea, glaucoma and absent frontal sinuses: a family study. J Pediatr 1969;74:968.

117. Holmes RD, Wilson GN, Hajra AK. Peroxisomal enzyme deficiency in the Conradi–Hunermann form of chondrodysplasia punctata. N Engl J Med 1987;316:1608.

118. Huang S, Steel H, Kumar G, et al. Ultrastructural changes of elastic fibers in pseudoxanthoma elasticum: a study of histogenesis. Arch Pathol 1967;83:108.

119. Hull DS, Aaberg TM. Fluorescein study of a family with angioid streaks and pseudoxanthoma elasticum. Br J Ophthalmol 1974;58: 738–745.

120. Hunermann C. Chondrodystrophia calcificans congenita als abortive Form der Chondrodystrophie. Z Kinderheilkd 1931;51:1.

121. Hyams SW, Dar H, Neumann E. Blue sclerae and keratoglobus. Ocular signs of a connective tissue disorder. Br J Ophthalmol 1969; 53:53–58.

122. Iqbal A, Alter M, Lee SH. PXE: a review of neurological complications. Ann Neurol 1978;4:18–20.

123. Izquierdo N, Traboulsi EI, Enger S, Maumenee IH. Glaucoma in the Marfan syndrome. Trans Am Ophthalmol Soc 1992;90:111–122.

124. Izquierdo N, Traboulsi EI, Enger C, Maumenee IH. Strabismus in the Marfan syndrome. Am J Ophthalmol 1994;117:632–635.

125. Jalali S, Boghani S, Vemuganti GK, Ratnakar KS, Rao GN. Penetrating keratoplasty in xeroderma pigmentosum. Case reports and review of the literature. Cornea 1994;13:527–533.

126. Jay B, Blach RH, Wells RS. Ocular manifestations of ichthyosis. Br J Ophthalmol 1968;52:217–226.

127. Jay B, Witkop CJ, King RA. Albinism in England. Birth Defects Orig Artic Ser 1982;18(6):319–329.

128. Jensen AD, Cross HE. Ocular complications in the Weill–Marchesani syndrome. Am J Ophthalmol 1974;77:261–269.

129. Jones EW, Heyl T. Naevus sebaceus. Br J Dermatol 1970;82:99–117.

130. Judisch GF, Martin-Casals A, Hanson JW, Olin WH. Oculodentodigital dysplasia: four new reports and a literature review. Arch Ophthalmol 1979;97:878.

131. Judisch GF, Waziri M, Krachmer FH. Ocular Ehlers–Danlos syndrome with normal lysyl hydroxylase. Arch Ophthalmol 1976;94: 1489–1491.

132. Kahler SG, Burns JA, Aylsworth AS. A mild autosomal recessive form of osteopetrosis. Am J Med Genet 1984;17:451.

133. Kainulainen K, Pulkinen L, Savolainen A, Kaitila I, Peltonen L. Location on chromosome 15 of the gene defect causing Marfan syndrome. N Engl J Med 1990;323:935–939.

134. Kaiser-Kupfer MI, McCain L, Shapiro JR, et al. Low ocular rigidity in patients with osteogenesis imperfecta. Investig Ophthalmol Vis Sci 1981;20:807–809.

135. Kadrnka-Lovrencic M, Jurkovic S, Reiner-Banovac Z, Najman E, Lovrencic M. Dysplasia oculodentodigitalis. Monatsschr Kinderheilkd 1973;121:595.

136. Katz B, Wiley CA, Lee VW. Optic nerve hypoplasia and the syndrome of nevus sebaceous of Jadassohn. A new association. Ophthalmology 1987;94:1570–1576.

137. Khalil M. Subhyaloid hemorrhage in osteogenesis imperfecta tarda. Can J Ophthalmol 1983;18:251–252.

138. King RA, Olds DP. Hairbulb tyrosinase activity in oculocutaneous albinism: suggestions for pathway control and block location. Am J Med Genet 1985;20:49–55.

139. Keith CG, Retinal atrophy in osteopetrosis. Arch Ophthlalmol 1968;79:234.

140. Key L, Carnes D, Cole S, et al. Treatment of congenital osteopetrosis with high-dose calcitriol. N Engl J Med 1984;310:409.

141. King RA, Mentnik MM, Oetting WS. Non-random distribution of missense mutations within the human tyrosinase gene in type I (tyrosinase-related) oculocutaneous albinism. Mol Biol Med 1991; 8:19–29.

142. Kinnear PE, Jay B, Witkop CJ Jr. Albinism. Surv Ophthalmol 1985; 30:75–101.

143. Kloepfer HW, Rosenthal JW. Possible genetic carriers in the spherophakia-brachymorphia syndrome. Am J Hum Genet 1955;7: 398–419.

144. Knobloch WH, Layer JM. Clefting syndromes associated with retinal detachment. Am J Ophthalmol 1972;73:517.

145. Kousseff BG. Cohen syndrome: further delineation and inheritance. Am J Med Genet 1981;9:25–30.

146. Kraemer KH, Lee MM, Scotto J. Xeroderma pigmentosum: cutaneous, ocular and neurologic abnormalities in 830 published cases. Arch Dermatol 1987;123:241–250.

147. Kraemer KH, et al. Prevention of skin cancer in xeroderma pigmentosum with the use of oral isotretinoin. New Engl J Med 1988; 318:1633–1637.

148. Kraemer KH, Slor H. Xeroderma pigmentosum. Clin Dermatol 1985;3:33–69.

149. Kraus JP, et al. Cloning and screening of nanogram amounts of immunopurified mRNAs: cDNA cloning and chromosomal mapping of cystathionine beta-synthase and the beta subunit of propionyl-CoA carboxylase. Proc Natl Acad Sci USA 1986;83:2047–2051.

150. Krupin T, Sly WS, Whyte MP, et al. Failure of acetazolamide to decrease intraocular pressure in patients with carbonic anhydrase II deficiency. Am J Ophthalmol 1985;99:396.

151. LaDu BN. Alcaptonuria. In: Scriver CR, Beaudet AL, Sly WS, Valle D (eds) The metabolic basis of inherited disease. New York: McGraw-Hill, 1989:775–790.

152. Lambert HM, Sipperley JO, Shore JW, et al. Linear nevus sebaceus syndrome. Ophthalmology 1987;94:278–282.

153. Lambert WC. Genetic diseases associated with DNA and chromosomal instability. Dermatol Clin 1987;5:85.

154. Le Saux O, Urban Z, Tschuch C, et al. Mutations in a gene encoding an ABC transporter cause pseudoxanthoma elasticum. Nat Genet 2000;25:223–227.

155. Lebwoh MG, Distefano D, Prioleau PG, et al. Pseudoxanthoma elasticum and mitral valve prolapse. N Eng J Med 1982;307:228–231.

156. Lebwohl M, Phelps RG, Yannuzzi L, Chang S, Schwartz I, Fuchs W. Diagnosis of pseudoxanthoma elasticum by scar biopsy in patients without characteristic skin lesions. N Engl J Med 1987;317:347–350.

157. Lee S-T, Nicholls RD, Bundey S, Laxova R, Musarella M, Spritz RA. Mutations of the P gene in oculocutaneous albinism, ocular albinism, and Prader–Willi syndrome plus albinism. N Engl J Med 1994;330:529–534.

158. Lehmann AR. Three complementation groups in Cockayne syndrome. Mutat Res 1982;106:347.

159. Lehmann AR, et al. Prenatal diagnosis of Cockayne syndrome. Lancet 1985;1:486.

160. Levin LS, Salinas CF, Jorgenson RJ. Classification of osteogenesis imperfecta by dental characteristics. Lancet 1978;1:332–333.

161. Levin PS, Green WR, Victor DI, MacLean AL. Histopathology of the eye in Cockayne syndrome. Arch Ophthalmol 1983;101:1093.

162. Levine RE, Snyder AA, Sugarman GI. Ocular involvement in chondrodysplasia punctata. Am J Ophthalmol 1974;77:851–859.

163. Liberfarb RM, Goldblatt A. Prevalence of mitral-valve prolapse in the Stickler syndrome. Am J Med Genet 1986;24:387–392.

164. Lowry RB. Early onset of Cockayne syndrome. Am J Med Genet 1982;13:209.

165. Macsai MS, Lemley HL, Schwartz T. Management of oculus fragilis in Ehlers–Danlos type VI. Cornea 2000;19:104–107.

166. Magid D, Pyeritz RE, Fishman EK. Musculoskeletal manifestations of the Marfan syndrome: radiologic features. Am J Radiol 1990;155:99–104.

167. Manzke H, Christophers E, Wiedemann H-R. Dominant sex-linked inherited chondrodysplasia punctata: a distinct type of chondrodysplasia punctata. Clin Genet 1980;17:97–107.

168. Marchesani O. Brachydaktylie und angeborene Kugellinse als Systemerk-rankung. Klin Monatsbl Augenheilk 1939;103:392–406.

169. Marfan AB. Un cas de deformation congenitale des quatres membres, plus prononcee aux extremites, characterisee par l'allongement des os, avec un certain degre d'amincissement. Bull Mem Soc Med Hop (Paris) 1896;13:220–226.

170. Marsalese DL, Moodie DS, Vacante M, et al. Marfan's syndrome: natural history and long-term follow-up of cardiovascular involvement. J Am Coll Cardiol 1989;14:422–428.

171. Maslen CL, Corson GM, Maddox BK, Glanville RW, Sakai LY. Partial sequence of a candidate gene for the Marfan syndrome. Nature (Lond) 1991;352:334–337.

172. Maumenee IH. The eye in the Marfan syndrome. Trans Am Ophthalmol Soc 1981;79:696–733.

173. Maumenee IH. Vitreoretinal degeneration: a sign of generalized connective tissue diseases. Am J Ophthalmol 1979;88:432–439.

174. Maumenee IH, et al. The Wagner syndrome versus hereditary arthroophthalmopathy. Trans Am Ophthalmol Soc 1982;80:349–365.

175. Maumenee IH, Traboulsi EI. The ocular findings in Kniest dysplasia. Am J Ophthalmol 1985;100:155–160.

176. Mayatepek E, Kallas K, Anninos A, Muller E. Effects of ascorbic acid and low-protein diet in alkaptonuria. Eur J Pediat 1998;157: 867–868

177. McDermott ML, Holladay J, Liu D, Puklin JE, Shin DH, Cowden JW. Corneal topography in Ehlers–Danlos syndrome. J Cataract Refract Surg 1998;24:1212–1215.

178. McGavic JS. Weill–Marchesani syndrome. Am J Ophthalmol 1966; 62:820–823.

179. McKusick VA. Multiple forms of the Ehlers–Danlos syndrome. Arch Surg 1974;109:475–476.

180. Mendez HMM, Paskulin GO, Vallandro C. The syndrome of retinal pigmentary degeneration, microcephaly, and severe mental retardation (Mirhosseini–Holmes–Walton syndrome): report of two cases. Am J Med Genet 1985;22:223–228.

181. Mevorah B, Frenk E, Muller CR, Propers HH. X-linked recessive ichthyosis in three sisters: evidence for homozygosity. Br J Dermatol 1981;105:711–717.

182. Meyer JC, Groh V, Giger V, Weiss H, Varbelow H, Schnyder VW. Rapid laboratory diagnosis of X-linked ichthyosis. Dermatologica 1982;164:249–257.

183. Meyer-Schwikerath G, Gruterch E, Weyers H. Mikrophthalmus-syndrome. Klin Monatsbl Augenheilkd 1957;131:18.

184. Migeon BR, Axelman J, Jan de Beur S, Valle D, Mitchell GA, Rosenbaum KN. Selection against lethal alleles in females heterozygous for incontinentia pigmenti. Am J Hum Genet 1989;4:100.

185. Mir S, Wheatley HM, Maumenee Hussels IE, Whittum-Hudson J, Traboulsi EI. A comparative study of the fibrillin microfibrillar system in the lens capsule of normal and Marfan syndrome patients. Investig Ophthalmol Vis Sci 1998;39:84–93.

186. Mirhosseini SL, Holmes LB, Walton DS. Syndrome of pigmentary retinal degeneration, cataract, microcephaly, and severe mental retardation. J Med Genet 1972;9:193–196.

187. Morgan JD. Incontinentia pigmenti (Bloch–Sulzberger syndrome) A report of four additional cases. Am J Dis Child 1971;122:294–300.

188. Morse RP, Rockenmacher S, Pyeritz RE, et al. Diagnosis and management of infantile Marfan syndrome. Pediatrics 1990;86:888–894.

189. Moyer DB, et al. Cockayne syndrome with early onset of manifestations. Am J Med Genet 1982;13:225–230.

190. Mudd SH, et al. Disorders of transulfuration. In: Scriver C, et al (eds) The metabolic basis of inherited disease. New York: McGraw-Hill, 1989:693–734.

191. Mueller RF, Crowle PM, Jones RAK, Davison BCC. X-linked dominant chondrodysplasia punctata: a case report and family studies. Am J Med Genet 1985;20:137–144.

192. Murdoch JL, Walker BA, Halpern BL, et al. Life expectancy and causes of death in the Marfan syndrome. N Engl J Med 1972;286:804–808.

193. Neldner KH. Pseudoxanthoma elasticum. Clin Dermatol 1988;6(1):83–92.

194. Newsome DA, Kraemer KH, Robbins JH. Repair of DNA in xeroderma pigmentosum conjunctiva. Arch Ophthalmol 1975;93:660–662.

195. Nik NA, Glew WB, Zimmerman LE. Malignant melanoma of the choroid in the nevus of Ota of a black patient. Arch Ophthalmol 1983;100:1641–1643.

196. Norio R, Raitta C. Are the Mirhosseini–Holmes–Walton syndrome and the Cohen syndrome identical? Am J Med Genet 1986;25:397–398.

197. Norio R, Raitta C, Lindahl E. Further delineation of the Cohen syndrome; report on chorioretinal dystrophy, leukopenia and consanguinity. Clin Genet 1984;25:1–14.

198. North C, Patton MA, Baraitser M, Winter RM. The clinical features of the Cohen syndrome: further case reports. J Med Genet 1985;22:131–134.

199. O'Donnell FE Jr, King RA, Green WR, Wilkope J Jr. Autosomal recessively inherited ocular albinism: a new form of ocular albinism affecting females as severely as males. Arch Ophthalmol 1978;96:1621–1625.

200. O'Donnell FE Jr, Hambrick GW Jr, Green WR, Iliff WJ, Stone DL: X-linked ocular albinism: an oculocutaneous macromelanosomal disorder. Arch Ophthalmol 1976;94:1883–1892.

201. O'Donnell FE Jr, Green WR, Fleischman JA, Hambrick GW. X-linked ocular albinism in blacks. Ocular albinism cum pigmento. Arch Ophthalmol 1978;96:1189–1192.

202. Ohdo S, et al. Association of ectodermal dysplasia, ectrodactyly, and macular dystrophy: the EEM syndrome. J Med Genet 1983;20:52–57.

203. Oorthuys JWE, Loewer-Sieger DH, Schutgens RBH, Wanders RJA, Heymans HSA, Bleeker-Wagemakers EM. Peroxisomal dysfunction in chondrodysplasia punctata, rhizomelic type. Ophthalmic Paediatr Genet 1987;8:183–185.

204. Opitz JM, France TD, Hermann J, Spranger JW. The Stickler syndrome. N Engl J Med 1972;286:546–547.

205. Ormerod AD, White MI, McKay E, Johnston AW. Incontinentia pigmenti in a boy with Klinefelter's syndrome. J Med Genet 1987;24:439–441.

206. Ota M. Nevus fusco-caeruleus ophthalmomaxillaris. Tokyo Med J 1939;63:1243–1245.

207. Otsuka F, Robbins JG. The Cockayne sydnrome. An inherited multisystem disorder with cutaneous photosensitivity and defective repair of DNA. Am J Dermatopathol 1985;7:387.

208. Patton MA, et al. Early onset Cockayne's syndrome: case reports with neuropathological and fibroblast studies. J Med Genet 1989;26:154–159.

209. Pearce WG. Ocular and genetic features of Cockayne's syndrome. Can J Ophthalmol 1972;7:435.

210. Pearce WG, Sauger R, Race RR. Ocular albinism and Xg. Lancet 1968;1:1282–1283.

211. Pedersen U. Bramsen T. Central corneal thickness in osteogenesis imperfecta and otosclerosis. J Otorhinolaryngol Relat Spec 1984;46:38–41.

212. Percival SPB. Angioid streaks and elastorrhexis. Br J Ophthalmol 1968;52:297–309.

213. Pope FM. Two types of autosomal recessive pseudoxanthoma elasticum. Arch Dermatol 1974;110:209–212.

214. Pope FM. Autosomal dominant pseudoxanthoma elasticum. J Med Genet 1974;11:152–157.

215. Pope FM. Historical evidence for the genetic heterogeneity of pseudoxanthoma elasticum. Br J Dermatol 1975;92:493–509.

216. Preus M, et al. Waardenburg syndrome: penetrance of major signs. Am J Med Genet 1983;15:383–388.

217. Pries C, Mittleman D, Miller M, et al. The EEC syndrome. Am J Dis Child 1974;127:840.

218. Pyeritz RE. Marfan syndrome: guidelines for recognizing an elusive disorder. J Musculoskel Med 1990;Dec:21–35.

219. Pyeritz RE, Fishman EK, Bernhardt BA, et al. Dural ectasia is a common feature of the Marfan syndrome. Am J Hum Genet 1988;43:726–732.

220. Pyeritz RE, McKusick VA. The Marfan syndrome: diagnosis and management. N Engl J Med 1979;300:772–777.

221. Rahi J, Hungerford J. Early diagnosis of the retinopathy of incontinentia pigmenti: successful treatment by cryotherapy. Br J Ophthalmol 1990;74:377–379.

222. Rainbow AJ, Howes MA. A deficiency in the repair of UV and gamma-ray damaged DNA in fibroblasts from Cockayne's syndrome. Mutat Res 1982;93:235.

223. Ramsey MS, Fine BS, Shields JA, et al. The Marfan syndrome. Am J Ophthalmol 1973;76:102–116.

224. Ramsey MS, Dickson DH. Lens fringe in homocystinuria. Br J Ophthalmol 1975;59:338–342.

225. Ramsey MS, Yanoff M, Fine BS. The ocular histopathology of homocystinuria. A light and electron microscopic study. Am J Ophthalmol 1972;74:377–385.

226. Rennert OM. The Marchesani syndrome. A brief review. Am J Dis Child 1969;117:703–705.

227. Resnick K, Zuckerman J, Cotlier E. Cohen syndrome with bull's eye macular lesion. Ophthalmic Paediatr Genet 1986;7:1–8.

228. Riedner ED, Levin LS, Holliday MJ. Hearing patterns in dominant osteogenesis imperfecta. Arch Otolaryngol 1980;106:737–740.

229. Riggs W Jr, Seibert J. Cockayne's syndrome. Roentgen findings. Am J Roentgenol 1972;116:623.

230. Ringpfeil F, Lebwohl MG, Christiano AM, Uitto J. Pseudoxanthoma elasticum: mutations in the MRP6 gene encoding a transmembrane ATP-binding cassette (ABC) transporter. Proc Natl Acad USA 2000;97:6001–6006.

231. Robbins JH, Kraemer KH, Lutzner MA, et al. Xeroderma pigmentosum: an inherited disease with sun sensitivity, multiple cutaneous neoplasms, and abnormal DNA repair. Ann Intern Med 1974; 80:221–248.

232. Roberts WM, Jenkins JJ, Moorhead EL, Douglass EC. Incontinentia pigmenti, a chromosomal instability syndrome, is associated with childhood malignancy. Cancer (Phila) 1988;62:2370.

233. Rodini ESO, Richieri-Costa A. EEC syndrome: report of 20 new patients, clinical and genetic considerations. Am J Med Genet 1990;37:42–53.

234. Rollnick BR, Hoo JJ. Genitourinary anomalies are a component of the ectodermal dysplasia, ectrodactyly, cleft lip/palate (EEC) syndrome. Am J Med Genet 1988;29:131–136.

235. Roper SS, Spraker MK. Cutaneous histiocytosis syndromes. Paediatr Dermatol 1985;3:19–30.

236. Rosen E. Fundus in pseudoxanthoma elasticum. Am J Ophthalmol 1968;66:236–244.

237. Rovin S, Dachi SF, Borenstein DB, Cotter WB. Mandibulofacial dysostosis. A familial study of five generations. J Pediatr 1964;65: 215–221.

238. Royce PM, Steinmann B, Vogel A, Steinhorst U, Kohlschuetter A. Brittle cornea syndrome: an heritable connective tissue disorder distinct from Ehlers–Danlos syndrome type VI and fragilis oculi,

with spontaneous perforations of the eye, blue sclerae, red hair, and normal collagen lysyl hydroxylation. Eur J Pediatr 1990;149:465–469.

239. Ruben JB, Morris RJ, Judisch GF. Chorioretinal degeneration in infantile malignant osteopetrosis. Am J Ophthalmol 1990;110:1–5.

240. Rudiger RA, Haase W, Passarge E. Association of ectrodactyly, ectodermal dysplasia, and cleft lip-palate. Am J Dis Child 1970;120:160–163.

241. Russell LJ, DiGiovanna JJ, Hashem N, Compton JG, Bale SJ. Linkage of autosomal recessive lamellar ichthyosis to chromosome 14q. Am J Hum Genet 1994;55:1146–1152.

242. Sakai LY, Keene DR, Engvall E. Fibrillin, a new 350-kD glycoprotein, is a component of extracellular microfibrils. J Cell Biol 1986;103:2499–2509.

243. Sanders RC, Broers CJM, Pyeritz RE. Sonography of the Marfan syndrome in utero. (Abstract). Am J Med Genet 1989;32:239.

244. Sanders TE. Intraocular juvenile xanthogranuloma. Trans Am Ophthalmol Soc 1960;58:59–74.

245. Secretan M, Zografos L, Guggisberg D, Piguet B. Chorioretinal vascular abnormalities associated with angioid streaks and pseudoxanthoma elasticum.Arch Ophthalmol 1998;116:1333–1336.

246. Seery CM, Pruett RC, Liberfarb RM, Choen BZ. Distinctive cataract in the Stickler syndrome. Am J Ophthalmol 1990;110:143–148.

247. Sefiani A, Abel L, Hellert ZS, et al. The gene for incontinentia pigmenti is assigned to Xq28. Genomics 1989;4:427–429.

248. Sefiani A, M'rad R, Simard L, et al. Linkage relationship between incontinentia pigmenti (IP2) and nine terminal X long arm markers. Hum Genet 1991;86:297–299.

249. Seguin LR, et al. Ultraviolet light-induced chromosomal aberrations in culture cells from Cockayne syndrome and complementation group C xeroderma pigmentosum patients: lack of correlation with cancer susceptibility. Am J Hum Genet 1988;42:468.

250. Shapiro LJ, Weiss R, Buxmann MM, et al. Enzymatic basis of typical x-linked ichthyosis. Lancet 1978;2:756–757.

251. Sheffield LJ, et al. Chondrodysplasia punctata: 23 cases of a mild and relatively common variety. J Pediatr 1976;89:916–923.

252. Sheffield LJ, Osborn AH, Hutchison WM, et al. Segregation of mutations in arylsulphatase E and correlation with the clinical presentation of chondrodysplasia punctata. J Med Genet 1998;35:1004–1008.

253. Shemen LJ, et al. Cockayne syndrome, an audiologic and temporal bone analysis. Am J Otolaryngol 1984;5:300.

254. Sherer DW, Bercovitch L, Lebwohl M. Pseudoxanthoma elasticum: significance of limited phenotypic expression in parents of affected offspring. J Am Acad Dermatol 2001;44:534.

255. Shimizu K. Mottled fundus in association with PXE. Jpn J Ophthalmol 1961;5:1–13.

256. Silengo MC, Luzzatti L, Silverman FN. Clinical and genetic aspects of Conradi–Hunermann disease. J Pediatr 1980;97:911–917.

257. Silengo MC, et al. Distinctive skeletal dysplasia in Cockayne syndrome. Pediatr Radiol 1986;16:264.

258. Sillence DO, Rimoin DL. Classification of osteogenesis imperfecta. Lancet 1978;1:1042.

259. Sillence DO, Barlow KK, Garber AP, Hall JG, Rimoin DL. Osteogenesis imperfecta type II: delineation of the phenotype with reference to genetic heterogeneity. Am J Med Genet 1984;17:407–423.

260. Sisk HE, Zahka KG, Pyeritz RE. The Marfan syndrome in early childhood: analysis of 15 patients diagnosed at less than 4 years of age. Am J Cardiol 1983;52:353–358.

261. Sjogren T, Larsson T. A clinical and genetic study of oligophrenia in combination with congenital ichthyosis and spastic disorders. Acta Psychiatr Neurol Scand 1957;32(suppl 113):1–112.

262. Skinner BA, Greist MC, Norins AL. The keratitis, ichthyosis, and deafness (KID) syndrome. Arch Dermatol 1981;117:285–289.

263. Sly WS, Whyte MP, Sundaram V, et al. Carbonic anhydrase II deficiency in 12 fmilies with the autosomal recessive syndrome of osteopetrosis with renal tubular acidosis and cerebral calcification. N Engl J Med 1985;313:139.

264. Snead MP, Yates JR. Clinical and molecular genetics of Stickler syndrome. J Med Genet 1999;36:353–359.

265. Sonada T, Hashimoto H, Enjoji M. Juvenile xanthogranuloma. Cancer (Phila) 1985;56:2280–2286.

266. Spallone A. Incontinentia pigmenti (Bloch–Sulzberger syndrome). Seven case reports from one family. Br J Ophthalmol 1987;71:629–634.

267. Spallone A. Stickler's syndrome: a study of 12 families. Br J Ophthalmol 1987;71:504–509.

268. Spranger JW, Opitz JM, Bidder U. Heterogeneity of chrondrodysplasia punctata. Humangenetik 1971;11:190–212.

269. Stevens AM, Johnson FC. A new eruptive fever associated with stomatitis and ophthalmia: report of two cases in children. Am J Dis Child 1922;24:526.

270. Stickler GB, Belu PG, Farrell FG, et al. Hereditary progressive arthroophthalmopathy. Mayo Clin Proc 1965;40:433–455.

271. Stickler GB, Pugh DG. Hereditary progressive arthroophthalmopathy: additional observations on vertebral abnormalities, a hearing defect, and a report of a similar case. Mayo Clin Proc 1967;42:495–500.

272. Struk B, Neldner KH, Rao VS, St Jean P, Lindpainter K. Mapping of both autosomal recessive and dominant variants of pseudoxanthoma clasticum to chromosome 16p13.1. Hum Mol Genet 1997;6:1823–1828.

273. Sugar HS. Oculodentodigital dysplasia syndrome with angle-closure glaucoma. Am J Ophthalmol 1978;86:36.

274. Sugar HS, Thompson JP, Davis JD. The oculo-dento-digital dysplasia syndrome. Am J Ophthalmol 1966;61:1448.

275. Sulzberger MB. Uber eine bisher nicht beschriebene congenitale Pigmentanomalie (incontinentia pigmenti). Arch Dermatol Syphilol (Berl) 1928;154:535–542.

276. Summers CG, Creel D, Townsend D, King RA. Variable expression of vision in sibs with albinism. Am J Hum Genet 1991;40:327–331.

277. Tahvanainen E, Norio R, Karila E, et al. Cohen syndrome gene assigned to the long arm of chromosome 8 by linkage analysis. Nat Genet 1994;7:201–204.

278. Tanaka K, Kawai K, Kumahara Y, Ikenaga M, Okada Y. Genetic complementation groups in Cockayne syndrome. Somatic Cell Genet 1981;7:445.

279. Teekhasaenee C, Ritch R, Rutnin U, Leelawongs N. Glaucoma in oculodermal melanocytosis. Ophthalmology 1990;97:562–570.

280. Temple IK. Stickler syndrome. J Med Genet 1989;26:119–126.

281. The International Incontinentia Pigmenti Consortium. Genomic rearrangement in NEMO impairs NF-kappa-B activation and is a cause of incontinentia pigmenti. Nature (Lond) 2000;405:466–472.

282. Traboulsi EI, Faris BM, Der Kaloustian VM. Persistent hyperplastic primary vitreous and recessive oculo-dento-osseous dysplasia. Am J Med Genet 1986;24:95.

282a. Traboulsi EI, Izin A, Massicotte SJ, et al. Posterior scleral choristoma in the organoid nevus syndrome (linear sebaceous of Jadassohn). Ophthalmology 1999;10:2126–2130.

283. Traboulsi EI, Maumenee IH. Bilateral melanosis of the iris. Am J Ophthalmol 1987;103:115–116.

284. Traboulsi EI, Maumenee IH, Kolsky M, Wilson D, Weleber R. Ophthalmologic findings in chondrodysplasia punctata (Abstract). Ophthalmology 1989.

285. Traboulsi EI, Parks MM. Glaucoma in oculo-dento-osseous dysplasia. Am J Ophthalmol 1990;109:310–313.

286. Traboulsi EI, DeBecker I, Maumenee IH. Ocular findings in Cockayne syndrome. Am J Ophthalmol 1992;114:579–583.

287. Traboulsi EI, Whittum-Hudson J, Mir S, Maumenee IH. Microfibril abnormalities of the lens capsule in patients with Marfan syndrome and ectopia lentis. Ophthalmic Genet 2000;21:9–15.

288. Tse K, Temple IK, Baraitser M. Dilemmas in counseling: the EEC syndrome. J Med Genet 1990;27:752–757.

289. Tsipouras P, Del Mastro R, Sarfarazi M, et al. Genetic linkage of the Marfan syndrome, ectopia lentis, and congenital contractural arachnodactyly to the fibrillin genes on chromosomes 15 and 5. N Engl J Med 1992;326:905–909.

290. Tucker K, Lipson A. Choanal atresia as a feature of ectrodactyly-ectodermal dysplasia-clefting (EEC) syndrome: a further case [Letter]. J Med Genet 1990;27:213.

291. Uitto AU, et al. Focal dermal hypoplasia: abnormal characteristics of skin fibroblasts in culture. J Invest Dermatol 1980;75:170–175.

292. van Dorp DB, Delleman JW, Loewer-Sieger DH. Oculocutaneous albinism and anterior chamber cleavage malformations. Not a coincidence. Clin Genet 1984;26:440–444.

293. Viljoen DL, Pope FM, Beighton P. Heterogeneity of pseudoxanthoma elasticum: delineation of a new form? Clin Genet 1987;32:100–105.

294. Vintiner GM, Temple IK, Middleton-Price HR, Baraitser M, Malcolm S. Genetic and clinical hetrogeneity of Stickler syndrome. Am J Med Genet 1991;41:44–48.

295. Vogel A, Holbrook A, Steinmann B, Gitzelmann R, Byers PH. Abnormal collagen fibril structure in the gravis form (type I) of Ehlers–Danlos syndrome. Lab Investig 1979;40:201–206.

296. Wachtel JG. The ocular pathology of Marfan's syndrome. Arch Ophthalmol 1966;76:512–522.

297. Wagner H. Ein bisher unbekanntes Erbleiden des Auges (degeneratio hyaloideo-retinalis hereditaria), beobachtet im Kanton Zurich. Klin Monatsbl Augenheilkd 1938;100:840–857.

298. Wanders RJA, Saelman D, Heymans HSA, et al. Genetic relation between the Zellweger syndrome, infantile refsum disease, and rhizomelic chondrodysplasia punctata. N Engl J Med 1986;314:787–788.

299. Warburg M, Pedersen SA, Horlyk H. The Cohen syndrome. Retinal lesions and granulocytopenia. Ophthalmic Paediatr Genet 1990;11:7–13.

300. Watzke RC, Stevens ST, Carney RG. Retinal vascular changes of incontinentia pigmenti. Arch Ophthalmol 1976;94:743–746.

301. Weill G. Ectopie des crystallins et malformations generales. Annu Oculist 1932;169:21–44.

302. Weintraub DM, Baum JL, Pashayan HM. A family with oculodentodigital dysplasia. Cleft Palate J 1975;12:323.

303. Wells RS, Kerr CB. Genetic classification of ichthyosis. Arch Dermatol 1965;92:1–6.

304. Wells RS, Kerr CB. Clinical features of autosomal dominant and sex-linked ichthyosis in an English population. Br Med J 1966;1:947–950.

305. Wenstrup RJ, Willing MC, Starman BJ, Byers PH. Distinct biochemical phenotypes predict clinical severity in nonlethal variants of osteogenesis imperfecta. Am J Hum Genet 1990;46:975–982.

306. Wheatley HM, Traboulsi EI, Flowers BE, Maumenee IH, Whittum-Hudson J. Immunohistochemical localization of fibrillin in human ocular tissues. Arch Ophthalmol 1995;113:103–109.

307. White JG, Clawson CC. The Chediak–Higashi syndrome: the nature of the giant neutrophil granules and their interactions with cytoplasm and foreign particulates. Am J Pathol 1980;98:151.

308. Wilkin DJ, Artz AS, South S, et al. Small deletions in the type II collagen triple helix produce Kniest dysplasia. Am J Med Genet 1999;85:105–112.

309. Willi M, Kut L, Cotlier E. Pupillary block glaucoma in the Marchesami syndrome. Arch Ophthalmol 1973;90:504–508.

310. Winterpracht A, Hilbert M, Schwarze U, Mundlos S, Spranger J, Zabel RU. Kniest and Stickler dysplasia phenotypes caused by collagen type II gene (COL2A1) defect. Nat Genet 1993;3:323–326.

311. Wright KM, Chrousos GA. Weill–Marchesani syndrome with bilateral angle-closure glaucoma. J Pediatr Ophthalmol Strabismus 1985;22:129–132.

312. Zimmerman LE. Ocular lesions of juvenile xanthogranuloma. Am J Ophthalmol 1965;60:1011–1035.

313. Zlotogora J, BenEzra D, Cohen T, Cohen E. Syndrome of brittle cornea, blue sclera, and joint hyperextensibility. Am J Med Genet 1990;36:269–272.

Neurocutaneous Syndromes

Maria A. Musarella

The neurocutaneous disorders are a group of clinically and genetically heterogeneous diseases that are characterized mainly by harmatomas and tumor growth, involving tissues derived by the embryonic germ layer. Older literature has called these disorders "phakomatoses" (mother-spot). The modern nomenclature and traditional eponyms of these entities are given in Table 6-1. Each of the neurocutaneous diseases is recognized as a distinct clinical disorder.

This chapter covers the ophthalmic aspects of these syndromes, as well as the numerous and varied multisystemic manifestations. Although Proteus syndrome and multiple endocrine neoplasia (MEN) 2B are considered separate from the neurocutaneous diseases, they are covered here because of the clinical resemblance to classic phakomatoses.

NEUROFIBROMATOSIS 1

Historical Perspective

Dr. Robert William Smith first described neurofibromatosis 1 (NF1) in 1849 in his treatise on *Pathology Diagnosis and Treatment of Neuroma*.[100] However, this work received little attention. Neurofibromatosis is most closely linked with the German pathologist, von Recklinghausen, who described the main features of this entity in his classic paper of 1882.[111]

Etiology

About 50% of cases of NF1 result from new mutations. The NF1 gene has been mapped to 17q11.2 and positionally cloned. The

TABLE 6-1. Neurocutaneous Syndromes.

Modern nomenclature	*Eponyms*
Neurofibromatosis 1	von Recklinghausen disease
	Peripheral neurofibromatosis
Neurofibromatosis 2	Central neurofibromatosis
Tuberous sclerosis	Bourneville disease
von Hippel–Lindau Disease	
Ataxia telangiectasia	Louis–Bar syndrome
Sturge–Weber	Encephalotrigeminal angiomatosis
Klippel–Trenaunay	Angiosteohypertrophy
Wyburn-Mason syndrome	Racemose angiomatosis
Multiple endocrine neoplasia 2B	Mucosal neuroma syndrome
	(Wagenmann–Froboese)
Proteus syndrome	

NF1 gene is one of the largest genes in which mutations lead to a disease in humans. It is approximately 350 kb in size, consists of 60 exons, and encodes for 11 to 13 transcripts with an open reading frame coding for 2818 amino acids.[14] In 1990, the NF1 gene and its protein product, neurofibromin, were identified. The gene product is as a tumor suppressor protein.[27,42,108] The protein encoded by NF1 has structural and functional similarity to a family of GTPase-activating proteins (GAPs) that down-regulate a cellular proto-oncogene, p21-*ras*. *ras* has been implicated in the control of cell growth and differentiation, and the capability of neurofibromin to down-regulate p21-*ras* suggests that the loss of neurofibromin may lead to uncontrolled cell growth and tumor formation.[4,40,73]

Incidence

NF1 is estimated to affect 1 in 3500 individuals.[46]

Ophthalmologic FEatures

Ophthalmologic features of NF1 are listed in Table 6-2. The most common uveal finding in NF1 is the Lisch nodule, which is a melanocytic harmatoma of the iris.[63] These harmatomas appear as elevated, smooth, clear to yellowish or brown, gelatinous, dome-shaped lesions (Fig. 6-1). Lisch nodules are usually multiple, bilateral, and discrete, measuring up to 2 mm in diameter. Lubs and associates examined the prevalence of Lisch nodules in children. Lisch nodules were found in only 5% of NF1 in children younger than 3 years of age, 42% among 3- to 4-year-olds, 55% among 5- to 6-year-olds, and in all adults over 21 years of age.[66] Lewis and Riccardi reported that Lisch nodules occur in 92% of patients over age 6 years and that the number of Lisch nodules is correlated to the age but not to the number of neurofibromas and café au lait spots.[59] Thus, Lisch nodules are specific for NF1 but their absence in children does not exclude the diagnosis. Lisch nodules have been described unilaterally in segmental neurofibromatosis with findings that include café au lait spots confined to one side or segment of the body.

Glaucoma is infrequent but may be present at birth or in early childhood. The most common cause is neurofibromatous infiltration and obstruction of the aqueous drainage pathways.[39] Neurofibromatous infiltration of the ciliary body may cause secondary angle closure; neovascular and synechiae closure of the angle may occur. Gluacoma is more likely in the presence of a plexiform neuroma of the ipsilateral upper eyelid.

Retinal astrocytic hamartomas occur in NF1, sometimes causing retinal dialysis and traction retinal detachment.[29] Other retinal manifestations include combined hamartomas of the retina and retina pigment epithelium (RPE), capillary hemangiomas, choroidal neourofibromas, congenital hypertrophy of the RPE, epiretinal membranes, sectoral retinitis pigmentosa, and myelinated nerve fibers.

Choroidal neurofibromas are flat yellow and are typically recognized in the posterior pole as single or multiple lesions; these occur in as many as half of affected patients.[29] Conjunctival hamartomas are painless lesions appearing as salmon-pink growths on the bulbar surface and may infiltrate corneoscleral limbus.[48] Prominent corneal nerves have been reported in up to 25% of patients. Plexiform neuromas typically enlarge the upper eyelid with an S-shaped deformity and ptosis (Fig. 6-2).[54] These lesions are difficult to excise satisfactorily because they are invested within the lid structures without defined margins. Regrowth is likely following excision.

Proptosis in NF1 signals orbital neurofibroma, optic glioma, or congenital absence/dysplasia of the greater wing of the sphenoid bone.[54] In the latter case, pulsatile proptosis may be evident. Optic pathway gliomas are the predominant central nervous system manifestation of NF1 (Figs. 6-3, 6-4). The natural history of the optic gliomas is an area of intense study and great clinical interest. However, the gliomas in NF1 are probably more indolent than sporadic ones.[64] Most develop in the first 6 years

TABLE 6-2. Ocular Manifestations of Neurofibromatosis Type 1 (NF1).

1. Orbital
   General
       Plexiform neurofibroma
       Neurilemoma (schwannoma)
       Proptosis
       Displacement of the globe
       Pulsation of the globe synchronous with pulse but no bruit
       Enlargement of the optic foramen
       Underdevelopment of the orbital bones
       Absence of the greater wing of sphenoid
       Optic nerve gliomas
       Neurofibromas and the ciliary nerves
   Lids
       Ptosis
       Café au lait spots
       Plexiform neuromas
       Neurofibroma of the eyelid
2. Extraocular
   Conjunctiva
       Neurofibroma
       Nodules
           Thickening of the conjunctival nerves
   Sclera
       Nodular swelling of the ciliary nerves
3. Intraocular
   Anterior segment
       Nodular swelling of the corneal nerves
       Medullated/myelinated corneal nerves
       Posterior embryotoxin
       Unilateral keratoconus
       Buphthalmos
       Dense abnormal tissue in the chamber angle
       Defects of Schlemm's canal
       Focal iris (Lisch) nodules/hamartomas
       Neurofibroma of the iris
       Congenital extropion uveae
       Iris neovascularization
   Media
       Cataract (rare)
       Anterior subcapsular cataract
       Neurofibroma of the ciliary body
   Choroid
       Choroidal ganglioneuromas
       Diffuse neurofibroma of choroid
       Diffuse and nodular involvement neurofibroma
       Uveal malignant melanoma
       Choroidal nevi
   Retina
       Hamartoma of the retina
       Café au lait spots on the retina

TABLE 6-2. (continued).

      Sectoral retinal pigmentation
      Sectoral chorioretinal scar
      Myelinated/medullated nerve fibers
      Typical peripheral retinoschisis
      Congenital hypertrophy of the retinal pigmented epithelium (RPE)
    Optic nerve
      Optic nerve drusen
      Hamartoma of the optic disc
      Primary optic atrophy due to tumor pressure
        Secondary atrophy due to papilledema
    Glioma of optic nerve head (rare)
  4. Other
    Extraocular muscle palsies
    Congenital glaucoma
    Secondary glaucoma
    Strabismus

of life, and 50% to 75% of patients are asymptomatic at diagnosis. Presenting symptoms depend on the location: Orbital tumors can cause proptosis, reduction in visual acuity, visual field defects, optic nerve dysfunction, relative afferent pupillary defect, optic disc edema (Fig. 6-2) or optic disc atrophy and strabismus. Chiasmal invasion and expansion may lead to hydrocephalus or, in 39% of patients, precocious puberty.[43,78]

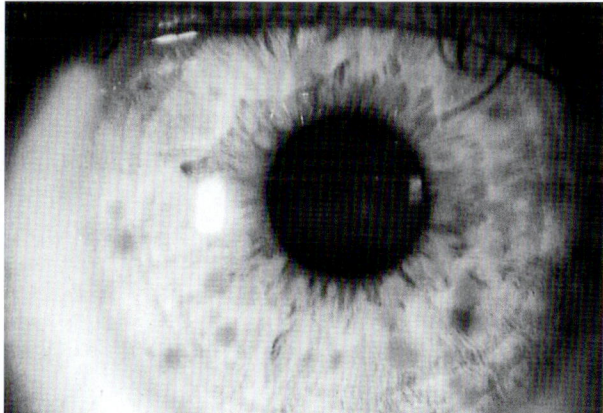

FIGURE 6-1. Numerous iris hamartomas on a lightly colored iris in a teenage boy.

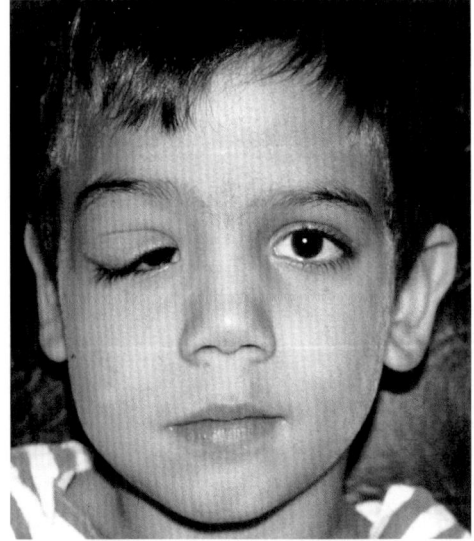

FIGURE 6-2. Plexiform neuroma is the right upper lid giving an S-shaped configuration in a 5-year-old boy with neurofibromatosis 1 (NF1).

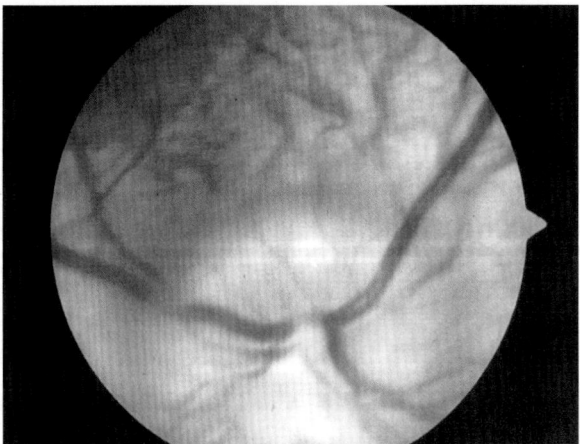

FIGURE 6-3. Optic disc edema from optic nerve glioma.

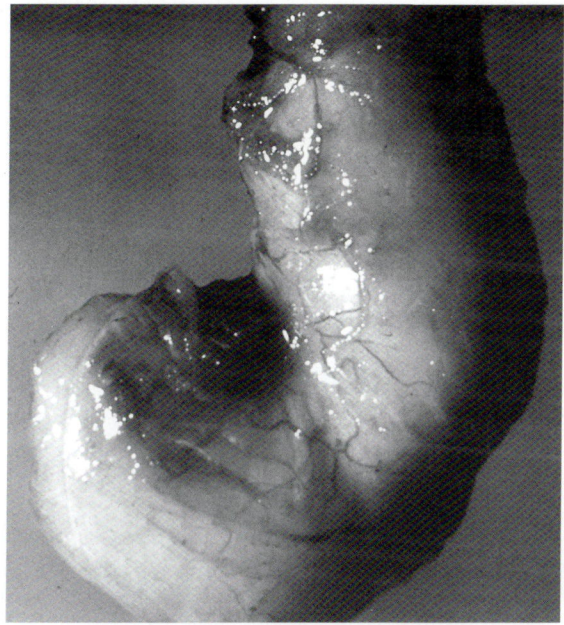

FIGURE 6-4. Optic glioma: gross pathology.

Clinical Assessment

Diagnostic criteria for NF1 developed by NIH Consensus Conferences are listed in Table 6-3.[78] The focus of the clinical assessment depends on the age of the patient. In the first 2 years of life, the presence and consequences of plexiform neuromas, glaucoma, sphenoid wing dysplasia, and pseudoarthroses are sought. Psychological assessment becomes important in preschool children. The possibility of hypertension from renal artery stenosis or pheochromocytoma demands annual measurement of blood pressure in all patients. Screening brain MRI scans in children with NF1 will detect optic nerve gliomas in 15%. In comparison to other conditions, the application of DNA testing in NF1 is relatively limited. The inability of present techniques to identify the numerous NF1 mutations limits their application. Even the most sensitive technique detects only 70% of mutations.[86] However, because clinical

TABLE 6-3. Diagnostic Criteria for Neurofibromatosis Type 1.

Diagnosis requires at least two of the following:
1. More than five café au lait macules
   Diameter: 5 mm or larger in prepubescent children, 15 mm or larger in adults
2. More than two neurofibromas (any type) or one plexiform neurofibroma
3. Axillary or inguinal freckling
4. Optic pathway glioma
5. More than two Lisch nodules (see text)
6. Osseous lesions (including sphenoid dysplasia or thinning of long bone cortex) + pseudoarthrosis
7. Affected first-degree relative

From Ref. 79, with permission.

diagnosis is usually straightforward, attempts at DNA testing are rarely required.

Systemic Associations

The principal cutaneous lesions are café au lait spots and neurofibromas (diffuse and plexiform); both lesions are found in 95% of patients. Café au lait spots are flat pigmented lesions, often with poorly defined, irregular borders; they are usually present on the trunk but may occur anywhere on the body. Neurofibromas are benign growths of Schawann cells, axons, fibroblasts, and perineural and epithelial cells. Multiple cutaneous neurofibromas develop in 90% of patients. Malignant peripheral nerve sheath tumors can occur in all types of neurofibromas. The overall risk is about 5%. Early diagnosis is hampered by frequent occurrence within preexisting large tumors, making new growth or change difficult to detect.[52]

Axillary and inguinal freckling is the presence of small café au lait spots in these areas.[24] Mild mental retardation and/or learning difficulties appear to affect about 30% to 40%.[86]

Recent studies show that the learning deficits caused by mutations that inactivate NF1 in mice and humans are caused by disruption of neurofibromin function in the adult brain, a finding with important implications for the development of a treatment for the learning disabilities with NF1.[23,116]

Other clinical features of NF1 include seizures, headaches, abdominal pain (caused by intestinal neurofibromas), vasculopathy, and possibly reduced platelet function. Some patients with NF1 have a phenotype overlapping Noonan's syndrome.[83]

Watson syndrome, a disease characterized by café au lait patches, mental retardation, and pulmonary stenosis, is thought to be allelic to NF1.[58]

Inheritance

NF1 is transmitted in an autosomal dominant fashion. Approximately 50% of cases are sporadic. There is no known racial, sexual, or ethnic predilection. Near-complete penetrance with variable phenotypic expression within and between families is typical.

Natural History

The majority of affected individuals have a benign course. Neurofibromas rarely develop in children younger than 6 years of age. Neurofibromas may increase in size and number during puberty, pregnancy, and the later decades. The complications of NF1 must be continuously sought and followed throughout the life of the patient.

Treatment

Specific treatments are available for some of the manifestations of NF1.[47] Tumors causing functional impairment or which are cosmetically objectionable may be treated with judicious surgical excision or debulking. A sympathetic plastic surgeon or ophthalmic plastic surgeon can benefit patient quality of life greatly. Obvious café au lait spots can be treated by dermabrasion. Neurofibromas causing pruritis can be treatment with ketotifen.[93] Optic gliomas in NF1 are treated conservatively, as their growth characteristics are typically most consistent with harmatomas rather than a true malignancy. Figure 6-4 shows an old specimen of optic nerve glioma treated surgically. Currently, aggressive and complicated cases are treated with radiation chemotherapy and surgical excision.[64]

Glaucoma in NF1 typically requires surgical intervention. Hypertension in NF1 can be caused by renal artery stenosis and pheochromocytomas and are treated with medication or surgery.[51] Orthopedic problems can be severe in NF1. Cervical kyphoscoliosis and tibial bowing are the two most common orthopedic problems. Spinal MRI is recommended to locate focal lesions in patients with kyphoscoliosis. Early treatment consists of braces and spinal fusion. Tibial bowing also is treated with braces to prevent factures and pseudoarthrosis.

Prognosis

The prognosis of NF1 patients varies widely. Surgical results depend on the site of the tumors. A new diagnosis of NF1 may be made in patients referred for the treatment of malignancy. Brain tumors tend to have a more indolent course in NF1 than in the general population and are managed more conservatively.

Future Research

New insights into the pathogenesis of NF1 may lead to the development of specific treatments with reduced toxicity and more precise molecular targeting. Improved understanding of the NF1 gene is needed to determine whether mechanisms other than *ras* regulation are important in pathogenesis. As new treatments are developed, improved methods to measure tumor growth and monitor outcomes will be needed. The ability to detect preclinical manifestations, as has been accomplished with MRI screening for optic pathway gliomas, will also become more important as treatments develop.

NEUROFIBROMATOSIS 2

Historical Perspective

The first documented case of neurofibromatosis 2 (NF2) was reported by J.H. Wishhart, who described a case of bilateral acoustic neuromas with multiple meningeal tumors.[113] NF2 was not established as a distinct entity until 1970.[115] NF2 was formally referred to as bilateral acoustic neuroma or central neurofibromatosis (the NIH Consensus Statement 1988).[78] As the tumors are histologically schwannomas arising on the vestibular branch of the eighth cranial nerve, the 1992 NIH Consensus Conference on Acoustic Neuromas recommended the use of the precise term vestibular schwannoma.[79]

Incidence

NF2 is much less common than NF1, with a prevalence of 1 in 33,000 to 40,000.[31]

Etiology

Cytogenetic study of meningiomas showing frequent loss of chromosome 22 provided the clue to the chromosome localization of NF2. The location of the NF2 gene was subsequently confirmed by linkage analysis.[32,96] Further studies identified flanking markers but showed no suggestion of locus heterogeneity.[77] The identification of a number of germline deletions in NF2 patients facilitated the cloning of the disease gene. The identified mutations include deletion of the entire gene or defective genes, which yields a truncated protein.[95] The gene product is called merlin or schwannomin, and is also a tumor supressor.

Ophthalmologic Features

The ocular signs in NF2 are extremely important because of the vision-threatening processes that may occur in affected children, who eventually become deaf. Posterior subcapsular cataracts (PSC) and posterior cortical cataracts occur in as many as 81% of patients.[87] These lesions caused significant visual disturbance in 2 of 47 patients with NF2. Retinal hamartomas (including combined pigment epithelium and retinal hamartomas, congenital hypertrophy of retinal pigment epithelium syndrome, and astrocytic hamartomas), epiretinal membranes, and optic disc meningiomas may lead to vision loss.[9] Additionally, intracranial tumors may cause papilledema with secondary optic atrophy. Cranial neuropathies can present with ocular motility disturbances.

Clinical Assessment

Clinical examinations continue to be important in the diagnosis of NF2. The diagnostic criteria for NF2 are listed in Table 6-3. Audiological testing may detect early sensorineural hearing loss, but contrast-enhanced MRI is required to identify or exclude small vestibular schwannomas.[10] Previously, at-risk individuals required biannual screening until 10 to 16 years of age and then yearly until 50 years of age. Molecular testing has altered traditional methods of clinical assessment. Molecular testing using linked genetic markers or direct mutational analysis can determine which at-risk individuals do not carry the disease mutation, freeing those patients from repeated clinical testing. Molecular testing permits earlier disease identification, allowing improved treatment.

A careful clinical examination with special attention to a dermatological evaluation, neurological symptomatology and ophthalmologic changes is mandatory. Initial radiographic evaluation of a patient known or suspected to have NF2 should include a cranial MRI scan with and without gadolinium enhancement.[30] Small intracanalicular tumors may not be seen on standard 5-mm slice thickness through the posterior fossa. Optimal evaluation includes 3-mm cuts overlapping by 1.5 mm on both axial and coronal postcontrast enhancement views through the internal auditory canals. CT scan may visualize large vestibular schwannomas and meningiomas. Audiological evaluation may show brainstem auditory evoked responds (BAER). Spinal MRI may be helpful in defining asymptomatic tumors. Genetic testing may be done on the basis of linkage when there is more than one affected individual. Because no mutation can be detected in at least one-third of individuals with typical NF2, mutational analysis is not useful for confirming a suspected diagnosis in a proband.

Systemic Associations

The hallmark of NF2 is the presence of bilateral vestibular schwannomas that occur in 85% of patients (Fig. 6-5).[71] In addition to the diagnostic criteria given in Table 6-4, if an individual with an affected first-degree relative has either a unilateral eighth nerve mass or any two of the following, then NF2 may be diagnosed: neurofibroma, hemangioma, glioma, schwannoma, or posterior subcapsular cataract or lens capacity at a young age.[32,79] Spinal tumors are a frequent manifestation of NF2.[74] There are often multiple tumors of variable types. Patients with NF2 tend to develop tumors of the neural coverings or linings such a meningiomas, optic nerve sheath meningiomas, schwannomas, and ependymonas.[18] Cutaneous and subcutaneous neurofibromas are found in NF2 but not nearly as frequently or severely as in NF1. Definitive genetic studies are useful in understanding patients with overlapping features of NF1 and NF2. Hearing loss in NF2 typically begins in the teens or twenties. However, it may present as early as the first or as late as the seventh decade. Schwannomas of the CNS are the most common type of tumor in NF2. In addition to the vestibular schwannomas already covered, other cranial nerves, especially the fifth, ninth, and tenth, frequently are involved. Spinal root and intramedullary schwannomas are also seen. Peripheral

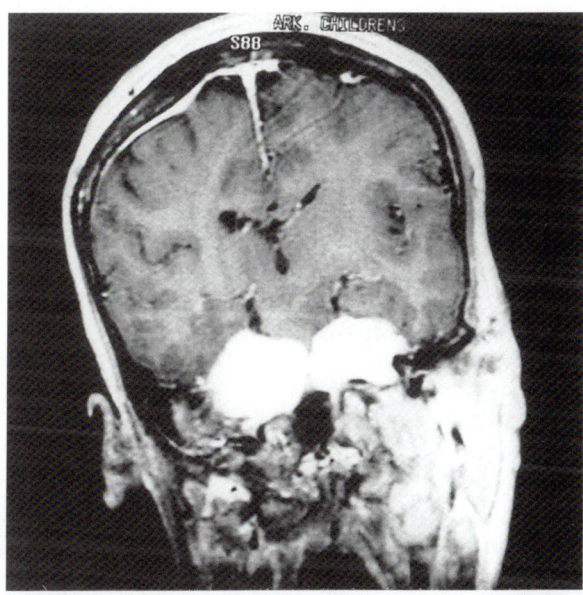

FIGURE 6-5. Bilateral vestibular schwannomas in a 20-year-old man.

nerve tumors are also very common in NF2. Peripheral neuropathy is seen in approximately 3% of patients with NF2. Patients with NF2 also show calcified subependymal deposits similar to those seen in tuberous sclerosis.[18]

TABLE 6-4. Diagnostic Criteria for Neurofibromatosis Type 2 (NF2).

1. Bilateral vestibular schwannomas, either proven histologically or seen by MRI with gadolinium enhancement
2. A parent, sibling, or child with NF2 and either of the following:
   a. Unilateral vestibular schwannoma or
   b. Any two of the following:
      Meningioma, glioma, schwannoma, posterior subcapsular lenticular opacities, cerebral calcification
3. Unilateral vestibular schwannoma and two or more of the following:
      Meningioma, glioma, schwannoma, posterior subcapsular lenticular opacities, cerebral calcification
4. Multiple meningiomas (two or more) and one or more of the following:
      Glioma, schwannoma, posterior subcapsular lenticular opacities, cerebral calcification

From Ref. 79, with permission.

Inheritance

NF2 is inherited in an autosomal dominant manner with almost complete penetrance by the age of 60 years.

Natural History and Prognosis

The mean age of first symptoms in the U.K. study[32] was 22.6 years (range, 2–52 years) and the median age of diagnosis was 27.6 years (range, 5–66 years). Ten percent of patients presented before the age of 10 years, and nearly all patients eventually developed symptoms related to the vestibular schwannomas, typically progressing to bilateral deafness. The mean age of death in the Evans study was 36.25 years; the mean duration of survival from diagnosis was 15 years.

Treatment

Therapy for vestibular schwannoma and other tumors remains primarily surgical.[41,67,82] Close neurological monitoring is mandatory for determining the timing of surgical intervention. Advances in hearing augmentation, such as auditory cochlear implants, may improve the quality of life for many patients. In addition, brainstem implants are now being developed for individuals with no cochlear nerve function.

TUBEROUS SCLEROSIS COMPLEX

History

In 1880, Bourneville described a case of a 15-year-old girl who had had seizures since childhood.[8] At autopsy, multiple sclerotic nodules were observed in the cerebral cortex, with similar tumors of the kidney and diffuse hamartomata of other tissues. He recognized the presence of skin lesions in his original case. Although tuberous sclerosis complex (TSC) has become the name used, the eponym Bourneville's disease is still recognized. It was not until 1908 that Vogt established the classic triad of epilepsy, mental retardation, and adenoma sebaceum of TSC.[109]

Incidence

The incidence of TSC is estimated at approximately 1 in 10,000 births.[57,84]

Etiology

TSC is a relatively common neurocutaneous syndrome caused by mutation in either of two genes, TSC1 or TSC2. The TSC1 gene is located at 9q34 and TSC2 is at 16p13.3.[88] The TSC1 and TSC2 genes encode novel proteins that have been termed hamartin and tuberin for which the cellular roles are largely unknown. Molecular genetic analysis of constitutional mutation in affected individuals and of somatic mutations in TSC-associated hamartomas has elucidated a tumor suppressor mechanism that underlies the phenotypic manifestations in many organs. It is now estimated that TSC1 and TSC2 each account for about 50% of the cases of TSC. TSC2 mutations are associated with more severe disease compared to TSC1 mutations.[25]

Ophthalmologic Features

Ocular lesions are shown in Table 6-5. The eye is involved in at least half of TSC patients. Glial hamartomas of the retina are present in 53% of patients.[80] Two types of retinal hamartoma have been recognized: (1) a more translucent, soft-appearing, relatively flat lesion usually located in the peripheral fundus and (2) an elevated, nodular, calcific mulberry lesion. The mulberry lesions are typically located in the posterior pole adjacent to the optic nerve but may be found anywhere in the fundus. An intermediate type may be encountered.[80] Most of these lesions remain static. Rarely, vitreous seeding may be associated with vitreous inflammation and hemorrhage. The retinal tumors are generally sparsely vascularized or nonvascularized.[89] Visual loss is an exception but may be caused by foveal involvement or continuing growth of nodular lesions. The appearance and has been compared with tapioca grains, fish eggs, or mulberries.

Retinitis pigmentosa has been associated with optic disc hamartomas; however, it is uncertain if any of these patients actually had TSC. Localized hypopigmented lesions of the fundus with ash leaf configurations have been described in TSC. Sectoral pigmentation of the iris has also been reported, along

TABLE 6-5. Ocular Manifestations of Tuberous Sclerosis.

1. Orbital
    General
        Proptosis
        Fibrous dysplasia of orbit
    Lids
        Adenoma sebaceum (angiofibroma)
        Poliosis (hypopigmented lashes)
        Nevus flammeus
2. Extraocular
    Small pedunculated whitish-gray tumors on palpebral conjunctiva
    Subconjunctival nodules
3. Intraocular
    Anterior segment
        Corneal opacities
        Lens opacities
        Cataract
        Depigmented sectors of iris
        Hypopigmented iris spots
        Coloboma of iris
        Coloboma of lens
        Megalocornea (single case)
        Posterior embryotoxin (single case)
    Media
        Vitreous often cloudy
        Vitreous hemorrhage (from hamartoma)
    Choroid
        Diffuse angiomatosis
        Coloboma of choroid
        Punched-out chorioretinal defects
    Retina
        Retinal mushroom-like tumor of grayish-white color
        Yellow-white plagues with small hemorrhages and cystic changes in retina
        Neurofibrilloma
        Neurocystoma
        Retinal glioneuroma
        Glial hamartoma of the retina in 53% of patients
        Pigmentary changes in the retina
        Ash leaf patches
        Atypical retinitis proliferans
        Retinal telangiectasia
        Retinal angioma
        Exophytic retinal astrocytoma
    Optic nerve
        Optic atrophy
        Papilledema
        Pseudopapilledema
        Disc drusen
        Glial hamartoma of the optic nerve (ON) anterior to the lamina cribosa
            (giant drusen)
4. Other
    Secondary glaucoma
    Glaucoma
    Nystagmus
    Strabismus
    Phthisis bulbi
    Progressive external ophthalmoplegia (single case)

with subtler hypopigmented iris spots. Poliosis of the eyelashes is common, present in 18% in one series. The ocular lesions of TSC do not normally interfere with visual function unless a large tumor is situated in the macula. Visual loss, however, may result from intracranial tumors disrupting the visual pathways. Tubers may directly compress the anterior visual pathways or disturb the geniculocalcarine radiations. Tumors in the posterior fossa can produce hydrocephalus with subsequent optic atrophy. Astrocytic hamartomas do not involve the orbital or intracranial portion of the optic nerve or chiasm, in contrast to gliomas in NF1. Orbital tumors are rare, and the incidence of glaucoma is not increased compared to normals. The ocular adnexa may be involved with angiofibromata, forming small salmon-colored nodules in the lid and under the conjunctiva. Lens colobomas with uveal colobomas of the iris have been reported. Isolated cases of progressive external ophthalmoplegia, megalocorneal, and posterior embryotoxin have been described in TSC patients.

Clinical Assessment

Diagnostic criteria for tuberous sclerosis are listed in Table 6-6.[94] Because of the variability of disease expression, it is recommended that parents and siblings and first-degree relatives of probands have a clinical evaluation; this should include dermatological examination (including ultraviolet lamp examination in a dark room), examination of the teeth for dental pits, and indirect ophthalmoscopy with dilated pupils to search for retinal astrocytomas. Cranial neuroimaging, cardiac and renal ultrasound, and skeletal surveys should also be done. Examination of the parents and siblings of apparently isolated cases, including ophthalmologic examination, is indicated. Cranial MRI of the patient and parents should be performed. MRI is the neuroimaging modality of choice. Cortical tubers are best imaged with T_2 weighting whereas subependymal nodules are better demonstrated with T_1 weighting. The cerebellum is involved in less than 15% of patients, and the spinal cord is rarely affected. Giant cell astrocytoma of the brain occurs in 2% of the patients.

The tubers of TSC occur predominantly at the gray–white matter interface; they are characterized by loss of normal cortical cytoarchitecture and the presence of abnormal neurons and glial cells. The subependymal nodules usually line the third ventricle and there are composed of densely segregated and uni-

TABLE 6-6. Diagnostic Criteria for Tuberous Sclerosis.

Major features
1. Facial angiofibromas or forehead plaques
2. Nontraumatic ungual or periungual fibromas
3. More than three hypomelanotic macules
4. Shagreen patch (connective tissue nevus)
5. Multiple retinal hamartomas
6. Cortical tuber
7. Subependymal nodule
8. Subependymal giant cell astrocytoma
9. Cardiac rhabdomyoma
10. Lymphangioleiomyomatosis
11. Renal angiomyolipoma

Minor features
1. Multiple randomly distributed pits in dental enamel
2. Hamartomatous rectal polyps
3. Bone cysts
4. Cerebral white matter "migration tracts"
5. Gingival fibromas
6. Nonrenal hamartoma
7. Retinal achromic patch
8. "Confetti" skin depigmentation
9. Multiple renal cysts

From Ref. 94, with permission.

formally appearing large, irregular cells. The nodules may grow to a size of 3 cm or more, appropriately termed by some subependymal giant cell astrocytoma. Also, some of the lesions may require histological confirmation of the diseases or radiologic confirmation. Next to central nervous system (CNS) hamartomas, renal involvement is the second most common source of morbidity. Regular monitoring for hypertension and renal ultrasounds, performed as frequently as yearly, have been recommended as surveillance measures.[94] Renal function should be monitored in those patients with structural renal abnormalities.

Systemic Associations

TSC can involve almost any organ, with propensity for the CNS, eyes, skin, heart, and kidney. Symptoms of TSC generally appear in the first 3 years of life. Infants usually present with seizures or infantile spasms, which carry a worse prognosis.

The CNS is involved in most cases of TSC. Seizures occur in 80% to 90%, and autism, other behavioral abnormalities, and mental retardation in more than 50%.[98] Adenoma sebaceum (angiofibromas) of the skin of the face occur in 83% of cases as small, flesh-colored papules of the malar area of the face; these are the only cutaneous sign in about one-third of patients. Adenoma sebaceum are in fact not tumors of the sebaceous glands but rather angiofibromas, histologically similar lesions that may be present in the subungual and periungual areas. Periungual fibromas are seen in the late teens in 20% of tuberous sclerosis patients and are pathognomonic.[82] Approximately two-thirds of patients have ash leaf spots, which are hypopigmented melanotic macules; these appear as oval lesions, usually present on the trunk, and may be detected using the Woods lamp. These hypopigmented lesions are usually present at birth and thus are often the earliest neurocutaneous sign of TSC. Unlike the other neurocutaneous disorders, approximately one-fourth of patients have shagreen patches, which are fibrous yellow elevated plaques, usually located in the lumbar region.

Following CNS hamartomas, renal involvement is the second most important source of morbidity. Renal cysts predominate in children and may cause failure and hypertension if large. Multiple vascular angiomyolipomas of the kidneys are usually asymptomatic but can be fatal if hemorrhage occurs. They are detectable by ultrasonography. Multiple cardiac rhabdomyomas in infancy are often asymptomatic but maybe responsible for embolism, cardiac arrythmia, or heart failure.

Inheritance

TSC is transmitted as an autosomal dominant trait with very high and possibly complete penetrance. Some 60% to 70% of cases are sporadic and appear to represent new mutations.

Natural History

Morbidity and mortality in TSC is dictated by the presence or absence of the various features, their severity, and their location. Hamartomas usually become evident in early childhood and may increase at adolescence. Facial nodular lesions are present in 50% of children by 5 years, whereas ash leaf spots or white macules are present at birth or in early infancy in almost all. Six percent of patients develop brain tumors such as periventricular nodules. However, malignant transformation of the periventricular nodules is rare. Seizures, which tend to develop in early childhood, may initially be myoclonic and later grand mal in type; control may be difficult. An EEG abnormality is found in 87% of patients, in an hypsarrhythmic pattern.[99] The seizures and mental defect seem to be related to the extent of the hamartomatous change in the brain. For those with mental deficiency, 100% have seizures, 88% by 5 years of age; in contrast, of those without serious mental deficiency, 69% have seizures, 44% by 5 years of age. Mental deterioration is unusual, except with intractable seizures.

The commonest cause of death is renal disease (renal failure, renal cell carcinoma), and this risk increases with age.[50] The next most frequent cause of death is subependymal giant cell astrocytoma. These tumors occur most frequently in the teens. Lymphangiomyomatosis of the lung is a more frequent cause of death in patients older than 40 years. Patients with severe mental handicap often die of status epilepticus and bronchopneumonia. Cardiovascular deaths usually occur in early childhood from cardiac rhabdomyomas and ruptured thoracic aortic aneurysms.

Treatment

Poor intellectual function is associated with early onset and intractability of seizures, and particularly with infantile spasms. Urgent control of generalized seizures in an infant or young child with TSC is a priority. Vigabatrin is widely used in Europe and has proven to be the most effective drug for treatment of infantile spasms in TSC. It has been recommended that treatment be continued for at least 3 years in patients who become seizure free. Vigabatrin has been associated with visual field defects, and visual fields should be monitored where possible. Carbamazepin is frequently used in the treatment of focal seizures in older children and adults, but may precipitate the recurrence of infantile spasms in very young patients.

Medically uncontrollable seizures call for neurosurgical assessment. However, only a small minority of patients will be found to have sufficiently focal epileptogenic foci to be good candidates for epilepsy surgery. Giant cell astrocystomas are histologically benign, but locally invasive, tumors that develop in approximately 6% of patients, usually in childhood and early adult life. They are often located near the foramen of Munro, leading to hydrocephalus. Recognition of raised intracranial pressure is frequently delayed in patients with intellectual disability. Therefore, some authors have suggested regular neuroradiologic surveillance. Developmental and behavioral problems are a major concern for the families of many patients with TSC. Early recognition facilitates appropriate referral to educational, psychological, and social agencies. Deterioration in development or behavior should prompt assessment to exclude underlining medical problems including brain tumor, subclinical epilepsy, pain from renal disease, and side effects of antiepileptic medications.

Vascular facial angiofibromas can be effectively treated using a dye laser or VerPulse laser. Argon laser treatment appears to carry a high risk of causing hypopigmentation. Skin-resurfacing lasers, such as the ultrapulse CO_2 or erbium/YAG, are required for more fibrotic lesions. Regular monitoring for hypertension and yearly renal ultrasounds are recommended as surveillance measures. Renal function should be monitored in those patients with structural renal abnormalities. Large (greater than 3.5 cm) angiomyolipomas are more likely to hemorrhage than smaller lesions, but absolute criteria for intervention in the asystemic patient have not been agreed upon.

Those patients with polycystic kidney disease caused by contiguous deletion of the TSC2 and PKD1 gene are at high risk of renal failure. Respiratory symptoms, particularly in the postpubertal female patient, should prompt investigation for lymphangioleiomomatosis by computerized tomography of the chest and pulmonary function testing. Echocardiography for the detection of cardiac rhabdomyomas may prove helpful diagnostically in the infant with suspected TSC. Routine follow-up is not required in the asymptomatic patient, and surgical resection of cardiac rhabdomyomas is very rarely indicated. The possibility of arrhythmia masquerading as a seizure disorder should be considered in patients with unexplained loss of consciousness.

VON HIPPEL–LINDAU DISEASE

Historical Perspective

von Hippel–Lindau's eponymous name originates from the contributions made by Eugene von Hippel (1904)[110] and Arvid Lindau (1926).[61] von Hippel studied the retinal lesions, concluded that they were hemangioblastomas and coined the term "angiomatosis retinae." Lindau, in a study of cerebellar cysts, concluded that most were associated with an angioblastic tumors of the CNS, retina, and kidneys.

Incidence

The incidence of von Hippel–Lindau (VHL) disease is 1 in approximately 40,000 to 53,000 of the general population.[68]

Etiology

VHL is a classic heritable tumor suppressor gene syndrome predisposing affected individuals to hemangioblastomas of the retina and CNS, renal cell carcinomas, pheochromocytomas, and renal, pancreatic, and epididymis cysts.[62] The gene for VHL disease was identified in 1993, 5 years after its localization to chromosome 3p25–3p26. The cloned coding sequence of VHL gene is represented in three exons with a predicted open reading frame of 213 amino acids. Molecular genetic studies of germ line mutations in VHL kindred have detected mutations in 70% to 75% of affected patients. Approximately 20% of patients have germ line deletions. Intragenic mutations can be detected in a further 50% of patients, almost half of which are missense mutations. Amino acid substitutions at codon 167 occur in up to 10% of patients and are associated with a high risk of pheochromocytoma and renal cell carcinoma. Kindreds with a missense mutation at codon 98 appear to have a high incidence of pheochromocytoma and a low incidence of renal cell carcinoma. In patients with germ line deletions, insertions, or nonsense mutations, the risk of pheochromocytoma is low (however, most VHL patients with pheochromocytoma have missense mutations). The VHL protein may be a nuclear protein, possibly with some capability of moving between the nucleus and cytosol. It may function by forming specific multiprotein complexes in the cytosol. Furthermore, it may act as a controller of the cellular transcription factor, elongin, which activates transcription elongation.[62]

Ophthalmic Features

Retinal hemangioblastomas (retinal angiomas or hemangiomas) (Fig. 6-6) are the most common presenting findings in patients with VHL disease.[44] The consequences of these lesions occur throughout the eye (Table 6-7). The mean age of diagnosis of retinal hemangioblastomas is VHL disease is 25 years.[71] Between 25% and 80% of patients with retinal hemangioblastomas will have VHL disease.[70] All patients with a retinal hemangioblastoma

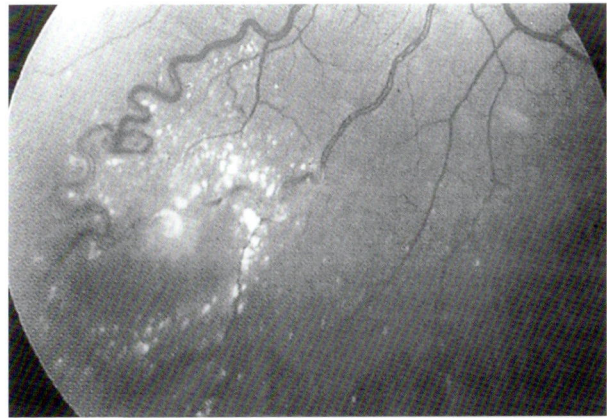

FIGURE 6-6. Peripheral hemangioblastoma in von Hippel–Lindau disease with exudation. Note large feeding arteriole and draining venule.

TABLE 6-7. Ocular Manifestations of von Hippel–Lindau Disease.

1. Orbital
     General
         Proptosis
     Lids
2. Intraocular
     Anterior segment
         Angiomatosis of the iris
     Media
         Vitreous hemorrhage and vascular proliferation
         Vitreous membrane formation
     Choroid
         The choroid is not usually invaded
     Retina
         Angiomatosis retinae, with tortuosity of dilated retinal artery and vein
             (feeder vessels)
         Juxtapapillary retinal angiomatosis
         Secondary retinal hemorrhages and exudates
         Retinitis proliferans (less frequent)
         Retinal detachment is late sequelae
         Macular star: lipid-like material in macula
         Cystic degeneration
         Twin retinal vessels
     Optic nerve
         Angiomata of the optic nerve
         Papilledema
3. Other
     Secondary glaucoma

and their first-degree relatives should be screened for VHL.[75] The younger the age of presentation in a patient with a retinal hemangioblastoma, the greater the likelihood of VHL. Multiple retinal hemangioblastomas are diagnostic of VHL. Two clinical types of hemangioblastomas of retinal and optic head are recognized: an endophytic and the less common exophytic tumor.[36] The endophytic hemangioma projects into the vitreous. Early lesions are minute reddish nodules with afferent and efferent vessels. Peripheral tumors are recognized by a smooth, elevated, round contour and are white to orange or reddish in color. More advanced large peripheral tumors are fed by a markedly dilated tortuous arteriole, with a dilated, efferent venule draining the lesion. Indirect ophthalmoscopy fluorescein angiography may be necessary to identify early small hemangiomas that resemble capillary dilations. Patients remain asymptomatic until visual loss occurs, usually in the second to third decade.

Visual loss can be a result from exudative or traction retinal detachment, macular edema or holes, epiretinal membranes, vitreous hemorrhages, neovascular glaucoma, uveitis, or postpapilledema optic atrophy. Exophytic tumors arise from the outer retina and occur most commonly in the peripapillary region. Their blood supply is from the retinal and posterior ciliary circulation.[36] On fluorescein angiography there is early filling of the angiomas during the arteriole phase. Twin vessels, the closely paired feeding arteriole and draining venule of larger, peripheral tumors, are clearly depicted with angiography. Hemangioblastomas may involve the optic disc, or the peripapillary retina, or occur within the optic nerve itself. Hemangioblastomas of the optic nerve causing progressive and compressive optic neuropathy are rare and may be confused with optic nerve tumors. Discordance between the retinal appearance and signs of optic nerve dysfunction may suggest the diagnosis. Surgical excision of the hemangioblastoma to preserve vision may be possible because the tumor does not infiltrate the optic nerve.

Clinical Assessment

The features of VHL disease, which can cause significant morbidity and mortality, are all potentially treatable if diagnosed early. This realization has led to development of screening protocols for the follow-up of affected individuals and at-risk relatives. Screening guidelines for affected individuals and at-risk family members are given in Table 6-8.[75]

TABLE 6-8. Screening Protocol for von Hippel–Lindau Disease in Affected Patients and At-Risk Relatives.

Affected patient
1. Annual physical examination and urine testing
2. Annual direct and indirect ophthalmoscopy
3. MRI brain scan every 3 years to age 50 and every 5 years thereafter (not mandatory)
4. Annual renal ultrasound scan, with CT scan every 3 years (more frequent if multiple renal cysts present)
5. Annual 24-h urine collection for VMA and metanephrines

At-risk relative
1. Annual physical examination and urine testing
2. Annual direct and indirect ophthalmoscopy from age 5
   Annual fluorescein angioscopy or angiography from age 10 until age 60
3. MRI brain scans every 3 years from age 15 to 40, and then every 5 years until age 60
4. Annual renal ultrasound scans, with abnormal CT scan every 3 years from age 20 to 65
5. Annual 24-h urine collection for VMA and metanephrines

Genetic testing is also available. Clinical heterogeneity exists in families with VHL, particularly concerning the occurrence of pheochromocytoma. The prognosis for the lifetime risk of pheochromocytoma can be estimated by determination of the underlying mutation.[16,34]

Systemic Associations

As many as 60% of patients develop hemangioblastomas of the CNS (cerebellum, medulla and spinal cord) (Table 6-9). Hemangioblastomas are diagnosed at a younger age (mean, 29 years) in patients with VHL disease compared to sporadic isolated cases (mean, 45 years).[71] Multiple or bilateral tumors are found frequently. Spinal hemangioblastomas are associated with VHL disease in 80% of cases.[16] Symptoms depend on tumor size and location. Suprasellar involvement can present with a chiasmal

TABLE 6-9. Classification of von Hippel–Lindau (VHL) Disease.

Type I	VHL without pheochromocytoma
Type II	VHL with pheochromocytoma
Type IIA	Pheochromocytoma, CNS hemangioblastomas, and retinal angiomas
Type IIB	VHL IIA plus pancreatic involvement and renal manifestations (tumors, cysts)

From Ref. 71, with permission.

syndrome. Some patients require emergent treatment for life-threatening CNS disease. The benign vascular tumors can hemorrhage, causing obstructive hydrocephalus, and are difficult to remove surgically because of their vascularity. Early detection permits treatment, which lessens the risk of spinal cord compression and sudden death in VHL patients. However, surgical excision is difficult because of tumor vascularity, and recurrence is likely.

Clear cell carcinoma of the kidney is the presenting illness in 10% of patients with VHL disease. The cumulative risk of developing renal cell carcinoma is more than 70% by age 60 years and it is the leading cause of death in VHL disease. Ultrasonographic (or even MRI) screening of asymptomatic patients is therefore advised. Pheochromocytoma is another visceral manifestation of VHL disease that is found in 7% to 18% of all VHL patients.[71] Approximately 19% of newly diagnosed pheochromocytomas are caused by VHL disease. As with other tumors, VHL-associated pheochromocytomas occur at an earlier age than nonfamilial cases and are multifocal in 55% of cases. Cysts of the kidneys, pancreas, and epididymis are common and do not appear to undergo malignant transformation. Papillary adenocarcinoma of the endolymphatic sac with bony erosion and hearing loss is believed to occur in 8% of patients. Polycythemia caused by tumor erythropoietin production occurrs in 5% to 20% of cases and is usually related to cerebellar hemangioblastomas and renal cell carcinomas.[45] Cutaneous lesions are rare in VHL disease.

Clinical Assessment

Guidelines for screening for von Hippel–Lindau disease in affected patients and at-risk relatives are given in Table 6-8.

Inheritance

von Hippel–Lindau disease is an autosomal dominantly inherited condition.

Natural History

The mean age at presentation of the symptomatic cases in the Cambridge series was 27 ± 12.6 years.[69] As in other neurocutaneous syndromes, the national history depends on which lesions develop. In unscreened populations, the disease is associated with significant morbidly and mortality. Screening should prevent the premature deaths of many VHL patients and avoid significant morbidity in others. In the Cambridge series, 51 of 152 patients had died, at a mean age of 41 years.[69] Renal carcinoma was the most common cause of death, followed by cerebellar hemangioblastoma.

The management of retinal hemangioblastomas depends on their location in size. Generally, hemangioblastomas progressively enlarge. Spontaneous regression of retinal hemangioblastomas has been described but is exceptional. Often there are no symptoms until a serious complication occurs, such as hemorrhage, retinal detachment, or macula edema. Several treatment modalities have been used, including cryotherapy, xenon arc photocoagulation, diatheramy, laser photocoagulation, radiotherapy, and local resections. Small peripheral tumors are best treated with argon laser photocoagulation, and cryotherapy can be applied to larger peripheral tumors.

Early detection of renal tumors by MRI screening has allowed small localized renal tumors to be removed. Most centers employ a conservative renal sparing approach to the management of renal cell carcinoma in VHL disease with local excision of tumor or partial nephrectomy. Such a strategy recognizes that VHL patients are at high risk of developing further primary tumors and aims to conserve functioning renal tissue. Nevertheless, bilateral nephrectomy may be necessary, and although relatively few patients have undergone renal transplantation, limited data suggest that renal transplantation is an effective therapy for anephric disease patients. The efficiency of screening protocols can be enhanced by molecular genetic diagnosis. Individuals at high risk of VHL can be frequently screened, with renal imaging beginning at age 15; relatives demonstrated to be at low risk on genetic linkage analysis could be screened less frequently. In kindreds in which a germ line mutation has been identified, relatives who have not inherited the mutation can be spared further following up. Cerebellar hemangioblastomas are usually not treated until they become symptomatic. Therefore, some centers reserve cranial imaging for symptomatic patients rather than applying it as a screening tool. Pancreatic carcinoma is best detected with MRI.

Prognosis

Prognosis is totally dependent on the early detection of tumors in retinal, CNS, retina cell carcinoma, and pheochromocytoma and pancreatic tumors. The outcome of treatment, usually surgical, depends on the stage at which these vascular tumors become symptomatic, as well as their location.

Treatment

Surgical removal of tumors, when possible, is the primary treatment available. (See Natural History section for further discussion.)

ATAXIA-TELANGIECTASIA

Ataxia-telangiectasia (A-T) is an autosomal recessive disorder characterized by neurological and immunogical symptoms, radiosensitivity, and cancer predisposition. This disease was initially described by Louis-Bar in 1941.[65]

Incidence

The incidence of A-T is estimated at 1 per 40,000 live births. The carrier frequency is approximately 1%.[37]

Etiology

A-T is a very pleiotropic syndrome that stems from the defective functioning of a mutated ATM gene. ATM belongs to a large molecular weight family of protein kinases. Delayed or reduced expression of p53 in radiation-damaged A-T cells suggests that ATM interacts with proteins upstream of p53 sensing double-strand break DNA damage. Seventy percent of ATM mutations result in a short truncated protein. These mutations are found over the entire gene.[37]

Ophthalmologic Features

This disorder presents in early childhood with the onset of ataxia at the time the child is learning to walk. Conjunctival telangiectasia develops between the ages of 4 and 7 (Fig. 6-7). The telangiectasias are a hallmark of A-T. The ocular telangiectasia consists of dilated and corkscrew, bulbar conjunctival vessels located in the interpalpebral zone of both eyes. Ocular motor apraxia with head thrusts and the inability to generate

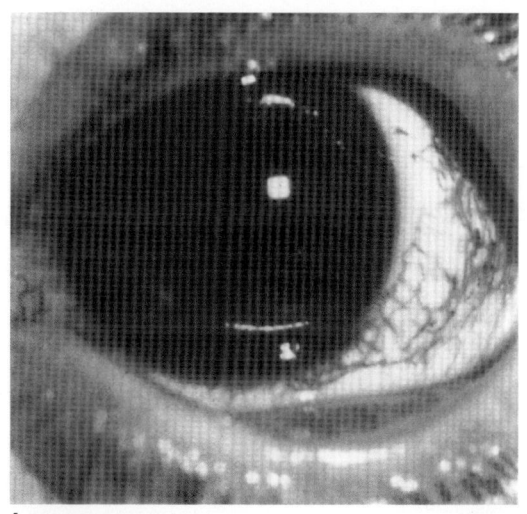

A

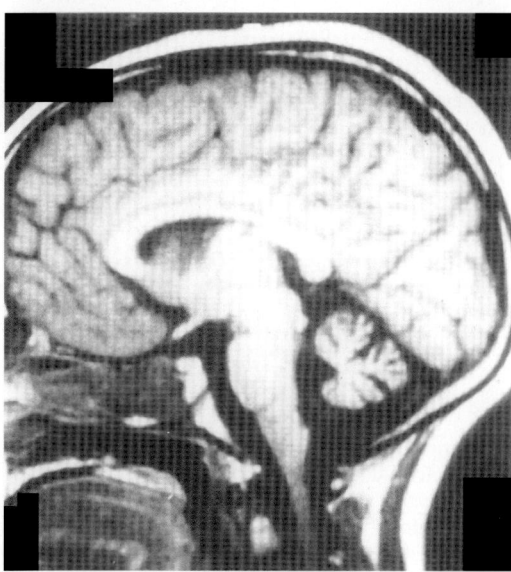

B

FIGURE 6-7A,B. (**A**) Marked conjunctival telengectasia in older patient with ataxia telengectasia. (**B**) Cerebellar atrophy in same patient as in (**A**).

saccades and loss of optokinetic responses develop at a later age.[37]

Clinical Assessment

Every A-T homozygote has a small embryonic-like thymus; 60% to 80% of A-T of the homozygotes manifest an IgA, IgE, or IgG2 deficiency. Serum alpha-fetoprotein (AFP) levels are elevated in 95% of A-T patients. AFP levels should be determined after 2 years of age. The gene for A-T is located at 11q23.1. Karyotyping, if successful, reveals translocations involving chromosomes 14q11, 14q32, 7q35, and 7p14. MRI of the cerebellum will usually show marked atrophy in children over 4 years of age (Fig. 6-7B). Newer techniques for imaging the cerebellum are also being evaluated such as functional MRI. DNA testing, now that the gene was positionally cloned from 11q23.1, can be used for prenatal testing.[37]

Systemic Associations

Progressive neurological dysfunction includes truncal ataxia, choreoathetosis, dystonia, and myoclonus, slurring of speech, and drooling. Oculocutaneous telangiectasias, usually present by 6 years of age, affect the malar region, nose, and ears. Premature aging occurs, and endocrine dysfunction causes hyperglycemia, hypogonadism, and growth retardation. Frequent, recurrent sinopulmonary and skin infections are caused by serum and immunodeficiencies. A-T patients have susceptibility to cancer, usually leukemia or lymphoma. Their hypersensitivity to ionizing radiation calls for modified dosing of radiation therapy for cancer.[37]

Natural History

Growth deficiency may be prenatal in onset, but more commonly becomes evident in later infancy or in childhood. Ataxia usually develops during infancy and eventually is accompanied by choreoathetosis, slurring of speech, drooling, ocular motor apraxia, stooped posture, presence of a dull, sad facies, and, occasionally, seizures. Ataxia often becomes so severe that ambulation is no longer possible in later childhood. Death is usually a consequence of lung infections, neurological deficit, or malignancy.[37]

Treatment

No effective therapy exists for halting the progression of the ataxia. Clinical trials are under way to test the efficacy of myoinositol, *N*-acetylcystine, and L-dopa on general symptoms. To date, preliminary data have been disappointing. Vitamin E, alpha-lipoic acid, and coenzme Q10 may also slow the deterioration. Folic acid may help to minimize chromosomal fragility and the formation of double-strand DNA breaks. Pulmonary or sinus infections may be treated conventionally because the normal spectrum of microbes is present. If possible, neurotoxic chemotherapeutic agents should be avoided. Patients with bronchiectasis are best treated in a similar fashion to patients with cystic fibrosis. In older patients, pulmonary infections are the major cause of failing health and death. In addition to appropriate antibiotics, intravenous gamma globulin every 3 to 4 weeks may reduce the frequency of infections.[37] Of paramount importance is an aggressive and engaging physical exercise program aimed at enhancing lung function, preventing contractures, and avoiding positional kyphoscoliosis.

Various agents can partially relieve some of the neurological symptoms, such as ataxia, drooling, and tremors. Buspirone is active in some types of cerebellar ataxia. Amantadine improves balance and coordination and minimizes drooling.[37] When radiation therapy is planned for treating a malignancy the dose should be reduced by approximately 30%. Some chemotherapeutic agents, especially alkylating agents, should also be given in reduced doses.[37]

Prognosis

Most A-T patients in the United States now live well beyond 20 years of age. Unfortunately, this major improvement from just a few years ago has not been universal. The improved survival in the United States may be related to better nutrition, better diagnostics, better treatment of pulmonary infections and malignancies, and more aggressive physical therapy. The application of an effective treatment given before neurological decline would represent a great advance.

STURGE–WEBER SYNDROME

Sturge–Weber syndrome (SWS) is a neurocutaneous disorder characterized by cutaneous facial angiomas, leptomeningeal angiomas, and seizures and other neurological complications, including mental retardation and glaucoma.

Incidence

The SWS occurs sporadically. Facial angiomas (port-wine stains, nevus flammeus) occur in 3 per 1000 births; however, only 5% of patients demonstrate the full features of SWS.[47]

Etiology

There are no reports of familial occurrence of Sturge–Weber syndrome. The condition may be more prevalent in Caucasians than in other races. There has been one report of a chromosomal abnormality at fragile site 10q24 in a young boy with this syndrome[106] and a supernumerary bisatellited chromosome. The family had several unaffected members.[28]

It is hypothesized that the primary lesion in Sturge–Weber is a maldevelopment of vasculature at 4 to 8 weeks gestational age. This flaw leads to fibrosis, hyaline degeneration, dilation and calcification of the vascular wall with venous wall stasis, recurrent thrombotic events, transient ischemic attacks, and gradual neurological deterioration. Another possible embryologic basis for this syndrome is a defective migration and differentiation of the promesencephalic neural crest, leading to abnormal proliferation of blood vessels and goniodysgenesis.[91]

Ophthalmologic Features

The ocular manifestations of SWS are listed in Table 6-10. The area of the ophthalmic division of the trigeminal nerve is often affected with nevus flammeus, including the upper eyelid and the conjunctiva (Fig. 6-8). Up to 30% of SWS patients have bilateral facial lesions (Fig. 6-9); 40% of patients with SWS may have choroidal hemangioma, and 50% of all choroidal hemangiomas occur in SWS patients. Choroidal hemangiomas may be discrete, appearing as yellowish, elevated, circular areas, which disappear or decrease in visibility with scleral depression. The diffuse type occurs more commonly in SWS patients and the age on onset of

TABLE 6-10. Ocular Manifestations of Sturge–Weber Syndrome (SWS).

1. Orbital
   General
      Exophthalmos
   Lids
      Ptosis
      Port-wine stain of eyelid
2. Extraocular
   Sclera
      Nevoid marks or vascular dilation of the episclera
      Telangiectasia of the episclera
      Large, anomalous vessels in the conjunctiva
      Oculocutaneous melanosis
3. Intraocular
   Anterior segment
      Increased corneal diameter
      Reduced corneal reflex
      Iris discoloration
      Telangiectasia of the iris with heterochromia
      Dilation and tortuosity of iris vessels
      Sluggish pupils
      Anisocoria or other disturbances in pupil reaction
      Coloboma of the iris
      Deep anterior chamber angle
      Buphthalmos
   Media
      Ectopia lentis
      Spontaneous dislocation of the lenses
   Choroid
      Choroidal angiomata
      Choroidal hemangioma
   Retina
      Dilation and tortuosity of retinal vessels
      Retinal arteriovenous aneurysm
      Varicosity of retinal veins
      Retinitis pigmentosa
      Glioma
      Retinal detachment
      Central retinal vein occlusion
   Optic nerve
      Arteriovenous angiomas
      Papilledema
      Optic atrophy
      Optic nerve cupping
      Optic nerve coloboma
      Optic nerve drusen
4. Other
   Strabismus
   Nystagmus
   Loss of vision (any degree)
   Cortical blindness
   Abnormal visual field caused by lesion in optic tract
   Hemianopia
   Secondary glaucoma (late)
   Anisometropia

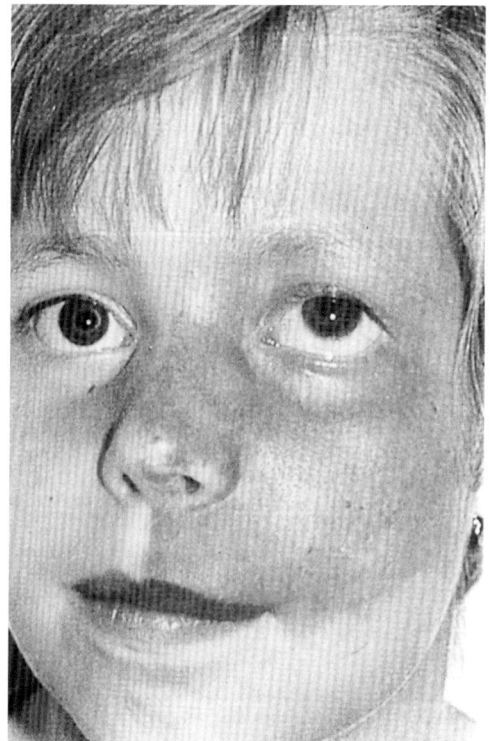

FIGURE 6-8. A child with Sturge–Weber syndrome (SWS) has nevus flammeus and glaucoma on left side of the face and eye.

ocular symptoms with the diffuse hemangioma (7.6 years) is earlier than with the solitary type (38.7 years).

Fluorescein angiography may illustrate early filling with late staining. Diffuse hemangiomas may be difficult to detect. Sometimes the color change at the change at the border of the lesion may be visualized. The appearance of an optic nerve buried in a sea of "tomato catsup" is the pathognomonic picture in a child with SWS.[104] As one alternately views the fundi of the involved and the normal eye, the primary finding is simply one of the dramatic color differences in the two fundi. The involved eye has a bright red fundus reflex compared to the normal eye. Fluorescein angiography may illustrate early filling with late

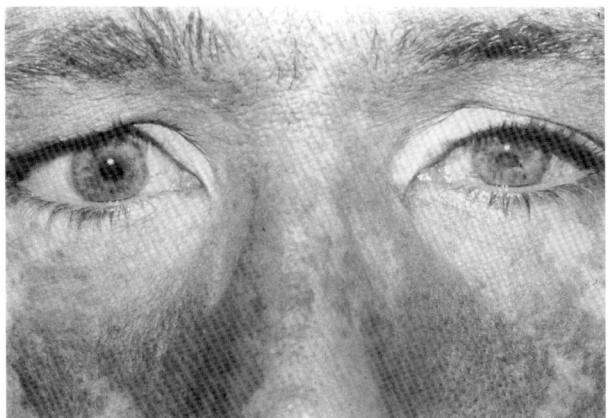

FIGURE 6-9. A 17-year-old patient with bilateral nevus flammeus and bilateral episcleral vessels OU.

staining. Other vascular anomalies of the eye include telangectasias of the conjunctiva, episclera, or iris, which may result in heterochromia.

Glaucoma occurs in approximately 71% of patients and is more common when the cutaneous hemangioma involves the eyelid and when prominent conjunctival or episcleral hemangiomas are present.[103] In a large retrospective study, SWS glaucoma had a bimodal onset, beginning before 2 years of age or after 5 years.[103] The early-onset group has trabeculodysgenesis with a flat, anterior iris insertion. Their presentation resembles that of primary infantile glaucoma (Fig. 6-10). Later-onset glaucoma is secondary to elevated episcleral venous pressure, although anomalous angle structures may play a role as well.[17,103]

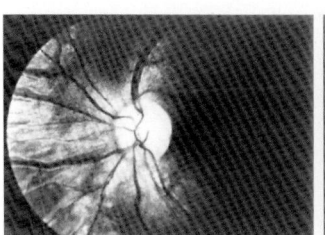 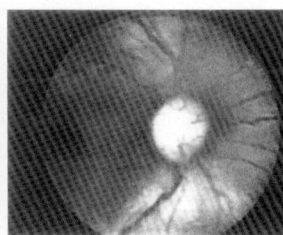

FIGURE 6-10. Cupped disc of girl in Figure 6-8.

Several cases of SWS have been associated with ocular cutaneous melanosis

Clinical Assessment

Evaluation includes examination for choroidal hemangioma and for glaucoma. Radiologic studies are helpful in assessing meningeal and cerebral involvement. MRI delineates parenchymal atrophy and ischemic changes, and gadolinium-enhanced MRI demonstrates the vascular abnormalities.[72]

Systemic Associations

The facial hemangiomas, referred to as either port-wine stain or nevus flammeus, typically occur along the trigeminal dermatome. However, they may involve part or all of the face down to the neck and chest areas. The lesions can be unilateral or bilateral; some unilateral lesions partially cross the midline. Pathologically, the flat angioma consists of ectatic dermal capillary to venule-sized blood vessels that may become nodular with age. These lesions do not regress.

The neurological features of SWS are caused by vascular malformations of the pial vessels of the occipitoparietal area. Impaired blood flow leads to hypoxia, encephalomalacia, cortical atrophy, and, ultimately, calcification.

The characteristic "tramline calcification" appearance, of parallel, linear radiodensities on CT, results from gyriform calcification of the cerebral cortex and usually develops after 2 years of age. Seizures, mental retardation, and hemiparesis may occur. Developmental delay occurs in approximately 50% of affected individuals. Delay is much less likely if there are no seizures and more likely if seizures began in the first year of life.[102] The seizures may be generalized or focal, affecting the contralateral side of the body; they occur in 75% to 90% of children.

Inheritance

This condition occurs sporadically.

Natural History

Sunjansky and Contrady (1995) performed a long-term study of 52 adults with SWS aged 18 to 63 years. Cranial port-wine stains were present in 98% and extracranial ones in 52%. The prevalence of glaucoma was 60%, with an age of onset from 0 to 41 years. Seizures were present in 83% (onset, 0–23 years), and neurological deficit occurred in 65%. A younger age of onset of seizures was associated with a worse prognosis.[102]

Treatment and Prognosis

There is some tendency for the facial angioma to become darker and more nodular with increasing age. Past treatments aimed at disguising the lesions were entirely unsatisfactory. In adolescents with well-controlled seizures and normal intelligence, the facial nevus flammeus is a great problem. Prior treatment with dermabrasion or surgical resection with split-thickness skin grafting often resulted in unacceptable scarring. Tunable dye laser therapy is the current preferred modality for treating nevus flammeus.

Worsening seizures and progressive intellectual deterioration present the major neurological problem in SWS. Most authorities favor drug therapy for management of the epilepsy, reserving neurosurgical procedures (hemispherectomy, lobectomy) for patients refractory to medical management.[55,81] Management of the choroidal hemangiomas brings similar therapeutic dilemmas for treating ophthalmologists. Prominent episcleral or choroidal hemangiomas increase the risk of choroidal effusion and expulsive hemorrhage at surgery. Most of these vascular malformations can cause exudative retinal detachment, leading to intractable secondary glaucoma. Treatment with laser photocoagulation has produced favorable results when initiated before the development of significant exudation, but the ultimate success rate is low. Low-dose external beam radiotherapy or plaque radiotherapy over the area of the tumor are effective in reducing or eliminating associated exudative retinal detachment.

Management of glaucoma is tailored to the individual case. Initial management of glaucoma is usually with aqueous suppressants. Lantanoprost has not been useful in SWS patients with glaucoma.[1] Goniotomy or trabeculectomy may be safe, initial alternatives to conventional filtration surgery. Preventive measures such as preplaced scleral sutures to allow rapid wound closure and prophylactic posterior sclerostomies are advocated by some. Multiple procedures including placement of drainage devices and cycloablation may be necessary to adequately control intraocular pressure.

KLIPPEL–TRENAUNAY SYNDROME

Klippel–Trenaunay syndrome (KTS) consists of a cutaneous hemangioma involving an extremity, along with varicosities and hypertrophy of the bone and soft tissue of the affected limb.

Historical Perspective

In 1869, Trelat-Monod recognized the association between limb hypertrophy and vascular dilation. Klippel and Trenaunay, in 1900, reported the triad of cutaneous hemangiomata, hemihypertrophy, and varicosities, calling it "naevus variqueux osteohypertrophique."[53]

Incidence

The incidence of KT syndrome is not established.

Etiology

The etiology of KTS is unknown.

Ophthalmic Manifestations

Most of the ocular findings result from vascular malformations through the eye and orbit. The affected eye is generally ipsilateral to the affected limb. Vascular malformations include orbital varices and retinal varicosities. Glaucoma, cataracts, heterochromia, and Marcus-Gunn pupil and have been reported.[60,92] Ocular manifestations of KTS are listed in Table 6-11.

Clinical Assessment

In addition to clinical examination, laboratory evaluation utilizes color duplex ultrasonography, MRI, lymphoscintigraphy, and plain radiography.

Systemic Associations

Patients with KT syndrome may have cutaneous capillary malformations, abnormal development of the deep and superficial veins, and mixed vascular malformations including capillary, venous, arteriolar, and lymphatic systems. Cutis marmorata

TABLE 6-11. Ocular Manifestations of Klippel–Trenaunay Syndrome (KTS).

1. Orbital/external
    General
        Venous angioma (congenital varix)
        Exophthalmos
        Enophthalmos
        Regional hypertrophy of orbital contents
    Lids
        Ptosis
2. Extraocular
    Conjunctiva
        Telangiectasias
        Angioma
    Sclera
        Angioma
        Melanosis
3. Intraocular
    Anterior segment
        Anomalous angle structures
        Iris coloboma
        Heterochromic irides
    Lens
        Cataracts
        Central nuclear opacity
    Choroid
        Choroidal angioma
        Chorioretinal scar
    Retina
        Retinal varicosities
        Tortuosity of retinal vessels
        Central retinal vein occlusion
        Retinal holes
        Retinal dysplasia
        Astrocytic proliferations of the retinal NFL
    Optic nerve
        Optic nerve enlargement
        Optic nerve hypoplasia
        Optic nerve variant
            Tilted disc with telangiectatic vessels
4. Other
    Glaucoma
        POAG (primary open angle)
        Congenital
    Strabismus
        Exotropia
    Esotropia

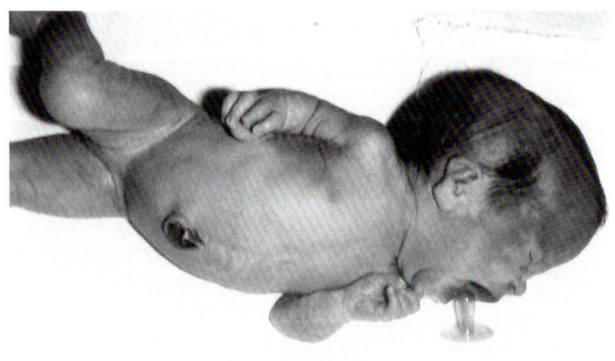

FIGURE 6-11. Ten-day-old infant girl with Klippel–Trehaunay (KT) syndrome. Note lesion on left arm, trunk, and abdomen. (Courtesy of R.A. Lewis.)

telangiectatica also occurs, with widespread reticulation of the skin from prominent veins and capillaries (Fig. 6-11).[101]

Inheritance

Most cases are sporadic.

Natural History

The prognosis is generally favorable; patients often need no treatment or elastic compression only. Disproportionate growth may require epiphyseal fusion or removal of the appropriate phalanx. Joint discomfort is not uncommon, and arthritic-type problems may develop. Leg swelling can be bothersome, and ulcers and other dermatological complications may occur. Clinically significant A-V shunting almost never occurs.

Treatment

Surgical intervention, rarely required, includes orthopedic procedures for overgrowth, pulse-dye laser treatment and reduction of A-V malformations are also done. Amputation may be needed if the patient develops Kasabach–Merritt syndrome with high output cardiac failure.[15] Some children may undergo resection of varicose veins.

WYBURN-MASON SYNDROME

Wyburn-Mason syndrome (WMS) is considered a neurocutaneous syndrome by many authors. It is characterized by arteriovenous malformations (AVM) of the brain, especially the midbrain, in conjunction with an AVM of the ipsilateral retina.

History

In the English literature, the association of the typical AVMs of the brain and central nervous system is attributed to Wyburn-Mason after his 1943 article.[114] However, 6 years earlier, Bonnet, Dechaume, and Blanc had reported the association of retinal vascular malformations with ipsilateral cerebral AVMS and facial nevi.[7]

Incidence

The incidence is unknown.

Etiology

WMS is a rare, sporadic syndrome with ophthalmologic and cerebral manifestations.

Ophthalmologic Features

The ocular manifestations of WMS are the most important clue to diagnosis (Table 6-12). However, retinal involvement is not essential for the diagnosis of WMS.[11] In Wyburn-Mason's original series, only 14 of 20 patients had both intracranial AVMs and retinal AVMs. The retinal lesion consists of a markedly dilated and torturous arteriole contiguous with a similar-appearing vein; there is no intervening capillary bed (Fig. 6-12). Many prefer the designation of racemose hemangioma instead of AVM, noting that a definite communication cannot always be demonstrated.[33] On fluorescein angiography there is a rapid transit of dye through the arteriolar and venous communication, typically without leakage. Thus, this condition is often asymptomatic and nonprogressive. If symptoms develop, they usually appear before age 30.

Vision may be normal or severely reduced depending on the location of the retinal lesions. Peripheral lesions usually cause little or no problem, in contrast to those situated near the posterior pole.[33] Children with posterior lesions may present with strabismus.

TABLE 6-12. Ocular Manifestations of Wyburn-Mason Syndrome (WMS).

1. Orbital
     General
          Pulsating proptosis
          Exophthalmos
          Intraorbital arteriovenous malformation (AVM)
          Enlarged optic foramen
          Proptosis
     Lids
          Ptosis
2. Extraocular
     Conjunctiva
          Congestion bulbar conjunctiva
          Abnormally dilated conjunctival vessels
3. Intraocular
     Anterior segment
          Reduced corneal reflex/corneal opacities
          Pupillary abnormalities (anisocoria, sluggish pupils, or other disturbances
               of pupil reaction)
          Abnormally dilated iris vessels
     Retina
          Retinal arteriovenous aneurysm
          Varicosity of retinal veins
          Tortuosity of retinal veins
     Optic nerve
          Optic nerve arteriovenous angioma
          Optociliary shunt vessels
          Papilledema
          Optic atrophy
4. Other
     Strabismus
          Esotropia
          Exotropia
          Nystagmus
          Loss of vision (any degree)
          Homonymous hemianopia
          External ophthalmoplegia
          Ocular ischemia
          Neovascular glaucoma

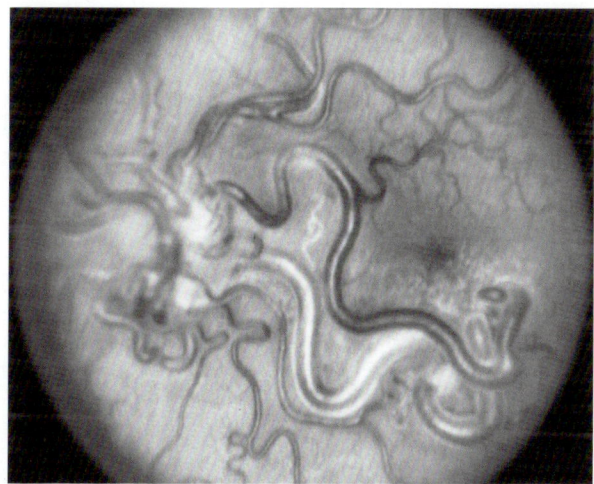

FIGURE 6-12. Arteriovenous malformation (AVM) in the fundus of a 19-year-old patient with Wyburn–Mason syndrome (WMS). (Courtesy of R.A. Lewis.)

The retinal AVMs range from small, unnoticeable shunts to large, markedly dilated and tortuous vessels. Visual loss occurs, rarely, from vascular growth, hemorrhage, and central retinal vein occlusion. AVMs may extend into the orbit from intracranial sites along the anterior visual pathways and cause proptosis.[114] Intracranial AVMs may cause cranial nerve palsies.

Clinical Assessment

Clinical assesment is made with indirect ophthalmoscopy, with MRI of the brain and orbits the main neuroimaging modality.

Systemic Associations

The syndrome may present with headaches, seizures, and subarachnoid hemorrhage. Obstructive hydrocephalus from aqueductal compression may occur. Signs and symptoms vary according to the size and location of the AVM. Vascular accidents usually begin in the second or third decade. The most common manifestations of the midbrain vascular malformations are seizures and intracranial hemorrhage, occurring in about 10% to 80% of cases.[2,3,33,105] Contralateral pyramidal deficits, mental disturbances, and contralateral homonymous hemianopia are common complications. Other complications include cranial nerve palsies, dorsal midbrain syndrome, internuclear ophthalmoplegia, nystagmus speech deficits, and mental retardation.

The cutaneous manifestations, present in half of patients, consist of a subtle nevus flammeus along the ipsilateral trigeminal distribution.[105] AVMs of the ipsilateral pterygoid fossa, mandible, and maxilla may hemorrhage following dental extraction and facial surgery.

Inheritance

WMS is a rare sporadic syndrome with no hereditary component.

Natural History

The natural history of WMS is unpredictable. Rare patients develop intravascular thrombosis with central vein occlusion and subsequent neovascular glaucoma. The neurological complications include headaches, seizures, and subarachnoid hemorrhages. These complications are the primary cause of morbidity and mortality in WMS.

Treatment

No treatment is required for the retinal lesions. The condition is congenital and nonprogressive. Recognition of the association between the retinal and intracranial lesions may allow early identification of cerebral AVMs. With newer techniques of endovascular embolization, the ability to eliminate the intracranial AVMs without compromise of the cerebral circulation is possible. A multidisciplinary management approach is recommended.

MULTIPLE ENDOCRINE NEOPLASIA TYPE 2B (MEN 2B, THE MUCOSAL NEUROMA SYNDROME)

MEN 2B or the mucosal neuroma syndrome is a hamartoneoplastic syndrome characterized by medullary thyroid carcinomas (MTC), pheochromocytomas, mucosal neuromas, ganglioneuromas of the intestinal tract, and skeletal and ophthalmic abnormalities. MEN 2B patients have a Marfanoid body habitus with a characteristic dysmorphic facies.[76]

Incidence

The incidence of MEN 2B has not been documented accurately.

Etiology

The MEN 2B phenotype is caused by a mutation in the RET proto-oncogene. A mutation in codon 918 causes the substitution of threonine for methionine in the tyrosine kinase domain of the RET protein. Recent biochemical evidence suggests that this mutation alters the substrate specificity of intracellular signal transduction.

Ophthalmic Features

The mucosal neuromas are seen at the eyelid margins, causing an anteverted eyelid (Fig. 6-13). Slit lamp examination can reveal subconjunctival neuromas (Fig. 6-14) and medullated nerve fibers in the cornea (Fig. 6-15).

Clinical Assessment

Regular biochemical testing and imaging, with surgery when necessary, has shown to be effective in preventing mortality and morbidity in MEN 2 families.

Screening for MTC in a RET mutation-positive child of a known MEN 2B patient probably should start at age 1 year.[97,107] However, normal calcitonin levels may be high in infants, and screening results may be difficult to interpret. In this situation some clinicians have advocated thyroidectomy on the basis of the MEN 2B phenotype alone. DNA testing for the MEN 2B mutation now provides greater certainty. In a family known to

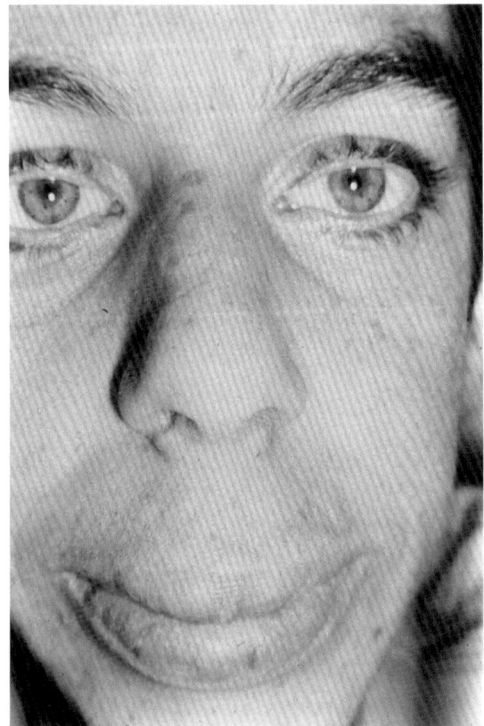

FIGURE 6-13. Face of patient with multiple endocrine neoplasia (MEN) 2B. Note anteverted lids secondary to neuroma of the lids, Marfanoid facies, and neuromas of the lips.

have MEN 2B in which the causative mutation can be identified, DNA testing of unaffected family members at risk will free those who do not have the mutation from the need for biochemical screening and simplfy surgical decision making in those with the mutation. Increasingly, opinion is moving toward a recommendation for thyroidectomy in childhood on the basis of DNA testing alone. Because 50% of MEN2 cases are sporadic, DNA testing plays an important role in determining which apparently sporadic cases have heritable disease. Somatostatin receptor scintigraphy is a sensitive method for assessing MTC and pheochromocytoma metastases.[56]

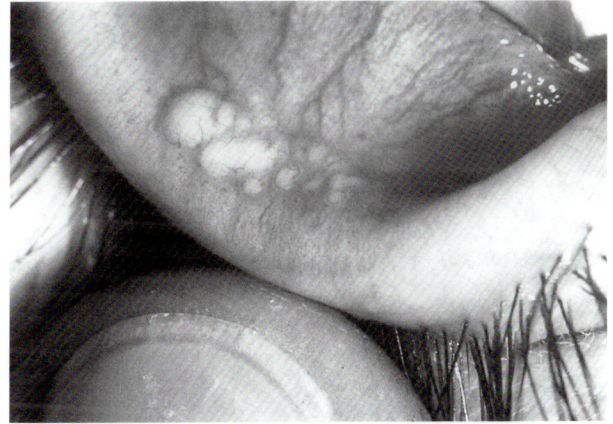

FIGURE 6-14. Subconjunctival neuroma in patient with MEN 2B.

Systemic Associations

MTC and pheochromocytoma are common and tend to present in young adulthood (18 and 24 years for MTC and pheochromocytoma). The main distinguishing features of MEN 2B are a characteristic facies with thick, blubbery lips and nodules on the

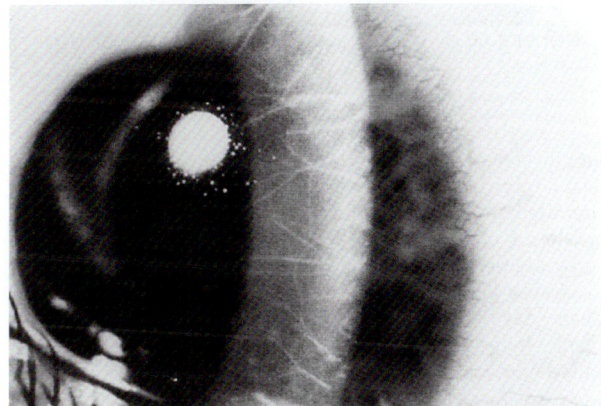

FIGURE 6-15. Prominent corneal nerves of patient in Figure 6-13.

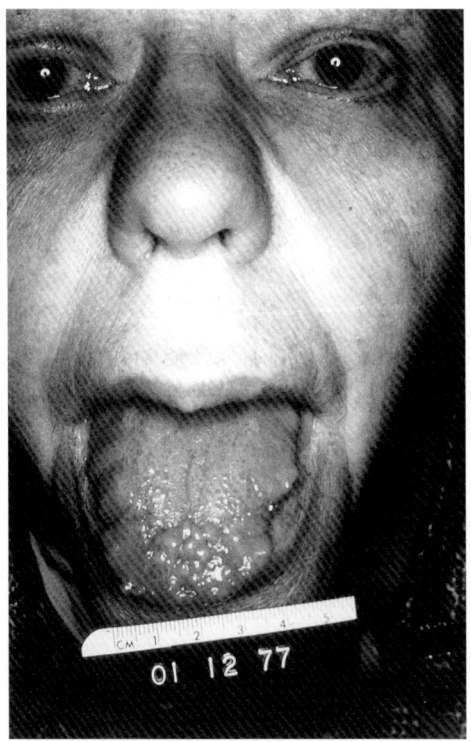

FIGURE 6-16. Diffuse nodular neuromas of the tongue in MEN 2 B.

interior tongue (Fig. 6-16). Hyperplasia of the autonomic ganglia in the intestinal wall leads to disordered gut motility,[12] which commonly presents in infancy or childhood as failure to thrive or alternating episodes of constipation and diarrhea. These abnormalities can be recognized on rectal biopsy. Generalized hypotonia (floppy baby) has been described in newborn infants.[35] There may be a variety of skeletal abnormalities including pes cavus, slipped femoral epiphyses, pectus excavatum, bifid ribs[13] and Marfanoid body habitus. Delayed puberty has been noted in a few girls with MEN 2B; the mechanism is unclear. Impotence in men is neurological in origin.

Inheritance

MEN 2B is inherited as an autosomal dominant gene, and 50% are de novo mutations.

Natural History

Oral neuromas are usually evident in childhood, with medullary thyroid carcinoma or pheochromocytoma becoming serious risks after adolescence. In MTC, total thyroidectomy is usually indicated as the lesion is often multicentric. Pheochromocytomas are often bilateral or even extrarenal. Severe constipation or diarrhea frequently develops before endocrine neoplasias are detected. An annual screening evaluation of all at-risk family members should be performed to identify and treat presymptomatic individuals.

Treatment

There is no medical treatment for MEN 2B. As mentioned earlier, thyroidectomy and adrenalectomy have been suggested even in presymptomatic patients.

Prognosis

The prognosis in MEN 2B depends on the early detection and treatment of the malignancies that occur.

PROTEUS SYNDROME

History

Initially described in 1979 by Cohen and Hayden,[22] this disorder was set forth as a clinical entity in 1983 by Wiedemann,[112] who utilized the term *proteus* (after the Greek god Proteus, the polymorphous), to capture the variable and changing phenotype of this condition. It has been suggested by Dr. Michael Cohen that John Merrick, the elephant man, most likely had the Proteus syndrome.[20]

Incidence

The disorder is rare, estimated to affect only several hundred patients in the United States and western Europe.[6]

Etiology

The etiology of Proteus syndrome is unknown. All cases have been sporadic in otherwise normal families. Recent reports have suggested that this disorder may be caused by somatic mutation during early development, resulting in mosaicism.[21]

Ophthalmic Features

Severe maldevelopment and malfunction of the retina lead to strabismus, nystagmus, and high myopia and retinal pigmentary abnormalities. In reviewing the literature, strabismus and epibulbar tumors were the most common abnormalities.[26] In another patient with multiple meningiomas and craniofacial hyperostosis, the retina showed diffuse disorganization with nodular gliosis, retinal pigmentary abnormalities, chronic papilledema, and optic atrophy.[38,114]

Clinical Assessment

At the present time, there are insufficient data to recommend periodic screening for specific tumors in Proteus syndrome. Instead, clinicians should be vigilant for clinical signs of neoplasia (see following) and initiate prompt and thorough evaluation.[5]

Systemic Associations

Proteus syndrome causes postnatal overgrowth of multiple tissues in a mosaic pattern. Diagnostic criteria are listed in Table 6-13. The overgrowth can involve skin, subcutaneous tissue, connective tissue (including bone), the central nervous system, and viscera. Complications of Proteus syndrome include, among others, progressive skeletal deformities, invasive lipomas, invasive benign and malignant tumors, and deep vein thrombosis with pulmonary embolism. The hyperostosis of the external auditory canal is a highly specific finding. Approximately 50% of reported cases have had intellectual disability.[5]

TABLE 6-13. Diagnostic Criteria for Proteus Syndrome.

General criteria:
    Mosiac distribution AND progressive course AND sporadic occurrence

Category A:
    Connective tissue nevus (see Fig. 6-1)

Category B:
    Epidermal nevus
    Disproportionate overgrowth of two of the following: limbs, skull, external
        auditory canal, vertebrae, or viscera (see Figs. 6-3, 6-4)
    Specific tumors before end of second decade: bilateral ovarian cystadenomas or
        paranoid monomorphic adenoma

Category C:
    Dysregulated adipose tissue (either lipoatrophy or lipomas)
    Vascular malformations: capillary, venous, or lymphatic
    Facial phenotype: long face, dolichocephaly, downslanted palpebral fissures,
        low nasal bridge, wide or anteveterted nares, open mouth at rest

The diagnosis of Proteus syndrome requires all three general criteria plus either
    one criterion from category A, two criteria from category B, or three criteria
    from category C

Inheritance

The majority of cases have been sporadic.

Natural History and Prognosis

Proteus syndrome patients are frequently normal at birth, although birth weight is usually increased. A few patients have had the characteristic features in the newborn period, but they typically become obvious over the first year of age. Generally progressive throughout childhood, growth of the hamartomas and the generalized hypertrophy usually ceases after puberty. Moderate mental deficiency is seen in 50% of cases. Caring for a child with Proteus syndrome is a major challenge for parents and physicians. These challenges relate to medical and psychosocial consequences of Proteus syndrome. Morbidity is significant. Of 11 patients evaluated by Clark et al., 2 required amputation of a leg, 6 had fingers or toes removed, and 2 women underwent breast reconstruction. Spinal stenosis may develop because of vertebral anomalies or tumor infiltration.[19]

    Cystic emphysematous pulmonary disease may be associated with severe morbidity and death. Affected individuals should be carefully monitored for the development of all types of neoplasms because the full spectrum of this disorder is not known.

Treatment

There is no specific medical treatment for Proteus syndrome. As already described, surgical treatment of neoplasms is frequently required.

Future Research

Although progress is being made in the clinical understanding of Proteus syndrome, much remains to be done. Surgical treatments for tissue overgrowth and deformity with careful follow-up of outcome should allow delineation of effective strategies.

Because Proteus syndrome is sporadic and hypothesized to be caused by somatic mutation, efforts are underway to characterize differences in gene expression or genomic abnormalities in paired affected and unaffected tissues from Proteus patients. Characterization of the molecular defect should allow accurate diagnosis and better understanding of the underlying pathophysiology. Although the progressive nature of the condition complicates management, this attribute suggests that there is an active hyperproliferative process that may be amenable to direct pharmacological intervention.[5]

References

1. Altuna JC, Greenfield DS, Wand M, et al. Lantanprost in glaucoma associated with Sturge–Weber syndrome: benefits and side effects. J Glaucoma 1999;8:199–203.
2. Bech K, Jenesen OA. Racemose haemangioma of the retina. Acta Ophthalmol 1958;36:769–781.
3. Bech K, Jenesen OA. On the frequency of coexisting racemose hemangiomata of the retina and brain. Acta Psychiatr Scand 1961;36: 47–56.
4. Bellester R, Marchuk DA, O'Connell P, et al. The NF1 locus encoded a protein functionally related to mammalian GAP and yeast IRA proteins. Cell 1990;63:851–859.
5. Biesecker LG. The multifaceted challenges of Proteus syndrome. JAMA 2001;285:2240–2243.
6. Biesecker LG, Peters KF, Darling TN, et al. Clinical differentiation between Proteus syndrome and hyperplasia: description of a distinct form of hemihyperplasia. Am J Med Genet 1998;79:311–318.

7. Bonnet P, Dechaume J, Blanc E. L'Aneury cirsoide de la retina (aneurysme racmeux); ses relations avec l'aneurysme cirsoide de la face et avec l'aneurysme cirsoide du cerveau. J Med Lyons 1937;18: 165–178.

8. Bourneville D. Scleros tubereuse des circonvolutions cerebrales idotie et epilepsy hemipelegique. Arch Ophthalmol 1880;1:181–191.

9. Bouzas EA, Parry DM, Eldridge R, et al. Familial occurrence of combined pigment epithelial and retinal hamartomas associated with neurofibromatosis 2. Retina 1992;12:103–107.

10. Briggs RJ, Brackman DE, Baser ME, et al. Comprehensive management of bilateral acoustic neuromas: current pespectives. Arch Otolaryngol Head Neck Surg 1994;120:1307–1314.

11. Brown DG, Hilal SH, Tenner HS. Wyburn–Mason syndrome: report of two cases without retinal involvement. Arch Neurol 1973;28:67–68.

12. Carney J, Go VLW, Sizemore GW, et al. Alimentary-tract ganglioneuromatomatosis: a major component of the syndrome of multiple endocrine neoplasia, type 2b. N Engl J Med 1976;295:1287–1291.

13. Carney JA, Bianco AJ, Sizeman GW, et al. Multiple endocrine neoplasia with skeletal manifestations. J Bone Joint Surg 1981;63A: 405–408.

14. Cawthon R, Weiss R, Xu G, et al. A major segment of neurofibromatosis type 1 gene: cDNA sequence, genomic structure and point mutations. Cell 1990;62:193–201.

15. Christenson L, Yankowitz J, Robinson R. Prenatal diagnosis of Kippel–Trenaunay–Weber syndrome as a cause for in utero heart failure and severe postnatal sequelae. Prenatal Diagn 1997;17:1176–1180.

16. Choyke PL, Glen GM, Walther MM, et al. von Hippel–Lindau disease: genetic, clinical and imaging features. Radiology 1995;194: 629–642.

17. Cibis G, Tripayhi R, Tripayhi B. Glaucoma in Sturge–Weber syndrome. Ophthalmology 1984;91:1061–1071.

18. Clarke A, Church W, Gardner-Medwin D, et al. Intracranial calcification and seizures: a case of central neurofibromatosis. Dev Med Child Neurol 1990;32:729–732.

19. Clark RD. Proteus syndrome. In: Neurofibromatoses. A pathogenetic and clinical review. London: Chapman & Hall, 1994.

20. Cohen MM Jr. The elephant man did not have neurofibromatosis. Proc Greenwood Genet Cent 1987;6:187–192.

21. Cohen MM Jr. Proteus syndrome: clinical evidence of somatic mosaicism and selective review. 1993;47:645–642.

22. Cohen MM Jr, Hayden PW. A newly recognized hamartomatous syndrome. In: O'Donnell JJ, Hall BD (eds) Birth defects: original article series, vol 15. White Plains, NY: March of Dimes, 1979:291–196.

23. Costa RM, Yang T, Huynh DP, et al. Learning deficits but normal development and tumor predisposition, in mice lacking exon 23a of NF1. Nat Genet 2001;27:354–355.

24. Crowe FW. Axillary freckling as a diagnostic aid in neurofibromatosis. Ann Intern Med 1964;61:1142–1143.

25. Dabora SL, Jozwaik S, Franz DN, et al. Mutational analysis in a cohort of 224 tuberous sclerosis patients indicates increased severity of TSC2, compared with TSC1, disease in multiple organs. Am J Hum Genet 2001;68:64–80.

26. De Becker I, Gajda DJ, Gilbert-Barness E, Cohen MM. Ocular manifestations in Proteus syndrome. Am J Med Genet 2000;92:350–352.

27. DeClue JE, Cohen BD, Lowy DR. Identification and characterization of the neurofibromatosis type 1 protein product. Proc Natl Acad Sci USA 1991;88:9914–9918.

28. DeGuttierrez A, Salamanca F, Lisker R, et al. Supernumeray bisatellited chromosome in a family acertained through a patient with Sturge–Weber syndrome. Ann Genet 1975;18:45–49.

29. Destro M, D'Amico DJ, Gragoudas ES, et al. Retinal manifestations of neurofibromatosis. Diagnosis and management. Arch Ophthalmol 1991;109:662–666.

30. Eldridge R, Martuza RL, Parry DM. Neurofibromatosis 2. In: Johnson RT (ed) Current therapy in neurologic diseases. New York: Dekker, 1990.

31. Evans DGR, Huson SM, Donnai D, et al. A genetic study of type 2 neurofibromatosis in the United Kingdom: prevalence, mutations rate, fitness, and confirmation of maternal transmission effect on severity. J Med Genet 1992;29:841–846.

32. Evans DGR, Huson SM, Neary W, et al. A clinical study of type 2 neurofibromatosis.Q J Med 1992;304:603–618.

33. Font RL, Freey AP. The phakomatoses. Int Ophthalmol Clin 1972;12:1–51.

34. Fredrich CA. Genotype-phenotype correlation in von Hippel–Lindau syndrome. Hum Mol Genet 2001;10:763–767.

35. Fryns JP, Chrzanowska. Mucosal neuromata syndrome [MEN type IIb (III)]. J Med Genet 1988;25:703–706.

36. Gass JDM, Brunstein R. Sessile and exophytic capillary angiomas of the juxtapapillary retina and optic nerve head. Arch Ophthalmol 1980;98:1790–11797.

37. Gatti RA. Ataxia-telangiectasia. In: Scriver CR, Beaudet AL, Sly WS, Valle D (eds). The metabolic and molecular bases of inherited disease. New York: McGraw-Hill, 2001:705–732.

38. Gilbert-Barness E, Cohen MM, Opitz JM. Mutiple meningiomas, craniofacial hyperostosis and retinal abnormalities. Am J Med Genet 2000;93:234–240.

39. Grant WM, Walton DS. Distinctive gonioscopic findings in glaucoma due to neurofibromatosis. Arch Ophthalmol 1968;79:127–137.

40. Gutman DH, Collins FS. Neurofibromatosis 1. In: Scriver CR, Beaudet AL, Sly WS, Valle D (eds) The metabolic basis of inherited disease. New York: McGraw Hill, 2001:877–896.

41. Gutmann GH, Ayisworth A, Carey JC, et al. The diagnostic evaluation and multidisciplinary management of neurofibromatosis 1 and neurofibromatosis 2. JAMA 1997;278:51–58.

42. Gutmann DH, Collins FS. The neurofibromatosis type 1 gene review and its protein product. Neuron 1993;10:335–343.

43. Habiby R, Silverman B, Listernick R. Precocious puberty in children with neurofibromatosis type 1. J Pediatr 1995;126:364.

44. Hardwig P, Robertson DM. von Hippel–Lindau disease: a familial, often lethal, multi-system phakomatoses. Ophthalmology 1984;91: 263–270.

45. Horton JC, Harsh GR IV, Fisher JW, et al. von Hippel–Lindau disease and erythrocytosis: radioimmunassay of erythropoietin in cysts fluid from a brainstem hemangioblastoma. Neurology 1991;41:753–754.

46. Huson S. Clinical and genetic studies of von Recklinghausen neurofibromatosis. MD thesis. Edinburgh: Edinburgh University, 1989.

47. Huson SM, Upadhyaya M. Neurofibromatosis I: clinical management and genetic counseling. In: The neurofibromatosis: a pathogenetic and clinical overview. London: Chapman & Hall, 1994.

48. Insler MS, Helm C, Napoli S. Conjunctival harmatoma in neurofibromatosis. Am J Ophthalmol 1985;99:731.

49. Jacobs AH, Walton RG. The incidence of birthmarks in the neonate. Pediatrics 1976;58:218–220.

50. Jones KL. Tuberous sclerosis. In: Smith's recognizable patterns of human malformation, 5th edn. San Diego: University of California, 1997:506–507.

51. Kalff V, Shapiro B, Lloyd R, et al. The spectrum of pheochromocytoma in hypertensive patients with neurofibromatosis. Arch Intern Med 1982;142:2092–2098.

52. King AA, DeBaun MR, Riccardi VM, et al. Malignant peripheral nerve sheath tumors in neurofibromatosis 1. Am J Med Genet 2000; 93:388–392.

53. Kippel M, Trenaunay P. Du naevus variqueux osteo-hypertrophique. Arch Gen Med 1900;85:641–672.

54. Korbin Jl, Blodi PC, Weingeist TA. Ocular and orbital manifestations of neurofibromatosis. Surv Ophthalmol 1979;24:45.

55. Kotagal P, Rothner D. Epilepsy in the setting of neurocutaneous syndrome. Epilepsia 1993;34:S71.

56. Krause Y, Rosler A, Guttmann H, et al. Somatostatin receptor scintigraphy for early detection of regional and distant metastases of medullary carcinoma of the thyroid. Clin Nucl Med 1999;24:256–260.

57. Kwiatowski DJ, Short MP. Tuberous sclerosis. Arch Dermatol 1994;130:348–354.

58. Leao M, da Silva ML. Evidence of central nervous system involvement in Watson syndrome. Pediatr Neurol 1995;12:252–254.

59. Lewis RA, Riccardi VM, von Recklinghausen neurofibromatosis: II. Incidence of iris harmatoma. Ophthalmology 1981;88:348–354.

60. Limaye SR, Doyle HA, Tang RA. Retinal varicosity in Kippel–Trenaunay syndrome. J Pediatr Ophthalmol Strabismus 1979;16: 371–373.

61. Lindau A. Studien uber Kleinhircysten: Bau, Pathogenes and Berziehungen zur Angiomatosis retinae. Acta Pathol Microbiol Scand Suppl 1926;1:1–128.

62. Linehan WM, Zbar B, Klausner. Renal cell carcinoma. In: Scriver CR, Beaudet AL, Sly WS, Valle D (eds) The metabolic and molecular bases of inherited disease. New York: McGraw-Hill, 2001:907–929.

63. Lisch K. Ueber Beteiligung der Augen, insbesondere das Vorkommen von Irisknotchen bei der Neurofiromatose (Recklinghausen). Z Augenheilkd 1937;93:137–143.

64. Listernick R, Charrow J, Greenwald M, et al. Natural history of optic pathway tumors in children with neurofibromatosis type I: a longitudinal study. J Pediatr 1994;125:63–66.

65. Louis-Bar D. Sur un syndrome progressif comprenant des telangiectasies cappillaires untanees et conjonctivales, a disposition naevpode et des troubles cerebelleux. Confin Neurol 1941;4:32–42.

66. Lubs MLE, Bauer MS, Formas ME, et al. Lisch nodules in neurofibromatosis type 1. N Engl J Med 1991;324:1264.

67. MaCollin M, Gusella J. Neurofibromatosis 2. In: Scriver CR, Beaudet AL Sly WS, Valle D (eds) The metabolic and molecular bases of inherited disease. New York: McGraw Hill, 2001:897–906.

68. Maher ER, Iselius L, Yates JRW, et al. von Hippel–Lindau disease: a genetic study. J Med Genet 1990;28:443–447.

69. Maher ER, Iselius L, Yates JR, et al. von Hippel–Lindau disease a genetic study. J Med Genet 1991;28:443–447.

70. Maher ER, Moore AT. von Hippel–Lindau disease. Br J Ophthalmol 1992;76:743–745.

71. Maher ER, Yates JR, Harris R, et al. Clinical features and natural history of von Hippel–Lindau disease. Q J Med 1970;77;1151–1163.

72. Marti-Bonmati L, Menor F, Mulas F. The Sturge–Weber syndrome: correlation between the clinical status and radiological and MRI findings. Child's Nerv Syst 1993;9:857–871.

73. Martin GA, Viskocil D, Bollaguski G, et al. The GAP-related domain of the neurofibromatosis type 1 gene product interacts with ras21. Cell 1990;63:843–849.

74. Mautner VF, Tagiba M, Lindenan M, et al. Spinal tumors in patients with neurofibromatosis type 2: MR imaging study, frequency, multiplicity, and variety. AJR (Am J Roentgenol) 1995;165:952–955.

75. Moore AT, Maher ER, Rosen, et al. Ophthalmological screening for von Hippel–Lindau disease. Eye 1992;5:723–728.

76. Morrison PJ, Nevin NC. Multiple endocrine neoplasia type 2B (mucosal neuroma syndrome, Wagenmann–Froboese syndrome). J Med Genet 1996;33:779–782.

77. Narod SA, Parry DM, Parboosingh J, et al. Neurofibromatosis type 2 appears to be genetically homogeneous disease. Am J Hum Genet 1992;51:486–496.

78. National Institutes of Health Consensus Development Conference. Neurofibromatosis: conference statement. Arch Neurol 1988;45: 575–578.

79. National Institute of Health Consensus Development Conference Statement. Acoustic neuroma. Neurofibromatosis Res Newsl 1992; 8:1–7.

80. Nyboer J, Robertson D, Gomez M. Retinal lesions in tuberous sclerosis. Arch Ophthalmol 1976;94:1277–1280.

81. Ogunmekan A, Hwang P, Hoffman H. Sturge–Weber–Dimitri disease. Role of hemispherectomy in prognosis. Can J Neurol Sci 1989;16:78.

82. Ojemann RG. Management of acoustic neuromas (vestibular schwannomas). Clin Neurosurg 1993;40:489–495.

83. Opitz JM, Weaver DDL. The neurofibromatosis–Noonan syndrome. Am J Med Genet 1985;21:477–490.

84. Osborne JP, Fryer A, Webb D. Epidemiology of tuberoses sclerosis. Ann NY Acad Sci 1991:615:125–127.

85. Ozonoff S. Cognitive impairment in neurofibromatosis type 1. Am J Med Genet 1999;89:45–52.

86. Park VM, Pivnick EK. Neurofibromatosis type 1 (NF1): a protein truncations assay yielding identification of mutations in 73% of patients. J Med Genet 1998;35:813–820.

87. Pearson-Webb MA, Kaiser-Kupfer MI, Elbridge R. Eye finding in bilateral acoustic (central) neurofibromatosis: association with presenile lens opacity and cataracts but absence of Lisch nodules. N Engl J Med 1986;315:1553–1554.

88. Povey S, Burley MW, Attwood J, et al. Two loci for tuberous sclerosis: one on 9q34 and one on 16p13. Ann Hum Genet 1994;58:107–127.

89. Ragge NK, Traboulsi EI. Phakomatoses. In: Traboulsi EI (ed) Genetic disease of the eye. New York: Oxford University Press, 1998:753–756.

90. Ragge NK, Traboulsi EI. Phakomatoses. In: Traboulsi EI (ed) Genetic disease of the eye. New York: Oxford University Press, 1998:750–753.

91. Ragge NK, Traboulis EI. Phakomatoses. In: Traboulsi EI (ed) Genetic disease of the eye. New York: Oxford University Press, 1998:756–759.

92. Reynolds JD, Johnson BL, Gioster S, et al. Glaucoma and Kippel–Trenaunay–Weber syndrome. Am J Ophthalmol 1988;196:494–496.

93. Riccardi VM. In: Gutmann DH, MacColin M, Riccardi VM (eds) Neurofibromatosis: phenotype, natural history, and pathogenesis. Baltimore: Johns Hopkins University Press, 1999:162–189.

94. Roach ES, Gomez MR, Northeup H. Tuberous sclerosis complex consensus conference: revised clinical diagnostic criteria. J Child Neurol 1998;13:624–628.

95. Rouleau GA, Merel P, Lutchmam M, et al. Alterations in a new gene encoding a putative membrane organizing protein causes neurofibromatosis type 2. Nature (Lond) 1993;363:515–521.

96. Rouleau GA, Seizinger BR, Ozelius LG, et al. Genetic linkage analysis of bilateral acoustic neurofibromatosis to DNA markers on chromosome 22. Nature (Lond) 1987;329:246–248.

97. Samaan NA, Drazian MB, Halpin RE, et al. Multiple endocrine syndrome type IIb in early childhood. Cancer (Phila) 1991;68:1832–1835.

98. Sampson JR. Tuberous sclerosis. In: Scriver CR, Beaudet AL Sly WS, Valle D (eds) The metabolic and molecular bases of inherited disease. New York: McGraw-Hill, 2001:5857–5873.

99. Shepherd CW, Gomez MR, Lie JT, et al. Causes of death in patients with tuberous sclerosis. Mayo Clin Proc 1991;66:792–796.

100. Smith RW. A treatise on the pathology, diagnosis and treatment of neuroma. Dublin: Hodges and Smith, 1849.

101. South D, Jacobs A. Cutis marmorata telangiectatica congenital (congenital generalized phlebectasia). J Pediatr 1978;93:944–949.

102. Sujansky E, Conradi S. Outcome of Sturge–Weber syndrome in 52 adults. Am J Med Genet 1995;22:35–45.

103. Sullivan T, Clarke M, Morin J. The ocular manifestations of the Sturge–Weber syndrome. J Pediatr Ophthalmol Strabismus 1992;29:349–356.

104. Susac JO, Smith JL, Scelfo RJ. The "tomato-catsup" fundus in Sturge–Weber syndrome. Arch Ophthalmol 1974;92:69–73.

105. Theron J, Newton TH, Hoyt WF. Unilateral retinocephalic vascular malformations. Neuroradiology 1974;7:185–196.

106. Traboulsi EI, Dudin G, To'mey, et al. The association of a fragile site on chromosome 10 with Sturge–Weber syndrome and congenital glaucoma. Ophthalmic Paediatr Genet 1983;3:135–140.

107. Vasen HFA, van der Feltz M, Rare F, et al. The natural course of multiple endocrine neoplasia type IIb. Arch Intern Med 1992;251:1250–1255.

108. Viskochil D, White R, Cawthon R. The neurofibromatosis type 1 gene. Annu Rev Neurosci 1993;10:183–205.

109. Vogt H. Zur Diagnostik der Tubersen Sklerose. Z Erforch Behandl Jugendl Schwaschisinns 1908;2:1–12.

110. von-Hippel E. Ubereine sehr seltene Erlranking der Netzhaut klinische Becobachtungn. Albrecht von Graefe's Arch Ophthalmol 1904;59:83–106.

111. von Recklinghausen F. Uber die multiplen Frome der Haut und ibre Beziehung zu den multiplen Neuromen. Berlin: Hirschwald, 1882.

112. Wiedemann HR, Burgio GR, Aldenhoff P, et al. The proteus syndrome: partial gigantism of the hands and/or feet, nevi, hemihypertrophy, subcutaneous tumors, macrocephaly or other skull anomalies and possible accelerated growth and visceral affections. Eur J Pediatr 1983;140:5–12.

113. Wishart JH. Case of tumors in the skull, dura mater, and brain. Edinb Med Surg J 1882;18:393–397.

114. Wyburn-Mason R. Arteriovenous aneurysm of mid-brain, facial naevi and mental changes. Brain 1943;66:162–203.
115. Young DF, Eldridge R, Gardner WJ. Bilateral acoustic neuromas in a large kindred. JAMA 1970;214:347–253.
116. Zhu Y, Parada LF. A particular GAP in mind. Nat Genet 2001;27: 354–355.

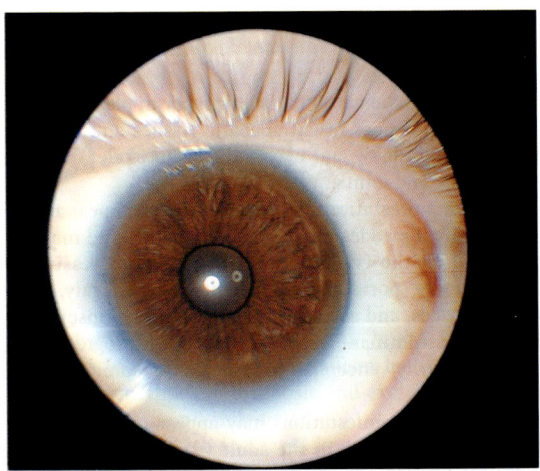

FIGURE 7-1. Kayser–Fleischer ring of Wilson's disease.

The Kayser–Fleischer ring is present in virtually all patients with neurological manifestations of Wilson's disease and is commonly present in those with nonneurological signs, although it is often absent in patients who present with acute liver disease; it is also often absent in asymptomatically affected siblings of patients with Wilson's disease.[63] (Note: A similar ring can be seen in patients with non-Wilsonian liver disease.[282])

A less frequent manifestation of Wilson's disease is sunflower cataract ("scheinkataract"), composed of fine copper pigment deposits beneath the anterior and posterior lens capsule that form a disclike opacity axially with radiating spoke-or petal-like extensions.[266,282] On slit lamp examination, the opacities appear to be of various colors, including reds, blues, greens, yellows, and browns. The opacities reportedly do not impair vision. (Note: Similar cataracts can be caused by exogenous copper.[266])

Ocular motor functions usually are spared in Wilson's disease, although jerky oscillations of the eyes, gaze paresis, involuntary gaze movements, impairment of accommodation and convergence, infrequent or absent blinking and apraxia of lid opening have occasionally been noted.[61,104,141,149] Night blindness and retinal changes have been reported in some cases.[104,202,217,232]

Wilson's disease is an autosomal recessive disorder. It occurs worldwide with an incidence of approximately 1 in 30,000.[60] The gene has been localized to chromosome 13q 14.3.[60] Heterozygotes do not exhibit clinical manifestations; approximately 20% have decreased levels of ceruloplasmin. Prenatal diagnosis is possible, provided DNA is available from the index case.[63]

Laboratory confirmation of the diagnosis of Wilson's disease involves demonstration of decreased serum ceruloplasmin, increased urinary copper, and elevated hepatic copper concentration.[60]

Wilson's disease can be effectively treated with penicillamine, a chelating agent that reduces body stores of copper. Both the Kayser–Fleischer ring and sunflower cataract may regress with treatment.[31,254,282] Changes in the eye can be used to monitor efficacy of treatment and compliance with treatment. Ocular complications of penicillamine therapy, particularly optic neuritis and retinal changes, have been reported.[74,108] Treatment alternatives are trientene or orally administered zinc salts. Liver transplantation has a place in the treatment of patients with advanced liver disease and can be successful in fulminant cases. Disappearance of the Kayser–Fleischer ring after liver transplantation has been documented.[227]

Menkes' Disease

In Menkes's disease, there is widespread disturbance in the cellular transport of copper. There is defective intestinal absorption of copper, resulting in copper deficiency, and defective synthesis of copper enzymes, with severe neurological and connective tissue consequences.[63] Major manifestations are abnormal hair, a distinctive facies, hypopigmentation, progressive neurological deterioration, lax skin, arterial degeneration, bone changes, urinary tract diverticulae, and hypothermia. Laboratory findings include very low levels of serum copper and ceruloplasmin, grossly reduced copper content in the liver, and greatly increased copper content in the intestinal mucosa.

The disorder is X-linked recessive, characteristically affecting hemizygous males; some heterozygous females show manifestations. The gene location is Xq 13.2–13.3.[60] The estimated incidence of the disease is 1 in 250,000 live births.[60] Prenatal diagnosis and heterozygote detection are possible.

Manifestations develop in infancy; some may be evident at birth. The hair is pale, lusterless, brittle, often stubby, giving rise to the descriptive term "steely hair." The face is distinguished by pudgy cheeks and sagging jowls. By age 3 months, infants show developmental delay and regression. Seizures develop. There is progressive psychomotor deterioration from widespread neuronal destruction and gliosis, especially in the cerebral cortex and cerebellum. Vascular abnormalities can be found in brain, viscera, and limbs; complications such as thrombosis and rupture occur. Subdural hematomas are common. Osteoporosis and fractures are common. Diverticulae of the bladder or ureters may rupture or predispose to infection. Death commonly occurs by age 3 years, although some patients survive longer, severely incapacitated.

The eyes often appear sunken because of paucity of orbital fat. The eyebrows typically are pale and "steely," often stubby and sparse. The eyelashes may be better preserved, somewhat more pigmented, curly or long and straight. The irides usually are light blue or gray with a delicate stromal pattern, but do not transilluminate. There may be photophobia. Generalized hypopigmentation of the fundus with increased visibility of the choroidal pattern is common (Fig. 7-2). There may be tortuosity of the retinal arterioles. Often the macular landmarks are poorly defined. Disc pallor develops with time. Visual function deteriorates with progression of the disease. Degeneration of retinal

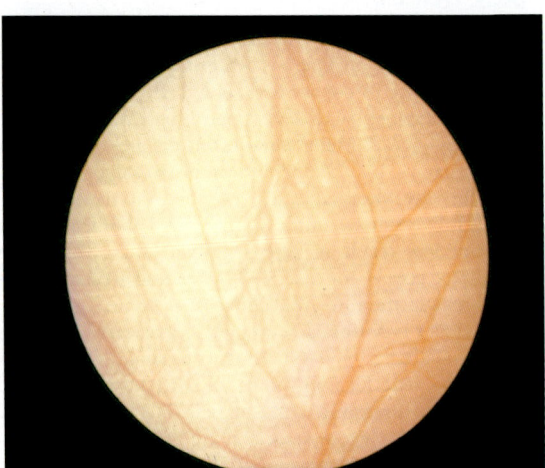

FIGURE 7-2. Fundus hypopigmentation in Menkes' disease.

ganglion cells with loss of nerve fibers and atrophic changes of the optic nerve have been documented by light and electron microscopy.[231,289] In addition, microcysts of the iris pigment epithelium and irregularity of melanin granules in the retinal pigment epithelium were found.[231,289] Electroretinogram (ERG) and visual evoked potential (VEP) responses diminish.[22,85,161,240,278] Nystagmus and strabismus are common. There may be blepharitis, dacryostenosis, and possibly tear deficiency.[168] Aberrant lashes have been noted.[85] In addition, cataracts, possibly incidental, have been reported.[218]

As yet there is no truly affective treatment for Menkes' disease.[60] Various forms of copper replacement therapy have been tried. Presymptomatic treatment with copper histidine injections can modify the disease, but no treatment has been found to significantly alter the course once brain damage has occurred.

THE MUCOPOLYSACCHARIDOSES

The group of syndromes generically referred to as the mucopolysaccharidoses (MPS) are caused by deficiency of specific lysosomal enzymes involved in the metabolic degradation of dermatan sulfate, heparan sulfate, and keratan sulfate, either singly or in combination; chondroitin sulfate also may be affected.[185] Incompletely degraded mucopolysaccharides (glycosaminoglycans) accumulate in various tissues and organs throughout the body and are excreted in the urine.

The mucopolysaccharidoses are characterized by a rather distinctive spectrum of clinical manifestations. Bone abnormalities (dysostosis multiplex), joint contractures, skeletal deformity, and dwarfing are prominent features. There is a characteristic facies with coarse, often somewhat grotesque features. Visceromegaly, cardiovascular disease, respiratory problems, hearing impairment, and mental deficiency occur within the group. Hypertrichosis is common. The principal ocular manifestations of the various mucopolysaccharidoses are progressive corneal clouding, pigmentary retinal degeneration, optic atrophy, sometimes papilledema, and in certain cases glaucoma (Table 7-1). The familiar prototype of the mucopolysaccharidoses is Hurler syndrome (MPS I-H).

All the mucopolysaccharidoses are autosomal recessive disorders with the exception of Hunter syndrome (MPS II), which

TABLE 7-1. The Systemic Mucopolysaccharidoses (MPS).

The disease	General manifestations	Ophthalmologic manifestations
MPS IH: Hurler syndrome α-L-Iduronidase deficiency (autosomal recessive)	Marked dysmorphism, coarse facial features Severe dysostosis multiplex, skeletal deformity Visceromegaly, pulmonary and cardiac disease Mental deficiency Hearing impairment Death in childhood, usually by age 10 years	Progressive corneal clouding Retinal degeneration Optic atrophy Nervehead swelling Vision loss In some cases, megalocornea and/or glaucoma
MPS IS: Scheie syndrome α-L-Iduronidase deficiency (autosomal recessive)	Less severe somatic and visceral signs than in Hurler prototype Prominent joint stiffness Aortic valve disease Normal or nearly normal intellect Hearing impairment Relatively normal lifespan	Corneal clouding Retinal degeneration Vision loss In some cases, glaucoma
MPS I H/S: Hurler–Scheie syndrome α-L-Iduronidase deficiency (autosomal recessive)	Phenotype intermediate between that of Hurler and Scheie Dwarfing, joint stiffness, coarse facial features, micrognathia Hepatosplenomegaly Cardiovascular disease Intellectual impairment Hearing impairment Survival into teens or twenties	Corneal clouding Retinal degeneration Vision loss In some cases, glaucoma
MPS II: Hunter's syndrome Iduronate sulfatase deficiency (X-linked recessive)	Dysmorphism, skeletal deformities and dwarfing Hepatosplenomegaly, cardiac and respiratory disease Hydrocephalus Hearing impairment Pebbly skin lesions In severe form, rapid psychomotor deterioration and early death In milder form, slower deterioration and longer survival into adulthood	Progressive retinal degeneration and vision loss Disc pallor Often nervehead swelling Clinically clear cornea; possibly microscopic changes Glaucoma in some cases
MPS III: Sanfilippo's syndrome Heparan N-sulfatase deficiency in type A	Similar clinical manifestations in all four biochemical forms Severe progressive mental deterioration	Corneas clinically clear; possibly microscopic changes

TABLE 7-1. (continued).

The disease	General manifestations	Ophthalmologic manifestations
α-N-Acetyl-glucosaminidase deficiency in type B Acetyl-CoA: α-glucosaminide acetyl transferase deficiency in type C N-Acetylglucosamine 6-sulfatase deficiency in type D All forms autosomal recessive	Less severe somatic changes Coarse facial features, megalocephaly, moderate skeletal changes Hepatosplenomegaly Survival into third decade	Some signs of retinal degeneration Vision impairment Possibly optic atrophy Rarely nervehead swelling
MPS IV: Morquio syndrome N-Acetylgalactosamine-6-sulfatase deficiency in deficiency in type A β-Galactosidase deficiency in type B Both forms autosomal recessive	In classic form (type A), distinctive skeletal deformities: severe dwarfing, kyphosis, sternal bulging, prominent joints, semicrouching stance, waddling gait Joint laxity rather than stiffness Odontoid hypoplasia, atlantoaxial instability; spinal cord and medullary compression, long tract signs, and respiratory paralysis may occur Hearing impairment Intellect normal or mildly impaired In milder form (type B), similar but less severe findings	Mild corneal clouding, fine haze, in types A & B Subcortical lens opacities in A In some cases, optic atrophy, disc blurring, retinal arteriolar attenuation Glaucoma
MPS V: no longer used (formerly Scheie)		
MPS VI: Maroteaux–Lamy syndrome N-Acetylgalactosamine 4-sulfatase deficiency (autosomal recessive)	Dysostosis multiplex, skeletal deformities and dwarfism, coarse facial features Visceromegaly and cardiac disease In some cases atlantoaxial subluxation, spinal cord compression, hydrocephalus Normal intellect Milder variants recognized	Corneal clouding Papilledema, abducent palsy secondary to hydrocephalus Optic atrophy Retinal vascular tortuosity Occasionally signs of retinal degeneration in milder form Glaucoma in some cases
MPS VII: Sly syndrome β-Glucuronidase deficiency (autosomal recessive)	Variable, often moderate Coarse facial features, skeletal deformity Hepatosplenomegaly Cardiovascular and respiratory problems Intellectual impairment	Corneal clouding in some cases Possibly nervehead swelling

is an X-linked recessive disorder.[185] Diagnosis of the various mucopolysaccharidoses is made on the basis of the distinguishing clinical features, the presence of excessive mucopolysaccharide substances in tissue and urine, and demonstration of the enzyme deficiency in fibroblasts, leukocytes, or serum. Prenatal diagnosis is possible by analysis of cultured amniotic fluid cells or chorionic villi. Identification of heterozygotes also is becoming increasingly available.

Enzyme replacement therapy is being investigated.[186] There has been some success in altering the course of certain of the mucopolysaccharidoses with bone marrow and stem cell transplantation.[186] Some improvement in the ocular findings after marrow transplantation has been documented.[115,253]

Hurler Syndrome: MPS IH

In Hurler syndrome, there is profound deficiency of α-L-iduronidase with excessive urinary excretion of both dermatan sulfate and heparan sulfate. The gene encoding this enzyme has been mapped to chromosome 4p 16.3.[186] There is accumulation of acid mucopolysaccharide in virtually every system of the body, producing marked somatic and visceral abnormalities beginning in infancy or early childhood, progressing with age, and leading to early death, usually by age 10 years.

The head tends to be large and misshapen; on radiologic examination the calvarium is thickened, there is premature closure of lamboid and sagittal sutures, the sella is enlarged and J-shaped, there is hypertelorism, the orbits are shallow, and the optic foramina may be enlarged. The facial features characteristically are coarse, the expression dull (Fig. 7-3). The eyes appear wide-set and prominent, the lids are puffy, the brows are prominent, and the lashes coarse. The nose is broad with wide nostrils and a flat bridge. The ears may be large and low-set. The lips usually are patulous, the tongue large and protuberant. The teeth generally are small, stubby, and widely spaced, the gums hyperplastic. The skin tends to be thick. Generalized hypertrichosis is common.

Moderate dwarfism, short neck, kyphoscoliosis, and gibbus are typical. On X-ray, the vertebral bodies, particularly those of the lower dorsal and upper lumbar region, are wedge shaped with an anterior hooklike projection referred to as beaking. The extremities are short, the hands and feet are broad, the phalanges short and stubby. Radiologically, the tubular bones show expan-

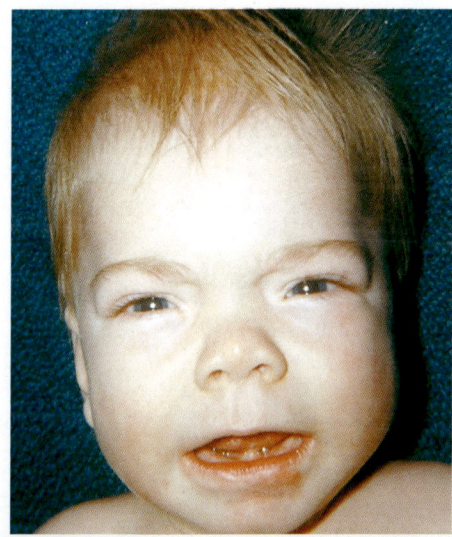

FIGURE 7-3. Coarse facial features of Hurler syndrome.

sion of the medullary cavity and thinning of the cortex, and the terminal phalangeal bones commonly appear hypoplastic. The joints are stiff and flexion contractures develop; clawlike deformity of the hands is especially characteristic. The posture is semicrouching, the gait awkward. There is thoracic deformity; the chest appears wide and large, with flaring of the lower ribs over the abdomen. On X-ray, the ribs appear spatulate or saber shaped, and the medial end of the clavicle is widened. The constellation of skeletal abnormalities and radiologic findings in MPS is described by the term dysostosis multiplex.

The abdomen is protuberant owing to visceromegaly and abnormalities in supporting tissues. As a rule, there is enlargement of both liver and spleen. Diastasis recti, umbilical hernia, and inguinal hernias are common. Pathological changes in the heart due to mucopolysaccharide deposition can be extensive; the great vessels and peripheral vessels also are affected. Cardiac manifestations include murmur, angina, myocardial infarction, and congestive heart failure. Respiratory problems, particularly recurrent upper respiratory tract infection, bronchitis, and chronic nasal congestion are common. The patients almost always are noisy mouth breathers. Contributing factors include deformity of the facial and nasal bones, narrowing of the passages, abnormalities of the tracheobronchial cartilage, and deposition of mucopolysaccharide in the lungs.

The principal neurological manifestation is mental deficiency. There may be motor signs. Pathologic changes can be found throughout the nervous system. Hydrocephalus may develop. Leptomeningeal cysts develop in some cases. Deafness is frequent; it may be of mixed, conductive or sensory neural type. Middle ear infections are common.

The ocular hallmark of Hurler syndrome, long recognized as a prominent feature of the disorder, is progressive corneal clouding[18,56,78] (Fig. 7-4). It is usually evident by age 2 to 3 years, often by age 1 year; it may be present at birth. Photophobia is a common early symptom. With time there is progression from generalized haziness to dense, milky ground glass opacification.

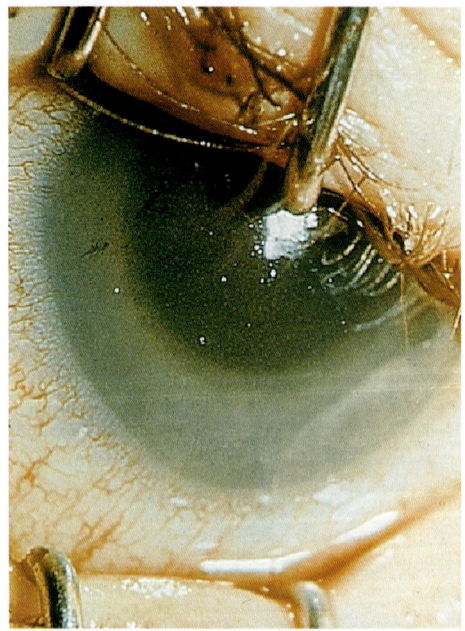

FIGURE 7-4. Ground glass corneal haze of Hurler syndrome.

Slit lamp examination reveals fine granular opacities, often increasing in density from the anterior stroma and subepithelial region to the posterior stromal layers of the cornea.[18,56] Corresponding histopathological and ultrastructural changes of mucopolysaccharide accumulation in the cornea have been well documented.[18,128,188]

Although corneal clouding may impair visualization of the fundus, signs of retinal degeneration, nerve head swelling, and optic atrophy are found in Hurler syndrome.[54,98] The ERG usually is markedly reduced.[35,98] Related histopathological and ultrastructural changes, including the presence of inclusions in retinal pigment epithelium, retinal ganglion cells, and optic nerve astrocytes, have been well documented.[37,188] Pathological evidence of mucopolysaccharide accumulation in virtually all ocular tissues has been found.[37,143]

Megalocornea has been described in many reports; in most cases the intraocular pressure has been normal, but glaucoma has been documented in some patients with Hurler syndrome.[18,56,78,188,191,247] Involvement of the trabecular meshwork has been found.[247] Normalization of ocular pressure after marrow transplantation for MPS IH has been reported.[41]

Progressive impairment of vision is usual, due to corneal clouding, retinal degeneration, and optic atrophy, singly or in combination; glaucoma, cerebral mucopolysaccharide accumulation, and hydrocephalus also may contribute. Considering all factors, corneal transplantation in an effort to improve vision has not generally been recommended in the past. Now, however, the possibility of altering the course of Hurler syndrome with treatment may alter the prospects for keratoplasty.[186]

Scheie Syndrome: MPS IS

In Scheie syndrome, there is deficiency of α-L-iduronidase and urinary excretion of both dermatan sulfate and heparan sulfate as in Hurler syndrome, but the clinical picture is somewhat different. The major manifestations are corneal clouding, joint stiffness, claw-hand deformity, carpal tunnel syndrome, and aortic valve disease, principally aortic stenosis and regurgitation. The facial features are coarse; the mouth is broad. Other somatic and visceral changes tend to be minimal. Stature is normal. The intellect is normal or nearly normal, although psychiatric disturbances have been reported. There may be hearing impairment. The lifespan is relatively normal.

Corneal clouding is a prominent feature of Scheie syndrome.[225] Evident early in life, sometimes at birth, the corneal clouding usually worsens with age and may ultimately interfere with vision. It is diffuse but tends to be most dense peripherally. The hazy cornea may appear enlarged, edematous, and thickened, initially raising suspicion of glaucoma, particularly when somatic signs of MPS are minimal. Reported histopathological and ultrastructural findings in cornea and conjunctiva are similar to those of Hurler syndrome.[143,225] Corneal transplants have been tried with little success in the past.[225] Glaucoma has been documented in some patients with Scheie syndrome.[152,205]

Although retinal changes have not been found in all cases,[225] retinal degeneration is a recognized feature of Scheie syndrome.[35,98,205] Manifestations include vision impairment, particularly progressive night blindness, field changes such as ring scotoma, retinal pigmentary changes, and diminished or extinguished ERG responses.

Hurler–Scheie Syndrome: MPS IH/S

Patients having features intermediate between those of the Hurler and Scheie syndrome have been described. They show deficiency of α-L-iduronidase and urinary excretion of dermatan sulfate and heparan sulfate. The prominent clinical manifestations are skeletal, with dwarfing and progressive joint stiffness, scaphocephaly, hypertelorism, and progressive coarsening of facial features. In addition, a receding chin or micognathia appears to be a distinctive feature. Other significant manifestations include hepatosplenomegaly, pulmonary and cardiovascular involvement, mental retardation, and hearing impairment. Destruction of the sella, cerebrospinal fluid rhinorrhea, and loss of vision related to the presence of arachnoid cysts have also been reported. Patients with Hurler–Scheie syndrome may survive into their teens or twenties.

Corneal clouding occurs in MPS IH/S.[137,250] The haze is diffuse, sometimes more dense peripherally, and progressive; it may be evident in childhood and in time may interfere with vision. Keratoplasty has been tried with some success.[137]

Retinal degeneration also occurs in MPS IH/S. There may be decreased acuity, night blindness, field constriction, retinal pigmentary changes, and ERG changes.[40,98] Optic nerve head swelling and optic atrophy have been reported.[54]

Chronic open-angle glaucoma in a child with MPS IH/S has been reported; ultrastructural changes consistent with mucopolysaccharide deposition were found in tissue obtained at trabeculectomy.[180]

Hunter's Syndrome: MPS II

In Hunter's syndrome, the only X-linked MPS, there is deficiency of iduronate sulfatase, with urinary excretion of dermatan sulfate and heparan sulfate. The gene for this defect has been mapped to Xq 28.[186]

Phenotypic manifestations of Hunter's syndrome closely resemble those of Hurler syndrome, but are generally less severe, and Hunter's syndrome is distinguished clinically by longer survival and the absence of gross corneal clouding. The features are coarse. Dwarfing and joint stiffness are prominent findings. There is usually hepatosplenomegaly; the abdomen is protruberant. Hernias are common. Cardiac involvement is a regular feature of MPS II, and respiratory disability is evident in most patients. Neurological manifestations vary. Spastic quadriplegia may develop from impingement on the cervical spinal cord. Hydrocephalus may develop. Mental deterioration may occur. Progressive deafness is common. Nodular or pebbly ivory-colored skin lesions are a distinctive feature of Hunter's syndrome. Adults also tend to have a rosy or ruddy complexion.

Based on severity, Hunter's syndrome can be classified into subtypes. Patients with the more severe form, type A, show more rapid neurological deterioration and usually die before age 15 years. The milder form, type B, is characterized by slower mental deterioration and is compatible with survival into the fifth or sixth decade.

The major ophthalmologic manifestation of MPS II is progressive retinal degeneration with impairment of vision.[98] Fundus signs include retinal pigmentary changes, sometimes spicule formation, retinal arteriolar attenuation, and disc pallor. The ERG usually is reduced or extinguished.[35,98] Bilateral epiretinal membranes with tortuosity of the retinal vessels have been reported as an unusual finding in siblings with type B Hunter's syndrome.[184]

Swelling of the optic nervehead, attributed to increased intracranial pressure or mucopolysaccharide deposition in and around the optic nerve, and potentially leading to optic atrophy, is a frequent finding.[16,54,236]

Obvious corneal clouding is not a feature of Hunter's syndrome. However, slight corneal changes may be detected by slit lamp examination in older patients, and histological and ultrastructural evidence of corneal mucopolysaccharide accumulation has been reported.[262] In addition, clinically visible corneal opacities have been documented in a child with severe MPS II, and fine corneal opacities have been seen on slit lamp examination in a young patient with mild MPS II.[249] Glaucoma has been reported in some patients with Hunter's syndrome.[133,249]

Light and electron microscopic studies have documented widespread changes in the eye in both severe and mild forms of MPS II.[170,262]

Sanfilippo's Syndrome: MPS III

Four biochemically different but clinically indistinguishable forms of Sanfilippo's syndrome occur: in type A there is deficiency of heparan N-sulfatase, the gene for which has been localized to 17q 25.3; in type B, deficiency of α-N-acetylglucosaminidase, which has been localized to 17q 21; in type C, deficiency of acetyl-CoA: α-glucosaminide-N-acetyltransferase; and in type D, deficiency of N–acetyl glucosamine 6-sulfatase, which has been localized to 12q 14.[186] In all forms, there is urinary excretion of heparan sulfate.

Mental retardation, the predominant clinical manifestation of MPS III, usually becomes evident in the first 3 years of life. There is progressive deterioration of intellect and behavior with increasing age. Somatic abnormalities tend to be mild or inconspicuous. There is some coarseness of facial features. Synophrys is common. Generalized hirsutism may be marked. Dwarfing, joint stiffness, and claw-hand deformity are usually evident but not as severe as in Hurler syndrome. Slight to moderate hepatosplenomegaly develops. The abdomen tends to be protuberant. Respiratory problems are common. Heart involvement may occur. Hearing loss occurs in moderate to severely affected patients. Hydrocephalus may develop.

Corneal clouding is not a feature of MPS III, although fine opacities were noted on slit lamp examination in one of Sanfilippo's patients, and histological and ultrastructural corneal and scleral changes have been reported in other cases.[132,223]

Retinal involvement and progressive vision loss may occur in MPS III. Narrowing of retinal vessels and pigmentary changes have been noted.[35,98,155] Decreased ERG responses have been recorded in type A and type B.[35,98] Optic atrophy may develop.[54] In addition, papilledema has been found in some cases.[54] Corresponding histopathological and ultrastructural changes of the retina and optic nerve have been documented in type A and type B Sanfilippo's syndrome.[36,68,158] There is evidence for mucopolysaccharide accumulation in virtually every ocular tissue.[36,86,158]

Morquio Syndrome: MPS IV

Clinically similar but enzymatically different forms of Morquio syndrome occur. In the classic form of Morquio syndrome, designated MPS IV-A, there is deficiency of *N*-acetylgalactosamine 6-sulfatase; the gene encoding this enzyme has been localized to chromosome 16q 24.3.[186] In the later-onset variant of Morquio syndrome, designated MPS IV-B, there is deficiency of *α*-galactosidase, which has been localized to chromosome 3p 21.33.[186] Both mild and severe forms of MPS IV-A and MPS IV-B occur. There is excessive urinary excretion of keratan sulfate in all forms.

Morquio syndrome is characterized by severe dwarfism and skeletal deformity, often with neurological complications, and a number of extraskeletal abnormalities. Patients appear normal in the first months of life, although radiologic signs may be present. During the early years, abnormalities such as retarded growth, knock-knees, prominent joints, dorsal kyphosis, sternal bulging, flaring of the rib cage, and awkward gait become evident, and worsen with age. Joint stiffness, however, is not a feature; rather joints may be abnormally loose, causing instability. The face is abnormal with somewhat coarse features, a broad-mouthed appearance, prominent jaw, and widely spaced teeth. Aortic regurgitation may develop. Progressive hearing loss is common. Invariably there is absence or hypoplasia of the odontoid process and usually ligamentous laxity of the spinal column. Atlantoaxial subluxation and spinal cord and medullary compression are frequent complications; signs may range from minimal long-tract signs to spastic paraplegia, respiratory paralysis, and death. Intellect usually is normal or mildly impaired. The course is one of progressive incapacitation.

Corneal clouding is a feature of Morquio syndrome, occurring in both MPS IV-A and MPS IV-B.[11,265,273] It is relatively mild, having the appearance of a fine haze. It may not become clinically evident to the unaided eye for several years, often not before age 10 years. The slit lamp appearance is that of diffuse involvement of the stroma with punctate or granular opacities, usually with sparing of epithelium, Bowman's layer, and endothelium. Histopathological and ultrastructural studies of the eye in Morquio syndrome have documented evidence of MPS accumulation in cornea, and also in conjunctiva and sclera.[11,97,130]

Fundus abnormalities have been reported infrequently in Morquio syndrome. Optic atrophy has been noted.[64] There has been mention of blurring of the discs.[62] Narrowing of retinal arterioles and ERG changes have been documented.[4,62] In most cases the fundi and ERG are normal.

Cataracts have been reported in siblings with MPS IV-A.[196] Mesodermal anomalies have been described in one patient with MPS IV.[273] Glaucoma may occur.[30] In addition, mydriasis attributed to sympathetic involvement in Morquio syndrome has been noted.[62]

Maroteaux–Lamy Syndrome: MPS VI

In this MPS, there is deficiency of *N*-acetylgalactosamine-4-sulfatase, with urinary excretion of predominantly dermatan sulfate. The gene encoding this enzyme has been localized to chromosome 5q13–q14.[186] Metachromatic granulation of circulating leukocytes is a characteristic finding in MPS VI. In addition to the classic severe form of Maroteaux–Lamy, milder variants with the same enzyme deficiency occur.

In the classic form of MPS VI, there is severe dwarfism. Growth retardation affecting both the trunk and limbs is usually evident by age 2 or 3 years. Genu valgum, lumbar kyphosis, and anterior sternal protrusion develop. The lower ribs are flared. Joint movement is restricted. Claw-hand deformity develops. Carpal tunnel syndrome is common. The head appears relatively large. Facial features tend to be coarse. There is often mild hypertrichosis. Hepatomegaly usually develops in patients older than 6 years, splenomegaly develops in many, and the abdomen usually is protruberant. Cardiac involvement, particularly valve lesions, may develop. Deafness occurs in some patients. The principal neurological manifestations are hydrocephalus and spinal cord compression from atlantoaxial subluxation consequent to hypoplasia of the odontoid process. Survival is variable; most patients with the severe form of MPS VI die by their second or third decade.

The principal ophthalmologic manifestation of MPS VI is progressive corneal clouding, usually evident within the first few years of life. The appearance is that of ground glass haziness throughout the stroma, sometimes more dense peripherally, and usually evident grossly.[103,141] In addition to stromal opacities, some epithelial and endothelial changes may be seen on slit lamp examination.[141] Corneal opacities have been found in the mild variant of MPS VI as well as in the severe form.[198] A decrease in corneal clouding after bone marrow transplantation has been reported.[154]

Papilledema in association with hydrocephalus in MPS VI has been reported.[54,103,236] Optic atrophy may develop.[54] Retinal vessel tortuosity also has been noted.[103] As a rule patients with MPS VI do not develop signs of retinal degeneration, and the ERG usually is normal.[144,204] However, pigmentary alteration and ERG abnormalities have been reported in an adult with a mild form of MPS VI.[73] Glaucoma has been described in several patients.[32]

The ocular pathology of MPS VI has been well documented.[144,204]

Sly Syndrome: MPS VII

In Sly syndrome, there is deficiency of β-gluc-uronidase, with urinary excretion of both dermaten sulfate and heparin sulfate. The gene encoding β-gluc-uronidase has been localized to chromosome 7q 21.11.[186]

A variable spectrum of clinical manifestations occurs, including short stature, progressive skeletal deformity and radiologic signs of dysostosis multiplex, coarse facial features, hypertelorism, hepatosplenomegaly, diastasis recti, protruberant abdomen, hernias, cardiovascular involvement and respiratory problems, and intellectual impairment. Coarse inclusions are found in circulating lymphocytes. A severe neonatal form associated with fetal hydrops has been described.

In many patients with Sly syndrome, the corneas are clear.[66,233,242] With phenotypic variation, however, corneal clouding may occur; it may be evident grossly or only on slit lamp examination.[15,271]

Optic nerve swelling, without increased intracranial pressure or hydrocephalus, has been reported.[54]

THE GANGLIOSIDOSES

Gangliosides are sialic acid-containing glycosphingolipids normally present in neural and extraneural tissues throughout the body; they are found in highest concentration in gray matter of the brain. Defects in lysosomal degradation of gangliosides can result in abnormal accumulation of these lipids and related products in brain and other tissue, producing a spectrum of clinical manifestations. Two major types of ganglioside storage disease occur: GM_1 and GM_2 gangliosidoses (Table 7-2).[109,257]

The GM_1 gangliosidoses are caused by deficiency of acid β-galactosidase; the gene for this enzyme has been localized to chromosome 3p21.33.[256] There is storage of GM_1 ganglioside in the nervous system and abnormal accumulation of galactose-containing oligosaccharide and keratan sulfate degradation products in somatic cells. Infantile, late infantile/juvenile and adult/chronic variants of GM_1 gangliosidoses occur.[257] The most familiar of these is the acute infantile form (GM_1 type I), commonly referred to as generalized gangliosidosis. This disorder affects patients of various ethnic groups.[257]

The various GM_2 gangliosidoses are due to a number of enzymatic variants; there may be deficiency of hexosaminidase A, deficiency of hexosaminidase A and B, or deficiency of the GM_2 activator protein that is needed for degradation of GM_2 by hexosaminidase A.[109] There is an underlying defect in one of three genes: HEXA, which encodes the α subunit of hexosaminidase A; HEXB, which encodes the β-subunit of hexosaminidase A and B; or GM_2 A, which encodes the GM_2 activator.[109] HEXA has been mapped to chromosome 15; HEXB and GM_2 A have been mapped to chromosome 5.[109] Phenotypic variability of the GM_2 gangliosidoses ranges from infantile-onset rapidly progressive disease to later-onset subacute or chronic forms.[109] The most familiar of the GM_2 gangliosidoses is Tay–Sachs disease (GM_2 type I). The incidence of Tay–Sachs disease has been reported to be highest in patients of Ashkenazic Jewish descent, but it does occur in other ethnic groups.[109]

The GM_1 and GM_2 gangliosidoses are autosomal recessive conditions.[109,257] Diagnosis can be confirmed by enzyme assay of tissues, body fluids, and cells. The heterozygote state also can be detected by these methods. Prenatal diagnosis is possible by assay of cultured amniotic cells and chorionic villi. As yet there is no specific treatment, such as enzyme replacement or effective cell therapy, for the gangliosidoses.[110,256]

TABLE 7-2. The Major Gangliosidoses (GM).

The disease	General manifestations	Ophthalmologic manifestations
Infantile GM$_1$ gangliosidosis; generalized gangliosidosis (β-galactosidase deficiency)	Dysmorphism, skeletal abnormalities, visceromegaly, psychomotor retardation, seizures, rapid neurological deterioration, and early death, usually by age 2 years	Cherry-red spot, optic atrophy, early vision loss Mild corneal clouding in some cases Retinal and conjunctival vascular abnormalities
Late infantile/juvenile GM$_1$ gangliosidosis (β-galactosidase deficiency)	Later onset, slower course, milder somatic abnormalities than infantile form Progressive psychomotor deterioration Seizures Death usually by age 3 to 10 years	Vision loss in later stages Optic atrophy Clinical absence of cherry-red spot Strabismus
Adult/chronic GM$_1$ gangliosidosis (β-galactosidase deficiency)	Range of onset from childhood to adulthood Protracted course Dystonia, progressive spasticity, ataxia Mild if any somatic abnormalities	Corneal clouding in some cases
Acute infantile GM$_2$ gangliosidosis: Tay–Sachs disease (hexosaminidase A deficiency)	Onset in infancy Psychomotor retardation Seizures Exaggerated startle response Megencephaly Progressive neurological deterioration leading to decerebrate rigidity, blindness, deafness Death usually by age 3 to 4 years	Cherry-red spot, optic atrophy, progressive vision loss Nystagmus, deterioration of eye movements
Infantile GM$_2$ gangliosidosis: Sandhoff variant (hexosaminidase A & B deficiency)	Clinical features resemble those of Tay–Sachs	Cherry-red spot, optic atrophy, vision loss Corneal opalescence in one case
Subacute GM$_2$ gangliosidosis: late infantile and juvenile forms (HEXA or HEXB mutations)	Onset between 2 to 10 years Ataxia developmental regression, spasticity Deterioration to vegetative state by age 10 to 15 years, followed by death within a few years	Cherry-red spot in some patients Retinal pigmentary changes in some cases Optic atrophy Vision loss in later stages Strabismus
Chronic GM$_2$ gangliosidosis	Range of onset from childhood to adulthood Spectrum of clinical presentations, including dystonia, spinocerebellar degeneration, lower motor neuron disease, psychiatric disorders Usually slowly progressive with long-term survival	Ocular motor abnormalities, including impairment of convergence, horizontal and vertical gaze defects Vision and fundi usually normal

Generalized Gangliosidosis: Infantile GM₁ Gangliosidosis

In generalized gangliosidosis (GM₁ type I), there is both neuronal lipidosis and visceral histiocytosis as a result of profound deficiency of acid β-galactosidase. Manifestations can be evident at birth or appear in the early months of life. The disease is characterized by dysmorphism, prominent bony abnormalities, visceromegaly, and neurological degeneration in infancy.[257] Signs include coarse facial features, frontal bossing, depressed nasal bridge, large low-set ears, gingival hypertrophy and macroglossia, and hirsutism of the forehead and neck. There may be edema of the extremities. Hepatomegaly usually develops within the first months of life. Dorsolumbar kyphoscoliosis is common. The hands are broad, the fingers short. Joint contractures develop. Firm nontender enlargement of the epiphyseal joints occurs. Radiologic findings are those of dysostosis multiplex, with deformities of vertebral bodies and long bones. Seizures commonly develop. There is rapidly progressive neurological deterioration, often to a state of decerebrate rigidity, spastic quadriplegia, blindness, deafness, and unresponsiveness. Death usually occurs by age 2 years.

Macular cherry-red spots occur in approximately 50% of patients with generalized gangliosidosis (Table 7-3).[193] There may be tortuosity of retinal vessels, retinal hemorrhages, and optic atrophy.[82] The cornea usually is clear, but mild diffuse corneal clouding has been documented in some cases.[82,281] Histopathological evidence for ganglioside accumulation in the retina and mucopolysaccharide accumulation in the cornea has been well documented.[50,82] Loss of vision occurs.[193] Strabismus and nystagmus are common.[193] Tortuosity and saccular microaneurysms of conjunctival vessels have been noted in some cases.[23]

Late Infantile/Juvenile GM₁ Gangliosidosis

In late infantile/juvenile GM₁ gangliosidosis (GM₁ type 2), as in the infantile form (GM₁ type 1), there is deficiency of β-galactosidase.[257] The onset, however, is later, the course is slower, and skeletal abnormalities are milder; in most cases there is no dysmorphism or visceromegaly. Neurological manifestations usually appear by age 1 year or so. Common early signs are generalized weakness, locomotor ataxia, strabismus, and loss of

TABLE 7-3. Cherry-Red Spot and Related Macular Signs in Metabolic Disorders.

Gangliosidoses
    Infantile GM_1 gangliosidosis: generalized gangliosidosis
        Classic cherry-red spot in 50% of cases
    Late infantile/juvenile GM_1 gangliosidosis
        Atypical cherry-red spot a rare finding
    Acute infantile GM_2 gangliosidosis: Tay–Sachs disease and Sandhoff variant
        Classic cherry-red spot in most cases.
    Subacute GM_2 gangliosidosis
        Cherry-red spot or diminished foveal light reflex
Niemann–Pick Disease
    Type A: sphingomyelin lipidosis
        Cherry-red spot in many cases, often extension of retinal haze beyond
        macula
    Type B: sphingomyelin lipidosis
        Macula halo syndrome; infrequently a cherry-red spot
    Type C: cholesterol lipidosis
        Cherry-red-like spot in some cases
Gaucher's Disease
    Type 3: subacute neuronopathic form
        Macular grayness in some cases
Metachromatic leukodystrophy
    Infantile form
        Macular grayness; cherry-red-like spot in some cases
Krabbe's Disease
    Infantile onset variant
        Cherry-red-like spot
Farber disease
    Macular grayness or cherry-red-like spot in some cases
Sialidosis
    Type I and Type II
        Cherry-red spot
Galactosialidosis
    Cherry-red spot
Neuronal ceroid lipofuscinosis
    Juvenile form: Spielmeyer–Sjögren
        Bull's-eye maculopathy
Fucosidosis
    Bull's-eye maculopathy

speech. Progressive mental and motor deterioration, spasticity, seizures, and in time decerebrate rigidity follow. Recurrent infections, particularly bronchopneumonia, are common. The life span usually is only 3 to 10 years.

Ocular abnormalities, particularly cherry-red spots, are not a feature of infantile/juvenile GM_1 gangliosidosis. Atypical cherry-red spots, however, have been described in one case.[260] Disc pallor has been noted.[101,256] In another case, microscopic and ultrastructural signs of lysosomal storage in the retina in the absence of clinically evident cherry-red spots were reported, and atrophic changes of the optic nerve were documented.[101] Loss of vision can occur late in the course of the disease.[194]

Adult/Chronic GM$_1$ Gangliosidosis

Patients with β-galactosidase deficiency classified as having adult/chronic GM$_1$ gangliosidosis (GM$_1$ type 3) have a protracted course, with variable age of onset, ranging from childhood to adulthood.[257] Dystonia and progressive pyramidal or extrapyramidal disease are the principal neurological manifestations. Intellectual deterioration is not remarkable. Dysmorphism is not obvious. Slight vertebral changes are described. Visceromegaly is not observed.

Ocular abnormalities are not a feature of chronic GM$_1$ gangliosidosis. Corneal clouding has been reported in some cases.[256]

Tay–Sachs Disease: Acute Infantile GM$_2$ Gangliosidosis

In Tay–Sachs disease (GM$_2$ type I), there is nearly total deficiency of hexosaminidase A, leading to abnormal accumulation of ganglioside GM$_2$.[107] Pathological changes of lipidosis are seen throughout the nervous system. Neurons become distended. Axonal degeneration, demyelination, and gliosis occur. Visceral changes, however, are not a feature of this disorder.

Clinical manifestations appear in infancy, often insidiously with listlessness, hypotonia, feeding difficulties, or irritability. The startle reaction, an extensor response to sudden sharp sound, is a characteristic early sign. Psychomotor development is retarded. Increasing weakness and decreasing attentiveness become evident in the early months. After age 18 months, spasticity and seizures develop. There is progressive deterioration to a state of decerebrate rigidity, deafness, and blindness. Death usually occurs by age 3 to 4 years.

Many affected patients have a doll-like facial appearance with pale translucent skin, delicate pink coloring, fine hair, and long eyelashes.

Macular cherry-red spots develop in virtually all cases of Tay–Sachs disease.[109] This characteristic finding was first described by the British ophthalmologist Warren Tay in 1881.[261] With accumulation of lipid, there is loss of transparency of the multilayered macular ganglion cells, producing a creamy-white, yellow, or hazy gray halo around the fovea, accentuating the red blush of the ganglion cell-free central region (Fig. 7-5A).[119] The macular haze is usually evident by the time other neurological signs appear in infancy. The distinctive features of a cherry-red spot may fade as ganglion cell destruction progresses (Fig. 7-5B).[150] Pathological changes in the retina are similar to those in the brain; there is lipid loading and degeneration of ganglion cells, and the presence of membranous cytoplasmic inclusions has been documented.[6,47,49,119] Deficiency of hexosaminidase A in the retina and optic nerve has been reported.[57] There is demyelination and degeneration of the optic nerves, chiasm, and tracts.[47] Optic atrophy is often clinically evident. Progressive loss of vision is common early; blindness is usually complete by age 2 years.[109] VEP responses are altered early, whereas the ERG is not affected until late in the course of the disease.[109] There may be deterioration of eye movements.[131] The enzyme defect can be detected in tears, a finding potentially useful in diagnosis and heterozygote detection.[34,239]

Sandhoff Variant of Infantile GM$_2$ Gangliosidosis

In this variant of Tay–Sachs disease, there is severe deficiency of both hexosaminidase A and hexosaminidase B activity, with neuronal lipidosis of GM$_2$, and some visceral accumulation of a globoside, due to HEXB mutation.[109] The clinical features of Sandhoff disease are like those of Tay–Sachs.

The principal ophthalmologic manifestations of Sandhoff disease are macular cherry-red spot, optic atrophy, and progressive vision loss leading to blindness.[194] Evidence of ganglioside storage in the retina and optic nerve has been documented by histopathological and ultrastructural examination.[27,75,96,189,263] Storage cytosomes also have been found in corneal keratocytes.[27,263] The corneas usually are clear clinically, but in one case appeared slightly opalescent.[263]

Subacute GM$_2$ Gangliosidosis

Patients with later-onset (late infantile or juvenile) subacute forms of GM$_2$ gangliosidosis may have HEXA or HEXB mutations.[109] The pathological findings are those of neuronal lipidosis with abnormal storage of GM$_2$; cytoplasmic inclusions like those of Tay–Sachs disease and other inclusions called pleo-

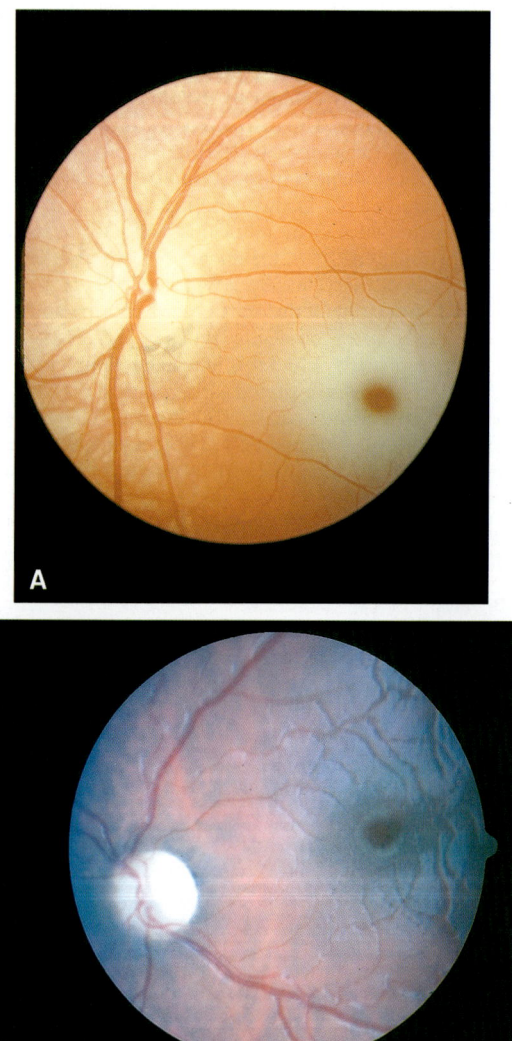

FIGURE 7-5A,B. (A) Classic macular cherry-red spot of Tay–Sachs disease. **(B)** Degenerated cherry-red spot of Tay–Sachs disease.

morphic lamellar bodies are present. Clinical signs generally appear between 2 and 10 years of age. Ataxia and incoordination develop. There is progressive psychomotor deterioration, with increasing spasticity and development of seizures in the first decade, leading to a vegetative state with decerebrate rigidity and death within a few years, often due to intercurrent infection.

Ophthalmologic signs vary somewhat from those of the infantile onset GM$_2$ gangliosidoses. Vision loss occurs later in the subacute form.[24,109,173] Macular cherry-red spot may develop but is not a consistent feature.[24] Pigmentary retinal changes may develop.[24,194] Optic atrophy develops in some cases.[24,173] There may be strabismus.[24]

Chronic GM$_2$ Gangliosidosis

The spectrum of later-onset, more slowly progressive or chronic forms of GM$_2$ gangliosidosis includes a variety of clinical presentations, reflecting predominant involvement of one or another part of the central nervous system.[109] Patients may exhibit primarily dystonia; signs of spinocerebellar degeneration; motor neuron disease; or psychiatric abnormalities. Onset may range from childhood to adulthood. These chronic forms generally are compatible with long-term survival.

Vision is rarely affected and the fundi usually are normal, but abnormalities of eye movement occur.[182,210] These problems include impairment of convergence, loss of optokinetic nystagmus, and vestibular nystagmus.[210] Defects of horizontal smooth pursuit movements, varying defects in vertical gaze (hypometric and hypermetric saccades), and inability to suppress the vestibulo-ocular reflex by fixation have been documented.[182]

The chronic variants of GM$_2$ gangliosidosis are more commonly caused by hexosaminidase A deficiency (HEXA mutations) then by combined hexosaminidase A and B deficiency (HEXB mutations); GM$_2$ activator defects in this group are rare.[109]

METACHROMATIC LEUKODYSTROPHY

Melachromic leukodystrophy is an inherited disorder of myelin metabolism characterized by lysosomal accumulation of glycolipids, predominantly sulfatides, in white matter of the central nervous system and in peripheral nerves, with progressive degeneration of myelin and progressive deterioration of mental and motor function.[151] In histological preparation, the accumulated lipid granules exhibit metachromasia, giving rise to the descriptive term metachromatic leukodystrophy (MLD).

Based on variation in clinical and biochemical features, several forms of MLD are described (Table 7-4).[151] Most common is the late infantile form. Presenting by age 1 to 2 years, this form is characterized by relatively rapid deterioration, leading to death within 1 to 7 years. Major manifestations are devopmental retardation and regression, generalized weakness, ataxia, progressive spastic quadriparesis, and bulbar and pseudobulbar palsies. Optic atrophy is common, often developing as the disease progresses.[51,53,166,230] There may be grayness of the macular region, in some cases a cherry-red-like spot.[51,166] Progressive loss of vision and impairment of the pupillary response to light have been documented.[166,230] VEP changes can be detected as the disease progresses.[69] Strabismus and nystagmus may develop.[51,166,230]

Histopathological and ultrastructural studies of the eye in late infantile MLD have documented atrophy of the optic nerve

TABLE 7-4. Forms of Metachromatic Leukodystrophy (MLD).

Classification	General features	Ophthalmologic manifestations
Late infantile MLD (arylsulfatase A deficiency)	Infantile onset, rapid psychomotordeterioration, death in childhood	Optic atrophy, macular grayness or cherry-red-like spot Vision loss
Juvenile MLD (arylsulfatase A deficiency)	Onset in childhood Protracted course into teens or beyond Intellectual deterioration Progressive ataxia Seizures	Optic atrophy
Adult MLD (arylsulfatase A deficiency)	Presents in teens or adult years Progressive mental deterioration Progressive pyramidal, extrapyramidal signs Seizures in some cases	Optic atrophy
Mucosulfatidosis (multiple sulfatase deficiency)	Manifestations similar to infantile MLD, with somatic and visceral features resembling MPS	Pigmentary retinal degeneration, macular grayness, optic atrophy, vision loss, corneal clouding, lens opacities

and degeneration of the myelin sheaths, with accumulation of metachromatic material between nerve fibers and the presence of inclusions in glial cells[51,53,99,166,230]; the presence of metachromatic material and a variety of cytoplasmic inclusions within the retinal ganglion cells and other retinal layers[51,53,99,166,230]; vacuolization of nonpigmented epithelial cells of the ciliary body and accumulation of metachromatic material in Schwann cells of the ciliary nerves[166]; and the presence of inclusions within corneal epithelial and endothelial cells, in keratocytes, lens fibers and epithelial cells, trabecular meshwork, and peripheral iris macrophages.[230]

The juvenile form presents usually by age 4 to 6 years, sometimes later. The course tends to be protracted, lasting 20 years or more, but some patients do not live beyond their teens. Early signs include decline in school performance, confusion, abnormal behavior, clumsiness, and incontinence. Progressive ataxia, spasticity, pseudobulbar palsy, and seizures develop. Optic atrophy is common.[166] The pupillary response to light may be diminished.[166] Macular changes have not been documented.[166] Histopathological and ultrastructural study of the eye in juvenile MLD has documented degeneration of the optic nerve and myelin sheaths and alteration of the ciliary nerves as in the late infantile form, and some depletion of retinal ganglion cells, but no evidence of abnormal retinal ganglion cell storage.[166]

Adult-onset MLD can manifest in the teens, twenties, thirties, or later. This form is characterized by progressive mental deterioration, progressive pyramidal and extrapyramidal signs, and in some cases seizures. Optic atrophy and nystagmus can develop, and in time vision may decrease.[102,203] Studies of the eye by light and electron microscopy in the adult form of MLD have shown loss of optic nerve axons and myelin sheaths and the presence of inclusions in glial cells of the optic nerve,[203] loss of retinal ganglion cells and retinal nerve fibers,[203] and the presence of membranous lysosomal residual bodies in retinal ganglion cells.[102]

In the late infantile, juvenile, and adult forms of MLD, there is profound deficiency of arylsulfatase A, the heat-labile component of cerebroside sulfate sulfatase.[151] Galactosyl sulfatide (cerboside sulfate), a constituent of myelin and cellular membranes, accumulates in the central and peripheral nervous system. Galactosyl sulfatide, and to a lesser extent lactosyl sulfatide, also accumulate in kidney, gallbladder, and other organs and are excreted in excessive amounts in urine. The arylsulfatase A gene has been mapped to the long arm of chromosome 22 band q13.[272] A number of disease-related mutations have been identified.

Several patients having many features of juvenile MLD, including sulfatiduria, but having normal arylsulfatase activity have been described. These patients have deficiency of the cebroside activator protein, saposin B, necessary in the hydrolysis of sulfatide.[151]

The classification of MLD also includes a rare variant resembling the infantile form, but having in addition features of mucopolysaccharidosis, including coarse facies, deafness, hepatosplenomegaly, skeletal abnormalities, and mucopolysacchariduria. In this variant, at least nine different sulfatases are deficient.[151] The condition is referred to as mucosulfatidosis or multiple sulfatase deficiency (MSD). Ocular manifestations in this variant include degenerative retinal pigmentary changes, macular grayness, optic atrophy and vision loss, strabismus, nystagmus, and other abnormal eye movements.[14,51,113,117,166,212] Corneal clouding has been reported but is uncommon.[51,268] Circumferential opacities of the peripheral anterior lens capsule have been noted.[14] ERG and VEP abnormalities have been documented.[14,117,212]

Light and electron microscopic study of the eye in MSD has shown partial demyelination of the optic nerve; accumulation of metachromatic material in the interstices of the optic nerve fibers, mostly within macrophages; similar changes of ciliary nerves; accumulation of metachromatic material in retinal ganglion cells; and the presence of numerous inclusions within retinal ganglion cells.[51]

All forms of MLD are autosomal recessive.[151] In the major forms, heterozygotes can be identified by assay of leukocytes or cultured skin fibroblasts for arylsulfatase or cebroside sulfate sulfatase activity, and prenatal diagnosis can be made by enzyme assay of cultured amniotic fluid cells or chorionic villus cells. Arylsulfatase deficiency also can be detected in tears.[166]

As yet there is no effective specific treatment for MLD. Vigabatrin, an inhibitor of GABA-aminotransferase, can be used to reduce spasticity and ataxia in children, but the drug does not alter the progression of the disease process. The possible benefits of bone marrow transplantation and gene replacement therapy are being investigated.[272]

NIEMANN–PICK DISEASE

The term Niemann–Pick disease (NPD) describes a group of biochemically and clinically distinct lipid storage disorders characterized by abnormal accumulation of predominantly sphingomyelin and cholesterol, the presence of foamy histiocytes in affected tissues and organs, and a broad spectrum of visceral and neurological manifestations.[228] The current classification includes two primary sphingomyelin lipidoses, designated NPD types A and B, and a cholesterol lipidosis, designated NPD type C (see Table 7-3).

Types A and B Niemann–Pick Disease

In types A and B NPD, there is deficiency of acid sphingomyelinase, a hydrolase important in metabolic degradation of sphingomyelin; this phospholipid is a common constituent of plasma membranes, subcellular organelles, endoplasmic reticulum, and mitochondria and a major lipid of myelin sheaths and erythrocyte stroma.[228] The enzyme defect leads to lysosomal accumulation of sphingomyelin, cholesterol, and other metabolically related lipids throughout the body.

The histopathological hallmark of NPD types A and B is a large lipid-laden foam cell referred to as the Niemann–Pick cell, found particularly in tissues and organs of the monocyte-macrophage system. In types A and B NPD there is infiltration of spleen and lymph nodes, marrow, liver, lung and kidney; endocrine glands and heart also may be affected. In addition, neuronal lipidosis occurs in type A, but not in type B.

Clinically type A NPD is characterized by failure to thrive, hepatosplenomegaly, and rapidly progressive neurological deterioration and debilitation in infancy, leading to death by age 2 to 3 years. Type B is characterized primarily by hepatosplenomegaly in childhood with little or no neurological involvement, and survival into adulthood. Progressive pulmonary infiltration can be a major problem in more severely affected type B patients.

Ocular manifestations are more frequent in type A NPD than in type B. Macular cherry-red spots occur in up to 50% of patients with type A[58,228,276]; a distinguishing feature in many cases is extension of retinal haze far beyond the parafoveal region. Cherry-red spots are infrequent in type B, but a distinctive "macula halo syndrome" has been described; this is characterized by a ring of crystalloid or granular opacities around the fovea, sometimes haziness of the macula.[43,86,169,248] Mild corneal haze and fine lens deposits may be clinically evident in patients with type A NPD.[86] In addition, periorbital fullness has been noted in patients with type B NPD.[86] Vision loss occurs late in the course of type A NPD; the retinal changes in type B are not usually associated with vision loss.[43]

Evidence of widespread lipid storage in the eye has been well documented by light and electron microscopy in type A NPD.[107,127,157,165,215] Granular cytoplasmic birefringence has been demonstrated in keratocytes, corneal endothelial and epithelial cells, and sclerocytes; in lens epithelium; in nonpigmented ciliary epithelium, fibrocytes of choroid, and endothelial cells of ciliary, choroidal, and retinal vessels; and in retinal ganglion cells, plexiform and nerve fiber layers, and retinal pigmented epithelium. Membranous cytoplasmic inclusion have been found in similar distribution, particularly in retinal ganglion cells and axons.

The inheritance of types A and B NPD is autosomal recessive. Type A NPD is more frequent in Ashkenazic Jews. The acid sphingomyelinase gene has been mapped to chromosome region 11p 15.1–p 15.4[229]; 18 mutations have been identified that cause types A and B NPD. Diagnosis is confirmed by assay of sphingomyelinase activity in cells and tissue extracts. Heterozygote detection requires molecular studies. Prenatal diagnosis by enzymatic or molecular assay of cultured amniocytes or chorionic villus cells is possible. As yet there is no effective specific treatment for NPD types A and B, although enzyme replacement and gene therapy have been under investigation.[229]

Type C Niemann–Pick Disease

This form of NPD is distinguished by a unique cellular disorder of cholesterol processing associated with abnormal lysosomal accumulation of unesterified cholesterol and other lipids.[200] The underlying molecular defect has not yet been defined. The pathological features are those of visceral and neuronal storage; characteristic inclusion-laden histiocytes referred to as foam cells and sea-blue histiocytes are found in affected tissues and organs.

Clinical manifestations of type C NPD vary. The "classic" phenotype is characterized by progressive dementia, ataxia, dystonia, gaze paresis, and hepatosplenomegaly. Manifestations appear in late childhood. There is gradual worsening of physical and intellectual disabilities, eventually leading to incapacitation. Death occurs in the teens. Other type C NPD presentations include self-limited or rapidly fatal liver disease in the newborn, hypotonia and delayed motor development in infancy, and late-onset variants with progressive neurological deterioration and cognitive and psychiatric disturbances in adolescents and adults.

The ophthalmologic hallmark of type C NPD is progressive supranuclear vertical gaze palsy.[45,58,111,187,190] There may be associated blinking or head thrusting on attempted upward or downward gaze. Horizontal gaze movements and convergence also may be affected. Macular cherry-red-like spots occasionally occur in type C NPD.[81,174] VEP abnormalities have been noted in type C NPD.[122] Electron microscopic examination of the eye from a child with presumed type C NPD demonstrated intracytoplasmic inclusions in conjunctival cells, keratocytes, lens epithelium, nonpigmented ciliary epithelium, retinal ganglion cells, choroidal fibrocytes, and optic nerve astrocytes,[197] whereas there was no evidence of intraocular lipid storage in another well-studied case.[81] Conjunctival inclusions, however, have been found in other patients with type C NPD.[163,174]

The inheritance of type C NPD is autosomal recessive. Linkage of type C to an 18p genomic marker, D 18S 40, has been found in some patients.[199] Diagnosis of type C NPD requires demonstration of abnormal intracellular cholesterol esterification and documentation of intralysosomal accumulation of unesterified cholesterol. Generalized screening for type C is not yet available. Prenatal diagnosis is possible in some cases. Currently there is no specific treatment for type C NPD.[199] Symptomatic treatment of seizures, dystonia, and catoplexy may be helpful.

Type C NPD is panethnic, but genetic isolates have been described in the French Acadians of Nova Scotia (formally NPD type D) and in Spanish Americans in southern Colorado.[200]

GAUCHER'S DISEASE

Gaucher's disease a lysosomal storage disease in which there is abnormal accumulation of glucosylceramide (glucocerebroside), primarily in cells of the reticuloendothelial system. The underlying defect is impaired intracellular hydrolysis of the glycolipid glucosylceramide and related glucosphingolipids due to deficiency of β-glucosidase (glucocerebrosidase).[19] The gene encoding this enzyme has been localized to chromosome 1.[19] A variety of mutations have been found to cause Gaucher's disease.

A hallmark of the disease is the presence of distinctive lipid-laden cells of the monocyte-macrophage system throughout the body; these so-called Gaucher cells are distinguished by cytoplasmic inclusions having a twisted tubular appearance.[19] The condition affects predominantly spleen, liver, and bone marrow, and in certain forms of the disease, the nervous system. Many patients develop ocular manifestations. Based on clinical variation, three major forms of Gaucher's disease are described: a chronic nonneuronopathic form, type 1; an acute neuronopathic form, type 2; and a subacute neuronopathic form, type 3 (Table 7-5).[20] All forms are autosomal recessive. The disease is paneth-

---

TABLE 7-5. Forms of Gaucher's Disease.

Type 1: Nonneuronopathic form
- Visceral and skeletal involvement without primary neurological involvement
- Onset in childhood or adulthood
- Broad spectrum of severity
- Ocular lesions resembling pingueculae in some patients
- Ashkenazi Jewish predilection

Type 2: Acute neuronopathic form
- Severe neurological involvement, extensive visceral and skeletal involvement
- Paralytic strabismus, conjugate gaze impairment
- Infantile onset, early death
- Panethnic

Type 3: Subacute neuronopathic form
- Neuronopathic involvement of later onset, more gradual progression, and lesser severity than type 2
- Usually visceral involvement
- Three subtypes:
  - 3a
    Progressive neurological disease dominated by myoclonus and dementia
    Of Northern Swedish predilection
  - 3b
    Aggressive visceral and skeletal disease
    Neurological manifestations largely limited to horizontal supranuclear gaze palsy
    Panethnic
  - 3c
    Neurological manifestations largely limited to horizontal supranuclear gaze palsy
    Cardiac valve calcifications and corneal opacities
    Generally little visceral involvement
    Panethnic

nic, but type 1 is more frequent in Ashkenazic Jews. Estimates of the disease incidence vary widely.

Diagnosis can be made by demonstration of Gaucher cells in marrow aspirates, by measurement of glucosylceramide in tissue samples, and by measurement of β-glucosidase activity in leukocyte or cultured skin fibroblasts of affected patients. Heterozygotes can be identified by enzyme assay, and prenatal detection is possible by amniocentesis.[19]

A variety of treatment modalities, including splenectomy, can be helpful. Accumulation of glucosylceramide and the associated clinical manifestations can be reversed by repeated infusions of modified β-glucosidase (alglucerase).[19] Results of bone marrow transplantation have been encouraging in some cases.[19]

Type 1 Gaucher's Disease: Chronic Nonneuronopathic Form

This form is characterized primarily by visceral and skeletal involvement.[19] Age of onset and severity vary widely. Manifestations may appear in childhood or in the adult years. The course may be rapid, slowly progressive, or protracted. The initial sign usually is splenomegaly; frequently there is hypersplenism with thrombocytopenia, anemia, and leukopenia. There may be hepatomegaly; there can be evidence of hepatic dysfunction. Osteoporotic erosions, aseptic necrosis of the femoral head, vertebral collapse, and pathological fractures of long bones are common. Patients may suffer episodic bone pain, sometimes accompanied by fever. Pulmonary hypertension and cor pulmonale may develop. Also, pulmonary involvement can predispose to pneumonia, a major cause of death in young patients. In older patients, yellowish pallor or yellow-brown pigmentation of the skin of the face and lower extremities may be noted. Primary neurological manifestations are not a feature of type 1 Gaucher's disease, but secondary neurological signs due to vertebral collapse, fat emboli, and coagulopathy may develop. There is an increased incidence of neoplastic disease in this disorder.[19]

Ocular lesions resembling pingueculae have been noted in patients with type 1 Gaucher's disease.[33,77,201] These lesions are described as yellow or brownish triangular areas of infiltration and thickening of the bulbar conjunctiva adjacent to the limbus nasally and temporally. Although some lesions have been reported to contain foamy histiocytes, other studies have not confirmed the presence of Gaucher cells.[33,42,77] Gaucher cells have been found in choroid.[201] Occasional reference has been made to macular or perimacular abnormalities.[46,201] Progressive retinal degeneration with optic atrophy and vision loss has been reported in an adult.[171] Retinal hemorrhages and retinal edema may occur.[33] Impairment of eye movements in association with seizures and mental deterioration has been reported in adult siblings,[175] although neurological involvement characteristically does not occur in type 1 Gaucher's disease.

Type 2 Gaucher's Disease: Acute Neuronopathic Form

Also referred to as the classic, infantile, or cerebral form, type 2 Gaucher's disease is characterized by severe neurological involvement and extensive visceral involvement.[19] The average age of onset is 3 months, with a range from birth to 18 months. Hepatosplenomegaly is an early presenting feature. Neurological manifestations develop within a few months, usually by age 6 months. Most patients show signs of cranial nerve and extrapyramidal tract involvement. The triad of trismus, strabismus, and retroflexion of the head is classic. Feeding problems and difficulty handling secretions are common. Progressive spasticity, hyperreflexia, and pathological reflexes develop. Seizures may occur. Osseous lesions may develop. The course is rapidly progressive. Death occurs early, often between age 1 month and 2 years, usually as the result of pulmonary infection or anoxia.

The principal ocular manifestation of type 2 Gaucher's disease is paralytic strabismus due to cranial nerve involvement.[19] Progressive impairment of conjugate movements has been noted.[45,112] The report of keratoconus in a family with Gaucher's disease is of interest.[219]

Type 3 Gaucher's Disease: Subacute Neuronopathic Form

In this form, sometimes referred to as the juvenile form, neurological involvement is of later onset than in type 2 and the course is more chronic.[19] There is usually marked visceral involvement; hepatosplenomegaly occurs as in types 1 and 2. Major neurologic manifestations are spasticity, ataxia, retardation, and seizures. An important neuro-ophthalmic manifestation is progressive disorder of horizontal gaze.[45,264] The signs may simulate those of congenital ocular motor apraxia, including impairment of voluntary horizontal saccades with retention of slow pursuit movements, compensatory head thrusting, and contraversive deviation of the eyes during rotation of the body. In some patients with type 3 Gaucher's disease, ocular motor abnormalities are the primary or only neurological manifestations of the disorder.[237]

Retinal abnormalities also may occur. Multiple small white spots situated superficially in the retina or on the surface of the retina in the posterior region of the fundus have been described,[44,216] and histopathological changes also have been documented.[44,216] Cherry-red spots are not a feature of Gaucher's disease, but grayness of the macular region has been noted.[44] Discrete stromal opacities of the cornea have been reported in some patients who may have had a variant of type 3 Gaucher's disease.[5,83,267] Myopia is a finding in many patients with Gaucher's disease.[84]

KRABBE'S DISEASE

Also referred to as globoid cell leukodystrophy, Krabbe's disease is a rare metabolic neurodegenerative disease that affects predominantly white matter, leading to rapidly progressive mental and motor deterioration and early death. The underlying defect is profound deficiency of galactosylceramidase (galactocerebrosidase-β-galactosidase); this enzyme normally catalyzes degradation of galactosylceramide (galactocerebroside), a sphingolipid involved in myelination.[258] A number of related galactolipids including galactosylsphingosine (psychosine) also are substrates for this enzyme, and it is postulated that accumulation of a toxic metabolite (psychosine) leads to destruction of oligodendroglia, the cells that produce myelin. Characteristically there is widespread loss of myelin and oligodendrocytes, and degeneration of axons and severe gliosis in the brain; spinal cord and peripheral nerves also are affected. The histopathological hallmark of he disease is the presence of distinctive multinucleated macrophages that contain undegraded galactosylceramide; these are referred to as globoid cells.

Clinical manifestations usually appear by age 3 to 6 months, sometimes later in infancy, childhood, or even adulthood. The clinical course of classic infantile-onset Krabbe's disease is often described as occurring in three stages.[258] The early stage is characterized by irritability, hypersensitivity to external stimuli, and some stiffness of the limbs; episodic fevers of unknown etiology, feeding difficulties, vomiting, and seizures may develop, and slight retardation or regression of psychomotor development may be evident. The next stage is characterized by rapidly progressive mental and motor deterioration, hypertonicity, hyperreflexia, and seizures. In the final or "burnt-out stage," the infant is decerebrate, often blind and deaf. The final stage may last years, but affected infants rarely survive beyond 2 years.

The major ophthalmologic manifestations of Krabbe's disease are optic atrophy, attendant impairment of the pupillary reaction to light, and progressive loss of vision, leading to blindness.[258] Loss of the foveal reflex may be evident.[84,255] In addition, subtle cherry-red-like macular changes have been reported in a child with an unusual variant of Krabbe's disease.[183] Histopathological and ultrastructural studies of the optic nerve have shown loss of axons, loss of myelin, gliosis, and the presence of globoid cells.[26,84,118] Degenerative changes of the retinal nerve fibers and ganglion cell layers also have been well documented.[26,84,118] Some patients with Krabbe's disease may exhibit an abnormality of saccadic eye movements resembling ocular motor apraxia.[120]

The inheritance of Krabbe's disease is autosomal recessive. Diagnosis is confirmed by assay of galactosylceramidase activity in leukocytes or cultured fibroblasts. Carriers also can be detected by enzyme assay, and prenatal diagnosis is possible by enzyme assay of amniotic fluid cells or chorionic villi.[258] The galactosylceramidase gene has been mapped to chromosome 14.[258]

Bone marrow transplantation offers some hope in the treatment of Krabbe's disease.[279]

FABRY'S DISEASE

Also referred to as angiokeratoma corporis diffusum universale, Fabry's disease is characterized by angiectatic lesions of the skin, cerebrovascular abnormalities, peripheral neuropathy, and autonomic symptoms related to lipid deposits throughout the body.[70] Vascular lesions of the eye and distinctive opacities of the cornea and lens are important signs of the disease.

This disease is an X-linked disorder of glycosphingolipid catalolism resulting from deficient activity of the lysosomal hydrolase, α-galactosidase A.[70] There is profound deficiency of enzymatic activity in the plasma and tissues of affected hemizygous males, and partial deficiency in heterozygous females, resulting in progressive systemic accumulation of neutral glycosphingolipids with terminal β-galactosyl moieties, predominantly trihexosylceramide (globotriaosylceramide), and to a lesser degree, galabiosylceramide and blood group B substances in most tissues, organs, and fluids of the body.[70] Birefringent lipid crystals are found in the lysosomes of blood vessels; in reticuloendothelial, connective tissue, and myocardial cells; and in epithelial cells of kidney, the adrenal glands, and eye. Lipid also accumulates in ganglion cells of the brain and peripheral nervous system and in peripheral cells of the autonomic system. Vascular changes are prominent throughout the nervous system.

Clinical manifestations of Fabry's disease usually develop during childhood or adolescence in hemizygous males; heterozygous females can be asymptomatic or show attenuated manifestations of the disease.

Characteristic flat or elevated angiectatic lesions of the skin, referred to as angiokeratomas, develop early and increase in size and number with age. The lesions tend to be most numerous between the umbilicus and knees. Mucosal areas, particularly the oral mucosa and conjunctiva, are commonly involved. Paroxysmal episodes of severe burning pain in the extremities are typical; crises may last minutes to days, and may be accompanied by low-grade fever. Patients may also experience parasthesias of the hands and feet. Hypohidrosis is common. With increasing age there is progressive involvement of the cardiovascular and renal systems. Angina, myocardial infarction, arrhythmias, valvular disease, cardiac enlargement, and heart failure may develop. Albuminuria, uremia, and systemic hypertension are common. Cerebrovascular complications including aneurysms, thromboses, and hemorrhage are frequent; patients may develop seizures, hemiplegia, aphasia, and personality or behavioral changes. Death usually occurs in adult life from renal failure or cardiovascular or cerebrovascular complications.

Distinctive corneal opacities resulting from accumulation of lipid in the epithelial cells are the ocular hallmark of Fabry's disease.[91,167,234,244] They are seen in almost all affected males and in many carrier females and may develop early in childhood or in infancy. On slit lamp examination, the typical appearance is that of a fine stippling of intra-or subepithelial opacities arranged in a whorl-like pattern of radiating lines, often more prominent inferiorly. The opacities may appear brownish, tan, or cream colored. The opacities do not seem to interfere with vision.

Lens changes also occur in Fabry's disease. Granular anterior capsular or subcapsular opacities arranged in a radiating wedge-shaped or "propeller" pattern may be seen in affected males.[91,234] In addition, fine whitish opacities arranged in a linear spokelike pattern on or near the posterior lens capsule may be seen in affected males and in some carrier females.[91,234,244]

Numerous ocular signs of vascular involvement occur in Fabry's disease. Some patients develop orbital and lid edema.[91,234,244] In the conjunctiva, aneurysmal dilatation, vessel tortuosity, sludging, and telangiectasis are common.[91,234,244] In the retina one may see tortuosity and segmental dilatation of retinal vessels.[91,234,244] There may be retinal edema, retinovascular signs of systemic hypertension, and in some patients papilledema.[91,244] Central retinal artery occlusion can occur as a severe complication of the disease.[234,235] Central retinal artery occlusion and ischemic neuropathy have been documented in female carriers as well as in males with Fabry's disease.[3,8] Internuclear ophthalmoplegia, presumably related to cerebrovascular involvement, has been reported.[123] Other neuro-ophthalmic manifestations such as nystagmus, ocular motor palsy, and strabismus also have been documented.[91] Optic atrophy has been noted in some cases.[234]

Pathological examination of the eye by light and electron microscopy and by histochemical study in Fabry's disease has documented accumulation of lipid material primarily within smooth muscle cells in the media of arterioles in choroid, retina, ciliary body, iris, limbus, and conjunctiva; similar deposits in endothelial cells and pericytes of small vessels and capillaries throughout the choroid, ciliary body, and iris; and in the basal cell layers of corneal epithelium, in the pigmented epithelium of the iris, and in the epithelium of the lens.[89] On light and electron microscopic examination of the eye of a female carrier, the whorl-like corneal lesion was found to consist of a series of subepithelial ridges composed of bands of reduplicated basement membrane and deposits of amorphous material between the basement membrane and Bowman's membrane, with intracellular deposits in the corneal epithelium above the ridges.[280] The demonstration of lipid inclusions by conjunctival biopsy can be useful in the diagnosis of the disease and the carrier state.[164]

The diagnosis of Fabry disease is confirmed by demonstration of deficient α-galactosidase A activity in plasma, leukocytes, or tears, or increased levels of globotriosylceramide in plasma or urinary sediment.[67,70,164] Heterozygote detection and prenatal diagnosis are possible.[70] The gene encoding α-galactosidase A has been localized to the X-chromosomal region Xq22.[70]

Management of Fabry's disease includes the use of medication for pain and discomfort, anticoagulants for stroke-prone patients, and renal dialysis and transplantation for end-stage renal disease. Enzyme replacement therapy is being investigated.[71]

FARBER DISEASE

The familiar descriptive term for Farber disease is disseminated lipogranulomatosis. The disorder is characterized by accumulation of lipid-laden macrophages and granuloma formations in many organs and tissues.[177] There is usually prominent involvement of periarticular tissues, skin, and larynx, with variable involvement of lung, heart, liver, spleen, lymph nodes, and other sites. Painful and progressive joint deformity, subcutaneous nodules, and progressive hoarseness are major manifestations of the disease. There also may be signs of neuronal lipid storage.

The underlying defect is deficiency of lysosomal acid ceramidase leading to accumulation of ceramide.[177] Ceramide plays a key role in sphingolipid metabolism; it is an intermediate for synthesis and degradation of gangliosides, myelin constituents, and membrane components such as sphingomyelin and complex glycolipids. The human acid ceramidase gene has been mapped to chromosomal region 8p 21.3/22; several mutations have been identified.[178]

The classical form of Farber disease presents in infancy. Signs include painful swelling of joints and, in time, joint contractures; palpable subcutaneous nodules, particularly in relation to affected joints and over pressure points, sometimes involving the mouth, nostrils, external ear, or conjunctiva; hoarseness that may progress to aphonia; feeding difficulties, vomiting, and poor weight gain; and respiratory distress and intermittent fever. There may be lymphadenopathy, hepatomegaly, splenomegaly, or cardiac disease. In some cases there are neurological manifestations including psychomotor retardation or deterioration, seizures, peripheral neuropathy, and myopathy. The disease is progressive, often leading to death early in childhood, although in some cases the course is protracted. There is considerable phenotypic variability and several subtypes of Farber disease have been described, differing in severity and site of involvement.[177]

A number of ocular abnormalities are associated with Farber disease, including xanthoma-like conjunctival lesions, corneal opacities, lenticular opacities, retinal changes, and vision loss.[177,290] There may be parafoveal grayness or cherry-red-like spots of the maculae.[52,290] Retinal pigmentary changes and disc pallor also have been noted.[52] Evidence for lipid storage in various tissues of the eye has been well documented, including the presence of inclusions of various morphological types in retinal ganglion cells, glia of the optic nerve, fibrocytes of sclera, epithelial cells and keratocytes of the cornea, endothelial cells of the trabecular meshwork, fibrocytes of the iris, nonpigmented epithelial cells of the ciliary body, some epithelial cells of the lens, epithelial and stromal cells of the conjunctiva, and in some nonmuscle cells of the extraocular muscles.[52,290]

Farber disease is rare. The inheritance is autosomal recessive. The diagnosis is confirmed by demonstration of the enzyme defect in cultured skin fibroblasts or white blood cells. Heterozygotes usually show reduced ceramidase activity. Prenatal diagnosis by enzyme assay of cultured amniotic fluid cells is possible. Although there is no specific treatment for the disease, corticosteroids may provide some relief, and surgery for the granulomas may be helpful.[177] The possible benefit of bone marrow transplantation has been under investigation.[178] Gene therapy also has been studied.[178]

NEURONAL CEROID-LIPOFUSCINOSES

The neuronal ceroid-lipofuscinoses (NCL) are a group of disorders in which the characteristic pathological findings are (1) accumulation of autofluorescent lipopigments (ceroid and lipofuscin) in neural and nonneural cells, (2) the presence of distinctive membrane-bound cytoplasmic inclusions having granular, curvilinear, or fingerprint patterns, and (3) progressive neuronal degeneration, particularly in the cerebral cortex and cerebellum; there is also demyelination of white matter with reactive gliosis.[211] The underlying biochemical defects have not yet been fully delineated. However, a number of genes for NCL have been identified; these genes encode either lysosomal enzymes or lysosomal membrane proteins.[124]

The familiar eponym applied to this group of disorders is Batten disease. Infantile, late infantile, and juvenile forms occur, referred to respectively as Santavuori–Haltia, Jansky–Bielschowsky, and Spielmeyer–Sjögren disease; there is also an adult form of NCL referred to as Kufs' disease. All are autosomal recessive. Occurring worldwide, the NCL are probably the most frequent of the hereditary neurodegenerative disorders of childhood. By some, the eponym Batten is reserved for juvenile-onset NCL, alternatively referred to as Batten–Spielmeyer–Vogt disease.

The principal clinical manifestations of the childhood forms of NCL are developmental retardation and progressive psychomotor deterioration, ataxia, seizures, and progressive vision loss with signs of retinal degeneration and optic atrophy (Fig. 7-6).[211] Atrophy of the brain is often evident on computed tomography and magnetic resonance imaging.

Confirmation of the diagnosis is often dependent on demonstration of the distinctive cytosomes by biopsy, usually of skin, sometimes conjunctiva. Enzymatic assays are available for the infantile and classical late infantile forms.[124] Prenatal diagnosis is possible in many cases. There is no specific treatment for the neuronal lipofuscinoses.[124]

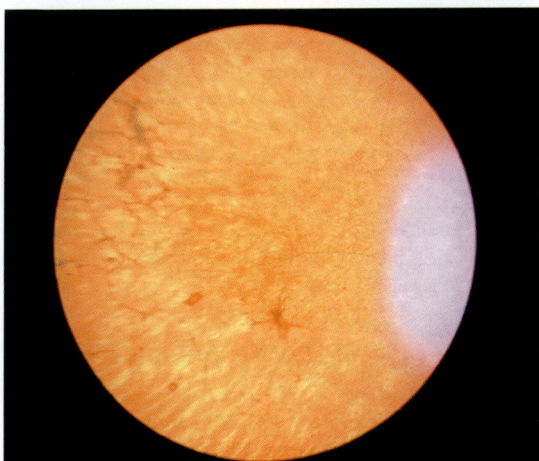

FIGURE 7-6. Pigmentary retinal degeneration of neuronal ceroid lipofuscinosis.

Santavuori–Haltia Disease: Infantile NCL

Beginning by age 12 to 18 months, sometimes as early as 8 months, affected children show mental and motor regression, hypotonia, ataxia, myoclonus, and micrencephaly. There is progressive deterioration to a vegetative state within several years. Death occurs usually by age 5 to 10 years. Vision loss, ultimately leading to blindness, is an early and prominent manifestation. There is retinal degeneration characterized by pigmentary changes (hypopigmentation and/or pigment aggregation), attenuation of retinal vessels, and optic atrophy (see Fig. 7-6).[13,207] The ERG is reduced or extinguished and the VEP is diminished.[207,211] Histopathological studies have documented atrophic changes of the retina and optic nerve.[211]

In infantile NCL there is deficiency of lysosomal palmitoyl-protein thioesterase, which removes fatty acids attached in thioester linkage to cystine in proteins. The gene has been localized to chromosome 1p32.[124]

Jansky–Bielschowsky Disease: Late Infantile NCL

Clinical signs usually appear between age 2 and 4 years, sometimes as early as 1 year. Seizures are a prominent manifestation of the disease. Ataxia develops early, followed by rapidly progressive motor and mental regression. Death occurs usually by age 8 to 14 years. Visual symptoms are not prominent early, but blindness occurs later in the course of the disease. Signs of retinal degeneration may be evident, including pigmentary changes, attenuation of retinal vessels, optic atrophy, and diminished ERG.[211,226] Photoreceptor degeneration and lipopigment storage in the retina have been documented by light and electron microscopy.[226]

In late infantile NCL there is deficiency of a lysosomal protease, pepinase.[124] The gene location for classical late infantile NCL is 11p15.[124]

Spielmeyer–Sjögren Disease: Juvenile NCL

Clinical manifestations usually appear between 5 and 10 years of age. The course is protracted, with survival into the second or third decade. Early signs include intellectual deterioration, decline in school performance, behavioral changes, and in time motor dysfunction. Seizures occur later in most patients.

Decreasing vision is often the presenting sign.[211] In time there is progression to blindness. Maculopathy, frequently described as bull's-eye maculopathy, is an important early finding.[245] Other signs of retinal degeneration, including pigmentary changes (granularity, clumping, spicule formation), vascular attenuation, and optic atrophy, often develop.[100,245] The ERG is reduced or extinguished early.[100,211] Accumulation of lipopigments in the retina has been documented.[100]

The presence of vacuolated lymphocytes in peripheral blood is an important diagnostic finding in juvenile NCL.[211] Battenin, a lysosomal membrane protein, is defective in juvenile NCL.[124] Its function is unknown. The gene location for juvenile NCL is 16p12.[124]

Kufs' Disease: Adult NCL

Mental and motor changes may appear in the second or third decade. Personality changes, ataxia, and myoclonus are common. Vision loss is not a prominent feature of adult NCL, but evidence of retinal degeneration and storage of lipopigment has been documented.[76]

ALBINISM

The term albinism describes a group of genetic disorders of melanin synthesis characterized by congenital hypopigmentation that can involve the skin, hair, and eyes (oculocutaneous albinism) or can be limited to the eye (ocular albinism) (Table 7-6). Essential to the diagnosis of all forms of albinism are ocular abnormalities, particularly retinal hypopigmentation, foveal hypoplasia, and misrouting of optic nerve fibers at the chiasm, with altered visual function; other common features are iris hypopigmentation and translucency, photophobia, nystagmus, strabismus, and high refractive errors.[145,148]

The melanins, which account for virtually all visible pigmentation in the skin, hair, and eyes, are produced by subcellular organelles called melanosomes within melanocytes. The melanocytes are derived from two embryonic tissues, the neural crest and the optic cup. Melanocytes originating in the neural crest migrate to the skin (at the epidermal–dermal border), the eyes (in the choroid and iris stroma), and the hair follicles. Melanocytes of the retinal pigment epithelium are derived from

TABLE 7-6. Forms of Albinism.

Oculocutaneous albinism (OCA)
  OCA1: TYR gene mutations, tyrosinase deficient
    OCA1A
      • No tyrosinase activity
      • Classic OCA phenotype with white hair, milky skin, pale irides
    OCA1B
      • Some residual tyrosinase activity
      • Minimal pigment, platinum or yellow OCA
  OCA2: P gene mutations, tyrosinase positive
      • Spectrum of pigmentation
      • Includes brown OCA
  OCA3: TYR P1 gene mutations
      • Rufous or red OCA
Ocular albinism (OA)
  OA1: X-linked
      • Nettleship–Falls

neuroectoderm as cells originating from the outer layer of the optic vesicle. Two types of melanin can be produced: eumelanins, which are black or brown, and pheomelanins, which are yellow or red. Normal pigmentation requires a number of critical steps during development, and a large number of genes have been shown to participate in the process. The enzyme critical to melanin production is tyrosinase, although there are also a number of posttyrosinase factors and enzymes that regulate the quantity and quality of melanin produced.[145]

Oculocutaneous Albinism (OCA)

This condition is the most common inherited disorder of generalized hypopigmentation. It has been described in all ethnic groups. The estimated frequency is 1 in 20,000 in most populations.[145]

The classification of oculocutaneous albinism includes three major genetic types, designated OCA 1, OCA 2, and OCA 3. All are autosomal recessive. Also important in the classification of OCA is a related syndrome, the Hermansky-Pudlak syndrome.

OCA 1 is tyrosinase-related (or tyrosinase-deficient) oculocutaneous albinism, resulting from mutations of the tyrosinase (TYR) gene, which has been mapped to chromosome 11q14–q21.[145] Two subtypes occur: in OCA 1A, there is no tyrosinase activity; in OCA 1B there is some residual tyrosinase activity. Individuals with OCA 1A (classic tyrosinase-negative oculocutaneous albinism) do not synthesize melanin in the skin, hair, or eyes at any time during life; they have white hair, milky skin, and translucent blue or gray irides from birth (Fig. 7-7). The phenotype of OCA 1B, sometimes referred to as yellow albinism, varies. Most individuals with OCA 1B have very little or no pigment at birth, and develop varying amounts of melanin in the hair and skin in the first to second decade. The hair color changes from white to yellow or golden blonde, and may darken with age. The irides, generally blue, can develop light tan or brownish pigment; some degree of iris translucency usually is present. Many individuals with OCA 1B will tan on exposure to sun.

Visual acuity is markedly reduced, usually 20/200 or worse. Severe photophobia, nystagmus, and strabismus are common.[148]

OCA 2 results from mutations of the P gene, which has been mapped to chromosome 15q11–q12.[145] This is the most common type of oculocutaneous albinism in the world. A broad range of phenotypic variability occurs. In Caucasian individuals with OCA 2, the hair can be lightly pigmented at birth, having a light yellow or blonde color, or more pigmented with a golden-blonde or even red color; it may darken with time. The skin is white and usually does not tan on exposure to sun. The iris is blue-gray or lightly pigmented; the degree of translucency varies with

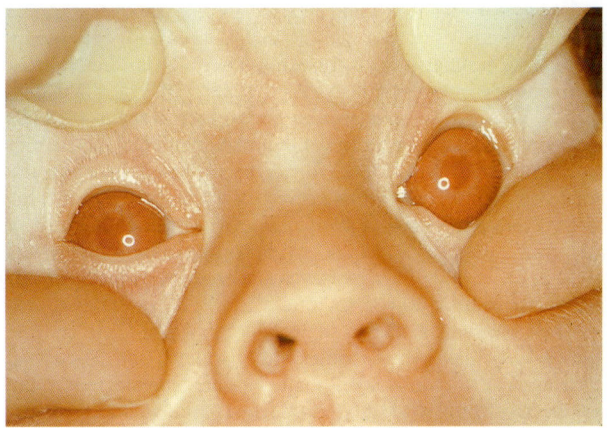

FIGURE 7-7. Iris transillumination in oculocutaneous albinism.

the amount of iris pigmentation. In African or African-American individuals with OCA 2, the hair is yellow at birth and remains yellow or may turn darker. The skin is creamy-white at birth, changes little with time, and usually does not tan. The irides are blue-gray or lightly pigmented, appearing hazel or tan. This is the common "tyrosinase-positive" OCA phenotype. Tyrosinase-negative and tyrosinase-positive forms of albinism can be distinguished by a hair bulb incubation test.[147]

Another variant of OCA 2 caused by mutation of the P gene is "brown OCA."[145,146] In this condition, the amount of eumelanin in the skin and hair is reduced but not absent. In African and African-American individuals with "brown OCA," the hair and skin color are light brown, the irides gray-blue to tan or brown. In time the hair may turn darker and the irides may accumulate more pigment. There is iris translucency. The skin will tan on exposure to sun.

OCA 3, also called rufous or red OCA, results from mutations of the tyrosinase-related protein-1 (TYRP1) gene.[145] Occurring in African or African-American individuals, the phenotype of OCA 3 includes individuals with red or reddish-brown skin, ginger or reddish hair, and hazel or brown irides. All ocular features of albinism, however, are not always present; many do not have iris translucency, foveal hypoplasia, or misrouting of optic nerve fibers, raising some questions of definition and classification.[145,155]

Hermansky–Pudlak syndrome (HPS) is a complex autosomal recessive disorder characterized by the triad of OCA, a bleeding diathesis, and a ceroid storage disease.[145,252] It occurs more often in Puerto Rican than non-Puerto Rican individuals; its frequency in Puerto Rico is approximately 1 in 1,800.[284] The gene responsible for most HPS in Puerto Rico maps to 10q24.[145]

Hypopigmentation of the skin and hair in HPS varies from marked to moderate. Freckles may be present in sun-exposed areas, but tanning does not occur. Iris color varies from blue to brown; there is iris translucency. Other ocular features of albinism including retinal hypopigmentation and foveal hypoplasia are present; nystagmus and strabismus are frequent; acuity varies from 20/400 to 20/60.[252]

The bleeding diathesis in HPS is related to deficiency of storage granules (dense bodies) in platelets, and associated deficiency of serotonin, adenine nucleotides, and calcium in the platelets.[145] Platelets do not show irreversible secondary aggregation in response to stimulation. Manifestations include easy bruiseability, epistaxis, hemoptysis, gingival bleeding; sometimes major, even life-threatening, hemorrhages occur.

The third component of the HPS triad is production of autofluorescent ceroid material, a yellow waxy substance that can be found in urine and many tissues throughout the body, particularly in the lung and gastrointestinal tract, and also in kidney and heart.[145] Manifestations include pulmonary fibrosis and granulomatous colitis, which can be severe.

Ocular Albinism (OA)

In ocular albinism (OA), hypopigmentation clinically is limited to the eye, although changes in the cutaneous pigment system also may be present when the ultrastructure of these tissues is examined.[145]

The OA 1 phenotype, also known as the Nettleship–Falls type of ocular albinism, is X-linked recessive. It is produced by the OA 1 gene on Xp22.[145] In OA 1, melanocytes are normal, but cutaneous and ocular melanocytes contain both normal-sized and giant or macro-melanosomes. Histopathological study of the skin is useful in the diagnosis in both the affected and carrier state.[195,259] Variable expression has been documented in both affected males and Caucasian females.[259] Affected Caucasian males have blue to brown irides with variable translucency, and the other ocular abnormalities of albinism are present. The skin and hair are normally pigmented. In African-American males, the iris color is usually brown, with little translucency. Many African-American males have scattered hypopigmented maculae of the skin.

Heterozygous females often have ocular pigment changes of mosaicism from X-inactivation. Many have a variegated pattern of retinal pigmentation and punctate areas of iris translucency. Some have ocular abnormalities of albinism, including reduced acuity and nystagmus. Occasionally unilateral changes are observed. Detection of the carrier state can be difficult, affecting reliable genetic counseling.[38]

Ocular Features of Albinism: Summary

The ocular abnormalities essential to the definition and diagnosis of all forms of albinism appear to be related to the reduction in melanin during embryonic development and postnatal life.[145,238] Reduction of melanin in the stroma and in the poste-

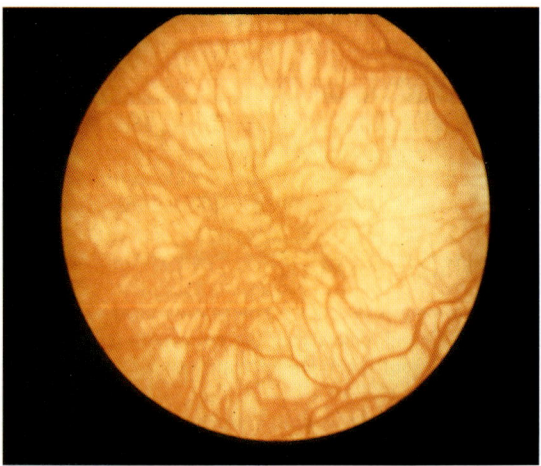

FIGURE 7-8. Fundus hypopigmentation in oculocutaneous albinism.

rior epithelial layer of the iris results in translucency of the iris.[148,252] Reduction of melanin in the retinal pigment epithelium results in varying degrees of hypopigmentation and translucency of the retina, sometimes frank transparency of the macula, allowing increased visibility of the choroidal vessels (Fig. 7-8).[148,252] The fovea in albinism is hypoplastic with a reduced or absent foveal reflex.[93,252] The cone density of the central retina is reduced.[283] Retinal vessels may course into the macular area.[246,252] The optic nerve may appear hypoplastic.[246] Visual acuity is subnormal, ranging from 20/400 to 20/40, commonly 20/200 to 20/100.[88,145] Color vision, however, usually is normal.[148] The ERG in most cases is normal or near normal.[274]

A critical abnormality of the visual system in albinism is abnormal decussation and misrouting of optic nerve fibers at the chiasm.[114] In normal individuals, nerve fibers of the nasal retina cross in the chiasm to terminate in the contralateral geniculate body, and nerve fibers of the temporal retina remain uncrossed to terminate in the ipsilateral geniculate body; in albinism, however, the nerve fibers of the temporal retina project to the contralateral geniculate body. In normal individuals, the ratio of crossed to uncrossed fibers is approximately 55:45; in albinism, the proportion of crossed fibers probably exceeds 90%.[145] Corresponding abnormalities in the size and configuration of the afferent visual pathways have not been documented by magnetic resonance imaging.[25] The visual evoked response is asymmetrical and distinctively diagnostic.[9,10,87,116,153] Stereopsis usually is reduced.[116,159] Nystagmus is present in most individuals with albinism, and many exhibit compensatory posturing.[1,2,148,252] Strabismus is common.[148] Many individuals with albinism have high refractive errors[88,252]; there is some evidence that the type of refractive error is reflective of the type of albinism.[138] Also, image quality may affect refractive development.[72] Compounding the effect of the neuroanatomic abnormalities of the afferent visual pathways, the nystagmus, high refractive errors, and light scatter all adversely affect retinal image quality.[1]

Axenfeld anomaly, other signs of anterior segment dysgenesis, and developmental glaucoma have been reported in patients with albinism.[156,252]

In the management of patients with albinism, all efforts should be made to improve visual function with appropriate refractive correction and whatever low-vision aids are found to be helpful and acceptable to the patient. Tinted lenses can provide relief from glare. Protection from ultraviolet effects must be advised. Extraocular muscle surgery for nystagmus may improve vision and compensatory posturing.[65] When strabismus presents a cosmetic problem, surgical correction can be offered.

When assessing an albino child's visual function for educational purposes, it is important to measure acuity binocularly at both distance and near, allowing compensatory posturing, in addition to testing acuity monocularly, as the measurements may vary in the presence of nystagmus. Young albino patients also should be allowed and encouraged to hold things close for maximal performance. As might be expected, intellectual capabilities and educational attainment in patients with albinism vary.[92]

TYROSINEMIA

A semiessential amino acid, tyrosine is derived from dietary sources and from hydroxylation of phenylalanine. It is incorporated into protein, and it is important in the synthetic pathways leading to catecholamines, thyroid hormone, and melanin pigments. Its degradation occurs primarily in hepatocytes, and under most circumstances the rate of its degradation is determined by

TABLE 7-7. Disorders of Tyrosine Metabolism.

Fumarylacetoacetate hydrolase (FAH) deficiency
　Hepatorenal tyrosinemia (tyrosinemia type 1)
　　Variable symptoms, including acute liver failure, cirrhosis, hepatocellular
　　　carcinoma, Fanconi's syndrome, peripheral neuropathy
Tyrosine aminotransferase (TAT) deficiency
　Oculocutaneous tyrosinemia (tyrosinemia type II)
　Palmoplantar keratoses and keratopathy
4-Hydroxyphenylpyruvate dioxygenase (4-HPPD) Dysfunction
　Hereditary 4-HPPD deficiency (tyrosinemia type III)
　Neurological signs, mental retardation, ataxia
Hawkinsinuria
　Metabolic acidosis and failure to thrive in infancy
Transient tyrosinemia of the newborn
　In most cases, no symptomatology
　In some infants, lethargy, reduced motor activity
　Possibly adverse developmental effects

the activity of tyrosine aminotransferase.[176] One of the least soluble of the amino acids, tyrosine at high concentration forms characteristic crystals.

A number of inherited and acquired disorders can cause hypertyrosinemia (Table 7-7).[176] Of these, tyrosinemia type II, referred to as oculocutaneous tyrosinemia, is of special importance in pediatric ophthalmology.

Oculocutaneous Tyrosinemia

Commonly known as Richner–Hanhart syndrome, this disorder is characterized by painful keratopathy, palmoplantar keratoses, and mental retardation.[176] It is caused by autosomal recessive deficiency of cytoplasmic tyrosine aminotransferase (TAT), the first enzyme of the tyrosine catabolic pathway.[176] In humans, this enzyme is located on chromosome 16q22.1–q22.3.[176]

Ocular manifestations usually develop in the first years of life, often in infancy, but can begin later.[29,105,220,221] Key signs and symptoms are photophobia, lacrimation, pain and redness of the eyes, often with exacerbations and partial remissions. On slit lamp examination the typical ocular lesion is a dendritiform or pseudodendritic opacity of the central or paracentral cornea, involving primarily epithelium, sometimes the subepithelial region, Bowman's layer, or anterior stroma.[7,39] The corneal changes characteristically are bilateral, although often asymmetrical.[7] Superficial punctate keratopathy, painful corneal erosions and ulcerations occur.[29,39] Neovascularization and corneal scarring may develop.[29,106] The hypothesis is that tyrosine crystalizes in the corneal epithelial cells, disrupting the lysosomes and initiating an inflammatory response.[7] Light microscopy of a corneal specimen showed some birefringent crystals in the corneal stroma, and on electron microscopy vacuolar degeneration of keartocytes with electron-dense particles in the vacuoles was found.[224] It is known that patients who have undergone keratoplasty can develop recurrent lesions in the graft.[12,224] There may also be conjunctival involvement including thickening, papillary hypertrophy, and microfollicular conjunctivitis; vacuoles and inclusion bodies have been found on pathological examination.[21,105] Subcapsular lens opacities have been noted in some cases.[29,106] Long-term consequences of oculocutaneous tyrosinemia include cornea plana, vision loss, associated nystagmus, and strabismus.[176]

It should be emphasized that affected children may be symptomatic before significant corneal changes can be detected, and the diagnosis of tyrosinemia type II should be considered in patients with unexplained photophobia, tearing, pain, and redness of the eyes.[206] Also, the ocular signs must be differentiated from those of herpetic infection.[39] The corneal lesion of tyrosinemia is thicker and more plaquelike, lacking the fine branching pattern and club-shaped edges of a true herpetic dendrite, and usually stains poorly if at all with fluorescein or rose bengal; also, corneal sensation is intact and viral cultures are negative.[39]

Fortunately the corneal manifestations of tyrosinemia can be reversed, and often prevented, by dietary restriction of tyrosine and phenylalanine[17,39,105,106,121]; early diagnosis and treatment are key. Symptomatic treatment with topical lubricants can be helpful for patients with keratopathy.

Cutaneous manifestations usually begin after age 1 year, but may begin in infancy.[176] Painful hyperkeratotic plaques develop in the soles, palms, and plantar surfaces of the digits.[105] Other areas, such as elbows, knees, and ankles, occasionally are involved, and leukokeratosis of the tongue has been reported.[176] The skin lesions improve with dietary treatment.[105,129,176]

Mental retardation occurs in less than 50% of patients.[176] Other neurological findings including seizures, microcephaly, extinguished visual evoked potentials, and behavioral problems have been reported in some cases.[7,176] Early dietary treatment may prevent mental retardation.[106]

CYSTINOSIS

Cystinosis is a rare metabolic disease characterized by intracellular lysosomal accumulation of free nonprotein cystine, with crystal formation in many tissues and organs, particularly kidney and eye. The underlying defect is impaired transport of the amino acid cystine across the lysosomal membrane.[95]

Several forms of cystinosis occur, ranging from a benign nonnephropathic variant presenting with corneal crystals, to classic early-onset nephropathic cystinosis characterized by life-threatening progressive renal disease and potentially debilitating ocular involvement (Table 7-8).[95] The most frequent is classic nephropathic cystinosis; its incidence in North America is approximately 1 in 100,000 to 1 in 200,000 live births. All forms are autosomal recessive. The cystinosis gene, CTNS, has been mapped to chromosome 17p; a number of mutations have been identified.[95] Heterozygotes for cystinosis, regardless of type, are clinically normal.

Infants with classic nephropathic cystinosis appear normal at birth, although in Caucasian families, the hair and skin

---

TABLE 7-8. Forms of Cystinosis.

Nephropathic:
  Infantile
  • Classic form, presenting at 6 to 18 months
  • Most common and devastating variant, with Fanconi syndrome, renal failure, and extrarenal complications
  • Extensive ocular involvement, particularly crystalline keratopathy and progressive retinopathy, possibly glaucoma

  Late onset
  • Range of presentation from 2 to 26 years, most commonly 12 to 15 years (adolescent form)
  • Usually not full Fanconi's syndrome; possibly late-onset renal deterioration
  • Cystine crystals in marrow aspirates
  • Crystalline deposits in cornea and conjunctiva; variable retinal involvement

Nonnephropathic:
  Ocular
  • Formerly adult or benign form
  • Crystalline deposits in cornea and conjunctiva, often discovered in teens to adult years
  • No retinopathy
  • Usually asymptomatic with possible exception of photophobia
  • Crystalline deposits in marrow
  • No renal disease

pigmentation of affected infants may be lighter than that of their siblings. Beginning usually between 6 and 12 months of age, signs of impaired renal tubular reabsorption (Fanconi's syndrome) develop, with excessive urinary losses of water, glucose, amino acids, calcium, phosphorus, sodium, potassium, bicarbonate, and other metabolites. Affected infants may be fussy, feed poorly, urinate and drink excessively, vomit, and suffer episodes of acidosis, dehydration, and electrolyte imbalances. They fail to grow and gain weight. They develop rickets, sometimes tetany, arrhythmias, and muscle weakness. Untreated, the natural course is one of progressive glomerular damage with renal failure and uremia, requiring dialysis or kidney transplantation usually by age 6 to 12 years; in some cases renal failure occurs as early as 1 to 3 years of age. Accumulation of cystine in other tissues and organs produces a variety of additional clinical manifestations. Primary hypothyroidism is common. Some patients develop insulin-dependent diabetes mellitus. Males may exhibit hypogonadism, delayed puberty. Some patients develop hepatomegaly, occasionally hypersplenism. Accumulation of cystine in the intestinal tract and appendix may contribute to nausea and vomiting. Continued accumulation in muscle can lead to impaired function; this may contribute to swallowing difficulties in older patients. There may be decreased ability to sweat. Neurological manifestations, such as seizures, tremor, or mental retardation, occur occasionally.

Involvement of the eye in cystinosis is extensive. Studies have documented accumulation of crystals within keratocytes; throughout subepithelial tissues of conjunctiva; in sclera and episclera; in epithelium and stroma of iris; in pigmented and nonpigmented epithelium and connective tissue of ciliary body; in choroid, mainly within fibrocytes and histiocytes; in retinal pigment epithelium; in meninges and fibrovascular pial septae of the optic nerves; and in extraocular muscles.[48,90,142,222,287]

Clinically, the pathognomonic ocular sign of cystinosis is a distinctive crystalline keratopathy (Fig. 7-9). Slit lamp examination reveals myriads of scintillating iridescent crystals within the corneal stroma, usually by age 1 year.[286] Deposition of the corneal crystals appears to begin in the anterior stroma and progress posteriorly, and to advance from the periphery of the cornea to the center, in time involving the full extent of the stroma.[172] Crystals may be found at or near the endothelial surface, but epithelium usually is spared.[172] In time the cornea may become diffusely hazy.[134] Punctate keratopathy, painful

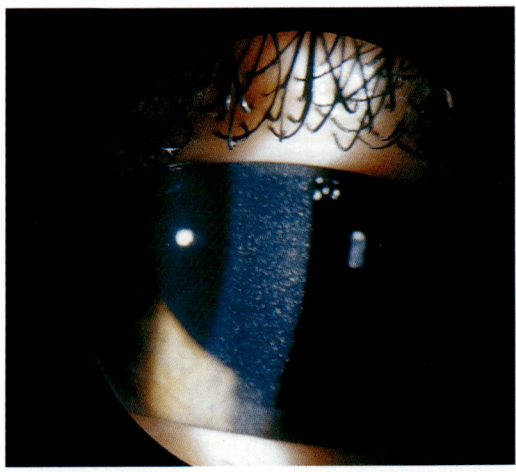

FIGURE 7-9. Iridescent corneal crystals of cystinosis.

recurrent corneal erosions, and band keratopathy may develop in time.[134,214] Photophobia, an early and prominent symptom, and blepharospasm, can be significant problems.[134,214] Glare disability has been documented.[140] Corneal sensitivity may be reduced.[139] On slit lamp examination, refractile crystals also can be detected within the conjunctiva, on the iris, and sometimes overlying the lens.[134,286]

Another major clinical ocular manifestation of cystinosis is progressive retinopathy, which is characterized by depigmentation and mottling of the fundus, often in a patchy distribution, involving predominantly the periphery, extending from the equatorial region to the ora serrata, often with fine to coarse pigment clumps distributed over the light background; there also may be granularity or fine pepper-like stippling of the posterior fundus (Fig. 7-10).[213,288] Conspicuous yellow mottling of the macula in association with generalized disturbance of the retinal pigment epithelium also has been described.[222] Retinal changes can be seen as early as infancy and can precede the development of corneal signs.[222] Glistening crystal-like deposits may be evident on fundus examination.[134,213] In young patients, visual function and ERG responses often are normal, but older surviving patients whose retinas have accumulated cystine for one to three decades commonly suffer progressive visual impairment, reduced acuity, color vision, dark adaptation, and ERG responses.[94,134,288]

Pupillary-block glaucoma, attributed to thickening and rigidity of the iris related to accumulation of crystals in iris stroma, can occur in childhood-onset cystinosis.[277] Posterior synechiae may contribute.[134] Narrowing of the anterior chamber angle and altered ciliary body configuration, which may contribute to the predisposition to glaucoma, has been demonstrated by ultrasound biomicroscopy.[181] Primary open-angle glaucoma also has been reported in the benign adult form of cystinosis.[285]

The diagnosis of cystinosis is confirmed by demonstrating elevated cystine content in polymorphonuclear leukocytes or cultured fibroblasts. At birth, measurements can be made of placenta or white cells of cord blood. Prenatal diagnosis can be made using cultured amniocytes or chorionic villi.[95] Heterozygote detection also is possible.[95]

Treatment of cystinosis includes management of renal losses, renal dialysis, and kidney transplantation for renal failure.[95] Cystine accumulation does not occur in the donor kidney, but continues in other sites, contributing to extrarenal complications in long-term survivors. Chronic therapy with a

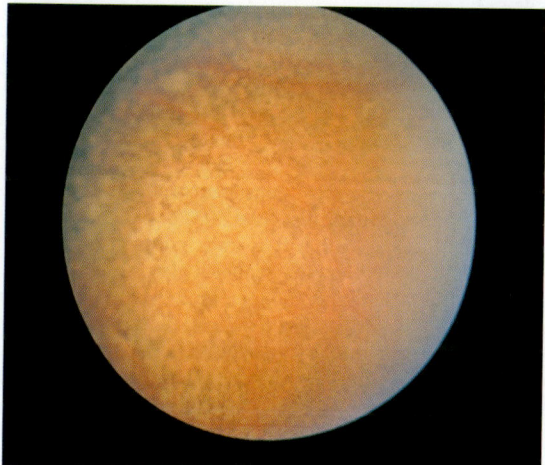

FIGURE 7-10. Pigmentary retinopathy of cystinosis.

cystine-depleting agent, cysteanine (β-mercaptoethylamine), taken orally can forestall renal failure and improve growth but does not reverse the ocular changes.[134] The use of cysteamine eyedrops can help prevent and reverse corneal crystal deposition.[135,136]

HOMOCYSTINURIA

The condition known as homocystinuria is caused by deficiency of cystathionine β-synthase.[179] Important in the complex scheme of methionine metabolism, this enzyme catalyzes conversion of homocysteine to cystathionine. The defect results in intracellular accumulation of homocysteine, increased serum levels of methionine, homocysteine, and homocystine, and excretion of these metabolites in urine. Cystathionine levels, particularly in brain, and cystine levels in urine, plasma, and red blood cells, are decreased.

The disorder affects predominantly the skeletal, vascular, and central nervous systems and the eye; other organs including liver, skin, and hair also may be involved.[179] Major clinical manifestations are osteoporosis, thromboembolism, mental retardation, and ectopia lentis.

The locus for cystathionine β-synthase has been mapped to 21q22.3.[179] The enzyme deficiency is inherited as an autosomal recessive condition. Direct enzyme assay confirms the diagnosis of the disorder; liver biopsy specimens, cultured skin fibroblasts, phytohemagglutinin-stimulated lymphocytes, or long-term established lines of such cells can be used. Identification of heterozygotes can be difficult. Prenatal diagnosis is feasible.

Osteoporosis is the most consistent skeletal manifestation of homocystinuria, found in at least 50% of patients by the end of the second decade of life; it is most common in the spine, followed by the long bones.[179] Scoliosis also is frequent. Other skeletal manifestations include increased length of long bones, arachnodactyly, biconcave "codfish" vertebrae, pes cavus, genu valgum, pectus carinatum or excavatum, various abnormalities of the metaphyses, epiphyses, carpal and metacarpal bones, and high arched palate.

Thromboembolism is a major cause of morbidity and the most frequent cause of death in patients with homocystinuria.[179] Vascular occlusion can occur at any age, including infancy. The risk of thromboembolism appears to increase with age, with pregnancy and the postpartum state, and possibly in the postoperative state. Other vascular manifestations of homocystinuria are malar flush and livedo reticularis.

The principal neurological manifestations of homocystinuria are mental retardation and psychiatric disturbances.[179] Seizures, EEG abnormalities, and extrapyramidal signs are less frequent. Focal neurological signs may occur with cerebrovascular occlusion.

Additional findings in patients with homocystinuria include fair brittle or sparse hair, thin skin, fatty liver changes, inguinal hernia, myopathy, endocrine abnormalities, and reduced clotting factors.[179]

The characteristic ocular manifestation of homocystinuria is ectopia lentis (Fig. 7-11).[59,243] Partial or complete dislocation of the lens has been found in almost all cases[59,243]; it is usually evident by age 10 years.[59,209] The dislocation is bilateral, progres-

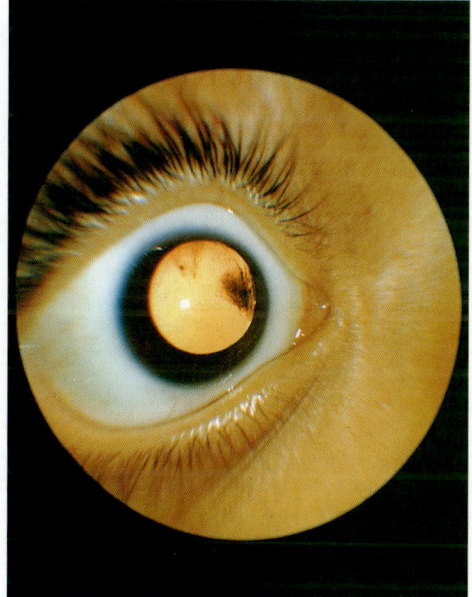

FIGURE 7-11. Ectopia lentis with cataract in homocystinuria.

sive, and commonly occurs in the inferior or nasal direction, although it may occur in any direction[59,179,243]; in some cases the lens may dislocate into the anterior chamber or vitreous.[59] An important clinical sign of ectopia lentis is iridodenesis. The ectopia is attributed to progressive fraying and disruption of the zonular fibers.[179] On slit lamp examination, a fringe of zonular remnants may be found attached to the anterior lens capsule.[208] It has been postulated that an abnormality of zonular fibrillin, like that in Marfan syndrome, is responsible for the ectopia lentis in homocystinuria.[179]

Myopia commonly develops as the lens loosens and becomes more spherical.[179] Significant myopia in the very young child should raise suspicion of ectopia lentis and the possibility of an underlying metabolic disorder such as homocystinuria.

Glaucoma, often pupillary block glaucoma,[59,243] is a frequent complication in patients with homocystinuria.[59,243] Cataracts have been noted in some cases.[243] A variety of other ocular abnormalities including optic atrophy, cystic and pigmentary changes of the peripheral retina, retinal detachment, keratitis, iritis, and strabismus have been described in patients with homocystinuria.[59,209,243] In many cases the iris stroma is lightly pigmented.[243]

Light and electron microscopic studies of the eye in homocystinuria have shown the zonular fibers to be deficient at the border of the lens and retracted to the surface of the ciliary body, forming a matted layer of filaments along a thickened basement membrane of the nonpigmented ciliary epithelium.[209] Zonular remnants attached to the lens capsule also have been found to be composed of short filaments in disarray, with occasional bundles of normal-appearing fibers.[208] In addition, peripheral degeneration of the retina has been documented on histopathological examination.[209] Note: Investigation into the nature of zonules has documented certain characteristics, particularly their elasticity and propensity to recoil, and their cysteine content, of great interest with regard to the pathological findings in homocystinuria.[251]

Treatment of patients with homocystinuria involves (1) management of the biochemical abnormalities in an effort to prevent or ameliorate clinical manifestations of the disease, and (2) management of complications that do occur as a result of the disease. Most patients detected in infancy are treated with a low-methionine, cystine-supplemented diet. Early dietary management can be effective in preventing mental retardation and ectopia lentis, and may possibly reduce the occurrence of initial thromboembolic events and the incidence of seizures.[179] In some patients, treatment with pyridoxine can be effective in reducing, but not completely normalizing, the biochemical abnormalities. In vitamin B_6-responsive patients, pyridoxine may be used alone or in conjunction with less stringent methionine dietary restriction. B_6-responsive patients generally have milder and more slowly developing manifestations that those who are not responsive to pyridoxine. Betaine can be useful for vitamin B_6-nonresponsive patients for whom dietary management is unsatisfactory.

Surgery for ectopia lentis can be complicated by vitreous loss and adhesions.[59] Visual results from removal of the lens vary.[59] It should be noted that some patients with homocystinuria have died of thromboembolism following ocular surgery.[59,179]

GALACTOSEMIA

Galactose is an essential source of energy in infants. Although some galactose is produced by endogenous synthesis from glucose, the main source of galactose is ingested milk and milk products containing lactose. Under normal circumstances, ingested galactose, a disaccharide, is hydrolyzed into its constituent monosaccharides, galactose and glucose; these monosaccharides are rapidly absorbed from the intestine, and galactose is then converted to glucose. The enzymes involved in the principal metabolic pathway for conversion of galactose to glucose are (1) galactokinase (GALK), (2) galactose-1-phosphate uridyltransferase (GALT), and (3) uridine diphosphate galactose-4′ epimerase (GALE).[126] The enzymes are found in many cell types and tissues, although the liver is the major organ of galactose metabolism. Genetic defects in galactose metabolism result in abnormally high concentrations of galactose and its metabolites in body tissues and fluids, with a variety of clinical manifestations, including cataracts. Prenatal screening for all three enzyme defects is available. All are autosomal recessive.

GALT Deficiency

Classical galactosemia results from deficiency of galactose-1-phosphate uridyltransferase (GALT). The gene encoding this enzyme has been localized to the short arm of chromosome 9 in the 9p13 region.[126] The disorder presents in the first weeks of life with poor feeding, vomiting, diarrhea, weight loss, lethargy, and hypotonia. There may be signs of liver dysfunction, including jaundice and hepatomegaly, with elevated liver transaminases and elevated plasma amino acids, coagulopathy, and hemolytic anemia, and there may be signs of renal tubular disease, including metabolic acidosis, galactosuria, glycosuria, albuminuria, and aminoaciduria. Septicemia is not uncommon.

The characteristic ocular manifestation of galactosemia is cataract. Galactosemic cataracts typically are bilateral and develop in the first weeks or months of life[55]; pathological changes of the lens have even been found in a fetus.[270] The clinical appearance of the galactosemic cataract in its early stages is often likened to that of an oil droplet within the lens; the nucleus is sharply demarcated from the surrounding perinuclear zone by a difference in refractive state.[270] In other cases there may be a distinct zonular opacity, lamellar cataract, or dense nuclear cataract, sometimes with fine punctate opacities in the periphery of the lens, or dense cortical or subcapsular opacities[270] (Fig. 7-12). The cataract formation has been attributed to accumulation of

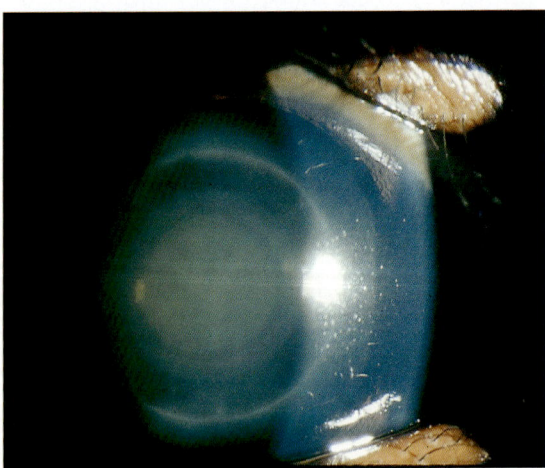

FIGURE 7-12. Nuclear and concentric lamellar cataract formation in galactosemia.

galactitol (dulcitol) in the lens.[126,269] There may be secondary nystagmus and strabismus.[55]

A less well recognized ocular manifestation of galactosemia is vitreous hemorrhage, probably related to coagulopathy.[160] Retinal scarring and pigmentary changes may follow. There may be significant visual impairment.

With early diagnosis of galactosemia and timely treatment with a galactose restricted diet, the systemic effects of galactosemia can be reversed, even prevented. However, even with early dietary treatment there may be long-term effects, including impaired cognitive development, speech and language defects, verbal apraxia, visual perceptual dysfunction, ataxic neurological disease, and ovarian failure.[126] Neuroimaging of the brain in patients with neurological manifestation has shown abnormal white matter, cortical atrophy and ventricular enlargement, cerebellar atrophy, and involvement of basal ganglia and brainstem.[126] Cataract formation also can be reversed, or even prevented, with early diagnosis and prompt dietary treatment.[28,55]

GALK Deficiency

In patients with deficiency of galactokinase (GALK), the only consistent clinical finding is cataract.[162] The cataracts are bilateral and morphologically like those of classic galactosemia (GALT deficiency).[162,192] They may be seen in the first weeks of life[162] and may be reversible with early diagnosis and timely treatment with a galactose-restricted diet.[162]

Pseudotumor cerebri has been found in some patients with GALK deficiency.[126] Other reported abnormalities such as macular deposits, mild retardation, complement deficiency, and seizures with neurological deterioration may be coincidental.[126]

The gene encoding galactokinase has been localized to chromosome 17p24.[126]

It is of interest that in studies of adult patients with idiopathic cataracts, some had diminished galactokinase levels.[79,241] Reduced galactokinase activity may increase the risk of developing presenile cataracts requiring surgery by the fourth decade.

GALE Deficiency

In most cases of uridine diphosphate galactose-4' epimerase deficiency, the enzyme defect is confined to the erythrocytes; most patients are asymptomatic and require no treatment.[126]

Cataracts are not a feature of this disorder. Generalized GALE deficiency is rare; a few patients with GALE deficiency have presented with manifestations similar to those of classic galactosemia and may have long-term complications.[126] These patients respond to galactose-restricted diets. The enzyme encoding uridine diphosphate galactose-4' epimerase has been localized to the short arm of chromosome 1 at 1p36.[126]

References

1. Abadi RV, Dickinson CM, Pascal E, Papas E. Retinal image quality in albinos. A review. Ophthalmic Paediatr Genet 1990;11:171–176.

2. Abadi RV, Pascal E. Visual resolution limits in human albinism. Vision Res 1991;31:1445–1447.

3. Abe H, Sakai T, Sawaguchi S, et al. Ischemic optic neuropathy in a female carrier with Fabry's disease. Ophthalmologica 1992;205:83–88.

4. Abraham FA, Yatziv S, Russell A, et al. A family with two siblings affected by Morquio syndrome (MPS IV): electrophysiological and psychophysical findings in the visual system. Arch Ophthalmol 1974;91:265–269.

5. Abrahamov A, Elstein D, Gross-Tsur V, et al. Gaucher's disease variant characterized by progressive calcification of heart valve and unique genotype. Lancet 1995;346:1000–1003.

6. Adachi M, Schneck L, Volk BW. Ultrastructural studies of eight cases of fetal Tay–Sachs disease. Lab Investig 1974;30:102–112.

7. Al-Hemidan AI, Al-Hazzaa SAF. Richner–Hanhart syndrome (tyrosinemia type II). Case report and literature review. Ophthalmic Genetics 1995;16:21–26.

8. Anderson MUN, Dahl H, Fledelius H, Nielson NV. Central retinal artery occlusion in a patient with Fabry's disease documented by scanning laser ophthalmoscopy. Acta Ophthalmol 1994;72:635–638.

9. Apkarian P. A practical approach to albino diagnosis. VEP misrouting across the age span. Ophthalmic Paediatr Genet 1992;13:77–88.

10. Apkarian P, Reits D, Spekreijse H, Van Dorp D. A decisive electrophysiological test for human albinism. Electroencephalogr Clin Neurophysiol 1983;55:513–531.

11. Arbisser AI, Donnelly KA, Scott CI, et al. Morquio-like syndrome with β-galactosidase deficiency and normal hexosamine sulfatase activity: mucopolysaccharidosis IV B. Ann J Med Genet 1977;1:195–205.

12. Bardelli AM, Borgogni P, Farnetani MA, et al. Familial tyrosinemia with eye and skin lesions. Presentation of two cases. Ophthalmologica 1977;175:5–9.

13. Bateman JB, Philippart M. Ocular features of the Hagberg–Santavuori syndrome. Am J Ophthalmol 1986;102:262–271.

14. Bateman JB, Philippart M, Isenberg SJ. Ocular features of multiple sulfatase deficiency and a new variant of metachromatic leukodystrophy. J Pediatr Ophthalmol Strabismus 1984;21:133–139.

15. Beaudet AL, DiFerrante NM, Ferry GD, et al. Variation in the phenotypic expression of β-glucuronidase deficiency. J Pediatr 1975; 86:388–394.

16. Beck M, Cole G. Disc oedema in association with Hunter's syndrome: ocular histopathologic findings. Br J Ophthalmol 1984;68: 590–594.

17. Benoldi D, Orsoni JB, Allegra F. Tyrosinemia type II: a challenge for ophthalmologists and dermatologists. Pediatr Dermatol 1997;14: 110–112.

18. Berliner ML. Lipin keratitis of Hurler's syndrome (gargoylism or dysostosis multiplex): clinical and pathologic report. Arch Ophthalmol 1939;22:97–105.

19. Beutler E, Grabowski GA. Gaucher disease. In: Scriver CR, Beaudet AL, Sly WS, Valle D, et al. (eds) The metabolic and molecular bases of inherited disease. New York: McGraw-Hill, 1995:2641–2670.

20. Beutler E, Grabowski GA. Gaucher disease. In: Scriver CR, Beaudet AL, Sly WS, Valle D, et al. (eds) The metabolic and molecular bases of inherited disease. New York: McGraw-Hill, 2001:3635–3668.

21. Bienfang DC, Kuwabara T, Pueschel SM. The Richner–Hanhart syndrome. Report of a case with associated tyrosinemia. Arch Ophthalmol 1976;94:1133–1137.

22. Billings DM, Degnan M. Kinky hair syndrome. A new case and a review. Am J Dis Child 1971;212:447–449.

23. Boniuk V, Ghosh M, Galin M. Conjunctival eye signs in GM$_1$ type 1 gangliosidosis. Birth Defects 1976;XII:543–551.

24. Brett EM, Ellis RB, Hass L, et al. Late onset GM$_2$-gangliosidosis. Clinical, pathological, and biochemical studies on eight patients. Arch Dis Child 1973;48:775–785.

25. Brodsky MC, Glasier CM, Creel DJ. Magnetic resonance imaging of the visual pathways in human albinos. J Pediatr Ophthalmol Strabismus 1993;30:382–385.

26. Brounstein S, Meagher-Villemure K, Polomeno RC, et al. Optic nerve in globoid leukodystrophy (Krabbe's disease). Ultrastructural changes. Arch Ophthalmol 1978;96:864–870.

27. Brownstein S, Carpenter S, Polomeno RC, Little JM. Sandhoff's disease (GM$_2$ gangliosidosis type 2). Histopathology and ultrastructure of the eye. Arch Ophthalmol 1980;98:1089–1097.

28. Burke JP, O'Keefe M, Bowell R, Naughten ER. Ophthalmic findings in classical galactosemia—a screened population. J Pediatr Ophthalmol Strabismus 1989;26:165–168.

29. Burns RP. Soluble tyrosine aminotransferase deficiency: an unusual cause of corneal ulcers. Am J Ophthalmol 1972;73:400–402.

30. Cahane M, Treister G, Abraham FA, Melamed S. Glaucoma in siblings with Morquio syndrome. Br J Ophthalmol 1990;74: 382.

31. Cairns JE, Wilson HP, Walshe JM. "Sunflower cataract" in Wilson's disease. Br Med J 1969;3:95–96.
32. Cantor LB, Disseler JA, Wilson FM. Glaucoma in the Marteaux–Lamy syndrome. Am J Ophthalmol 1989;108:426–430.
33. Carbone AO, Petrozzi CF. Gaucher's disease. Case report with stress on eye findings. Henry Ford Hosp Med J 1968;16:55–60.
34. Carmody PJ, Rattazzi MC, Davidson RG. Tay-Sachs disease. The use of tears for the detection of heterozygotes. N Engl J Med 1973;28: 1072–1074.
35. Caruso RC, Kaiser-Kupfer MI, Muenzer J, et al. Electroretinographic findings in the mucopolysaccharidoses. Ophthalmology 1986;93: 1612–1616.
36. Ceuterick C, Martin JJ, Libert J, Farriaux JP. Sanfilippo. A disease in the fetus: comparison with pre- and postnatal cases. Neuropediatrie 1990;11:176–185.
37. Chan CC, Green WR, Maumenee IH, et al. Ocular ultrastructural studies of two cases of the Hurler syndrome (systemic mucopolysaccharidosis I-H). Ophthalmol Pediatr Genet 1983;2:3–19.
38. Charles SJ, Moore AT, Grant JW, Yates JR. Genetic counseling in X-linked ocular albinism: clinical features of the carrier state. Eye 1992;6:75–79.
39. Charlton KH, Binder PS, Wozniak L, Digby DJ. Pseudodendritic keratitis and systemic tyrosinemia. Ophthalmology 1981;88:355–360.
40. Chijiiwa T, Inomata H, Yamana Y, et al. Ocular manifestations of Hurler–Scheie prototype in two sibs. Jpn J Ophthalmol 1983;27: 54–62.
41. Christiansen SP, Smith TJ, Henslee-Downey PJ. Normal intraocular pressure after a bone marrow transplant in glaucoma associated with mucopolysaccharidosis type I-H. Am J Ophthalmol 1990;109:230–231.
42. Chu FC, Rodrigues MM, Cogan DG, Barranger JA. The pathology of pingueculae in Gaucher's disease. Ophthalmic Paediatr Genet 1984; 4:7–11.
43. Cogan DG, Chu FC, Barranger JA, Gregg RE. Macula halo syndrome. Variant of Niemann–Pick disease. Arch Ophthalmol 1983;101:1698–1700.
44. Cogan DG, Chu FC, Gittinger J, Tychsen L. Fundal abnormalities of Gaucher's disease. Arch Ophthalmol 1980;98:2202–2203.
45. Cogan DG, Chu FC, Reingold D, et al. Ocular motor signs in some metabolic diseases. Arch Ophthalmol 1981;99:1802–1808.
46. Cogan DG, Federman DD. Retinal involvement with reticuloendotheliosis of unclassified type. Arch Ophthalmol 1964;71:489–491.
47. Cogan DG, Kuwabara T. Histochemistry of the retina in Tay-Sachs disease. Arch Ophthalmol 1959;61:415–423.
48. Cogan DG, Kuwabara T. Ocular pathology of cystinosis, with particular reference to elusiveness of the corneal crystals. Arch Ophthalmol 1960;63:51–57.

49. Cogan DG, Kuwabara T. The sphingolipidoses and the eye. Arch Ophthalmol 1968;79:437–451.

50. Cogan DG, Kuwabara T, Kolodny E, Driscoll S. Gangliosidoses and the fetal retina. Ophthalmology 1984;91:508–512.

51. Cogan DG, Kuwabara T, Moser H. Metachromatic leukodystrophy. Ophthalmologica 1970;160:2–17.

52. Cogan DG, Kuwabara T, Moser H, et al. Retinopathy in a case of Farber's lipogranulomatosis. Arch Ophthalmol 1966;75:752–757.

53. Cogan DG, Kuwabara T, Richardson EP, et al. Histochemistry of the eye in metachromatic leucoencephalopathy. Arch Ophthalmol 1958;60:397–402.

54. Collins MLZ, Traboulsi EI, Maumenee IH. Optic nerve head swelling and optic atrophy in the systemic mucopolysaccharidoses. Ophthalmology 1990;97:1445–1449.

55. Cordes FC. Galactosemia cataract; a review. Report of a case. Am J Ophthalmol 1960;50:1151–1158.

56. Cordes FC, Hogan MJ. Dysostosis multiplex (Hurler's disease; lipochondrodysplasia; gargoylism). Report of the ocular findings in five cases, with a review of the literature. Arch Ophthalmol 1942;27:637–664.

57. Cotlier E. Tay Sachs' retina: deficiency of acetyl hexosaminidase A. Arch Ophthalmol 1971;86:352–356.

58. Crocker AC, Farber S. Niemann–Pick's disease: a review of 18 patients. Medicine (Baltim) 1958;37:1–95.

59. Cross HE, Jensen AD. Ocular manifestations in the Marfan syndrome and homocystinuria. Am J Ophthalmol 1973;75:405–420.

60. Culotta VC, Gitlin JD. Disorders of copper transport. In: Scriver CR, Beaudet AL, Sly WS, Valle D, et al. (eds) The metabolic and molecular bases of inherited disease. New York: McGraw-Hill, 2001:3105–3161.

61. Curran RE, Hedges TR, Boger WP. Loss of accommodation and the near response in Wilson's disease. J Pediatr Ophthalmol Strabismus 1982;19:157–160.

62. Dangel ME, Tsou B H-P. Retinal involvement of Morquio's syndrome (MPS IV). Ann Ophthalmol 1985;17:349–354.

63. Danks DM. Disorders of copper transport. In: Scriver CR, Beaudet AL, Sly WS, Valle D, et al. (eds) The metabolic and molecular bases of inherited diseases. New York: McGraw-Hill, 1995:2211–2235.

64. Davis DB, Currier FP. Morquio's disease: Report of two cases. JAMA 1934;102:2173–2176.

65. Davis PL, Baker RS, Piccione RJ. Large recession nystagmus surgery in albinos. Effects on acuity. J Pediatr Ophthalmol Strabismus 1997;34:279–285.

66. deKremer RD, Girorgi I, Agaranna CE, et al. Mucopolysaccharidosis type VII (β-glucuronidase deficiency): a chronic variant with an oligosymptomatic severe skeletal dysplasia. Am J Med Genet 1992;44:145–152.

67. Del Monte MA, Johnson DL, Cotlier E, et al. Diagnosis of inherited enzymatic deficiencies with tears: Fabry disease. Birth Defects 1976; 12:209–219.

68. Del Monte MA, Maumenee IH, Green WR, Kenyon KR. Histopathology of Sanfilippo's syndrome. Arch Ophthalmol 1983;101:1255–1262.

69. DeMeirleir LJ, Taylor MJ, Logan WJ. Multimodal evoked potential studies in leukodystrophies of children. Can J Neurol Sci 1988;15: 26–31.

70. Desnick RJ, Ioannou YA, Eng CM. α-Galactosidase A deficiency: Fabry disease. In: Scriver CR, Beaudet Al, Sly WS, Valle D, et al. (eds) The metabolic and molecular bases of inherited disease. New York: McGraw-Hill, 1995:2741–2784.

71. Desnick RJ, Ioannou YA, Eng CM. α-Galactosidase A deficiency: Fabry disease. In: Scriver CR, Beaudet AL, Sly WS, Valle D, et al. (eds) The metabolic and molecular bases of inherited disease. New York: McGraw-Hill, 2001:3733–3774.

72. Diether S, Schaffer F. Local changes in eye growth induced by imposed local refractive error despite active accommodation. Vision Res 1997;37:659–668.

73. DiFerrante N, Hyman BH, Klish W, et al. Mucopolysaccharidosis VI (Maroteaux–Lamy disease): clinical and biochemical study of a mild variant case. Johns Hopkins Med J 1974;135:42–53.

74. Dingle J, Havener WH. Ophthalmoscopic changes in a patient with Wilson's disease during long-term penicillamine therapy. Ann Ophthalmol 1978;10:1227–1230.

75. Dolman CL, Chang E, Duke RJ. Pathologic findings in Sandhoff disease. Arch Pathol 1973;96:272–275.

76. Dom R, Brucher JM, Ceuterick C, et al. Adult ceroid-lipofuscinosis (Kufs' disease) in two brothers. Retinal and visceral storage in one; diagnostic muscle biopsy in the other. Acta Neuropathol 1979;45:67.

77. East T, Savin LH. A case of Gaucher's disease with biopsy of the typical pingueculae. Br J Ophthalmol 1940;24:611–613.

78. Ellis RWB, Sheldon W, Capone NB. Gargoylism (chondroosteodystrophy, corneal opacities, hepatosplenomegaly, and mental deficiency). Q J Med 1936;29:119–135.

79. Elman MJ, Miller MT, Matalon R. Galactokinase activity in patients with idiopathic cataracts. Ophthalmology 1986;93:210–215.

80. Emery JM, Green WR, Huff DS. Krabbe's disease. Histopathology and ultrastructure of the eye. Am J Ophthalmol 1972;74:400–405.

81. Emery JM, Green WR, Huff DS, et al. Niemann–Pick disease (type C). Histopathology and ultrastructure. Am J Ophthalmol 1972;74: 1144–1154.

82. Emery JM, Green WR, Wyllie RG, Howell RR. GM₁-gangliosidosis. Ocular and pathological manifestations. Arch Ophthalmol 1971;85: 177–187.

83. Erduran E, Mocan H, Gedik Y, et al. Hydrocephalus, corneal opacities, deafness, left ventricle hypertrophy, clinodactyly in an adoles-

cent patient. A new syndrome associated with glucocerebrosidase deficiency. Genet Counsel 1995;6:211–215.

84. Erikson A, Wahlberg I. Gaucher disease: Norrbottnian type. Ocular abnormalities. Acta Ophthalmol 1985;63:221–225.

85. Ferreira RC, Heckenlively JR, Menkes JH, Bateman B. Menkes disease. New ocular and electroretinographic findings. Ophthalmology 1998;105:1076–1078.

86. Filling-Katz MR, Fink JK, Gorin MB, et al. Ophthalmologic manifestations of type B Niemann-Pick disease. Metab Pediatr Syst Ophthalmol 1992;15:16–20.

87. Fitzgerald K, Cibis GW. The value of flash visual evoked potentials in albinism. J Pediatr Ophthalmol Strabismus 1994;31:18–25.

88. Fonda G, Thomas H, Gore GV. Educational and vocational placement, and low-vision corrections in albinism. A report based on 253 patients. Sight Sav Rev 1971;41:29–36.

89. Font RL, Fine BS. Ocular pathology in Fabry's disease. Histochemical and electron microscopic observations. Am J Ophthalmol 1972; 73:419–430.

90. Frazier PD, Wong VG. Cystinosis. Histologic and crystallographic examination of crystals in eye tissues. Arch Ophthalmol 1968;80:87–91.

91. Franceschetti AT. Fabry disease: ocular manifestations. Birth Defects 1976;12:195–208.

92. Fulcher T, O'Keefe M, Bowell R, et al. Intellectual and educational attainment in albinism. J Pediatr Ophthalmol Strabismus 1995;32: 368–372.

93. Fulton AB, Albert DM, Craft JL. Human albinism. Light and electron microscopy study. Arch Ophthalmol 1978;96:305–310.

94. Gahl WA, Kaiser-Kupfer MI. Complications of nephropathic cystinosis after renal failure. Pediatr Nephrol 1987;1:260–268.

95. Gahl WA, Thoene JG, Schneider JA. Cystinosis. A disorder of lysosomal membrane transport. In: Scriver CR, Beaudet AL, Sly WS, Valle D, et al. (eds) The metabolic and molecular bases of inherited disease. New York: McGraw-Hill, 2001:5085–5108.

96. Garner A. Ocular pathology of GM_2 gangliosidosis, type 2 (Sandhoff disease). Br J Ophthalmol 1973;57:514–520.

97. Ghosh M, McCulloch C. The Morquio syndrome: light and electron microscopic findings from two corneas. Can J Ophthalmol 1974;9: 445–452.

98. Gills JB, Hobson R, Hanley B, et al. Electroretinography and fundus oculi findings in Hurler's disease and allied mucopolysaccharidoses. Arch Ophthalmol 1965;74:596–603.

99. Goebel HH, Busch-Hettwer H, Bohl J. Ultrastructural study of the retina in late infantile metachromatic leukodystrophy. Ophthalmic Res 1992;24:103–109.

100. Goebel HH, Fix JD, Zeman W. The fine structure of the retina in neuronal ceroid-lipofuscinosis. Am J Ophthalmol 1974;77:25–39.

101. Goebel HH, Fix JD, Zeman W. Retinal pathology in GM₁ gangliosidosis type II. Am J Ophthalmol 1973;75:434–441.

102. Goebel HH, Shimokawa K, Argyrakis A, et al. The ultrastructure of the retina in adult metachromatic leukodystrophy. Am J Ophthalmol 1978;85:841–849.

103. Goldberg MF, Scott CI, McKusick VA. Hydrocephalus and papilledema in the Maroteaux–Lamy syndrome (mucopolysaccharidosis type VI). Am J Ophthalmol 1970;69:969–975.

104. Goldberg MF, von Noorden GK. Ophthalmologic findings in Wilson's hepatolenticular degeneration with emphasis on ocular motility. Arch Ophthalmol 1966;75:162–170.

105. Goldsmith LA, Kang E, Bienfang DC, et al. Tyrosinemia with plantar and palmar keratosis and keratitis. J Pediatr 1973;83:798–805.

106. Goldsmith LA, Reed J. Tyrosine-induced eye and skin lesions. A treatable genetic disease. JAMA 1976;236:382–384.

107. Goldstein I, Wexler D. Niemann–Pick's disease with cherry-red spots in the macula. Ocular pathology. Arch Ophthalmol 1931;5:704–716.

108. Goldstein NP, Hollenhorst RW, Randall RV, Gross JB. Possible relationship of optic neuritis, Wilson's disease, and DL-penicillamine therapy. JAMA 1966;196:734–735.

109. Gravel RA, Clarke JTR, Kaback MM, et al. The GM₂ gangliosidoses. In: Scriver CR, Beaudet AL, Sly WS, Valle D, et al. (eds) The metabolic and molecular bases of inherited disease. New York: McGraw-Hill, 1995:2839–2879.

110. Gravel RA, Kaback MM, Proia RL, et al. The GM₂ gangliosidoses. In: Scriver CR, Beaudet AL, Sly WS, Valle D, et al. (eds) The metabolic and molecular bases of inherited disease. New York: McGraw-Hill, 2001:3827–3876.

111. Grover WD, Naiman JL. Progressive paresis of vertical gaze in lipid storage disease. Neurology 1971;21:896–899.

112. Grover WD, Tucker SH, Wenger DA. Clinical variation in two related children with neuronopathic Gaucher's disease. Ann Neurol 1978;3:281–283.

113. Guerra WF, Verity A, Fluharty AL, et al. Multiple sulfatase deficiency: clinical neuropathological, ultrastructural and biochemical studies. J Neuropathol Exp Neurol 1990;41:406–423.

114. Guillery RW. Normal and abnormal visual field maps in albinos. Central effects on non-matching maps. Ophthalmic Paediatr Genet 1990;11:177–183.

115. Gullingsrud EO, Krivit W, Summers CG. Ocular abnormalities in the mucopolysaccharidoses after bone marrow transplantation. Longer follow-up. Ophthalmology 1998;105:1099–1105.

116. Guo S, Reinecke RD, Fendick M, Calhoun JH. Visual pathway abnormalities in albinism and infantile nystagmus. VECPs and stereoacuity measurements. J Pediatr Ophthalmol Strabismus 1989;26:97–104.

117. Harbord M, Buncic R, Chuang SA, et al. Multiple sulfatase deficiency with early severe retinal degeneration. J Child Neurol 1991;6:229–235.

118. Harcourt B, Ashton N. Ultrastructure of the optic nerve in Krabbe's leukodystrophy. Br J Ophthalmol 1973;57:885–891.

119. Harcourt RB, Dobbs RH. Ultrastructure of the retina in Tay–Sachs disease. Br J Ophthalmol 1968;52:898–902.

120. Harris CN, Shawkat F, Russell-Eggitt I, et al. Intermittent horizontal saccade failure (ocular motor apraxia) in children. Br J Ophthalmol 1996;80:151–158.

121. Heidemann DG, Dunn SP, Bawle EV, Shepherd DM. Early diagnosis of tyrosinemia type II. Am J Ophthalmol 1989;107:559–560.

122. Higgins JJ, Patterson MC, Dambrosia JN, et al. A clinical staging classification for type C Niemann–Pick disease. Neurology 1992;42: 2286–2290.

123. Ho PC, Feman SS. Internuclear ophthalmoplegia in Fabry's disease. Ann Ophthalmol 1981;13:949–951.

124. Hofmann SL, Peltonen L. The neuronal ceroid lipofuscinoses. In: Scriver CR, Beaudet AL, Sly WS, Valle D, et al. (eds) The metabolic and molecular bases of inherited disease. New York: McGraw-Hill, 2001:3877–3894.

125. Hogan MJ, Cordes FC. Lipochondrodystrophy (dysostosis multiplex: Hurler's disease): pathologic changes in the cornea in three cases. Arch Ophthalmol 1944;32:287–295.

126. Holton JB, Walter JH, Tyfield LA. Galactosemia. In: Scriver CR, Beaudet AL, Sly WS, Valle D, et al. (eds) The metabolic and molecular bases of inherited disease. New York: McGraw-Hill, 2001: 1553–1587.

127. Howes EL, Wood IS, Golbus M, et al. Ocular pathology of infantile Niemann–Pick disease. Study of a fetus of 23 weeks' gestation. Arch Ophthalmol 1975;93:494–500.

128. Huang Y, Bron AJ, Meek KM, et al. Ultrastructural study of the cornea in a bone marrow-transplanted Hurler syndrome patient. Exp Eye Res 1996;62:377–387.

129. Hunziker N. Richner–Hanhart syndrome and tyrosinemia type II. Dermatologica 1980;160:180.

130. Iwamoto M, Nawa Y, Maumenee IH, et al. Ocular histopathology and ultrastructure of Morquio syndrome (systemic mucopolysaccharidoses IV A). Graefe's Arch Ophthalmol 1990;228:342–349.

131. Jampel RS, Quaglio ND. Eye movements in Tay–Sachs disease. Neurology 1964;14:1013–1019.

132. Jensen OA. Mucopolysaccharidosis type III (Sanfilippo's syndrome): Histochemical examination of the eyes and brain with a survey of the literature. Acta Pathol Microbiol Scand 1971;78:257–273.

133. Kaiden JS, Schecter R, Bader BF, et al. Angle-closure glaucoma in a patient with Hunter's syndrome. J Ocul Ther Surg 1982;1:250–252.

134. Kaiser-Kupfer M, Caruso RC, Minkler DS, Gahl WA. Long-term ocular manifestations in nephropathic cystinosis. Arch Ophthalmol 1986;104:706–711.

135. Kaiser-Kupfer MI, Fujikawa L, Kuwabara T, et al. Removal of corneal crystals by topical cysteamine in nephropathic cystinosis. N Engl J Med 1987;316:775–779.

136. Kaiser-Kupfer MI, Gazzo MA, Datiles MB, et al. A randomized placebo-controlled trial of cysteamine eye drops in nephropathic cystinosis. Arch Ophthalmol 1990;108:689–693.

137. Kajii T, Matsuda K, Ohsawa T, et al. Hurler/Scheie genetic compound (mucopolysaccharidosis IH/IS) in Japanese brothers. Clin Genet 1974;6:394–400.

138. Kasman B, Kuprecht KW. Might the refractive state in oculocutaneous albinism patients be a clue for distinguishing between tyrosinase-positive and tyrosinase-negative forms of oculocutaneous albinism? Ger J Ophthalmol 1997;5:422–427.

139. Katz B, Melles B, Schneider JA. Corneal sensitivity in nephropathic cystinosis. Am J Ophthalmol 1987;104:413–416.

140. Katz B, Melles RB, Schneider JA. Glare disability in nephropathic cystinosis. Arch Ophthalmol 1987;105:1670–1671.

141. Keane JR. Lid-opening apraxia in Wilson's disease. J Clin Neuro-Ophthalmol 1988;8:31–33.

142. Kenyon KP, Sensenbrenner JA. Electron microscopy of cornea and conjunctiva in childhood cystinosis. Am J Ophthalmol 1974;78:68–76.

143. Kenyon KP, Quigley HA, Hussels IE, et al. The systemic mucopolysaccharidoses: ultrastructural and histochemical studies of conjunctiva and skin. Am J Ophthalmol 1972;73:811–833.

144. Kenyon KP, Topping TM, Green WR, et al. Ocular pathology of the Maroteaux–Lamy syndrome (systemic mucopolysaccharidosis type VI): histologic and ultrastructural report of two cases. Am J Ophthalmol 1972;73:718–741.

145. King RA, Hearing VJ, Creel DJ, Oetting WS. Albinism. In: Scriver CR, Beaudet AL, Sly WS, Valle D, et al. (eds) The metabolic and molecular bases of inherited disease. New York: McGraw-Hill, 2001: 5587–5627.

146. King RA, Lewis RA, Townsend DeW, et al. Brown oculocutaneous albinism. Clinical, ophthalmological, and biochemical characterization. Ophthalmology 1985;92:1496–1505.

147. King RA, Olds DP. Hairbulb tyrosinase activity in oculocutaneous albinism. Suggestions for pathway control and block location. Am J Med Genet 1985;20:49–55.

148. Kinnear PE, Jay B, Witkop CJ. Albinism. Survey Ophthalmol 1985; 30:75–101.

149. Kirkham TH, Kanin DF. Slow saccadic eye movements in Wilson's disease. J Neurol Neurosurg Psychiatry 1974;37:191–194.

150. Kivlin JD, Sanborn GE, Myers GG. The cherry-red spot in Tay–Sachs and other storage diseases. Ann Neurol 1985;17:356–360.

151. Kolodny EH, Fluharty AL. Metachromatic leukodystrophy and multiple sulfatase deficiency: sulfatide lipidosis. In: Scriver CR, Beaudet

AL, Sly WS, Valle D, et al. (eds) The metabolic and molecular bases of inherited disease. New York: McGraw-Hill, 1995;2693–2739.

152. Koshenoja M, Suvanto E. Gargoylism: report of adult form with glaucoma in two sisters. Acta Ophthalmol 1959;37:234–240.

153. Kriss A, Russel-Eggitt I, Harris CM, et al. Aspects of albinism. Ophthalmic Paediatr Genet 1992;13:89–100.

154. Krivit W. Maroteaux–Lamy syndrome (mucopolysaccharidosis type VI). Treatment by allogenic bone marrow transplantation in 6 patients and potential for autotransplantation bone marrow gene insertion. Int Pediatr 1992;7:42–52.

155. Kromberg JGR, Castle DJ, Zwane EM, et al. Red or rufous albinism in Southern Africa. Ophthalmic Paediatr Genet 1990;11:229–235.

156. Larkin DFP, O'Donoghue HN. Developmental glaucoma in oculocutaneous albinism. Ophthalmic Paediatr Genet 1988;9:1–4.

157. Larson HW, Ehlers N. Ocular manifestations in Tay–Sachs' and Niemann–Pick disease. Acta Ophthalmol 1965;43:286–293.

158. Lavery MA, Green WR, Jabs EW, et al. Ocular histopathology and ultrastructure of Sanfilippo's syndrome, type III-B. Arch Ophthalmol 1983;101:1263–1274.

159. Lee KA, King RA, Summers CG. Stereopsis in patients with albinism. Clinical correlates. J Am Assoc Pediatr Ophthalmol Strabismus 2001;5:98–104.

160. Levy HL, Brown AE, Williams SE, deJuan E. Vitreous hemorrhage as an ophthalmic complication of galactosemia. J Pediatr 1996;129:922–925.

161. Levy NS, Dawson WW, Rhodes BJ, et al. Ocular abnormalities in Menkes' kinky-hair syndrome. Am J Ophthalmol 1974;77:319–325.

162. Levy NS, Krill AE, Beutler E. Galactokinase deficiency and cataracts. Am J Ophthalmol 1972;74:41–48.

163. Libert J, Danis P. Diagnosis of type A, B and C Niemann-Pick disease by conjunctival biopsy. J Submicrosc Cytol 1979;11:143–157.

164. Libert J, Tondeur M, Van Hoof F. The use of conjunctival biopsy and enzyme analysis in tears for the diagnosis of homozygotes and heterozygotes with Fabry disease. Birth Defects 1976;12:221–239.

165. Libert J, Toussaint D, Guiselings R. Ocular findings in Niemann–Pick disease. Am J Ophthalmol 1975;80:1991–1002.

166. Libert J, Van Hoof F, Toussaint D, et al. Ocular findings in metachromatic leukodystrophy. An electron microscopic and enzyme study in different clinical and genetic variants. Arch Ophthalmol 1979;97:1495–1504.

167. Macrae WG, Ghosh M, McCulloch C. Corneal changes in Fabry's disease: a clinico-pathologic case report of a heterozygote. Ophthalmic Pediatr Genet 1985;5:213–218.

168. Martyn LJ. Unpublished personal observations.

169. Matthews JD, Weiter JJ, Kolodny EH. Macular halos associated with Niemann–Pick type B disease. Ophthalmology 1986;93:933–937.

170. McDonnell JM, Green WR, Maumenee IH. Ocular histopathology of systemic mucopolysaccharidosis, type II-A (Hunter syndrome, severe). Ophthalmology 1985;92:1772–1779.

171. McKeran RO, Bradbury P, Taylor D, Stern G. Neurological involvement in type 1 (adult) Gaucher's disease. J Neurol Neurosurg Psychiatry 1985;48:172–175.

172. Melles RB, Schneider JA, Rao NA, Katz B. Spatial and temporal sequence of corneal crystal deposition in nephropathic cystinosis. Am J Ophthalmol 1987;104:598–604.

173. Menkes JH, O'Brien JS, Okada S, et al. Juvenile GM$_2$ gangliosidosis. Biochemical and ultrastructural studies on a new variant of Tay–Sachs disease. Arch Neurol 1971;25:14:22.

174. Merin S, Livni N, Yatziv S. Conjunctival ultrastructure in Niemann–Pick disease type C. Am J Ophthalmol 1980;90:708–714.

175. Miller JD, McCluer R, Kanfer JN. Gaucher's disease. Neurologic disorder in adult siblings. Ann Intern Med 1973;78:883–887.

176. Mitchell GA, Grompe M, Lambert M, Tanguay RM. Hypertyrosinemia. In: Scriver CR, Beaudet AL, Sly WS, Valle D, et al. (eds) The metabolic and molecular bases of inherited diseases. New York: McGraw-Hill, 2001:1777–1805.

177. Moser HW. Ceramide deficiency: Farber lipogranulomatosis. In: Scriver CR, Beaudet AL, Sly WS, Valle D, et al. (eds) The metabolic and molecular bases of inherited disease. New York: McGraw-Hill, 1995:2589–2599.

178. Moser HW, Linke T, Fensom AH, et al. Acid ceramidase deficiency. Farber lipogranulomatosis. In: Scriver CR, Beaudet AL, Sly WS, Valle D, et al. (eds) The metabolic and molecular bases of inherited disease. New York: McGraw-Hill, 2001:3573–3588.

179. Mudd HS, Levy HL, Krause JP. Disorders of transsulfuration. In: Scriver CR, Beaudet AL, Sly WS, Valle D, et al. (eds) The metabolic and molecular bases of inherited disease. New York: McGraw-Hill, 2001:2007–2056.

180. Mullaney P, Abdulaziz HA, Millar L. Glaucoma in mucopolysaccharidosis I-H/S. J Pediatr Ophthalmol Strabismus 1996;33:127–132.

181. Mungen N, Nischal KK, Heon E, et al. Ultrasound biomicroscopy of the eye in cystinosis. Arch Ophthalmol 2000;118:1329–1333.

182. Musarella MA, Raab EL, Rudolph SH, et al. Oculomotor abnormalities in chronic GM$_2$ gangliosidosis. J Pediatr Ophthalmol Strabismus 1982;19:80–89.

183. Naidu S, Hofmann KJ, Moser HW, et al. Galactosylceramide β-galactosidase deficiency in association with cherry-red spot. Neuropediatrics 1988;19:46–48.

184. Narita AS, Russell-Eggitt II. Bilateral epiretinal membranes; a new finding in Hunter syndrome. Ophthalmic Genet 1996;17:75–78.

185. Neufeld EF, Muenzer J. The mucopolysaccharidoses. In: Scriver CR, Beaudet AL, Sly WS, Valle D, et al. (eds) The metabolic and molecular bases of inherited disease. New York: McGraw-Hill, 1995:2465–2494.

186. Neufeld EF, Muenzer J. The mucopolysaccharidoses. In: Scriver CR, Beaudet AL, Sly WS, Valle D, et al. (eds) The metabolic and molecular bases of inherited disease. New York: McGraw-Hill 2001: 3421–3452.

187. Neville BGR, Lake BD, Stephens R, et al. A neurovisceral storage disease with vertical supranuclear ophthalmoloplegia, and its relationship to Niemann–Pick disease: a report of nine patients. Brain 1973;96:97–120.

188. Newell FW, Koistinen A. Lipochondrodystrophy (gargoylism): pathologic findings in five eyes of three patients. Arch Ophthalmol 1955; 53:45–62.

189. Norby S, Jensen OA, Schwartz M. Retinal and cerebellar changes in early fetal Sandhoff disease (GM$_2$-gangliosidosis type 2). Metab Pediatr Ophthalmol 1980;4:115–1119.

190. Norman RM, Forrester RM, Tingey AH. The juvenile form of Niemann–Pick disease. Arch Dis Child 1967;42:91–96.

191. Nowaczyk MJ, Clarke JTR, Morin JD. Glaucoma as an early complication of Hurler's disease. Arch Dis Child 1988;63:1091–1093.

192. Oberman AE, Wilson WA, Frasier SD, et al. Galactokinase-deficiency cataracts in identical twins. Am J Ophthalmol 1972;74:887–892.

193. O'Brien J. Generalized gangliosidosis. J Pediatr 1969;75:167–186.

194. O'Brien JS, Okada S, Ho MW, et al. Ganglioside storage diseases. Fed Proc 1971;30:956–969.

195. O'Donnell FE, Hambrick GW, Green WR, et al. X-linked ocular albinism. An oculocutaneous macromelanosomal disorder. Arch Ophthalmol 1976;94:1883–1892.

196. Olsen H, Bargemen K, Sjolie AK. Cataracts in Morquio syndrome (mucopolysaccharidosis IV A). Ophthalmol Pediatr Genet 1993;14: 87–89.

197. Palmer M, Green WR, Maumenee IH, et al. Niemann–Pick disease: type C. Ocular histopathologic and electron microscopic studies. Arch Ophthalmol 1985;103:817–822.

198. Paterson DE, Rad M, Harper G, et al. Maroteaux–Lamy syndrome, mild form, MPS VI b. B J Ophthalmol 1982;55:805–812.

199. Patterson MC, Vanier MT, Suzuki K, et al. Niemann–Pick disease type C: a lipid trafficking disorder. In: Scriver CR, Beaudet AL, Sly WS, Valle D, et al. (eds) The metabolic and molecular bases of inherited disease. New York: McGraw-Hill, 2001:3611–3633.

200. Pentchev PG, Vanier MT, Suzuki K, Patterson MC. Niemann-Pick disease type C; a cellular cholesterol lipidosis. In: Scriver CR, Beaudet AL, Sly WS, Valle D, et al. (eds) The metabolic and molecular bases of inherited disease. New York: McGraw-Hill, 1995:2625–2639.

201. Petrohelos M, Tricoulis D, Kotsiras I, Vouzoukos A. Ocular manifestations of Gaucher's disease. Am J Ophthalmol 1975;80:1006–1010.

202. Pillat A. Change of the eyegrounds in Wilson's disease (pseudosclerosis). Am J Ophthalmol 1933;16:1–6.

203. Quigley HA, Green WR. Clinical and ultrastructural ocular histopathologic studies of adult-onset metachromatic leukodystrophy. Am J Ophthalmol 1976;83:472–479.

204. Quigley HA, Kenyon KR. Ultrastructural and histochemical studies of a newly recognized form of systemic mucopolysaccharidosis (Maroteaux–Lamy syndrome, mild phenotype). Am J Ophthalmol 1974;77:809–818.

205. Quigley HA, Maumenee AE, Stark WJ. Acute glaucoma in systemic mucopolysaccharidosis I-S. Ann J Ophthalmol 1975;80:70–72.

206. Rabinowitz LG, Williams LR, Anderson CE, et al. Painful keratoderma and photophobia: hallmarks of tyrosinemia type III. J Pediatr 1995;126.

207. Raitta C, Santavuori P. Ophthalmological findings in infantile type of so-called neuronal ceroid lipofuscinosis. Acta Ophthalmol 1973;51:755–763.

208. Ramsey MS, Dickson DH. Lens fringe in homocystinuria. Br J Ophthalmol 1975;59:338–342.

209. Ramsey MS, Yanoff M, Fine BS. The ocular histopathology of homocystinuria. A light and electron microscopic study. Am J Ophthalmol 1972;74:377–385.

210. Rapin I, Suzuki K, Suzuki K, et al. Adult (chronic) GM$_2$ gangliosidosis. Atypical spinocerebellar degeneration in a Jewish sibship. Arch Neurol 1976;33:120–130.

211. Rapola J. Neuronal ceroid-lipofuscinosis in childhood. In: Landing BH, Haust MD, Bernstein J, Rosenberg HS (eds) Genetic metabolic disease. Basel: Karger, 1993:7–44.

212. Raynaud EJ, Escourolle R, Beaumann N, et al. Metachromatic leukodystrophy. Ultrastructural and enzymatic study of a case of variant O form. Arch Neurol 1975;32:834–838.

213. Read J, Goldberg MF, Fishmann G, Rosenthal I. Nephropathic cystinosis. Am J Ophthalmol 1973;76:791–796.

214. Richler M, Milot J, Quigley M, O'Reagan S. Ocular manifestations of nephropathic cystinosis. The French-Canadian experience in a genetically homogeneous population. Arch Ophthalmol 1991;109:359–362.

215. Robb RM, Kuwabara T. The ocular pathology of type A Niemann–Pick disease. A light and electron microscopic study. Investig Ophthalmol 1973;12:366–377.

216. Rodriguez MJG, Conde HP, Nieto CL, et al. La participation rétinienne dans la maladie de Gaucher. J Fr Ophthalmol 1992;15:185–190.

217. Rossa V. Netzhautveranderungen bei M. Wilson. Fortschr Ophthalmol 1991;88:230–232.

218. Sakano T, Okuda N, Yoshimitsu K, et al. A case of Menkes syndrome with cataracts. Eur J Pediatr 1982;138:357–358.

219. Salgado-Borges J, Silva-Araujo A, Lemos MM, et al. Morphological and biochemical assessment of the cornea in a Gaucher disease carrier with keratoconus. Eur J Ophthalmol 1995;5:69–74.

220. Sammartino A, de Crecchio G, Balato G, et al. Familial Richner–Hanhart syndrome: genetic, clinical and metabolic studies. Ann Ophthalmol 1984;16:1069–1074.

221. Sandberg HO. Bilateral keratopathy and tyrosinosis. Acta Ophthalmol 1975;53:760–764.

222. Sanderson PO, Kuwabara T, Stark W, et al. Cystinosis. A clinical, histopathologic, and ultrastructural study. Arch Ophthalmol 1974; 91:270–274.

223. Sanfilippo SJ, Podosin R, Langer L, et al. Mental retardation associated with acid mucopolysacchariduria (heparitin sulfate type). J Pediatr 1963;63:837–838.

224. Sayar RB, von Domarus D, Schäfer HJ, Beckenkamp G. Clinical picture and problems of keratoplasty in Richner–Hanhart syndrome (tyrosinemia type II). Ophthalmologica 1988;197:1–6.

225. Scheie HG, Hambrick GW, Barness LA. A newly recognized form fruste of Hurler's disease (gargoylism). Am J Ophthalmol 1962;53: 753–769.

226. Schochet SS, Font RL, Morris HH. Jansky–Bielschowsky form of neuronal ceroid-lipofuscinosis. Ocular pathology of the Batten–Vogt syndrome. Arch Ophthalmol 1980;98:1083–1088.

227. Schoenberger M, Ellis PP. Disappearance of Kayser–Fleischer ring after liver transplantation. Arch Ophthalmol 1979;97:1914–1915.

228. Schuchman EH, Desnick RJ. Niemann-Pick disease types A and B: acid sphingomyelinase deficiencies. In: Scriver CR, Beaudet AL, Sly WS, Valle D, et al. (eds) The metabolic and molecular bases of inherited disease. New York: McGraw-Hill, 1995:2601–2624.

229. Schuchman EH, Desnick RJ. Niemann-Pick disease types A and B: acid sphingomyelinase deficiencies. In: Scriver CR, Beaudet AL, Sly WS, Valle D, et al. (eds) The metabolic and molecular bases of inherited disease. New York: McGraw-Hill, 2001:3589–3610.

230. Scott IU, Greene WR, Goyal AK, et al. New sites of ocular involvement in late-infantile metachromatic leukodystrophy revealed by histopathologic studies. Graefe's Arch Clin Exp Ophthalmol 1993; 231:187–191.

231. Seelenfreund NH, Gartner S, Vinger PF. The ocular pathology of Menkes' disease (kinky hair disease). Arch Ophthalmol 1968;80: 718–720.

232. Segal P, Ruszkowski M, Berger S, Masiak M. Abortive form of Wilson's syndrome with dark adaptation disturbance. Am J Ophthalmol 1957;44:623–629.

233. Sewell AC, Gehler J, Mittermaier G, Meyer E. Mucopolysaccharidosis type VII (β-glucuronidase deficiency): a report of a new case and a survey of those in the literature. Clin Genet 1982;21:366–373.

234. Sher NA, Letson RD, Desnick RJ. The ocular manifestations in Fabry's disease. Arch Ophthalmol 1979;97:671–676.

235. Sher NA, Reiff W, Letson RD, et al. Central retinal artery occlusion complicating Fabry's disease. Arch Ophthalmol 1978;96:815–817.

236. Sheridan M, Johnson I. Hydrocephalus in pseudotumor cerebri in the mucopolysaccharidoses. Child Nerv Syst 1994;10:148–150.

237. Sidransky E, Tsuji S, Stubblefield BK, et al. Gaucher patients with oculomotor abnormalities do not have a unique genotype. Clin Genet 1992;41:1–5.

238. Silver J, Sapiro J. Axonal guidance during development of the optic nerve: the role of pigmented epithelia and other extrinsic factors. J Comp Neurol 1981;202:521–538.

239. Singer JD, Cotlier E, Krimmer R. Hexosaminidase A in tears and saliva from rapid identification of Tay–Sachs disease and its carriers. Lancet 1973;2:1116–1119.

240. Singh S, Bresman MJ. Menkes' kinky-hair syndrome (trichopolyo-dystrophy). Low copper levels in the blood, hair and urine. Am J Dis Child 1973;125:572–578.

241. Skalka H, Prchal JT. Presenile cataract formation and decreased activity of galactosemic enzymes. Arch Ophthalmol 1980;98:269–273.

242. Sly WS, Quinton BA, McAlister WH, et al. Beta-glucuronidase deficiency: report of clinical, radiologic and biochemical features of a new mucopolysaccharidosis. J Pediatr 1973;82:249–257.

243. Spaeth GL, Barber GW. Homocystinuria: its ocular manifestations. J Pediatr Ophthalmol 1966;3:42–48.

244. Spaeth GL, Frost P. Fabry's disease. Its ocular manifestations. Arch Ophthalmol 1965;74:760–769.

245. Spalton DJ, Taylor DSI, Sanders MD. Juvenile Batten's disease: an ophthalmological assessment of 26 patients. Br J Ophthalmol 1980;64:726–732.

246. Spedick MJ, Beauchamp GR. Retinal vascular and optic nerve abnormalities in albinism. J Pediatr Ophthalmol Strabismus 1986;23:58–63.

247. Spellacy E, Bankes JLK, Crow J, et al. Glaucoma in a case of Hurler disease. Br J Ophthalmol 1980;64:773–778.

248. Sperl W, Bart G, Vanier MT, et al. A family with visceral course of Niemann–Pick disease, macular halo syndrome and low sphingomyelin degradation rate. J Inherit Metab Dis 1994;17:93–103.

249. Spranger J, Cantz M, Gehler J, et al. Mucopolysaccharidosis II (Hunter disease) with corneal opacities. Report on two patients at the extremes of a wide clinical spectrum. Eur J Pediatr 1978;129:11–16.

250. Stevenson RE, Howell RR, McKusick VA, et al. The iduronidase-deficient mucopolysaccharidosis: clinical and roentgenographic studies. Pediatrics 1976;57:111–122.

251. Streeten BW. The nature of the ocular zonule. Trans Am Ophthalmol Soc 1982;LXXX:824–854.

252. Summers CG, Knobloch WH, Witkop CJ, King RA. Hermansky–Pudlak syndrome. Ophthalmic findings. Ophthalmology 1988;95:545–554.

253. Summers CG, Purple RL, Krivit W, et al. Ocular changes in the mucopolysaccharidoses after bone marrow transplantation. A preliminary report. Ophthalmology 1989;96:977–985.

254. Sussman W, Scheinberg IH. Disappearance of Kayser–Fleischer rings. Effects of penicillamine. Arch Ophthalmol 1969;82:738–741.

255. Suzuki K, Grover WD. Krabbe's leukodystrophy (globoid cell leukodystrophy). An ultrastructural study. Arch Neurol 1970;22: 385–396.

256. Suzuki Y, Oshima A, Nanba E. β-Galactosidase deficiency (β-galactosidosis): GM$_1$ gangliosidosis and Morquio B disease. In: Scriver CR, Beaudet AL, Sly WS, Valle D, et al. (eds) The metabolic and molecular bases of inherited disease. New York: McGraw-Hill 2001:3775–3809.

257. Suzuki Y, Sakaraba H, Oshima A. β-Galactosidase deficiency (β-galactosidosis): GM$_1$ gangliosidosis and Morquio B disease. In: Scriver CR, Beaudet AL, Sly WS, Valle D, et al. (eds) The metabolic and molecular bases of inherited disease. New York: McGraw-Hill, 1995:2785–2823.

258. Suzuki K, Suzuki Y, Suzuki K. Galactosylceramide lipidosis: globoid-cell leukodystrophy (Krabbe disease). In: Scriver SR, Beaudet AL, Sly WS, Valle D, et al. (eds) The metabolic and molecular bases of inherited disease. New York: McGraw-Hill, 1995:2671–2692.

259. Szymanski KA, Boughman JA, Nance WE, et al. Genetic studies of ocular albinism in a large Virginia kindred. Ann Ophthalmol 1984; 16:183–196.

260. Takamoto K, Beppu H, Hirose K, Uono M. Juvenile β-galactosidase deficiency—a case with mental deterioration, dystonic movements, pyramidal symptoms, dysostosis and cherry red spot. Clin Neurol (Tokyo) 1980;20:339–344.

261. Tay W. Symmetrical changes in the region of the yellow spot in each eye of an infant. Trans Ophthalmol Soc UK 1881;1:55–57.

262. Topping TM, Kenyon KP, Goldberg MF, et al. Ultrastructural ocular pathology of Hunter's syndrome: systemic mucopolysaccharidosis type II. Arch Ophthalmol 1971;88:164–177.

263. Tremblay M, Szots F. GM$_2$ type 2 gangliosidosis (Sandhoff's disease). Ocular and pathological manifestations. Can J Ophthalmol 1974; 9:338–346.

264. Tripp JH, Lake BD, Young E, et al. Juvenile Gaucher's disease with horizontal gaze palsy in three siblings. J Neurol Neurosurg Psychiatry 1977;40:470–478.

265. Trojak JE, Ho C-K, Roesel RA, et al. Morquio-like syndrome (MPS IV B) associated with deficiency of α-galactosidase. Johns Hopkins Med J 1980;146:75–79.

266. Tso MOM, Fine BS, Thorpe HE. Kayser–Fleischer ring and associated cataract in Wilson's disease. Am J Ophthalmol 1975;79:479–488.

267. Uyama E, Takahashi K, Owada M, et al. Hydrocephalus, corneal opacities, deafness, valvular heart disease, deformed toes and leptomeningeal fibrous thickening in adult siblings: a new syndrome

associated with β-glucocerebrosidase deficiency and a mosaic population of storage cells. Acta Neurol Scand 1992;86:407–420.

268. Vamos E, Liebaers I, Bousark N, et al. Multiple sulfatase deficiency with early onset. J Inherit Metab Dis 1981;4:103–104.

269. van Heyningen R. Sugar alcohols in the pathogenesis of galactose and diabetic cataracts. Birth Defects 1976;XII:295–303.

270. Vannas A, Hogan MJ, Golbus M, Wood I. Lens changes in a galactosemic fetus. Am J Ophthalmol 1975;80:726–733.

271. Vogler C, Levy B, Kyle JW, et al. Mucopolysaccharidoses VII: postmortem biochemical and pathologic findings in a young adult with β-glucuronidase deficiency. Mod Pathol 1994;7:132–137.

272. von Figura K, Gieselmann V, Jaeken J. Metachromatic leukodystrophy. In: Scriver CR, Beaudet AL, Sly WS, Valle D, et al. (eds) The metabolic and molecular bases of inherited disease. New York: McGraw-Hill, 2001:3695–3724.

273. von Noorden GK, Zellweger H, Ponseti IV. Ocular findings in Morquio-Ulrich's disease: with report of two cases. Arch Ophthalmol 1960;64:585–591.

274. Wack MA, Peachy NS, Fishman GA. Electroretinographic findings in human oculocutaneous albinism. Ophthalmology 1989;96:1778–1785.

275. Walshe JM. The eye in Wilson's disease. In: Bergsma D, Bron AJ, Cotlier E (eds) The eye and inborn errors of metabolism. New York: Liss, 1976:187–194.

276. Walton DS, Robb RM, Crocker AC. Ocular manifestations of group A Niemann–Pick disease. Am J Ophthalmol 1978;85:178–180.

277. Wan WL, Minkler DS, Rao NA. Pupillary-block glaucoma associated with childhood cystinosis. Am J Ophthalmol 1986;101:700–705.

278. Watanabe I, Watanabe Y, Motomura E, et al. Menkes' kinky hair disease: clinical and experimental study. Doc Ophthalmol 1985;60:173–181.

279. Wegner DA, Suzuki K, Suzuki Y, Suzuki K. Galactosylceramide lipidosis: globoid cell leukodystrophy (Krabbe disease). In: Scriver CR, Beaudet AL, Sly WS, Valle D, et al. (eds) The metabolic and molecular bases of inherited disease. New York: McGraw-Hill, 2001: 3669–3694.

280. Weingeist TA, Blodi FC. Fabry's disease: ocular findings in a female carrier. Arch Ophthalmol 1971;85:169–176.

281. Weiss MJ, Krill AE, Dawson G, et al. GM₁ gangliosidosis type I. Am J Ophthalmol 1973;76:999–1004.

282. Wiebers DO, Hollenhorst RW, Goldstein NP. The ophthalmologic manifestations of Wilson's disease. Mayo Clin Proc 1977;52:409–416.

283. Wilson HR, Metz MB, Nagv SE, Kressel AB. Albino spatial vision as an instance of arrested visual development. Vision Res 1988;28:979–990.

284. Witkop CJ, Almadovar C, Piñeiro B, Babcock MN. Hermansky–Pudlak syndrome (HPS). An epidemiologic study. Ophthalmic Paediatr Genet 1990;11:245–250.

285. Wong VG. The eye in cystinosis. In: Schulman JD (ed) Cystinosis Publ NIH 72-249. Washington, DC: U.S. Department of Health, Education and Welfare, 1973:23–35.

286. Wong VG. Ocular manifestations in cystinosis. Birth Defects 1976; XII:181–186.

287. Wong VG, Kuwabara T, Brubaker R, et al. Intralysosomal cystine crystals in cystinosis. Investig Ophthalmol Vis Sci 1970;9:83–88.

288. Wong VG, Lietman PS, Seegmiller JE. Alteration of pigment epithelium in cystinosis. Arch Ophthalmol 1967;77:361–369.

289. Wray SH, Kuwabara T, Sanderson P. Menkes' kinky hair disease: a light and electron microscopic study of the eye. Investig Ophthalmol 1976;15:128–138.

290. Zarbin MA, Green WR, Moser HW, et al. Farber's disease. Light and electron microscopic study of the eye. Arch Ophthalmol 1985; 103:73–80.

8

Selected Genetic Syndromes with Ophthalmic Features

Natalie C. Kerr and Enikö Karman Pivnick

AICARDI'S SYNDROME

Aicardi's syndrome (AS) is a rare disorder characterized by the clinical triad of agenesis of the corpus callosum, infantile spasms, and chorioretinal lacunae. Since its description in 1965,[1] more than 200 cases have been reported.[26,123,191] With the exception of one XXY male,[79] all reported cases have been in female children.

Etiology

The etiology of AS is unknown. An infectious basis has not been found.[204] The more likely pathophysiological mechanism in AS is an arrest of fetal development between the 9th and 20th weeks of gestation.[9,44,81] Support for this theory comes from reports of persistent fetal vasculature in the eye[57] and unilateral aplasia of the cerebellum, which may result from a developmental defect in the posterior arterial system of Willis' polygon.[169] The frequent occurrence of hamartomas and other tumors in AS implicates faulty cell migration as an underlying event in AS.[103,157]

Clinical Features

The typical presentation of AS is flexion spasms at around 9 weeks of age.[47] Infantile spasms are a unique form of epilepsy characterized by myoclonic seizures and a hypsarrhythmic EEG pattern. The early signature of AS on EEG is bilateral independent bursts (BIBs). Hypotonia and psychomotor retardation are present.

Ophthalmic examination reveals pathognomonic chorioretinal lacunae (Fig. 8-1). These are typically bilateral, although they may be asymmetrical and/or unilateral.[23,26,81] They are typically clustered around the optic nerve,[202] and range in size from 0.1 to 3 disc diameters,[45,81] although lacunae larger than 5 disc diameters have been reported.[123] These lesions represent absent choroidal pigment and retinal pigment epithelium with intact overlying retina (although the retinal architecture may be abnormal).[153] These lesions are stable from birth, and visual prognosis is excellent unless the lesions involve the macula, in which case poor vision is likely. Large lacunae have been associated with low levels of cognitive and motor development.[123] The differential diagnosis for the chorioretinal lacunae includes toxoplasmosis lesions and chorioretinal colobomas.

Fifty percent of children with AS have optic nerve colobomas.[26,45] Mild to moderate optic nerve hypoplasia, microphthalmia, pupillary membrane, posterior synechiae, posterior polar cataract, and epipapillary and epiretinal gliosis have also been reported.[57] Previous reports of retro-orbital cysts in these eyes[172] actually represent optic nerve colobomas on MRI.

Electroretinography (ERG) and visual evoked potentials (VEP) are usually normal. The role of ERG and VEP in this entity is of limited predictive value for establishing visual function or diagnosis.[123]

Clinical Assessment and Systemic Associations

Clinical assessment of a patient suspected to have Aicardi's syndrome includes a dilated fundus examination for the typical chorioretinal lacunae, electroencephalography for hypsarrythmia, and neuroradiologic studies for characteristic malformations and tumors.

Neuroimaging typically reveals agenesis of the corpus callosum (total or partial), as well as cortical migration defects (heterotopic gray matter). Microgyria, cortical and subependymal heterotopias of gray matter, hemispheric asymmetry, ventriculomegaly, unilateral lissencephaly, absence of the pineal gland, cerebellar malformations, and Dandy–Walker cyst have all been identified in connection with AS.[151,169,172,179] Arachnoid cysts are a common finding in the posterior fossa as well as the supratentorial compartment. Papilloma of the choroid plexus is a

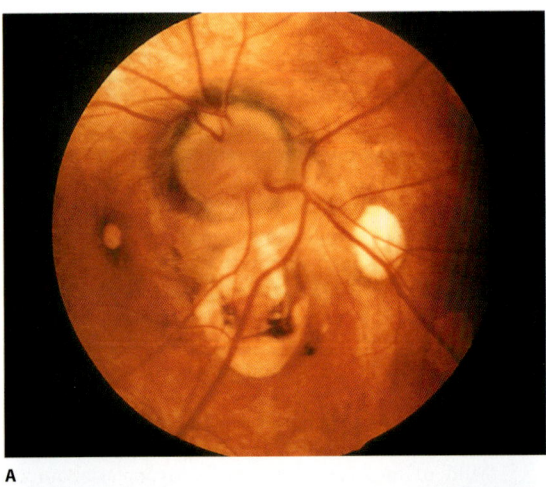

A

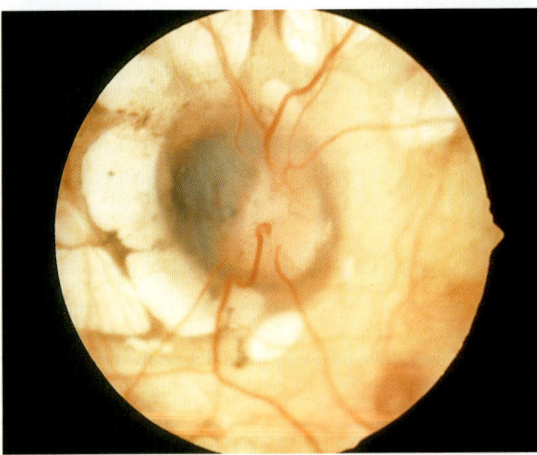

B

FIGURE 8-1A,B. (A) Typical chorioretinal lacunae and optic nerve anomaly in Aicardi syndrome. **(B)** Extensive chorioretinal lacunae in Aicardi's syndrome.

common brain tumor in AS.[157] Various other tumors have been reported, including embryonal carcinoma, hepatoblastoma, teratoma of the soft palate, angiosarcoma, lipoma, and palatal hemangioma.[47,103,120,172,182] Robinow et al. grouped AS with the genetic hamartoses,[157] and other diseases with central nervous system hamartomas might be considered in the differential diagnosis (tuberous sclerosis, neurofibromatosis, and von Hippel–Lindau disease).

Numerous other congenital abnormalities have been described in AS, including cleft lip and palate, costovertebral and vertebral abnormalities, and facial and skull asymmetry.

Inheritance

It is assumed that Aicardi's syndrome is an X-linked disease with fetal demise in affected males. All reported cases have been sporadic except one.[15] AS has been reported in several ethnic groups. Chromosomes in all patients have been normal with the exception of a case with an unbalanced X-autosomal translocation involving a breakpoint near Xp22. Two additional cases have had microdeletion at the Xp22 position of the X chromosome. This finding, however, has not been confirmed in other AS patients to date.[47,132]

Monozygotic twins discordant for Aicardi's syndrome have been reported, prompting supposition that the affected twin was probably the consequence of a postzygotic mutation in early embryonic development.[37] X inactivation has been studied, and unlike other X-linked dominant mutations, appears to be random in Aicardi's syndrome.[75]

Treatment

Symptomatic treatment of seizure disorders is indicated. ACTH appears to have the most beneficial effect in seizure control. In some cases, removal of the choroid plexus papillomas may also lead to significant improvement.[157] Monitoring for ophthalmic sequelae of the disease, including retinal detachments from colobomas, refractive errors, and ophthalmic signs of CNS tumors, is indicated. Barring any associated structural abnormality interfering with vision, such as a macular chorioretinal lacuna, retinal detachment, anisometropia, or optic nerve coloboma, vision is usually normal. Although optic nerve atrophy has not been reported with this entity,[123] hydrocephalus secondary to choroid plexus papillomas has been reported[180] and could predispose children with AS to progressive optic nerve atrophy.

Prognosis

The prognosis for children with AS is extremely poor, with severe developmental delay and little to no development of language, poor to no ambulatory ability, and a shortened lifespan. Intractable seizures are common. Death may occur within the first 5 years, usually from secondary respiratory infections, but patients may survive into their early teens.[159]

ALPORT'S SYNDROME

Alport's syndrome (AS), the most common type of hereditary nephritis syndrome, was first described during the early 1900s.[3] It affects 1 in 5000 individuals.[52] In AS, the hereditary nephritis is accompanied by high-tone sensorineural deafness and distinctive ocular signs.

Etiology

Alport's syndrome is caused by a genetic defect in the type IV collagen (COL4A3, COL4A4, COL4A5), which makes up the basement membranes in many body systems.[6] Marked variability is seen in the clinical presentation, natural history, histopathological abnormalities, and genetic patterns among patients with AS.

Clinical Features and Systemic Associations

Patients most commonly present in early childhood with asymptomatic, miscroscopic hematuria and recurrent episodes of gross hematuria that progress to renal failure in adulthood. In connection with one of the infectious diseases of childhood or a common cold in early childhood or adolescence, the affected individual will suddenly develop massive hematuria and/or proteinuria, often accompanied by cylindruria and leukocyturia. These urinary signs may vary in degree during the following months, and in some patients they may almost disappear. However, they may become more pronounced again during the next episode of infectious disease or physical strain. Hypertension may occur in affected individuals and worsen as renal function deteriorates.[84] In the X-linked form of AS (XL-AS), affected females have less obvious urinary findings and rarely develop uremia, whereas in the autosomal forms (AD-AS, AR-AS) males and females are equally affected.

Kidney biopsies obtained during the first decade of life may show changes by light microscopy. Later, the glomeruli develop mesangial proliferation and capillary wall thickening, leading to progressive glomerular sclerosis. Tubular atrophy, interstitial inflammation and fibrosis, and "foam" cells develop if the disease progresses.

Hearing loss in patients with AS is progressive, symmetrical, and sensorineural. The degree of hearing loss varies from subtle to profound. The onset of hearing loss is usually before the age of 10 years and is more severe in males in XL-AS.[8] The molecular composition of the basement membranes of the cochlea is specific, and changes in the component proteins can lead to sensorineural hearing loss. COL4A3, COL4A4, and COL4A5 are found in the basilar membrane parts of the spiral ligament and in the stria vascularis. Although the mechanism of hearing loss is not known, there is focal thinning and thickening in the glomerulus of the kidney with eventual basement membrane splitting. Extrapolating to the spiral sulcus of the ear, loss of integrity of the basement membrane might affect adhesion of the tectorial and basilar membrane and its junction with the spiral ligament, affecting translation of mechanical energy.[36]

The most common ophthalmic manifestations of Alport's syndrome are bilateral anterior lenticonus and perimacular retinal flecks,[65] reported in 24% to 37% of patients.[66,147,149,185] They are more likely found in affected adults than children,[186] presumably as a result of gradual accumulation of abnormal collagen.[58]

Anterior lenticonus is associated with Alport's syndrome in more than 90% of cases.[99] It is not present at birth, but appears during the second to third decade of life.[63,86,101,183] Electron microscopy shows a thinned basal lamina with basement membrane disruptions.[99,177] Spontaneous and traumatic ruptures of the anterior lens capsule have occurred.[142,177] Anterior and posterior subcapsular cataracts have been reported as frequent findings in AS,[63] but glucocorticoid medications are also commonly used by affected patients and may contribute to cataract formation.[147] Posterior lenticonus has been reported to occur infrequently in patients with anterior lenticonus and Alport's syndrome.[131]

Perimacular yellow flecks are the most common retinal finding, presumably caused by a toxic effect to or primary degeneration of the retinal pigment epithelium or Bruch's membrane.[76] Reddish macular patches and loss of the foveal reflex have been described.[147]

Reports of electrophysiological studies have largely been normal,[58,59,76,86,149,165] although abnormal electroretinography, electro-oculography, and/or fluorescein angiography have all been reported in affected patients.[188]

Corneal findings in AS include corneal arcus,[63,147] posterior polymorphous dystrophy,[76,183,185] and recurrent nontraumatic corneal erosions.[18,153]

Correlation between the type of mutation causing the disease and type or incidence of ocular finding has not been made,[147,188] and variation of ocular findings within pedigrees is common.[147]

Other features described in AS include thrombocytopenia, macrothrombocytopathia, hypoparathyroidism, polyneuropathy, ichthyosis, and thyroid abnormalities.[8]

Inheritance

Seventy-five percent of cases are transmitted through X-linked dominant inheritance, although autosomal dominant (15%) and recessive (10%) inheritance patterns have also been reported.[50] Accurate familial study is mandatory in patients with AS, as the identification of the different patterns of inheritance greatly affects genetic counseling.

The majority of AS patients have XL-AS, involving mutations in the COL4A5 gene located on the long arm of X chromosome (Xq22.3). Mutation of the COL4A3 and COL4A4 genes located on the long arm of chromosome 2 (2q36–2q37) causes AR-AS. Recently a dominant form of AS (AD-AS) was linked to the COL4A3/COL4A4 locus.[193] Cochat et al. in 1988 described the association of diffuse leiomyomatosis with a subtype of XL-AS.[30] Later, Zhou et al. in 1993 demonstrated that the leiomyomatosis-nephropathy syndrome represents a contiguous gene syndrome due to deletions that disrupt the COL4A5 and COL4A6 genes, two adjacent genes on the X chromosome.[208] Although the diagnosis of AS still relies heavily on histological studies, routine application of molecular genetic diagnosis will probably be available in the near future.

Treatment

There is no effective treatment for the glomerulonephritis. Peritoneal and hemodialysis may be necessary. Renal transplantation for AS is usually very successful. However, certain mutations within the type IV collagen genes carry an increased risk of developing specific antiglomerular basement membrane (anti-GBM) nephritis after renal transplantation. Anti-GBM nephritis of the allograft almost always results in graft loss.[109,125]

Prognosis

Dual sensory loss in AS patients creates an urgent need for appropriate vision and care and rehabilitation. Because of the high risk for developmental delay and decreased social integration, early intervention should be considered in the treatment plan. A multidisciplinary approach by the health care management team will enhance the quality of life and positive outcomes for AS patients.[121]

ALSTRÖM SYNDROME

A syndrome of retinal degeneration combined with obesity, diabetes mellitus, and sensorineural hearing loss was described in 1959 by C.H. Alström. It has since come to be known as a distinct syndrome, Alström syndrome.[4] As of 1997, 37 definite cases had been reported in the literature.[164]

Etiology

The etiology of Alström syndrome is unknown.

Clinical Features

Presentation is typically of an infant or young child with profound vision loss and nystagmus. Severe photophobia and nystagmus are common by 4 months of age and almost uniformly present by 1 year of age. Although the fundus is typically normal at birth, a narrowing of the retinal vessels can be seen early on with patchy diffuse atrophy of the retinal pigment epithelium and/or increased pigment in the midperiphery and a macular sheen. There is typically no "bull's-eye" maculopathy early on, as is commonly seen in Bardet–Biedl syndrome.[164] Also, bone spicule formation is not noted until the second or third decade. Posterior subcapsular cataracts have been reported in 100% of patients with Alström syndrome.[168]

Reported ophthalmic histopathological findings are consistent with diabetes, and include iris and ciliary body lacy vacuolization and asteriod hyalosis.[168] No sign of chorioretinal fusion or optic nerve atrophy has been seen in patients with Alström syndrome, in contrast to patients with retinitis pigmentosa. Large, superficial optic nerve drusen were found. Histopathology was indistinguishable from that of other secondary or pseudoretinitis pigmentosa syndromes.[168]

ERG is absent or attenuated, with rod function better preserved than cone function until later in childhood, when all visual function is extinguished.[187] This condition has created some confusion with Leber's congenital amaurosis. Russell-Eggitt and associates previously reported seven patients with infantile cardiomyopathy and atypical Leber's amaurosis in 1989,[163] who were subsequently found to have Alström syndrome.[104] The diagnosis of Alström syndrome should be considered in infantile cone and rod retinal dystrophy, particularly if the weight is above the 90th percentile, or if there is infantile cardiomyopathy.

Natural History

See Prognosis.

Systemic Associations

Infantile obesity, infantile cardiomyopathy, and hypogenitalism are typical. Sensorineural deafness is common by 7 years of age.[164] Normal secondary sexual characteristics are found, although gynecomastia and reduced fertility are typically seen later on. Noninsulin-dependent diabetes mellitus (NIDDM) occurs in the second or third decades. Polydactyly and mental retardation, central features of Bardet–Biedel syndrome, are not seen in Alström syndrome.

Because of a potentially fatal infantile cardiomyopathy at 2 weeks to 7 months of age, infants suspected of having Alström syndrome should be referred for cardiac evaluation in an urgent fashion.[164] Once the diagnosis is suspected, workup should begin for signs of renal or hepatic failure, hypothyroidism, growth hormone deficiency, hyperuricemia, hypercholesterolemia, hypertriglyceridemia, and kyphoscoliosis.

Inheritance

Alström syndrome probably has an autosomal-recessive pattern of inheritance. A large French Canadian kindred with an autosomal recessive pattern of inheritance has revealed a locus on 2p13, although a second locus may be associated with the Alström phenotype.[35] A mouse model candidate has a defective gene on mouse chromosome 7, with homologous human region 11p15.[135,136]

Treatment

There is no known treatment for the vision loss secondary to Alström syndrome. Management of the endocrine, cardiac, and kidney disease is critical, although a shortened lifespan is expected.

Prognosis

There is a rapid and progressive loss of visual function to less than 20/200 by 10 years of age and to no light perception by 20 years of age. In the final stages of the disease, affected individuals exhibit progressive chronic nephropathy with eventual renal failure, which is the most frequent cause of death.[62] The oldest surviving patient reported in the literature is 36 years of age.[164]

BRACHMANN–DE LANGE SYNDROME

Brachmann–de Lange syndrome (BDLS), often referred to as Cornelia de Lange syndrome or de Lange syndrome, is a phenotypically variable multisystem disorder involving congenital malformations, growth retardation, and neurodevelopmental delay. Although the first reported case in the literature was Brachmann's in 1916, Cornelia de Lange in 1933 suggested that these manifestations comprised a new malformation syndrome.[43,194] The incidence has been estimated at 1 in 10,000 live births, but is difficult to estimate because mild cases may go undiagnosed.[64,139]

Etiology

The etiology of BDLS is unknown.

Clinical Features

Brachmann–de Lange syndrome (BDLS) in its severe form is easily recognizable by the experienced examiner. The characteristic face, pre- and postnatal growth deficiency, feeding dysfunction, limb anomalies (when present), psychomotor delay, and distinctive behavioral pattern are diagnostic in a newborn or young infant.

Ocular features did not figure prominently in the original descriptions of BDLS. However, in 1990, Levin and associates reported a series of 22 children with BDLS detailing the ophthalmic findings.[110] Of the 21 children in this series with available histories, 17 (81%) had required previous ophthalmic care, highlighting the importance of ophthalmic features in this disease. The most common ophthalmic feature in CDLS is hypertrichosis of the eyebrows and eyelashes with synophrys. The synophrys is typically in a "V" configuration over the nasal bridge. Other tendencies include antimongoloid slant, hypertelorism, ptosis, nystagmus, high myopia, strabismus, amblyopia, and photophobia. Absent upper lacrimal puncta and canaliculi have been reported with BDLS.[196] A significant percentage of children with BDLS have a history of recurrent conjunctivitis, blepharitis, hordeola, and nasolacrimal duct obstructions. Treatment of high myopia and amblyopia with glasses and/or patching can prove difficult in patients with BDLS because of their defensive behavioral tendencies. Diagnostic examinations can also be challenging.

The facial features are perhaps the most diagnostic of all physical signs (Fig. 8-2). Microcephaly and brachycephaly, "penciled" eyebrows, synophrys, long eyelashes, anteverted nostrils, long philtrum, thin lips, crescent-shaped mouth, and widely spaced teeth are all typical features.[83] Hypertrichosis, including generalized hirsutism, as well as a low posterior hairline, and hair tufts on the neck or lower back are common.

By far, the two most common areas of involvement in BDLS are the gastrointestinal (GI) tract and the heart. GI abnormalities include gastrointestinal (GE) reflux and various forms of obstructions. Persistent vomiting and feeding problems result in failure to thrive.[194] Heart defects are widely variable from minor

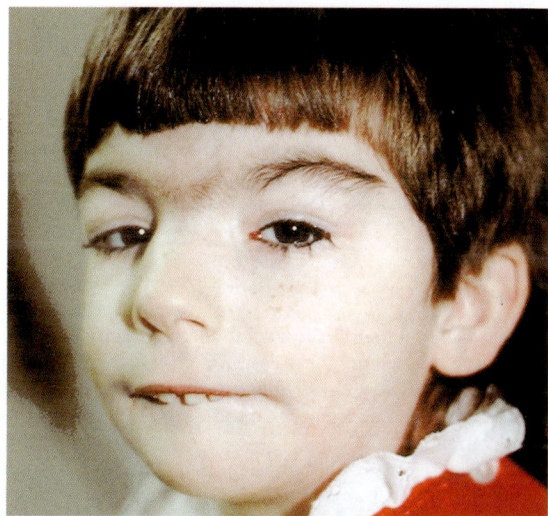

FIGURE 8-2. Five-year-old girl with Brachmann–de Lange syndrome. Note synophrys, epiphora secondary to nasolacrimal duct anomaly, short nose, anteverted nares, long philtrum, and thin upper lip. (Courtesy of Dr. J.C. Ward, Memphis, TN.)

to severe in their clinical consequences. Respiratory problems are usually limited to recurrent upper respiratory infections and pneumonias. Many respiratory difficulties are probably complicated or initiated by undetected GE reflux. Genitourinary anomalies are common in BDLS and include genital hypoplasia, hydronephrosis, and renal dysplasia or hypoplasia.[54]

Limb abnormalities usually associated with BDLS include oligodactyly or severe deficiencies of the arms. Relatively small hands and feet are frequently a striking feature.[12]

Significant speech delay has been noted in the majority of children with BDLS. The majority of the speech delay is attributed to hearing loss due to stenotic external auditory canals, and/or frequent ear infections.[85]

The BDLS has a range of severity from perinatal lethality with multiple congenital anomalies to almost imperceptible cases compatible with normal reproduction and normal intelligence.[139] The majority of patients with BDLS have severe mental retardation, with IQs generally ranging from 30 to 50.[88]

Mild mental retardation with milder phenotypic expression has been reported in some cases of BDLS.[64] Behavioral dysfunction is evident in every age group in the severe and moderate cases of BDLS. As an infant, tactile defensiveness, irritability, and opisthotonic posturing is common.[98] As children, BDLS patients prefer a structured environment. Activities stimulating the vestibular system are pleasurable to BDLS patients; these activities include swimming, swinging, and horseback riding.[194]

Inheritance

Most cases are sporadic. Autosomal dominant inheritance has been suggested based on a few cases in which a mildly affected parent and one or more children of his/hers was affected. Recurrence risk is negligible if, after careful evaluation, both parents are determined to be normal.[88]

It is well recognized that there is phenotypic similarity between BDLS and the duplication of q26–27 band region of chromosome 3.[49] The search for the candidate gene of BDLS has, however, failed to identify BDLS patient-specific mutations in a gene cluster located at 3q27.[173] Therefore, cautious chromosome studies are indicated in some atypical BDLS patients.

Treatment

Treatment of disease of the ocular adnexae, such as blepharitis and chalazia, may be required. However, successful treatment of myopia, strabismus, and amblyopia may be hindered by patient uncooperation.

Prognosis

Mortality in infants and older patients with BDLS is mainly due to apneic episodes, seizures, cardiac-related illnesses, or effects from other congenital malformations.[85]

BRANCHIO-OCULO-FACIAL SYNDROME

The branchio-oculo-facial syndrome was first described by Hall and colleagues in 1984.[69] The pathognomonic finding in this disorder is cervical infraauricular skin defects, which are often described as aplastic, "hemangiomatous," or otherwise abnormal skin overlying draining sinus fistulae. These defects are most often located at the superior head of the sternocleidomastoid. A variety of eye, ear, oral, and craniofacial anomalies are associated with this disorder. Renal malformations are common, although congenital heart and central nervous system defects are rare. Forty-three patients have been reported in the literature.[115]

Etiology

The underlying etiology is unknown.

Clinical Features and Assessment

Ophthalmic abnormalities include nasolacrimal duct stenosis, dermoids of the brow area, strabismus, ptosis, colobomas, cataracts, microphthalmia, myopia, hypertelorism, and upslanting palpebral fissures (Fig. 8-3A–E). Hemangiomatous orbital

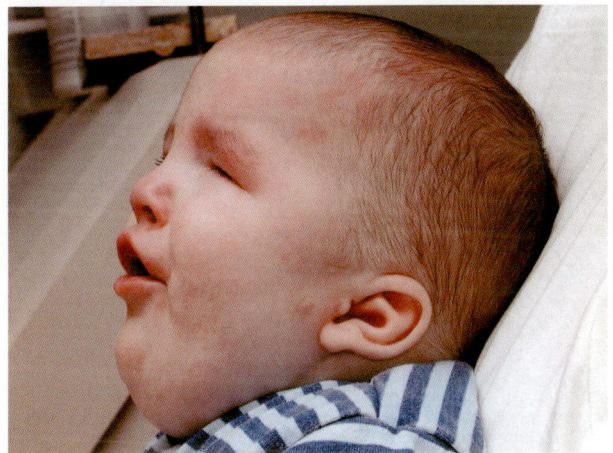

A

FIGURE 8-3A–E. (A) Face of child with features of branchio-oculo-facial syndrome, demonstrating hypertelorism, pseudocleft lip, and low-set, posteriorly rotated ears.

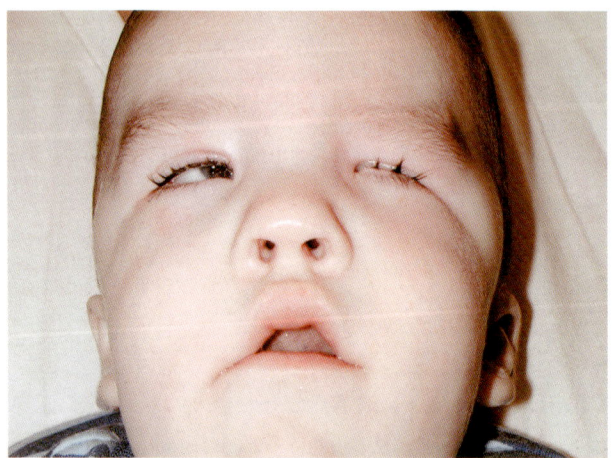

B

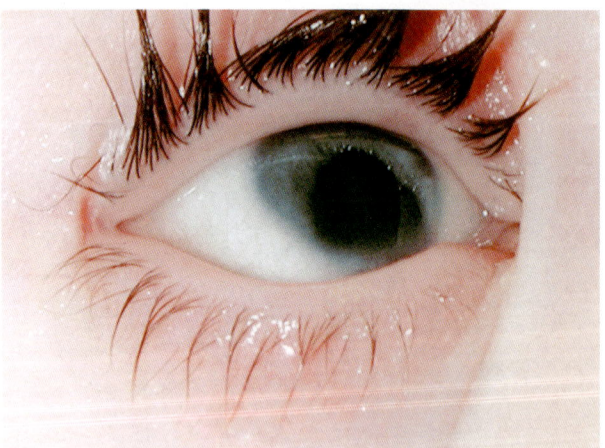

C

FIGURE 8-3A–E. (B) Face of child with features of branchio-oculo-facial syndrome, demonstrating hypertelorism, pseudocleft lip, and low-set, posteriorly rotated ears. **(C)** Right eye of child with branchio-oculo-facial syndrome showing iris coloboma.

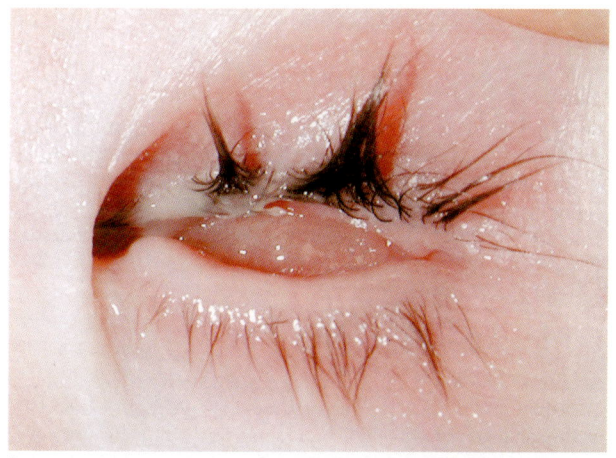

D

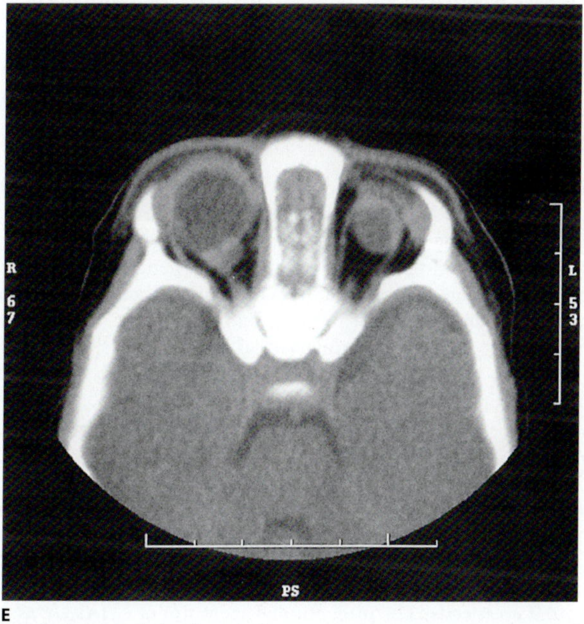

E

FIGURE 8-3A–E. (D) Left eye of same patient demonstrating microphthalmia. **(E)** Computed tomography of orbits demonstrating optic nerve and chorioretinal coloboma (*right eye*) and severe microphthalmos (*left eye*).

cysts have been reported in siblings.[51] Oral anomalies include a cleft lip and pseudocleft lip, lip pits, and cleft palate. The ears are typically low set and posteriorly rotated. Dolichocephaly has been noted, as well as premature graying of the hair. The differential diagnosis for this disorder includes Treacher Collins, branchio-oculo-renal syndrome, CHARGE association, Van der Woude's syndrome, Goltz–Gorlin syndrome, and Delleman syndrome.

Inheritance

An autosomal dominant inheritance has been reported, although most reported cases have been sporadic.[55,107] Although branchio-oculo-facial syndrome (BOF) and branchio-oto-renal syndrome (BOR) are thought to be distinct syndromes,[116] one father–son pair has been reported,[108] and we have observed a child with microphthalmia, a feature "distinctive" for BOF, but without the distinctive skin findings of BOF (Fig. 8-3).

CHARGE ASSOCIATION SYNDROME

The acronym CHARGE proposed by Pagon et al.[146] refers to a nonrandom clustering of malformations first described by Hall,[68] including ocular coloboma, heart malformation, atresia of choanae, retarded growth and development and/or central nervous system malformations, genital hypoplasia and/or hypogonadism, and ear abnormalities and/or deafness. In addition, facial palsy, esophageal and laryngeal abnormalities, renal malformations, and facial clefts have been observed with higher frequency in patients with CHARGE association.[46,68,184]

Etiology

The cause and exact prevalence of the CHARGE association remains unknown (Fig. 8-4A,B).[68] However, the combination of malformations observed in CHARGE association strongly evokes a polytopic developmental field defect involving the neural crest cells. The total clinical spectrum of CHARGE association is still waiting to be determined.

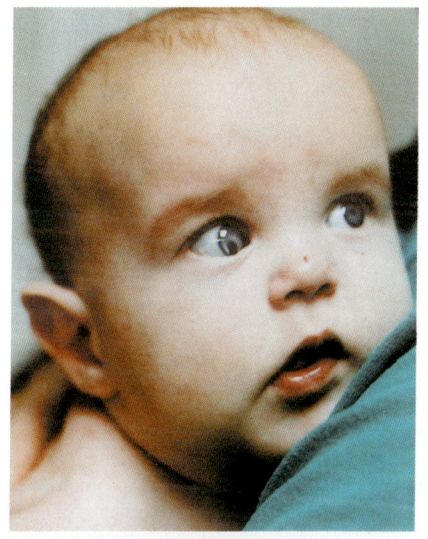

A

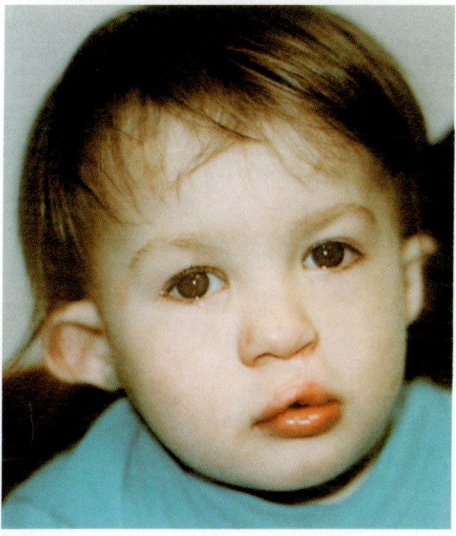

B

FIGURE 8-4A,B. (A) Young infant with CHARGE association. Note the abnormal ears, right iris coloboma, and left facial palsy. (Courtesy of Dr. Bryan D. Hall, University of Kentucky, Lexington, KY.) **(B)** A 27-month-old girl with CHARGE association, demonstrating a characteristic face, protruding cupped ears lacking earlobes, and repaired unilateral cleft lip. (Courtesy of Dr. B.D. Hall, Lexington, KY.)

Clinical Features and Systemic Associations

Colobomas found in the CHARGE association are indistinguishable from colobomas found in other genetic diseases (Fig. 8-4B). They range from iris colobomas and small choroidal colobomas with no visual impairments to colobomas with severe micropthalmos and poor to no vision. In the original report of CHARGE association by Roberta Pagon and associates,[146] the severity of the coloboma or visual impairment did not correlate with the severity of the other CNS anamolies and developmental delay. A review of 180 cases of CHARGE from the literature[71] documented ocular colobomas in 81.7% of cases. A majority of these were posterior colobomas of the choroid and/or optic nerve. When iris colobomas were present, they were usually accompanied by choroidal and optic nerve colobomas.[162] Colobomas are typically bilateral, but can be quite asymmetrical (personal observation). The large number of posterior colobomas highlights the need for careful dilated fundus examination in any child suspected of having CHARGE association, even when there is no outward sign of poor vision or eye malformation. The differential of *bilateral colobomas* includes an autosomal recessive isolated genetic disease, as well as trisomy 13, cat-eye syndrome, and 4p− syndrome (Wolf–Hirschorn syndrome).

Microphthalmia was observed in 49 of 129 cases reviewed.[71] Other ocular abnormalities reported include optic nerve hypoplasia,[162] persistent hypoplastic primary vitreous (PHPV), lacrimal canalicular atresia,[11] congenital glaucoma due to maldevelopment of the anterior chamber angle,[192] eyelid coloboma,[162] and bilateral Marcus-Gunn jaw winking phenomenon.[201]

Congenital heart defects were found in 85% of patients with CHARGE association in one large study.[184] There are conflicting data in the literature with regard to the frequency of specific cardiac malformations in CHARGE association. Tellier et al.[184] found that the most common malformations were atrial and ventricular septal defects, followed by patent ductus arteriosus (PDA), conotruncal heart defects, and outflow anomalies. Aortic arch anomalies were rare. However, another review reported that the most common malformations were conotruncal anomalies followed by aortic arch anomalies,[114] a pattern similar to DiGeorge sequence.

Choanal atresia is present in about 58% of the patients with CHARGE association. The atresia is unilateral or bilateral, and both bony and membranous.[89]

Growth deficiency is usually postnatal and affects all the body in a symmetrical fashion. Head circumference is proportional to length.[146,184] Growth hormone deficiency has been reported in a few patients.[184] Growth deficiency couples with failure to gain weight. The linear growth and weight curve of patients with CHARGE association usually shifts below the 3rd percentile during the first 6 to 9 months of age.[146]

Mental development is affected in most patients with CHARGE association. Mental retardation may range from mild to profound.[89] Axial hypotonia was found to be common (93%) in one large study.[114] In an extensive review, Lin et al.[117] found CNS malformations to be common in CHARGE association. These malformations may be due to aberrant development, migration, or interaction of the cephalic neural crest.[199] The following CNS malformations have been noted in patients with CHARGE association: holoprosencephaly, arhinencephalia, agenesis of corpus callosum and septum pellucidum, various forebrain and hindbrain defects, and various cranial nerve palsies (VI, VII, VIII, IX, and X).[117,184]

Genital hypoplasia is more prone to be recognized and reported in males than females. Hypogonadism in males with CHARGE association include micropenis, cryptorchidism, and rarely hypospadius. Central gonadotropin deficiency may account for some of these abnormalities.[184]

Characteristically, ear malformations in the CHARGE association include asymmetry and ears that are short, wide, and low set with small or absent lobes, ear tags, and malformed pinnae.[40] Asymmetrical or bilateral hearing loss is present in more than two-thirds of patients with CHARGE association. Both middle ear anomalies (ossicular malformation) and internal ear anomalies (semicircular canal hypoplasia) are common. Deafness can be mild to profound, sensorineural, or mixed sensorineural and conductive, and may progress over time.[41]

Other systemic findings include skeletal and GI anomalies. Skeletal anomalies of the vertebrae and ribs have been found in about one-half of patients with CHARGE association. Intestinal malformations include esophageal atresia, tracheoesophageal fistula, renal anomalies, velopharyngeal incompetence, and DiGeorge sequence.[184] On prenatal echography, the combination of intrauterine growth retardation, CNS anomalies, congenital heart disease, esophageal atresia, and renal anomalies may raise a suspicion for CHARGE association. These signs, however, could be observed in several other multiple congenital anomaly syndromes, such as VATER association.

Inheritance

The CHARGE association is usually a sporadic event of unknown cause.[170] However, some affected patients have had abnormal chromosomes, including a microdeletion of 22q11 (DiGeorge sequence). Because CHARGE association shares phenotypic features with recognized chromosomal syndromes such as trisomy 13, the cat-eye syndrome, and the 4p− syndrome, molecular and chromosome analysis should be performed in all patients with CHARGE association.[29]

Prognosis

Although the prognosis of CHARGE patients is poor, the clinical spectrum of this condition is variable. The presence of midline anomalies and esophageal and bilateral choanal atresia are frequently combined and carry a poor prognosis.[100,117] Severe phenotypic expression of CHARGE association in males has been noted in one large study.[184]

COCKAYNE'S SYNDROME

In 1936, E.A. Cockayne described two children with dwarfism, retinal atrophy, and deafness.[31] Cockayne's syndrome (CS) is a rare autosomal recessive disorder with postnatal growth failure, characteristic facies, atypical retinopathy, deafness, mental deterioration, UV light sensitivity, and premature aging. CS is a progressive disorder with an underlying leukodystrophy.[128]

Etiology

A defect in DNA metabolism has been documented in fibroblasts of CS patients that involves increased sensitivity of cells to UV light, decreased RNA synthesis following UV exposure, and abnormal excision repair.[17] The two genes involved in CS (CSI, CSII) are required for transcription-coupled repair (TCR), a subpathway of nucleotide excision repair. Alterations of these two genes are likely to be responsible for the two forms of CS.

Clinical Features

Pigmentary degeneration of the retina is one of the hallmarks of CS.[31] The fundus findings described in the original monograph were markedly narrowed arterioles with sparing of the veins, an absent macular reflex, and blackish dots concentrated in the posterior pole. Since then, the most common and pervasive ophthalmic abnormality described has been pigmentary retinopathy, with 55% of the diagnosed children being affected.[128] The pigmentary retinopathy is progressive, and normal fundus findings early in life may not exclude the diagnosis of Cockayne's syndrome. Other ophthalmic abnormalities reported in Cockayne's syndrome include decreased lacrimation, corneal infiltrates and opacities, band keratopathy, miotic pupils, iris hypoplasia, microphthalmos, cataracts, and optic atrophy or hypoplasia.[128]

Ocular pathology has been reported in one case.[111] Lipofuscin deposition was noted in the retinal pigment epithelium. The outer segments of the photoreceptors disintegrated, with loss of cells from the ganglion cell and outer nuclear layers. Marked thinning of the nerve fiber bundles was noted over the optic nervehead, with both axonal loss and partial demyelination. In the cornea, there were pigment-laden macrophages.

Systemic Associations

Growth and development usually proceed at a normal rate in early infancy. Profound growth failure, however, begins after 2 years of age. Weight is more affected than length, which has led to the term cachectic dwarfism for describing CS patients[128] (Fig. 8-5).

All patients with CS eventually develop neurological dysfunction, including the cerebellar signs of gait ataxia, tremor, incoordination and dysarthric speech, as well as peripheral neuropathy, autonomic dysfunction, and seizures.[127,128] Almost all patients with CS over 2 years of age have microcephaly. Cerebral imaging may demonstrate cerebral atrophy with calcifications in various parts of the brain. Cerebral histopathology of patients with CS commonly demonstrates a patchy "tigroid"

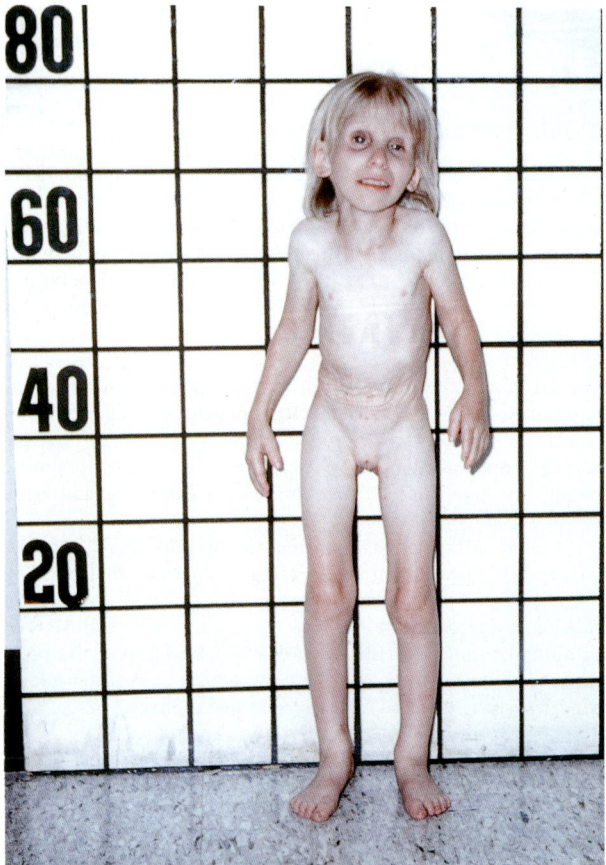

FIGURE 8-5. Ten-year-old girl with Cockayne's syndrome. Note the short stature, cachectic habitus, abnormal standing posture, flexion deformity of the joints, barrel-shaped chest deformity, deep-set eyes, and thin hair. (Courtesy of Dr. R.S. Wilroy, Memphis, TN.)

demyelination of the subcortical white matter with macroscopic and microscopic calcifications and neurofibrillary tangles.[178,181] Despite their mental deficiencies, patients with CS are described as friendly, interactive, happy, and social.

Sensorineural hearing loss occurs in about half of CS patients.[90] Dental complications (especially severe caries) are common. Photosensitive dermatitis is present in two-thirds of the patients with CS. Thin, dry, scaly skin with diminished adipose tissue, thin hair, and sunken eyes are responsible for the "aged" appearance of patients with CS.[128] Various renal complications, including renal vascular hypertension and structural anomalies of the kidneys, have been observed in about 10% of all reported cases.[74] In male patients, cryptorchidism and micropenis may be present. Females with CS may develop irregular menstrual cycles. Patients with CS have a characteristic appearance with kyphosis and progressive hip, knee, and ankle contractures.

CS is clearly a disorder with variability in type and severity of symptoms. The average age of death is about 12 years.[128] An early-onset "severe form" of CS has been reported in a subset of patients.[148] Cataracts noted at birth or within the first 3 years of life are a poor prognosticator in CS. Nance and Berry noted that only 2 of 22 reported cases of CS with cataracts less than 3 years old survived beyond the age of 7.[128]

In the differential diagnosis one must consider other conditions such as progeria (Hutchinson–Gilford syndrome), Werner syndrome, cerebro-oculo-facial syndrome, and Pena–Shokeir II syndrome.[91] The differential diagnosis for the pigmentary retinopathy seen with early neurological demise includes Pelizaeus–Merzbacher syndrome, Refsum's disease, and ceroid lipofuscinosis.

Inheritance

Inheritance is autosomal recessive. Parents should receive genetic counseling regarding the 25% risk of subsequent affected children.

Treatment

The management of CS is purely symptomatic.

Prognosis

The prognosis is poor, with an average lifespan of 12 years.

Kabuki Make-Up Syndrome

Kabuki make-up syndrome (KMS), also known as *Niikawa–Kuroki syndrome*, was first described in 1981,[134] and is a multiple congenital anomalies/mental retardation (MCA/ MR) syndrome characterized by a peculiar face (100%), dermatoglyphic abnormalities (93%), skeletal anomalies (92%), mental retardation (92%), and postnatal growth retardation (83%).[105,134] The name of the syndrome comes from the fact that the face of these patients resembles the mask used in the traditional Japanese "Kabuki" theater. More than 70 Japanese individuals and 100 non-Japanese individuals with this syndrome have been reported.[189,205]

Etiology

The etiology of KMS is unknown.

Clinical Features

The ophthalmic features diagnostic for KMS are long palpebral fissures, eversion of the lower eyelids, and laterally sparse, arched eyebrows (Fig. 8-6). The phenotype evolves over time, making the diagnosis difficult in infancy.[19] Ptosis, strabismus,[28] long eyelashes, epicanthal folds, hypotelorism,[67] cataracts,[145] blue sclerae, and uveitis[22] have all been reported.

Systemic Associations

Other facial features include a broad and depressed nasal tip, prominent and broad philtrum, malar hypoplasia, cup-shaped ears with large prominent earlobes, preauricular dimples, and a low posterior hairline. Patients with KMS commonly have retromicrognathia, cleft or high arched palate, deficient dentition, and widely spaced teeth.[67] The open mouth with tented upper lip gives a myopathic facial appearance to KMS patients.

Various skeletal abnormalities are prevalent in patients with KMS. Radiologic abnormalities include spinal deformities, sagittal cleft of the vertebrae, curved fifth fingers, and stubby short fingers (brachydactyly). Joint laxity and joint dislocations (hips, patella) have been reported in connection with KMS.[19,22] Other unusual findings in KMS include the persistence of fingertip pads, atypical dermatoglyphic pattern of the fingers and palms,

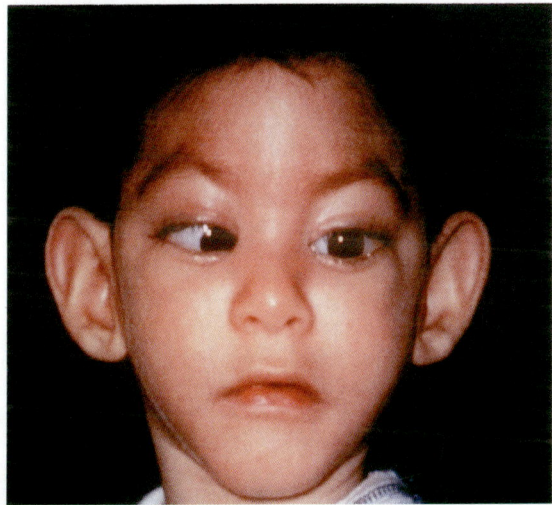

FIGURE 8-6. Child with Kabuki make-up syndrome. Note the long palpebral fissures, eversion of the lateral portion of the lower eyelids, arching eyebrows, strabismus, and protruding ears. (Courtesy of Dr. G.S. Oliveira, Campinas, Brazil.)

a simian crease, and an excess of the ulnar loop patterns on fingers.[67]

Among patients with KMS, recurrent otitis media is quite common. Igawa and associates demonstrated middle and inner ear malformations including hypodysplasia of the cochlea, vestibule, and semicircular canal with subsequent hearing deficits. Computerized tomography (CT) of the petrous bone and audiometry should be performed during early infancy in patients with KMS to optimize rehabilitation of the affected individuals.[82]

The primary manifestation of the CNS is microcephaly.[19,105,133] Structural CNS defects have been reported (arachnoid cyst,[28] ventriculomegaly[93]). Mental retardation is present in more than two-thirds of the patients. The mean developmental quotient is 52 in children and 62 in older patients. Severe mental retardation is uncommon. Occasional individuals have had normal intelligence.[93]

Postnatal growth deficiency usually manifests within the first year of life and becomes more obvious with advancing age.

Mean height in children 12 months and over is 2 standard deviations below average.[93]

In addition to the cardinal features of KMS, about 50% of the patients have congenital heart defects. Malformations associated with altered hemodynamics can occur, and include coarctation of the aorta, bicuspid aortic valve, mitral valve prolapse, membranous ventricular septal defect, pulmonary, aortic, mitral valve stenosis, tetralogy of Fallot, single ventricle with common atrium, double-outlet right ventricle, and transposition of the great vessels.[133]

Inheritance

Most patients with KMS represent a new mutation.[133] There are, however, a few examples of familial KMS cases in the medical literature. KMS in these families shows an autosomal dominant inheritance pattern with a variable expressivity.[67,171,190]

OPITZ G/BBB SYNDROME

Opitz G/BBB syndrome was first described in 1969 as two separate disorders, the G syndrome and the BBB syndrome.[140,141] The G syndrome, also known as Opitz–Frias syndrome, was characterized by ventral midline defects including hypertelorism, hypospadias, cleft lip and palate, and laryngo-tracheo-esophageal defects. The BBB syndrome was characterized by hypertelorism and hypospadias in males, with affected females having only hypertelorism. It has become clear that the BBB and G syndromes are in fact one entity, now named the Opitz G/BBB syndrome.[129]

Etiology

See Heredity section.

Clinical Features and Systemic Associations

Wide clinical variability, ranging from neonatal lethality to an asymptomatic form, has been well described in Opitz G/BBB, making diagnosis difficult in mild cases.[138] The most striking features of Opitz G/BBB are the facial manifestations, which may include ocular hypertelorism, telecanthus, upward or downward slanting palpebral fissures and epicanthal folds, broad nasal bridge with anteverted nostrils, cleft lip with or without cleft palate, short frenulum of the tongue, micrognathia, posterior rotation of the auricles, and widow's peak (Fig. 8-7).[94] Occasionally, bifid uvula, cleft tongue, dental anomalies, and ankyloglossia are observed in patients with Optiz G/BBB.[16]

Severe abnormalities may involve tracheo-esophageal-laryngeal cleft or fistula formation, and neuromuscular defects of the esophagus, leading to chronic dysphagia, regurgitation, and aspiration pneumonia. Although males tend to have more severe and more frequent laryngoesophageal defects, it is important to recognize that this disorder can express itself in both males and females with equal severity. Infants classically

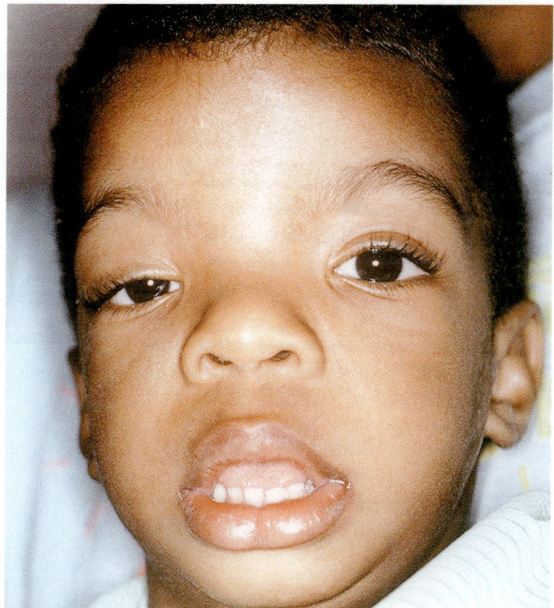

FIGURE 8-7. Face of a boy with Opitz (G/BBB) syndrome. Note hypertelorism, telecanthus, broad nasal bridge, and ptosis (*right eye*).

present with a weak, hoarse cry and stridor. Mildly affected patients may only manifest functional swallowing impairment, which improves with age.[80] Initial failure to thrive is followed by normal growth in survivors.[94] Frequently, patients with Optiz G/BBB have ectopic or imperforated anus.[16] Patients with Optiz G/BBB often have mild to moderate mental retardation.

A variety of midline brain anomalies including absence of corpus callosum, wide septum pellucidum, cerebellar vermal hypoplasia, and large cisterna magna have been described among those Optiz G/BBB patients who have had imaging studies.[118] The most common cardiac defects encountered are conotruncal lesions and have been observed in a subset of patients with Optiz G/BBB.[94]

In the differential diagnosis of Optiz G/BBB, one must consider Aarskog syndrome, Robinow's syndrome, and frontonasal dysplasia sequence. Individuals affected with Aarskog syndrome and Robinow's syndrome have abnormally wide-set eyes and midline facial and genital anomalies, but individuals affected with frontonasal dysplasia sequence have facial anomalies involving the midline but do not have genital anomalies.

Inheritance

Opitz syndrome (Optiz G/BBB) is a heterogeneous condition with both autosomal dominant and X-linked transmission.[119,176] Clinically indistinguishable forms have been mapped to Xp22 and to 22q11.2.[155] Based on clinical data, it appears that Optiz G/BBB is a condition distinct from DiGeorge/velo-cardio-facial (DGS/VCFS), which has also been mapped to 22q11.2. There is, however, some overlap among these conditions, especially in regard to the types of congenital heart defects.[156] The candidate gene at the Xp22.3 locus is called MID1. The transcript of this gene has been found in virtually all normal fetal tissues. No transcripts were detected however, in samples from affected males with Optiz G/BBB. The MID1 gene encodes a protein called midin, whose function is predicted to be important for development of midline structures.[167]

Prognosis

Progosis is highly variable because of the wide range of clinical severity.

PRADER–WILLI SYNDROME

In 1956, Prader, Labhart, and Willi described what has come to be known as Prader–Willi syndrome (PWS).[152] Also known as the Prader–Labhart–Willi syndrome, it is the most common dysmorphic form of human obesity (Fig. 8-8). The prevalence of PWS is estimated to be 1 in 15,000, with an incidence ranging from 1 in 16,000 to 1 in 25,000 births.[87]

Etiology

Prader–Willi syndrome is caused by a defect in the region of chromosome 15q11–q13 (see Inheritance section).

Clinical Features and Systemic Associations

Criteria for the clinical diagnosis of PWS were established in 1993, and include obesity, short stature, small hands and feet, hypotonia in infancy, hypogonadism, and mental retardation (Fig. 8-8).[77] Although several of the clinical features and endocrine abnormalities associated with PWS suggest a hypothalamic problem, examinations of the hypothalamus and pituitary gland by routine methods have failed to show pathological lesions.[13]

The ocular manifestations of Prader–Willi syndrome (PWS) include strabismus, almond-shaped eyes, and hypopigmentation of the uvea. Fifty percent to 95% of patients with PWS have strabismus,[5,25,73] with esotropia being the most common form of strabismus (Hered). Myopia is another relatively common finding, observed in 15% to 40% of PWS children.[25,73] Bilateral cataracts have been described, and may be associated with a metabolic etiology (an abnormal glucose tolerance test).[198] Telecanthus,[158] nystagmus,[38] nonspecific visual field defects, optic atrophy, congenital ectropion uveae, and glaucoma have been reported.[56]

Creel et al. reported an abnormal VEP in three of six patients tested with PWS.[38] The finding of VEP asymmetry typically seen in albinism has not been replicated in subsequent series when VEPs were conducted on known PWS patients.[158] A likely explanation for this discrepancy is that the *p* gene, which is important to normal pigmentation in humans and is the site for the most common form of albinism (OCA2), also contains the critical, distinct regions for the PWS and Angelman's syndrome.

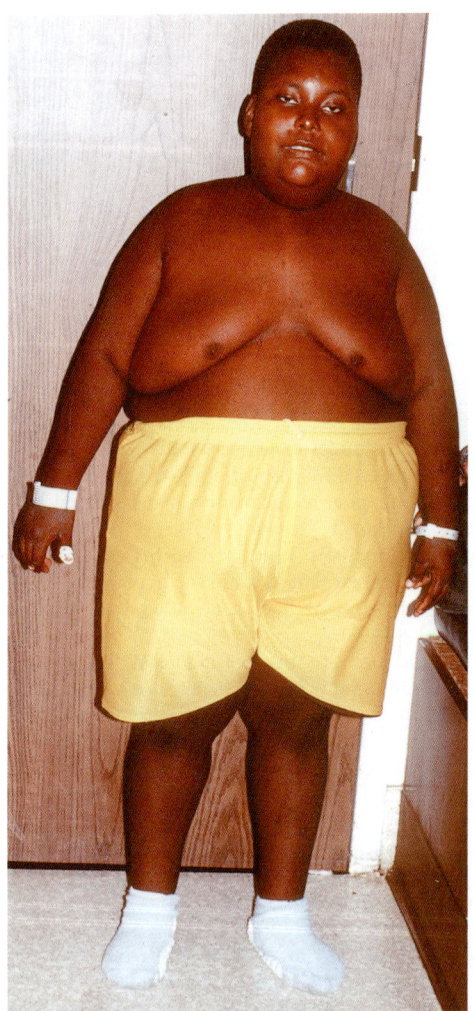

FIGURE 8-8. A 15-year-old boy with Prader–Willi syndrome. Note short stature, truncal obesity, small hands and feet, and typical facial features, including narrow bifrontal diameter and almond-shaped eyes.

Thus, a subset of patients with PWS and Angelman's also have OCA2.[14]

Characteristic facial features of PWS include almond-shaped appearance of palpebral fissures, which may be upslanting, narrow bifrontal diameter of the head, and thin upper lip.[87] Decrease in hand width with straight ulnar border is unique in PWS.[77] Fairer skin and lighter hair compared to other family members is present in about 50% of patients. Most hypopigmented children have a cytogenetic deletion.[20]

A typical pattern of growth has been demonstrated in PWS: normal length at birth, deceleration of linear growth during the first few months of life, relatively steady length growth during childhood, and falloff in growth in adolescence. Mean adult height is 155 cm for males (<3rd centile) and 147 cm for females (<3rd centile).[21]

Fetal and neonatal hypotonia, feeding problems, and failure to thrive in the newborn period are the earliest clinical features of PWS. Excessive weight gain follows the period of failure to thrive in early infancy in PWS. The onset of obesity is from 6 months to 6 years.[87] An increased caloric intake and decreased caloric expenditure are believed to account for the obesity. Diabetes mellitus is seen in patients with PWS and is probably related to the obesity. Children younger than 6 years of age show delayed motor, cognitive, and language development. Mental retardation is mild in 63%, moderate in 31%, and severe in the rest of PWS patients.[39]

A peculiar feature of PWS is the common presence of thick viscous saliva, which tends to crust at the corners of the mouth. A high threshold for vomiting is another odd, unexplained observation in many individuals with PWS.[77] Food-related behavior problems, including excessive appetite and an absent sense of satiation, are typical. Excessive daytime sleeping frequently occurs in older children and adults with PWS.[24] Sleep apnea may be obstructive or central or both.

The manifestations of hypogonadism vary in both sexes in PWS. The extent of sexual maturation is variable in PWS patients who are not treated with hormones.[87]

Patients with PWS are frequently described as stubborn. Verbal perseverance on favorite topics is one of the most common annoying behavioral features in PWS. Self-mutilating habits, especially picking at minor skin lesions, are common behaviors in older children with PWS. People with PWS have surprisingly high pain tolerances.[77] In many individuals with

PWS, strong visual-perceptional-motor skills have been documented. This exceptional skill may explain the proficiency of PWS patients with jigsaw puzzles.[77]

Early feeding difficulties may require alternative feeding regimens, such as gavage or even gastrostomy.[13] Life-threatening obesity was once thought inevitable and incurable in PWS. However, lowering caloric intake in persons with this syndrome has been successful.[78]

Inheritance

The PWS is caused by absence of a paternal contribution of the chromosome region 15q11–q13, resulting from paternal deletions (70%), maternal uniparental disomy (i.e., two maternal copies and no paternal copies of 15q), or rare imprinting mutations.[48,106,130] The deletion of the long arm of chromosome 15 at q11–q13 is detectable with either high-resolution chromosomal analysis or fluorescent in situ hybridization (FISH) using specific probes. In an individual patient with relatively certain clinical diagnosis of PWS, FISH analysis may be the most efficient diagnostic test, as approximately 70% of patients will have a deletion detectable by FISH.[61]

In cases where the diagnosis is in question, methylation analysis is the most efficient single test for ruling out a PWS diagnosis. Conventional cytogenetic analysis in parallel with methylation studies is advised to detect rare chromosomal translocation cases and also to detect other chromosomal abnormalities in patients who do not prove to have PWS.[61]

PROTEUS SYNDROME

The Proteus syndrome (PS) is a rare congenital hamartoneoplastic disorder, with markedly variable clinical expression, in which several systems are involved in an apparently haphazard process of overgrowth (Fig. 8-9). Cohen and Hayden were the first to delineate Proteus syndrome in 1979.[34] It has been suggested that Joseph Merrick, the Elephant Man, most likely had PS.[32] Fewer than 100 cases of PS have been recorded to date.

Etiology

Recent reports have suggested that this disorder results from a somatic alteration of a gene leading to mosaic effects that

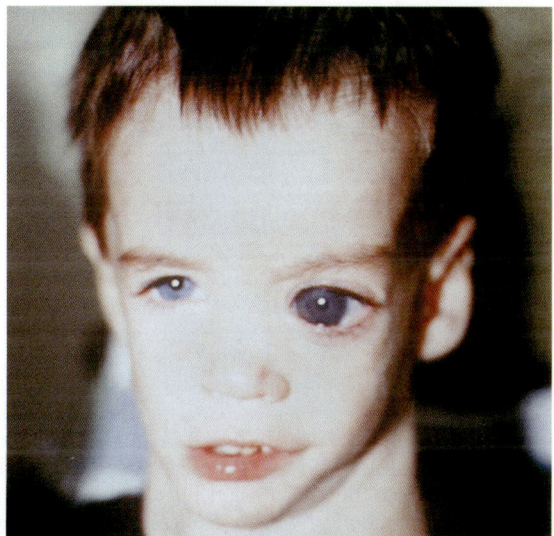

FIGURE 8-9. Five-year-old boy with Proteus syndrome. On the left, note large corneal diameter secondary to congenital glaucoma and large tumor of the neck. (Courtesy of Dr. R. Sid Wilroy, University of Tennessee, Memphis, TN.)

would be lethal if the mutation were carried in nonmosaic fashion.[70]

Clinical Features and Systemic Associations

A workshop on PS held in 1998 at the National Institute of Health developed guidelines for evaluation of patients with PS.[10] The general characteristics mandatory for diagnosis are a mosaic distribution of lesions, progressive course, and sporadic occurrence, regardless of specific manifestations in a given patient with PS.[10] A great variability of clinical findings is common in PS. Asymmetrical growth is perhaps the only constant feature of the syndrome.

The disorder, named after the Greek god Proteus (the polymorphous), is composed of hemihypertrophy, skull exostoses, digital overgrowth, and various soft tissue tumors. These tumors may include subcutaneous and internal fatty, fibrous tumors, as well as lymphatic and vascular malformations. The growth potential and behavior of these tumors and malformations are unpredictable. Other neoplasms may also occur. The spectrum of cutaneous lesions includes café au lait spots, pigmented skin nevi, and epidermal nevi. A unique feature of patients with PS is cerebriform convolutions of the volar skin of the soles and palms. These lesions are facultative but not obligatory. Histologically, they are connective tissue nevi and, when present, are almost pathognomonic for PS.[33,202]

Many of the ocular malformations seen in Proteus syndrome may be traced to "maldevelopment" and subsequent malfunction of the neuroretina.[42] The other ocular findings in Proteus syndrome that can be explained on the basis of neuroretinal abnormalities include strabismus, nystagmus, high myopia, retinal pigment abnormalities with vitreoretinal traction, cataracts secondary to ocular digital reflex or retinal detachment, and posterior segment hamartomas.[42] Pathological examination has revealed diffuse disorganization of the retina, with focal and diffuse retinal gliosis and retinal pits, focal absence and/or proliferation of the retinal pigment epithelium, and congenital absence of choroidal vessels.[60] An ERG on one patient has shown severe rod cone dysfunction.[42] Glaucoma, optic disc drusen, and optic atrophy have also been reported.[33,42,60,120]

Proteus syndrome should be differentiated from Klippel–Trenaunay–Weber syndrome (KTW), neurofibromatosis type 1 (NF1), Bannayan–Riley–Ruvalcaba syndrome, encephalocraniocutaneous lipomatosis (ECCL), and Maffucci syndrome.[96,154]

Inheritance

All cases have been sporadic events in otherwise normal families.

Prognosis

Characteristic features of PS become obvious over the first year of life and are generally progressive throughout childhood. The generalized hypertrophy usually ceases after puberty. Moderate mental retardation is present in 20% of cases.[96] Morbidity is significant. In some cases, overgrowth of legs, fingers, and toes may require amputation. Spinal stenosis and neurological sequelae may develop because of vertebral anomalies or tumor infiltration. Cystic emphysematous lung disease may be associated with severe morbidity and, in some cases, death.[96]

RUBINSTEIN–TAYBI SYNDROME

Originally described in 1963, Rubinstein–Taybi syndrome (RTS) is a multiple congenital anomaly mental retardation syndrome that combines distinctive craniofacial changes including a "beaked" nose with broad thumbs and broad big toes (Fig. 8-10).[161]

Etiology

The majority of cases of RTS are sporadic. The genetic locus of RTS appears to be at 16p13.3, a region that encodes the human cAMP-regulated enhancer-binding protein (CBP). About one-fourth of cases are caused by submicroscopic deletions detectable by fluorescent in situ hybridization (FISH). Various other alterations in the candidate gene of RTS have been reported in the medical literature.[15,161] However, RTS remains a clinical diagnosis.

Clinical Features and Assessment

Ophthalmic manifestations are common in patients with RTS. A review of 207 patients described in the literature found that 117 of these patients had ocular abnormalities.[195] External features contributing to the characteristic faces of RTS include downward slanting palprebral fissures, hypotelorism, epicanthal folds, long eyelashes, high arched eyebrows, ptosis, and strabismus (Fig. 8-10).[159] Additionally, lacrimal duct anomalies, corneal abnormalities, congenital glaucoma, congenital cataract, and colobomas (iris, lens, retinal, and/or optic nerve) were the most frequently described serious ocular abnormalities.

In a series of 571 affected individuals reported by Rubinstein in 1990,[160] refractive errors were found in 56%, strabismus in 71%, ptosis in 29%, and lacrimal duct anomalies in 37% of cases.

In a series reported in 2000,[195] high myopia was found to be present in 25% of individuals, and photophobia was found in 11 patients, with no demonstrable cause in 7 of these patients. Seventy-five percent of study patients had macular anomalies,

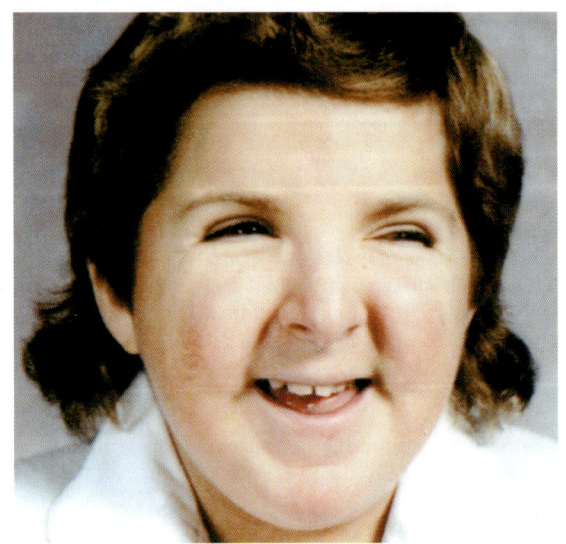

A

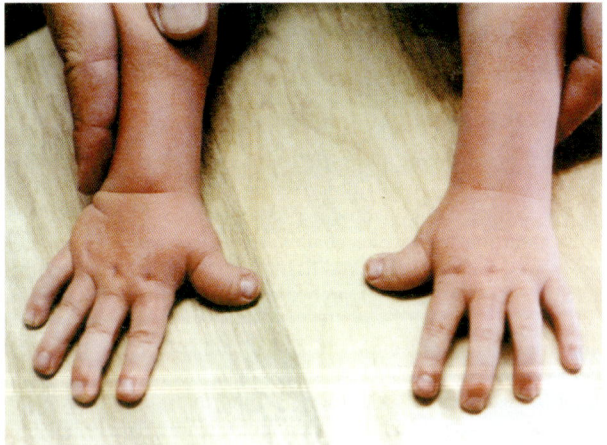

B
FIGURE 8-10A,B. (A) Face of a 14-year-old girl with Rubinstein–Taybi syndrome. Note puffy face, downward slanted palpebral fissures, hypertelorism, prominent nose with low nasal septum, and a grimacing smile. (Courtesy of Dr. Cathy A. Stevens, University of Tennessee, Chattanooga, TN.) **(B)** Hands of a patient with Rubinstein–Taybi syndrome. Note brachydactyly and proximally placed, broad, and short thumbs with radial angulation. (Courtesy of Dr. Cathy A. Stevens, University of Tennessee, Chattanooga, TN.)

including mild or absent foveal reflexes, increased reddening of the foveal area, or unusual distribution of pigmentation in the posterior pole. Of 18 ERGs recorded in these patients, 14 (78%) showed abnormalities, including decreased cone responses and combined decrease in cone and rod responses. Visual handicap was noted to occur in 20% of patients (visual acuity less than or equal to 0.3). Glaucoma has been reported associated with Rubinstein–Taybi syndrome and can be congenital or juvenile in onset.[113]

Systemic Associations

The most characteristic facial abnormality found in all patients is the abnormal shape of the nose: prominent, and/or beaked, with or without low nasal septum. In addition, the following anomalies are frequently described in regard to RTS patients: facial hirsutism, abundant scalp hair, small mouth, and a grimacing smile. The facial manifestations are less characteristic in early infancy than at a later age.[12,160]

Microcephaly is present in about one-third of the patients with RTS.[95] Palatal and dental abnormalities are frequent with cleft of soft and/or hard palate and overcrowding of teeth. Progressive distortion of the midface adds to the dysharmony of the upper and lower jaw, resulting in a grotesque facial appearance.

The broad thumbs are usually described as spatulate, short, stubby, clubbed, and large (Fig. 8-10B). Radial angulation of the distal phalanx of the thumb is common. Other fingers tend to be somewhat broad and short. Persistent fetal pad of the fingertip is a peculiar feature of RTS. The broadening of the hallux is often overlooked because of the great range of normal variation. Nail anomalies of the hallucies often reflect duplication of the underlying bony structures. While polydactyly of the hallux is common, duplication of the thumb is rare.

Most structural cardiac defects seen in RTS are flow lesions. The significant incidence and potential severity of cardiac anomalies warrant strong consideration of cardiac evaluation in patients with RTS.[174] Structural and functional urinary tract abnormalities in both genders and cryptorchidism in males have been reported.[95]

Hypotonia and various skeletal anomalies including atlantoaxial instability, vertebral anomalies, scoliosis and kyphosis, spina bifida occulta, and sternal and rib anomalies are present in nearly half of the patients with RTS.[160]

Stridor, hoarseness, husky voice, and laryngospasm have been repeatedly observed in patients with RTS. Keloid formation is increased in RTS. Certain tumors, including medulloblastoma, neuroblastoma, oligodendroglioma, pheochromocytoma, rhabdomyosarcoma, leiomyosarcoma, pinealoma, and angioblastic meningioma have all been reported in RTS.[124,175]

Prenatal growth appears to be normal, while postnatally the weight, height, and head circumference fall below the 5th percentile in the first few months of life. Height velocity is relatively normal, except for the lack of a pubertal growth spurt, which probably contributes to the short stature.[175]

Patients with RTS have an increased risk when undergoing general anesthesia because of their high arched palate, crowded teeth, laryngospasm, propensity for cardiac arrhythmias, and atlantoaxial instability. Sleep disturbances in RTS may result from these above abnormalities as well.[72,175]

The medical history of patients with RTS is often characterized by feeding difficulties, recurrent respiratory and ear infections, and severe chronic constipation.[175] The ages of puberty and menarche do not differ from those of the general population.

Inheritance

See Etiology.

Prognosis

In general, individuals with RTS have global developmental delay. They frequently experience speech difficulties. Mental retardation may vary from mild to severe. The average IQ score for RTS patients is 51. Patients with RTS usually display pleasant personality traits—happy, loving, and friendly. At the same time, they may engage in self-stimulatory behaviors.[175]

WALKER–WARBURG SYNDROME (WWS)

Walker–Warburg syndrome (WWS) is an autosomal recessive genetic disorder characterized by malformation of the brain and the eyes with muscular dystrophy. Walker published the first description of a lethal case with lissencephaly, hydrocephalus, microphthalmia, and retinal dysplasia.[197] Warburg reviewed similar cases and noted that most patients with this condition did not live past infancy.[200] WWS is also known as HARD+/−E, an abbreviation for hydrocephalus, agyria, and retinal dysplasia, with or without encephalocele, as well as COMS (cerebro-ocular-muscular dystrophy syndrome), and MEB (muscle–eye–brain disease).[46,143,186]

Etiology

The etiology of WWS is unknown.

Clinical Features and Assessment

Of the three minimal criteria required for the diagnosis of WWS, retinal dysplasia is the ophthalmic manifestation required to meet diagnostic criteria.[144] Retinal dystrophy often manifests as bilateral leukocoria and results from dysplastic retinae that are pale or elevated and unattached. This nonattachment of the retina can be used for prenatal ultrasound diagnosis.[27] Persistent hyperplastic primary vitreous and Peter's anomaly can also create the leukocoria noted in this syndrome. Microphthalmia and coloboma of the choroid and disc have been described. Postmortem examination of the eyes may be necessary to detect the full range of ocular involvement seen in these patients.[144] Total agenesis of the optic nerves and pathways has been reported.[206] Posterior lenticonus and ectopia lentis have all been described in postmortem examination.[112] A distinct "leopard spot" retinopathy has also been described in two sibling cases with the characteristic brain and muscle pathology found in WWS.[7]

Systemic Associations

Type II lissencephaly with widespread agyria and scattered areas of macrogyria and/or polymicrogyria are invariably present in patients with WWS. In addition to the typical neuronal migrational abnormalities, the cerebral cortex is abnormally thick and severely disorganized with absent white matter interdigitations. Various midline developmental abnormalities of the CNS may also be present.[46] Cerebellar malformations are present in all patients with WWS. Hypoplasia of the cerebellar vermis is often associated with enlargement of the fourth ventricle to form a retrocerebellar cyst, usually referred to as Dandy–Walker malformation.[203] Posterior encephaloceles are an important but inconstant (25%–50%) manifestation of WWS. Enlargement of the ventricular system with or without progressive hydrocephalus is very frequent (53%–95%).[46]

The other hallmark of WWS is a congenital muscular dystrophy; this presents with hypotonia at birth, variable congenital contractures, an elevated serum creatine kinase, "myopathic" changes on electromyography (EMG), and pathological changes in muscle tissue.[46] The disruption in the basal lamina may play a primary role in the degeneration of muscle fibers in WWS.[192] Occasionally patients with WWS may have cleft lip/palate, renal dysplasia, and genital anomalies in males.[97]

The spectrum of WWS was delineated by Dobyns et al.[46] and includes several disorders considered previously to be distinct: the cerebro-ocular-muscular syndrome (COMS) and muscle–eye–brain syndrome (MEB).[46] Patients with Fukuyama congenital muscular dystrophy (FCMD) may have features that overlap with WWS. However, haplotype analysis using polymorphic microsatellites flanking the FCMD locus on 9q31–q33 failed to demonstrate links between WWS and FCMD.[166] Clinical characteristics in WWS tend to be more severe than in FCMD. Molecular studies, however, have demonstrated a broader clinical spectrum of FCMD than it was previously presumed.[207] Therefore, it is possible that some of the severe cases of FCMD in the past may have been misclassified as WWS. The classification of these disorders will remain difficult until the molecular base of each of these conditions becomes available.

Inheritance

WWS is an autosomal recessive genetic defect, with 25% recurrence risk in families with an affected child. Prenatal diagnosis of eye and CNS malformations by fetal ultrasonography for at-risk families should be the standard of care. In cases with negative family history where brain dysgenesis is detected prenatally, the possibility of WWS should be raised.[27]

Prognosis

The majority of affected children with WWS usually die within the first 60 days of life.[46] However, 5% to 10% of affected infants with less severe retardation may survive more than 5 years. In these cases, severe psychomotor retardation, muscle hypotonia, visual impairment, and progressive seizure disorder are common.[104]

References

1. Aicardi J, Lefebvre J, Lerique-Koechlin A. A new syndrome: spasms in flexion, callosal agenesis, ocular abnormalities. Electroencephalogr Clin Neurophysiol 1965;19:609–610.

2. Allanson J. Rubinstein–Taybi syndrome: the changing face. Am J Med Genet Suppl 1990;6:38–41.

3. Alport A. Hereditary familial congenital haemorrhagic nephritis. Br Med J 1927;1:504–506.

4. Alström C, Hallgren B, Nilsson L, et al. Retinal degeneration combined with obesity, diabetes mellitus, and neurogenous deafness. A specific syndrome (not hitherto described) distinct from the Laurence–Moon–Bardet–Biedel syndrome. A clinical, endocrinological, and genetic examination based on a large pedigree. Acta Psychiatr Neurol Scand Suppl 1959;129:1–35.

5. Apkarian P, Spekreijse H, Swaay E, et al. Visual evoked potentials in Prader–Willi syndrome. Doc Ophthalmol 1989;71:355–367.

6. Barker D, Hostikka S, Zhou J, et al. Identification in the COL4A5 collagen gene in Alport syndrome. Science 1990;248:1224–1227.

7. Barth R, Pagon R, Bunt-Milam A. 'Leopard spot' retinopathy in Warburg syndrome. Ophthalmic Paediatr Genet 1986;7(2):91–96.

8. Bass H. Nephritis-deafness (sensorineural) hereditary type. In: Buyse ML (ed) Birth defect encyclopedia. Cambridge: Blackwell, 1990:1222.

9. Bertoni J, von Loh S, Allen R. The Aicardi syndrome: report of 4 cases and review of the literature. Ann Neurol 1979;5:475–482.

10. Biesecker L, Happle R, Mulliken J, et al. Proteus syndrome: diagnostic criteria, differential diagnosis, and patient evaluation. Am J Med Genet 1999;84:389–395.

11. Bowling B, Chandna A. Superior lacrimal canalicular atresia and nasolacrimal duct obstruction in the CHARGE association. J Pediatr Ophthalmol Strabismus 1994;31:336–337.

12. Braddock S, Lachman R, Charman C, et al. Radiological features in Brachmann–de Lange syndrome. Am J Med Genet 1993;47:1006–1013.

13. Bray G, Wilson W. Prader–Labhart–Willi syndrome: an overview. Growth Genet Horm 1986;2(3):1–5.

14. Brilliant M, King R, Francke U, et al. The mouse pink-eyed dilution gene: association with hypopigmentation in Prader–Willi and Angelman syndromes and with human OCA2. Pigment Cell Res 1994;7(6):398–340.

15. Breuning M, Dauwerse H, Fugazza G, et al. Rubinstein–Taybi syndrome caused by submicroscopic deletion within 16p13.3. Am J Med Genet 1993;52:249–254.

16. Brooks J, Leonard C, Coccaro P. Opitz (BBB/G) syndrome: oral manifestations. Am J Med Genet 1992;43:595–601.

17. Brosh R, Balajee A, Selzer R, et al. The ATPase domain but not the acidic region of Cockayne syndrome group B gene product is essential for DNA repair. Mol Biol Cell 1999;10(11):3583–3594.

18. Burke J, Clearkin L, Talbot J. Recurrent corneal epithelial erosions in Alport's syndrome. Acta Ophthalmol (Copenh) 1991;69:555–557.

19. Burke L, Jones M. Kabuki syndrome: underdiagnosed recognizable pattern in cleft palate patients. Cleft Palate Craniofac J 1995;32:77–84.

20. Butler M. Hypopigmentation: a common feature of Prader–Willi syndrome. Am J Hum Genet 1989;45:140–146.

21. Butler M, Meaney F. Standards for selected anthropometric measurements in Prader–Willi syndrome. Pediatrics 1991;88:853–860.

22. Carcione A, Piro E, Albano S, et al. Kabuki make-up (Niikawa–Kuroki) syndrome: clinical and radiological observations in two Sicilian children. Pediatr Radiol 1991;21:428–431.

23. Carney S, Brodsky M, Good W, et al. Aicardi syndrome: more than meets the eye. Surv Ophthalmol 1993;37:419–424.

24. Cassidy S, McKillop J, Morgan W. Sleep disorders in Prader–Willi syndrome. Dysmorph Clin Genet 1990;4:13–17.

25. Cassidy S. Prader–Willi syndrome. Curr Probl Pediatr 1984;14:1–55.

26. Chevrie J, Aicardi J. The Aicardi syndrome. In: Pedley TA, Meldrum BS (eds) Recent advances in epilepsy. New York: Churchill Livingstone, 1986:189–210.

27. Chitayat D, Toi A, Babul R, et al. Prenatal diagnosis of retinal nonattachment in the Walker–Warburg syndrome. Am J Med Genet 1995;56:351–358.

28. Chu D, Finley S, Young D, et al. CNS malformation in a child with Kabuki (Niikawa–Kuroki) syndrome: report and review. Am J Med Genet 1997;72:205–209.

29. Clementi M, Tenconi R, Turolla L, et al. Apparent CHARGE association and chromosome anomaly: chance or contiguous gene syndrome. Am J Med Genet 1991;42:246–250.

30. Cochat P, Guibaud P, Garcia-Torres R, et al. Diffuse leiomyomatosis in Alport syndrome. J Pediatr 1988;113:339–343.

31. Cockayne E. Dwarfism with retinal atrophy and deafness. Arch Dis Child 1936;11:1–8.

32. Cohen M. Understanding Proteus syndrome, unmasking the elephant man, and stemming elephant fever. Neurofibromatosis 1988; 1:260.

33. Cohen M Jr. Proteus syndrome: clinical evidence for somatic mosaicism and selective review. Am J Med Genet 1993;47:645–652.

34. Cohen M Jr, Hayden P. A newly recognized hamartomatous syndrome. In: Bergsma D (ed) Penetrance and variability in malformation syndromes. New York: Liss, 1979:291–296.

35. Collin G, Marshall J, Cardon L, et al. Homozygosity mapping at Alstrom syndrome to chromosome 2p. Hum Mol Genet 1997;6:213–219.

36. Cosgrove D, Rogers K, Meehan D, et al. Integrin alpha1beta 1 and transforming growth factor-beta1 play distinctive roles in Alport glomerular pathogenesis and serves as dual targets for metabolic therapy. Am J Pathol 2000;157(5):1649–1659.

37. Costa T, Greer W, Rysiecki G, et al. Monozygotic twins discordant for Aicardi syndrome. J Med Genet 1997;34:688–691.

38. Creel D, Bendel C, Wiesner G, et al. Abnormalities of the central visual pathways in Prader–Willi syndrome associated with hypopigmentation. N Engl J Med 1986;314:1606–1609.

39. Crnic K, Sulzbacher S, Snow J, et al. Preventing mental retardation associated with gross obesity in the Prader–Willi syndrome. Pediatrics 1982;66:787–789.

40. Davenport S, Hefner M, Mitchell J. The spectrum of clinical features in CHARGE syndrome. Clin Genet 1986;29:298–310.

41. Davenport S, Hefner M, Thelin J. CHARGE syndrome. External ear anomalies. Int J Pediatr Otorhinolaryngol 1986;12:137–141.

42. De Becker I, Gajda D, Gilbert-Barness E, et al. Ocular manifestations in Proteus syndrome. Am J Med Genet 2000;92:350–352.

43. de Lange C. Sur un type nouveau de generation (typus Amstelodamensis). Arch Med Enfant 1933;36:713–719.

44. Del Pero R, Mets M, Tripathi R, et al. Anomalies of retinal architecture in Aicardi syndrome. Arch Ophthalmol 1986;104:1659–1664.

45. Denslow G, Robb R. Aicardi's syndrome. A report of four cases and review of the literature. J Pediatr Ophthalmol Strabismus 1979;16: 10–15.

46. Dobyns W, Pagon R, Armstrong D, et al. Diagnostic criteria for Walker–Warburg syndrome. Am J Med Genet 1989;32:195–210.

47. Donnenfeld A, Packer R, Zackai E, et al. Clinical, cytogenetic, and pedigree findings in 18 cases of Aicardi syndrome. Am J Med Genet 1989;32:461–467.

48. Driscoll D, Waters M, Williams C, et al. A DNA methylation imprint, determined by the sex of the parent, distinguishes the Angelman and Prader–Willi syndromes. Genomics 1992;13:917–924.

49. Falek A, Schidt R, Jervis G. Familial de Lange syndrome with chromosome abnormalities. Pediatrics 1966;37:92–101.

50. Feingold J, Levy M, Broyer M, et al. Genetic heterogeneity of Alport syndrome. Kidney Int 1985;27:672–677.

51. Fielding D. Recurrence of orbital cysts in the branchio-oculo-facial syndrome. J Med Genet 1992;29:430–431.

52. Flinter F. Molecular genetics of Alport's syndrome. Q J Med 1993;96: 289–292.

53. Font R, Marines H, Cartwright J, et al. Aicardi syndrome: clinicopathological case report and electron microscopic observations. Ophthalmology 1991;98:1727–1731.

54. France N, Abraham J. Pathological features in the de Lange syndrome. Acta Paediatr Scand 1969;58:470–480.

55. Fujimoto A, Lipson M, Lacro R, et al. New autosomal dominant branchio-oculo-facial syndrome. Am J Med Genet 1987;27:943–951.

56. Futterweit W, Ritch R, Teekhasaenee C, et al. Coexistence of Prader–Willi syndrome, congenital ectropion uveae with glaucoma, and Factor XI deficiency. JAMA 1986;255(23):3280–3282.

57. Ganesh A, Mitra S, Koul R, et al. The full spectrum of persistent fetal vasculature in Aicardi syndrome: an integrated interpretation of ocular malformations [Letter]. Br J Ophthalmol 2000;84:227–228.

58. Gehrs K, Pollock S, Zilkha G. Clinical features and pathogenesis of Alport retinopathy. Retina 1995;15:305–311.

59. Gelisken Ö, Hendrikse F, Schröder C, et al. Retinal abnormalities in Alport's syndrome. Acta Ophthalmol (Copenh) 1988;66:713–717.

60. Gilbert-Barness E, Cohen M Jr, Opitz J. Multiple meningiomas, craniofacial hyperostosis and retinal abnormalities in Proteus syndrome. Am J Med Genet 2000;93:234–240.

61. Gillessen-Kaesbach G, Gross S, Kaya-Westerloh S, et al. DNA methylation based testing of 450 patients suspected of having Prader–Willi syndrome. J Med Genet 1995;32:88–92.

62. Goldstein J, Fialkow P. The Alstrom syndrome. Report of three cases with further delineations of the clinical pathophysiological, and genetic aspects of the disorder. Medicine (Baltim) 1973;52:53–71.

63. Govan J. Ocular manifestations of Alport's syndrome: a hereditary disorder of basement membranes? Br J Ophthalmol 1983;67:493–503.

64. Greenberg F, Robinson L. Mild Brachmann–de Lange syndrome: changes of phenotype with age. Am J Med Genet 1989;32:90–92.

65. Gubler M, Antignac C, Knebelmann B. Inherited glomerular disease. In: Holliday M, Barratt T, Avner E (eds) Pediatric nephrology, 3rd edn. Baltimore: Williams & Wilkins, 1994:515–536.

66. Gubler M, Levy M, Broyer M. Alport's syndrome: a report of 58 cases and a review of the literature. Am J Med 1981;70:493–505.

67. Halal F, Gledhill R, Dudkiewicz A. Autosomal dominant inheritance of the Kabuki make-up (Niikawa–Kuroki) syndrome. Am J Med Genet 1989;33:376–381.

68. Hall B. Choanal atresia and associated multiple anomalies. J Pediatr 1979;95:395–398.

69. Hall B, de Lorimier A, Foster L. A new syndrome of haemangiomatous branchial clefts, lip pseudoclefts, and abnormal facial appearance. Am J Med Genet 1984;14:135–138.

70. Happle R. Cutaneous manifestation of lethal genes. Hum Genet 1986;72:280.

71. Hayashi N, Valdes-Dapena M, Green W. CHARGE association: histopathological report of two cases and a review. J Pediatr Ophthalmol Strabismus 1998;35:100–106.

72. Hennekam R, Van Den Boogaard M, Sibbles B, et al. Rubinstein–Taybi syndrome in the Netherlands. Am J Med Genet Suppl 1990;6:17–29.

73. Hered R, Rogers S, Zang Y, et al. Ophthalmologic features of Prader–Willi syndrome. J Pediatr Ophthalmol Strabismus 1988;25:145–150.

74. Higginbottom M, Griswold W, Jones K, et al. The Cockayne syndrome: an evaluation of hypertension and studies of renal pathology. Pediatrics 1979;64:929–934.

75. Hoag H, Taylor S, Duncan A, et al. Evidence that skewed X inactivation is not needed for the phenotypic expression of Aicardi syndrome. Hum Genet 1997;100:459–464.

76. Hochgesand P, Steinbach P, Straub E. Augenveranderungen bei Alport-Syndrome. Klin Monatsbl Augenheilkd 1974;165:447–452.

77. Holm V, Cassidy S, Butler M, et al. Prader–Willi syndrome: consensus diagnostic criteria. Pediatrics 1993;91(2):398–402.

78. Holm V, Pipes P. Food and children with Prader–Willi syndrome. Am J Dis Child 1976;130:1063–1067.

79. Hopkins I, Humprey I, Keith C, et al. The Aicardi syndrome in a 47, XXY male. Aust Paediatr J 1979;15:278–280.

80. Howell L, Smith J. G syndrome and its otolaryngologic manifestations. Ann Otol Rhinol Laryngol 1989;98:185–190.

81. Hoyt C, Billson F, Ouvrier R, et al. Ocular features of Aicardi's syndrome. Arch Ophthalmol 1978;96:291–295.

82. Igawa H, Nishizawa N, Sugihara T, et al. Inner ear abnormalities in Kabuki make-up syndrome: report of three cases. Am J Med Genet 2000;92:87–89.

83. Ireland M, Donnai D, Burn J. Brachmann–de Lange syndrome. Delineation of the clinical phenotype. Am J Med Genet 1993;47:959–964.

84. Iversen U. Hereditary nephropathy with hearing loss: Alport's syndrome. Acta Paediatr Scand (Suppl) 1974;245:1–23.

85. Jackson L, Kline A, Barr M, et al. de Lange syndrome: a clinical review of 310 individuals. Am J Med Genet 1991;47:940–946.

86. Jacobs M, Jeffrey B, Kriss A, et al. Ophthalmologic assessment of young patients with Alport syndrome. Ophthalmology 1992;99(7):1039–1044.

87. Jones K. Recognizable patterns of human malformations, 5th edn. Philadelphia: Saunders, 1997:202–205.

88. Jones K. Smith's recognizable patterns of human malformation, 5th edn. Philadelphia: Saunders, 1997:88–91.

89. Jones K. Smith's recognizable patterns of human malformation, 5th edn. Philadelphia: Saunders, 1997:668–670.

90. Jones K. Smith's recognizable patterns of human malformation, 5th edn. Philadelphia, Saunders, 1997:144–145.

91. Jones K. Smith's recognizable patterns of human malformation, 5th edn. Philadelphia: Saunders, 1997:138–141.

92. Jones K. Smith's recognizable patterns of human malformation, 5th edn. Philadelphia: Saunders, 1997:174–175.

93. Jones K. Smith's recognizable patterns of human malformation, 5th edn. Philadelphia: Saunders, 1997:116–117.

94. Jones K. Smith's recognizable patterns of human malformation, 5th edn. Philadelphia: Saunders, 1997:132–135.

95. Jones K. Smith's recognizable patterns of human malformation, 5th edn. Philadelphia: Saunders, 1997:92–95.

96. Jones K. Smith's recognizable patterns of human malformation, 5th edn. Philadelphia: Saunders, 1997:512–513.

97. Jones K. Smith's recognizable patterns of human malformation. Philadelphia: Saunders, 1997:192–193.

98. Johnson H, Ekman P, Friesen W, et al. A behavioral phenotype in the de Lange syndrome. Pediatr Res 1976;10:843–850.

99. Junk A, Stefani F, Ludwing K. Bilateral anterior lenticonus: Scheimpflug imaging system documentation and ultrastructural confirmation of Alport syndrome in the lens capsule. Arch Ophthalmol 2000;118(7):895–897.

100. Kaplan L. Choanal atresia and its associated anomalies: further support for the CHARGE association. Int J Pediatr Otorhinolaryngol 1985;8:237–242.

101. Kashtan C, Michael A. Alport syndrome. Kidney Int 1996;50:1445–1463.

102. Katai N, Urakawa Y, Sato Y, et al. CHARGE association with congenital glaucoma due to maldevelopment of the anterior chamber angle. Acta Ophthalmol Scand 1997;75:322–324.

103. Kiristioglu I, Kilic N, Gurpinar A, et al. Aicardi syndrome associated with palatal hemangioma. Eur J Pediatr Surg 1999;9(5):325–326.

104. Korinthenberg R, Palm D, Schlake W, et al. Congenital muscular dystrophy, brain malformation and ocular problems (muscle, eye and brain disease) in two German families. Eur J Pediatr 1984;142:62–68.

105. Kuroki Y, Suzuki Y, Chyo H, et al. A new malformation syndrome of long palpebral fissures, large ears, depressed nasal tip, and skeletal anomalies associated postnatal dwarfism and mental retardation. J Pediatr 1981;99:570–573.

106. Ledbetter D, Riccardi V, Airhart S, et al. Deletion of chromosome 15 as a cause of the Prader–Willi syndrome. N Engl J Med 1981;304:325–329.

107. Lee W, Root A, Fenske N. Bilateral branchial cleft sinuses associated with intrauterine and postnatal growth retardation, premature aging and unusual facial appearance: a new syndrome with dominant transmission. Am J Med Genet 1982;11:345–352.

108. Legius E, Fryns J, Van der Burgt I. Dominant branchial cleft syndrome with characteristics of both branchio-oto-renal and branchio-oculo-facial syndrome. Clin Genet 1990;37:347–350.

109. Lemmink H, Schroder C, Monnens L, et al. The clinical spectrum of the type IV collagen mutations. Hum Mutat 1997;9:477–499.

110. Levin A, Seidman D, Nelson L, et al. Ophthalmologic findings in the Cornelia de Lange syndrome. J Pediatr Ophthalmol Strabismus 1990;27(2):94–102.

111. Levin P, Green W, Victor D, et al. Histopathology of the eye in Cockayne's syndrome. Arch Ophthalmol 1983;101:1093–1097.

112. Levine R, Gray D, Gould N, et al. Warburg syndrome. Ophthalmology 1983;90:1600–1603.

113. Levy N. Juvenile glaucoma in the Rubinstein–Taybi syndrome. J Pediatr Ophthalmol 1976;13(3):141–143.

114. Lin A, Chin A, Devine W, et al. The pattern of cardiovascular malformation in the CHARGE association. Am J Dis Child 1987;141: 1010–1013.

115. Lin A, Gorlin R, Lurie I, et al. Further delineation of the branchio-oculo-facial syndrome. Am J Med Genet 1995;56:42–59.

116. Lin A, Semina E, Daack-Hirsch S, et al. Exclusion of the branchio-oto-renal syndrome lLocus (EYA1) from patients with branchio-oculo-facial syndrome. Am J Med Genet 2000;91:387–390.

117. Lin A, Siebert J, Graham J. Central nervous system malformations in the CHARGE association. Am J Med Genet 1990;37:304–310.

118. MacDonald M, Schaefer G, Olney A, et al. Brain magnetic resonance imaging findings in the Opitz G/BBB syndrome: extension of the spectrum of midline brain anomalies. Am J Med Genet 1993;46: 706–711.

119. May M, Huston S, Wilroy R, et al. Linkage analysis in a family with the Opitz GBBB syndrome refines the location of the gene in Xp22 to a 4cM region. Am J Med Genet 1997;68:244–248.

120. Mayatepek E, Kurczynski T, Ruppert E, et al. Expanding the phenotype of the Proteus syndrome: a severely affected patient with new findings. Am J Med Genet 1989;32:402–406.

121. McCarthy P, Maino D. Alport syndrome: a review. Clin Eye Vis Care 2000;12(3–4):139–150.

122. McLaughlin E, Brown L, Weiss S, et al. VEGF and its receptors are expressed in a pediatric angiosarcoma in a patient with Aicardi's syndrome. J Investig Dermatol 2000;114(6):1209–1210.

123. Menezes A, Lewis T, Buncic J. Role of ocular involvement in the prediction of visual development and clinical prognosis in Aicardi syndrome. Br J Ophthalmol 1996;80:805–811.

124. Miller R, Rubinstein J. Tumors in Rubinstein–Taybi syndrome. Am J Med Genet 1995;56:112–115.

125. Milliner D, Pierides A, Holley K. Renal transplantation in Alport's syndrome: anti-glomerular basement membrane glomerulonephritis in the allograft. Mayo Clin Proc 1982;57:35–43.

126. Molina J, Mateos F, Merino M, et al. Aicardi syndrome in two sisters. J Pediatr 1989;115:282–283.

127. Moosa A, Dubowitz V. Peripheral neuropathy in Cockayne's syndrome. Arch Dis Child 1970;45:674–677.

128. Nance M, Berry S. Cockayne syndrome: review of 140 cases. Am J Med Genet 1992;42:68–84.

129. Neri G, Cappa M. The Opitz syndrome [Letter]. Am J Med Genet 1988;30:851.

130. Nicholls R. Genomic imprinting and candidate genes in the Prader–Willi and Angelman syndromes. Curr Opin Genet Dev 1993;3:445–456.

131. Nielsen C. Lenticonus anterior and Alport's syndrome. Acta Ophthalmol (Copenh) 1978;56:518–530.

132. Nielsen K, Anvert M, Flodmark O, et al. Aicardi syndrome: early neurological manifestations and results of DNA studies in one patient. Am J Med Genet 1991;38:65–68.

133. Niikawa N, Kuroki Y, Kajii T, et al. Kabuki make-up (Niikawa–Kuroki) syndrome: a study of 62 patients. Am J Med Genet 1988;31:565–589.

134. Niikawa N, Matsuura N, Fukushima Y, et al. Kabuki make-up syndrome: a syndrome of mental retardation, unusual facies, large and protruding ears, and postnatal growth deficiency. J Pediatr 1981;99:565–569.

135. Noben-Trauth K, Naggert J, North M, et al. A candidate gene for the mouse mutation tubby. Nature (Lond) 1996;380:534–538.

136. Ohlemiller K, Hughes R, Mosinger-Ogilvie J, et al. Cochlear and retinal degeneration in the tubby mouse.Neuroreport 1995;6:845–849.

137. Olitsky S, Was W, Wilson M. Rupture of the anterior lens capsule in Alport syndrome. J Am Assoc Pediatr Ophthalmol Strabismus 1999;3:381–382.

138. Opitz J. G syndrome (hypertelorism with esophageal abnormality and hypospadias, or hypospadias-dysphagia, or "Opitz-Frias" or "Opitz-G" syndrome): perspective in 1987 and bibliography. Am J Med Genet 1987;28:275–285.

139. Opitz J. The Brachmann–de Lange syndrome [Editorial]. Am J Med Genet 1985;22:89–102.

140. Opitz J, Frias J, Gutenberger J, et al. The G syndrome of multiple congenital anomalies. In: Bergsma D (ed) The clinical delineation of birth defects. Part II. Malformation syndromes, vol 5. New York: The National Foundation, 1969:5:95–101.

141. Opitz J, Summitt R, Smith D. The BBB syndrome. Familial telecanthus with associated congenital anomalies. In: Bergsma D (ed) The clinical delineation of birth defects. Part II. Malformation syndromes, vol 5. New York: The National Foundation, 1969:86–94.

142. Oto S, Aydin P. Spontaneous anterior capsular rupture in Alport syndrome. Eye 1998;12:152–153.

143. Pagon R, Chandler J, Collie W, et al. Hydrocephalus, agyria retinal dysplasia, encephalocele (HARD+/−E) syndrome: an autosomal recessive condition. Birth Defects Orig Artic Ser 1978;14(6B):232–241.

144. Pagon R, Clarren S, Milam D Jr, et al. Autosomal recessive eye and brain anomalies: Warburg syndrome. J Pediatr 1983;102:542–546.

145. Pagon R, Downing A, Ruvalcaba R. Kabuki make-up syndrome in a Caucasian. Ophthalmic Paediatr Genet 1986;7(2):97–100.

146. Pagon R, Graham J, Zonana J, et al. Coloboma, congenital heart disease and choanal atresia with multiple anomalies: CHARGE association. J Pediatr 1981;99:223–227.

147. Pajari H, Setälä K, Heiskari N, et al. Ocular findings in 34 patients with Alport syndrome: correlation of the findings to mutations in COL4A5 gene. Acta Ophthalmol Scand 1999;77:214–217.

148. Patton M, Giannelli F, Francis A, et al. Early onset Cockayne's syndrome: case reports with neuropathological and fibroblast studies. J Med Genet 1989;26:154.

149. Perrin D, Jungers P, Grunfeld J, et al. Perimacular changes in Alport's syndrome. Clin Nephrol 1980;13(4):163–167.

150. Petri F, Giles R, Dauwerse H, et al. Rubinstein–Taybi syndrome caused by mutations in the transcriptional co-activator CBP. Nature (Lond) 1995;376:348–351.

151. Phillips H, Carter A, Kennedy J, et al. Aicardi syndrome: radiologic manifestations. Radiology 1978;127:453–455.

152. Prader A, Labhart A, Willi H. Ein syndrom von adipositas, klein-wuchs, kryptorchismus und oligophrenie nach myotonieartigem zustand im neugeborenenalter. Schweiz Med Wochenschr 1956;86:1260–1261.

153. Rhys C, Snyers B, Pirson Y. Recurrent corneal erosion associated with Alport's syndrome. Rapid communication. Kidney Int 1997;52(1):208–211.

154. Riccardi VM. Von Recklinghausen neurofibromatosis. N Engl J Med 1981;305:1617–1626.

155. Robin N, Feldman G, Aronson A, et al. Opitz syndrome is genetically heterogeneous, with locus on Xp22, and second locus on 22q11.2. Nat Genet 1995;11:459–461.

156. Robin N, Opitz J, Muenke M. Opitz G/BBB syndrome: Clinical comparisons of families linked to Xp22 and 22q, and a review of the literature. Am J Med Genet 1996;62:305–317.

157. Robinow M, Johnson F, Minella P. Aicardi syndrome, papilloma of the choroid plexus, cleft lip, and cleft of the posterior palate. J Pediatr 1984;104(3):404–405.

158. Roy M, Milot J, Polomeno R, et al. Ocular findings and visual evoked potential response in the Prader–Willi syndrome. Can J Ophthalmol 1992;27(6):307–312.

159. Roy F, Summitt R, Hiatt R, et al. Ocular manifestations of the Rubinstein–Taybi syndrome. Case report and review of the literature. Arch Ophthalmol 1968;79:272–278.

160. Rubinstein J. Broad thumb-hallux (Rubinstein–Taybi) syndrome. 1957–1988. Am J Med Genet Suppl 1990;6:3–16.

161. Rubinstein J, Taybi H. Broad thumbs and toes and facial abnormalities. A possible mental retardation syndrome. Am J Dis Child 1963;105:588–608.

162. Russell-Eggitt I, Blake K, Taylor D, et al. The eye in the CHARGE association. Br J Ophthalmol 1990;74:421–426.

163. Russell-Eggitt I, Taylor D, Clayton P, et al. Leber's congenital amaurosis—a new syndrome with a cardiomyopathy. Br J Ophthalmol 1989;73:250–254.

164. Russell-Eggitt I, Clayton P, Coffey R. Alström syndrome. Report of 22 cases and literature review. Ophthalmology 1998;105:1274–1280.

165. Sabates R, Krachmer J, Weingeist T. Ocular findings in Alport's syndrome. Ophthalmologica 1983;186:204–210.

166. Sasaki M, Kondo E, Yamashita Y, et al. A patient of Walker–Warburg syndrome with a haplotype different from that in Fukuyama-type muscular dystrophy. No To Hattatsu 1999;31(5):445–451.

167. Schweiger S, Forester J, Lehmann T, et al. The Opitz syndrome gene product, MID1, associate with microtubules. Proc Natl Acad Sci U S A 1999;96(6):2794–2799.

168. Sebag J, Albert D, Craft J. The Alström syndrome: ophthalmic histopathology and retinal ultrastructure. Br J Ophthalmol 1984;68: 494–501.

169. Serrano Gonzalez C, Prats Vinas J. Unilateral aplasia of the cerebellum in Aicardi's syndrome. Neurologia 1998;13(5):254–256.

170. Siebert J, Graham J, McDonald C. Pathologic features of the CHARGE association. Support for involvement of the neural crest. Teratology 1985;31:331–336.

171. Silengo M, Lerone M, Seri M, et al. Inheritance of Niikawa–Kuroki (Kabuki makeup) syndrome [Letter]. Am J Med Genet 1996;66:368.

172. Smith C, Ryan S, Hoover S, et al. Magnetic resonance imaging of the brain in Aicardi's syndrome. Report of 20 patients. J Neuroimaging 1996;6(4):214–221.

173. Smith M, Herrell S, Lusher M, et al. Genomic organization of the human chordin gene and mutation screening of candidate Cornelia de Lange syndrome genes. Hum Genet 1999;105(1–2):104–111.

174. Stevens C, Bhakta M. Cardiac abnormalities in the Rubinstein–Taybi syndrome. Am J Med Genet 1995;59:346–348.

175. Stevens C, Carey J, Blackburn B. Rubinstein–Taybi syndrome: a natural history study. Am J Med Genet Suppl 1990;6:30–37.

176. Stevens C, Wilroy R. The telecanthus-hypospadias syndrome. J Med Genet 1988;25:536–542.

177. Streeten B, Robinson M, Wallace R, et al. Lens capsule abnormalities in Alport's syndrome. Arch Ophthalmol 1987;105:1693–1697.

178. Sugarman G, Landing B, Reed W. Cockayne syndrome: clinical study of two patients and neuropathologic findings of one. Clin Pediatr 1977;16(3)225–232.

179. Tagawa T, Mimaki T, Ono J, et al. Aicardi syndrome associated with an embryonal carcinoma. Pediatr Neurol 1989;5(1):45–47.

180. Taggard D, Menezes A. Three choroid plexus papillomas in a patient with Aicardi syndrome. A case report. Pediatr Neurosurg 2000; 33(4):219–223.

181. Takada K, Becker L. Cockayne's syndrome: Report of two autopsy cases associated with neurofibrillary tangles. Clin Neuropathol 1986;5:64–68.

182. Tanaka T, Takakura H, Takashima S, et al. A rare case of Aicardi syndrome with severe brain malformation and hepatoblastoma. Brain Dev 1985;7:507–512.

183. Teekhasaenee C, Nimmanit S, Wutthipan S. Posterior polymorphous dystrophy and Alport syndrome. Ophthalmology 1991;98:1207–1215.

184. Tellier A, Cormier-Daire V, Abadie V, et al. CHARGE syndrome: report of 47 cases and review. Am J Med Genet 1998;76:402–409.

185. Thompson S, Deady J, Willshaw H, et al. Ocular signs in Alport's syndrome. Eye 1987;1:146–153.

186. Towfighi J, Sassani J, Suzuki K, et al. Cerebro-ocular-dysplasia-muscular dystrophy (COD-MD) syndrome. Acta Neuropathol 1984; 65:110–123.

187. Tremblay F, LaRoche R, Shea S, et al. Longitudinal study of the early electroretinographic changes in Alström syndrome. Am J Ophthalmol 1993;115:657–665.

188. Tsilou E, Rubin B, Caruso R, et al. A case of Alport's syndrome and retinal degeneration. Retina 2001;21(1):89–92.

189. Tsukahara M, Kuroki Y, Imaizumi K, et al. Dominant inheritence of Kabuki make-up syndrome. Am J Med Genet 1997;73:19–23.

190. Tsukahara M, Kuroki Y, Imaizumi K, et al. Dominant inheritance of Kabuki make-up syndrome. Am J Med Genet 1997;73(1):19–23.

191. Umansky W, Neidich J, Schendel S. The association of cleft lip and palate with Aicardi syndrome. Plast Reconstr Surg 1994;93:595–597.

192. Vajsar J, Ackerley C, Chitayat D, et al. Basal lamina abnormality in the skeletal muscle of Walker–Warburg syndrome. Pediatr Neurol 2000;22(2):139–143.

193. van der Loop F, Heidet L, Timmer E, et al. Autosomal dominant Alport syndrome caused by a COL4A3 splice site mutation. Kidney Int 2000;58(5):1870–1875.

194. Van Ellen M, Fillipi G, Siegel-Bartelt J, et al. Clinical variability within Brachmann-de Lange syndrome: a proposed classification system. Am J Med Genet 1993;47(7):947–958.

195. van Genderen M, Kinds G, Riemslag F, et al. Ocular features in Rubinstein–Taybi syndrome: investigation of 24 patients and review of the literature. Br J Ophthalmol 2000;84:1177–1184.

196. Vila-Coro A, Arnoult J, Robinson L, et al. Lacrimal anomalies in Brachmann–de Lange's syndrome [Letter]. Am J Ophthalmol 1988; 106(2):235–237.

197. Walker A. Lissencephaly. Schweiz Arch Neurol Psychiatr 1942;48: 13–29.

198. Wang X, Norose K, Kiyosawa K. Ocular findings in a patient with Prader–Willi syndrome. Jpn J Ophthalmol 1995;39(3):284–289.

199. Warburg M. Ocular coloboma and multiple congenital anomalies: the CHARGE association. Ophthalmic Paediatr Genet 1983;2:189–199.

200. Warburg M. The heterogeneity of microphthalmia in the mentally retarded. Birth Defects Orig Artic Ser 1971;VII(3):136–154.

201. Weaver R Jr, Seaton A, Jewett T. Short subjects. Bilateral Marcus Gunn (jaw-winking) phenomenon occurring with CHARGE association. J Pediatr Ophthalmol Strabismus 1997;34(5):308–309.

202. Wiedemann H, Burgio G, Aldenhoff P, et al. The Proteus syndrome: partial gigantism of the hands and/or feet, nevi, hemihypertrophy, subcutaneous tumors macrocephaly or other skull anomalies and possible accelerated growth and visceral affections. Eur J Pediatr 1983;140:5–12.

203. Williams R, Swisher C, Jennings M, et al. Cerebro-ocular dysgenesis (Walker–Warburg syndrome) neuropathologic and etiologic analysis. Neurology 1984;34:1531–1541.

204. Willis J, Rosman N. The Aicardi syndrome versus congenital infection: diagnostic considerations. J Pediatr 1980;96(2):235–239.

205. Wilson G. Thirteen cases of Niikawa–Kuroki syndrome: report and review with emphasis on medical complications and preventive management. Am J Med Genet 1998;79:112–120.

206. Yanoff M, Rorke L, Allman M. Bilateral optic system aplasia with relatively normal eyes. Arch Ophthalmol 1978;96:97–101.

207. Yoshioka M, Toda T, Kuroki S, et al. Broader clinical spectrum of Fukuyama-type congenital muscular dystrophy manifested by haplotype analysis. J Child Neurol 1999;14(11):711–715.

208. Zhou J, Hertz J, Tryggvason K. Mutation in the alpha-5 (IV) collagen chain in juvenile-onset Alport syndrome without hearing loss or ocular lesions: detection by denaturing gradient gel electrophoresis of a PCR product. Am J Hum Genet 1992;50:1291–1300.

9

Infectious Diseases

R. Christopher Walton, Roger K. George, and Alissa A. Craft

A number of pediatric infectious diseases have significant ophthalmic manifestations. These infections include both congenital and acquired disorders affecting children and adolescents. Congenital infections result from infection in utero and are often described by the acronym TORCH. The TORCH infections include toxoplasmosis, "other," rubella, cytomegalovirus, and herpes simplex. The "other" category includes syphilis, varicella, and several newer pathogens such as lymphocytic choriomeningitis virus. Acquired infectious diseases affecting children and adolescents with potentially serious ophthalmic manifestations include cat scratch disease, Lyme disease, toxocariasis, measles, rubella, and varicella. The systemic and ocular manifestations of many of these diseases as well as their diagnosis and treatment are discussed in this chapter.

BACTERIAL DISEASES

Cat Scratch Disease

Cat scratch disease is a relatively benign, self-limited illness caused by the fastidious gram-negative bacillus, *Bartonella henselae*. The disease is typically transmitted via the scratch or bite of a cat or kitten. It is characterized by lymphadenopathy of local lymph nodes draining the site of infection. Common ocular manifestations include *Parinaud's oculoglandular syndrome*, neuroretinitis, and focal chorioretinitis.

INCIDENCE

Cat scratch disease has been estimated to affect 22,000 patients annually in the United States.[60] Children and young adults appear to be at increased risk for the disease, especially during the fall and early winter months.[39] Ocular manifestations develop in up to 10% of patients with cat scratch disease.

ETIOLOGY

Bartonella henselae is the etiological agent in cat scratch disease. Cats are the primary mammalian reservoir for *B. henselae*, and most infections are transmitted through the scratch or bite of a cat, especially cats less than 1 year of age.[64] Rates of cat infection are higher in kittens, free-ranging cats, and flea-infested cats.[28,64] Additionally, *B. henselae* seropositivity of cats is higher in warmer regions and areas with higher amounts of annual rainfall.

CLINICAL FEATURES

Ocular complications are not uncommon in cat scratch disease. Parinaud's oculoglandular syndrome is the most common ocular manifestation and typically develops within 1 to 2 weeks following exposure. The syndrome is characterized by unilateral granulomatous conjunctivitis with tender preauricular and sub-mandibular adenopathy.[18] Granulomatous nodules may occur on the palpebral or bulbar conjunctiva.[28]

Neuroretinitis characterized by optic disc edema with a partial or complete macular star occurs in up to 2% of patients with cat scratch disease (Fig. 9-1).[18,89] Most cases are unilateral although several cases have been reported with bilateral involvement.[127] Although most patients will develop a macular star, some manifest optic disc swelling alone or with subretinal and intraretinal exudates.[29,126]

Additional posterior segment manifestations of cat scratch disease have been described. Isolated foci of retinitis or choroiditis involving the outer retina or choroid or the superficial retina are not uncommon.[117] These areas of retinitis or choroiditis have also been described in patients with neuroretinitis.[46,128] Other posterior segment manifestations of cat scratch disease include serous retinal detachment, intermediate uveitis, retinal vascular occlusions, optic nerve granuloma, vitreous hemorrhage, and macular edema.[63,90,117]

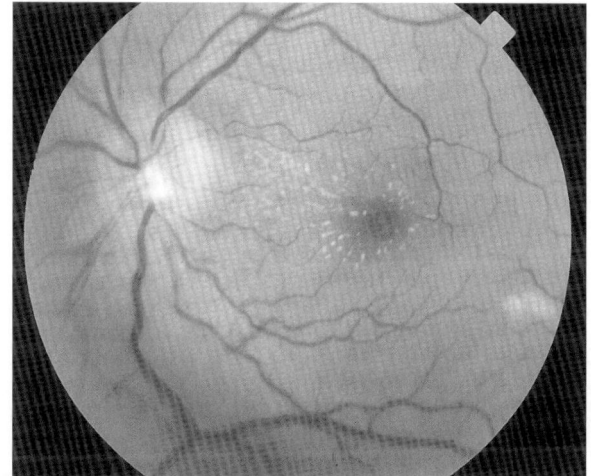

FIGURE 9-1. Eye of 16-year-old girl with cat scratch disease and neuroretinitis. Disc edema and macular star are present. There is a small area of retinitis temporal to the fovea.

CLINICAL ASSESSMENT

The diagnosis of cat scratch disease is established by the presence of specific clinical manifestations combined with serological testing for *B. henselae*. Currently available serologic tests include enzyme immunoassay, Western immunoblot, and indirect fluorescent antibody test. The enzyme immunoassay is the most sensitive and specific of the available tests.[69]

SYSTEMIC ASSOCIATIONS AND NATURAL HISTORY

Most patients with *B. henselae* infection develop a systemic flu-like illness. Typically, a papule or pustule develops at the site of inoculation approximately 3 to 10 days following a scratch or bite. One to 3 weeks later, patients develop constitutional symptoms including headache, nausea, vomiting, sore throat, anorexia, and tender regional lymphadenopathy.[119] In most patients, the systemic symptoms are relatively mild and resolve over several months.

INHERITANCE

No inheritance pattern.

TREATMENT

There are no clear treatment guidelines for the ocular complications of *B. henselae* infection. Some authors have advocated the use of antibiotics while others have recommended conservative, symptomatic treatment only.[55,68,98] The most effective antibiotics for *B. henselae* infection are rifampin, ciprofloxacin, intramuscular gentamicin, and trimethoprim-sulfamethoxazole.[71] When considering treatment of children with *B. henselae* infection, consultation with a pediatric infectious disease specialist should be obtained.

PROGNOSIS

In most cases, cat scratch disease is a relatively benign and self-limited infection. In general, patients with neuroretinitis have a good long-term prognosis although some may eventually develop a mild optic neuropathy.[98] Chorioretinal inflammatory foci typically resolve with no significant sequelae. Peripheral vascular occlusions also resolve without sequelae while vascular occlusions involving the macula may lead to visual impairment.[117]

Lyme Disease

Lyme borreliosis is a multisystem disease caused by the spirochete *Borrelia burgdorferi* which is transmitted by ticks of the *Ixodes* genus. Infection results in a progressive disease characterized by three stages: early, disseminated, and persistent. Ocular manifestations are not uncommon and can occur during any stage of Lyme disease.

INCIDENCE

In the United States, most cases of Lyme disease occur in the middle Atlantic states, southern New England, and the upper Midwest. Additional cases have been reported along the northern Pacific coast. Within these endemic areas, the annual incidence of Lyme disease ranges from 20 to 105 cases per 100,000 people.[110] Children from 5 to 10 years of age have the highest incidence of Lyme disease.

ETIOLOGY

Lyme disease is a zoonosis caused by the spirochete *Borrelia burgdorferi*. The disease is transmitted by infected ticks of the *Ixodes* genus. In the Middle Atlantic states and the upper Midwest, the deer tick *Ixodes scapularis* is the vector for Lyme borreliosis, whereas the western black-legged tick *Ixodes pacificus* is the vector for the disease along the northern Pacific coast.[110,120]

CLINICAL FEATURES

The ophthalmic manifestations of Lyme disease vary with the stage of the disease. Ocular manifestations during the early stage of Lyme disease include follicular conjunctivitis and episcleritis. Most of the ocular manifestations occur during disseminated disease and include cranial nerve palsies, optic nerve disorders, and uveitis. The most common cranial neuropathy is seventh cranial nerve palsy, which is bilateral in as many as one-third of cases.[25] Other cranial neuropathies include abducens nerve palsy, third, fourth, and fifth cranial nerve palsy, and multiple cranial nerve palsies. Optic nerve disorders include optic neuritis, papillitis, and papilledema.[67,116]

The spectrum of intraocular inflammation seen in Lyme disease includes intermediate uveitis, anterior uveitis, neuroretinitis, panuveitis, retinal vasculitis, and choroiditis.[62,130] Intermediate uveitis is one of the most common forms of uveitis and may be severe, with vitreous snowballs, vitreous cells, and marked vitreous haze.[16] Anterior uveitis may be nongranulomatous or granulomatous with mutton-fat keratic precipitates and iris nodules.

Stromal and subepithelial keratitis can occur during the persistent stage of the disease. Typically, bilateral focal infiltrates are located within the subepithelial layer and the stroma. Diffuse stromal keratitis may also occur in some patients.[6,37,65] The keratitis may be associated with keratic precipitates and corneal edema.

CLINICAL ASSESSMENT

Isolation of *B. burgdorferi* from a patient with specific clinical findings is considered diagnostic of Lyme borreliosis; however, positive cultures have been obtained only during the early stage of the disease.[11,110,120] Serological tests are insensitive during the first weeks of infection, and many of the commercial diagnostic kits for Lyme disease are inaccurate and may lead to misdiagnosis.[3,70] Therefore, the current recommendation for serological testing in patients suspected of Lyme borreliosis includes a two-step process to increase specificity. A quantitative enzyme-linked immunosorbent assay (ELISA) is used as the initial test for patients with a high probability of the disease. For patients with a positive or equivocal ELISA, a Western immunoblot should be performed to confirm the result.[22] The serological tests for Lyme borreliosis have a high rate of false-positive results and should not be used in patients with a low probability of the disease.[109,110] Instead, serological tests should be performed in selected patients with specific clinical findings suggestive of Lyme disease to ensure that the predictive value of the test is high.[84]

SYSTEMIC ASSOCIATIONS AND NATURAL HISTORY

Early infection manifests as localized erythema migrans, typically 7 to 10 days following the bite of an infected tick. This lesion is present in approximately 80% to 90% of patients and often begins as a red macule or papule that enlarges over weeks into an annular lesion if untreated. Patients often have associated symptoms including malaise, fatigue, headache, fever, arthralgias, myalgias, and regional lymphadenopathy during this stage.[110,120]

Disseminated disease develops several weeks following infection, and patients may develop skin, neurological, joint, and cardiac manifestations. Multiple *erythema migrans* may occur 3 to 5 weeks following the tick bite. Also during this period, neurological manifestations may develop including cranial nerve palsies, meningitis, papilledema, optic neuritis, and motor or sensory radiculoneuritis. As many as 60% of untreated patients develop intermittent arthritis that is typically monoarticular or oligoarticular. The arthritis usually affects the large joints, especially the knee.[120] Rarely, patients may develop cardiac complications, most commonly atrioventricular block and occasionally myocarditis or pericarditis.

INHERITANCE

No inheritance pattern.

TREATMENT

For children older than 8 years of age with early localized or disseminated disease, doxycycline for 14 to 21 days is recommended. For children less than 8 years of age, amoxicillin should be used.[120] Cefuroxime axetil may be used as a third choice in children allergic to either of these drugs. Children with neurological manifestations should be treated with intravenous ceftriaxone for 2 to 4 weeks. Lyme arthritis may be treated with doxycycline or intravenous ceftriaxone.

Currently, no specific guidelines have been established for the treatment of intraocular inflammation associated with Lyme borreliosis. Therapeutic options include oral doxycycline or intravenous ceftriaxone. Children with intraocular inflammation should undergo a neurological evaluation including cerebrospinal fluid examination. Intravenous ceftriaxone should be used in children with associated central nervous system manifestations. Isolated intraocular inflammation may be treated with doxycycline; however, the disease may recur after the antibiotic is discontinued.[130] In children with persistent or recurrent intraocular inflammation following doxycycline therapy, intravenous ceftriaxone may be useful.[122]

In addition to systemic antibiotic therapy, topical corticosteroids and cycloplegics are useful in the management of anterior uveitis. Topical corticosteroids are also useful for subepithelial and stromal keratitis. To avoid recurrence of keratitis, topical corticosteroids should be gradually tapered before discontinuation.

PROGNOSIS

The conjunctivitis and episcleritis seen during early disease are typically mild and self-limited.[120] Cranial nerve palsies also resolve in most patients with no long-term sequelae although they may recur in some cases. The keratitis responds to topical corticosteroid therapy, although recurrent cases have been described following abrupt cessation of therapy. Intraocular inflammation typically responds to systemic antibiotic therapy; however, some patients may develop chronic or relapsing uveitis despite appropriate antibiotic therapy.[122] Optic nerve involvement may result in optic atrophy in some patients.

Syphilis

Congenital syphilis continues to be an important cause of infant morbidity, especially in areas where prenatal care is inadequate. Children born to infected mothers acquire the disease through transplacental transmission or during passage through the birth canal. Approximately 50% of children born to infected mothers will develop congenital syphilis.[33] Acquired syphilis is also a significant public health problem for children and adolescents. The majority of cases of acquired syphilis in children and adolescents are sexually transmitted; however, children may also acquire syphilis during early childhood as a consequence of child abuse, breast-feeding, kissing, or handling.[104]

INCIDENCE

In 2000, 529 cases of congenital syphilis were reported to the Centers for Disease Control, resulting in a rate of 13.4 per 100,000 liveborn infants in the United States.[24] Minority populations and those in the southeastern United States have some of the highest rates of syphilis in the United States. The incidence of ocular manifestations in children infected with syphilis is uncertain.

ETIOLOGY

Syphilis is a systemic disease caused by the spirochete *Treponoma pallidum*. Sexual contact is the usual mode of transmission, although infection can occur by direct contact with infectious lesions.

CLINICAL FEATURES

Syphilis can affect most structures of the eye and adnexa in children. Clinical features seen in children with congenital infection include orbital periostitis, nasolacrimal duct stenosis, dacryoadenitis, papular skin rash of the eyelids, mucous patches of the conjunctiva, stromal keratitis, congenital cataract, acute iridocyclitis, glaucoma, chorioretinitis, chorioretinal scarring, and optic atrophy. In children with acquired syphilis, the ocular manifestations are similar to those seen in adults and vary by stage of the disease. In primary syphilis, chancres of the adnexa and conjunctiva may occur. Ocular manifestations of secondary syphilis include cranial nerve palsies associated with basilar meningitis, orbital periostitis, maculopapular rash of the eyelid skin, papillary conjunctivitis, episcleritis, marginal keratitis, granulomatous or nongranulomatous anterior uveitis, iris roseolae, lens subluxation, vitritis, diffuse or localized choroiditis or chorioretinitis, disc edema, exudative retinal detachment, neuroretinitis, retinal vasculitis, chorioretinal scars, optic neuritis, and optic perineuritis.[73]

CLINICAL ASSESSMENT

All pregnant women should be screened for syphilis at the time of their initial prenatal visit and at delivery. Nontreponemal tests such as the Venereal Disease Research Laboratory (VDRL) or rapid plasma regain (RPR) should be used as screening tests. Infants suspected of infection with *T. pallidum* should undergo a thorough evaluation for evidence of congenital infection that should include the following: physical examination, quantitative nontreponemal serological test for syphilis performed on the infant's serum, cerebrospinal fluid examination including VDRL, long bone X-rays, complete blood count with differential, platelet counts, and liver function tests. An ophthalmologic evaluation should be performed if there is evidence of infection. For those infants with no evidence of congenital syphilis following this evaluation, a specific antitreponemal IgM antibody test should be performed.[121]

Acquired syphilis in children is diagnosed using the methods for diagnosing syphilis in adults. Evaluation includes a direct fluorescent antibody test for *T. pallidum* in suspected lesions, as well as serological tests for syphilis. Children with a negative nontreponemal serological test for syphilis should have a treponemal test—fluorescent treponemal antibody absorption (FTA) or microhemagglutination treponema pallidum (MHA-TP)—performed.[97]

Neurosyphilis can occur during any stage of the disease. Ocular manifestations including syphilitic uveitis are often associated with neurosyphilis, and therefore children with these manifestations should have a cerebrospinal fluid examination.

SYSTEMIC ASSOCIATIONS AND NATURAL HISTORY

Congenital syphilis can be divided into early and late stages. Early congenital syphilis includes all the manifestations occurring from birth through the end of the second year of life. Clinical manifestations during early congenital syphilis include prematurity, low birth weight, respiratory symptoms, hepatosplenomegaly, generalized lymphadenopathy, mucocutaneous lesions, and skeletal abnormalities.[82] Snuffles is one of the earliest findings during early congenital syphilis. Copper-red macules and papules similar in appearance to acquired secondary syphilis may develop on the face, trunk, palms, soles, and genitalia. Other skin findings include condyloma lata and mucous patches. Skeletal abnormalities include osteochondritis, periostitis, and saddle-nose deformity. Ocular manifestations during this stage include chorioretinitis, uveitis, glaucoma, and optic atrophy. The chorioretinitis is typically bilateral and causes degeneration of the retinal pigment epithelium creating the "salt-and-pepper" appearance of the fundus.[112]

Late congenital syphilis occurs after the age of 2 years. This form of congenital syphilis may be difficult to differentiate from acquired syphilis. However, *Hutchison's triad* is still considered pathognomonic for late congenital syphilis and consists of notched, wide-spaced central incisors, eighth nerve deafness, and *interstitial keratitis*. Additional manifestations of late congenital syphilis include periostitis of the frontal and parietal bones as well as the long bones, synovitis of the knee, saddle nose, mental retardation, seizures, and gumma. Ocular manifestations include interstitial keratitis, uveitis, and glaucoma. Interstitial keratitis develops between the ages of 5 and 20 years.

Acquired syphilis during childhood and adolescence is similar to syphilis acquired during adulthood. Children may present with primary chancres or signs of secondary or latent syphilis.[97] Chancres seen in primary syphilis may occur on the genitalia similar to adults; however, children may develop lesions in other areas, depending on the site of inoculation.[41] Painless regional lymphadenopathy is also common during this stage of the disease. Chancres resolve within 3 to 6 weeks of onset with or without treatment.

Signs of secondary syphilis typically develop 6 to 8 weeks following the development of the chancre. Cutaneous manifestations are the most characteristic features of secondary syphilis and include macular, papular, follicular, pustular, or nodular lesions. Classic lesions are copper-red macular lesions found on the face, trunk, and the extremities, including the palms and soles.[91] This stage may include a prodrome of malaise, anorexia, fever, headache, sore throat, rhinorrhea, arthralgia, and lymphadenopathy. Other manifestations of secondary syphilis include patchy alopecia, asymptomatic central nervous system involvement or meningitis, uveitis, periostitis, polyarthritis, tenosynovitis, and glomerulonephritis. In most cases, the signs and symptoms of secondary syphilis resolve with or without treatment.

In patients with latent syphilis, serological tests are positive but no clinical signs or symptoms are present. Tertiary syphilis typically develops 10 to 20 years following the initial disease. Fortunately, tertiary syphilis is rare in children and adolescents and is not be discussed in this chapter.

INHERITANCE

No inheritance pattern.

TREATMENT

For children 4 weeks of age or younger, the current treatment recommendations are aqueous crystalline penicillin G 100,000 to 150,000 units/kg/day for 10 to 14 days (total dose divided and administered every 12 h during the first week of life and every 8 h thereafter) or daily intramuscular procaine penicillin G 50,000 units/kg/dose for 10 days.[23] Children older than 4 weeks of age with possible congenital syphilis should be treated with aqueous crystalline penicillin G 200,000 to 300,000 units/kg/day for 10 to 14 days (total dose divided and administered every 6 h).

Children with acquired primary or secondary syphilis should be treated with benzathine penicillin G 50,000 units/kg intramuscular, up to the adult dosage of 2.4 million units/kg as a single dose.[23] Children with clinical evidence of neurosyphilis or uveitis, neuroretinitis, or optic neuritis should be treated with intravenous aqueous crystalline penicillin G 18 to 24 million units daily, divided into 3 to 4 million units every 4 h for 10 to 14 days.[23] Topical corticosteroids and cycloplegics are also useful for children with anterior uveitis.

PARASITIC DISEASES

Toxocariasis

Toxocariasis is among the most common zoonotic infections affecting children in the United States. Ocular toxocariasis is an important cause of childhood uveitis and blindness.

INCIDENCE

Toxocariasis is the most common nematode infection affecting the eye in the United States; however, the exact incidence of ocular toxocariasis in unknown.

ETIOLOGY

Most cases of human toxocariasis are caused by infection with the dog intestinal roundworm *Toxocara canis* or, rarely, the cat roundworm *Toxocara catis*.[45,105] Ocular toxocariasis results from invasion of the eye by the second- or third-stage larva of the nematode. The dog is the definitive host and acquires the intestinal infection by several mechanisms including transplacental and transmammary transmission, ingestion of infective ova, ingestion of adults or larvae within feces or vomitus of infected puppies, and ingestion of larvae in tissues of paratenic hosts such as mice.[44,113]

Most puppies are infected in utero through transplacental migration of the larvae.[36] Children become infected after ingestion of eggs from contaminated soil, food, or other materials. Although most children acquire the infection by ingestion of contaminated soil, contact with puppies is a significant risk factor for the disease.

CLINICAL FEATURES

Approximately 80% of children with ocular toxocariasis are less than 16 years of age. A spectrum of ocular manifestations can occur in these children although several common ocular presentations have been described. The most common presentation is a unilateral granuloma of the posterior pole or peripheral retina. The posterior pole lesion is typically round, elevated, and up to two disc diameters in size (Fig. 9-2). Vitritis is relatively common and may be severe in some cases. Peripheral granuloma are hazy white elevated lesions located in the peripheral retina. Peripheral granuloma located in the inferior retina may resemble pars planitis in some children. Vitreous membranes are often visible radiating from the peripheral lesion and may form radial retinal folds extending to the optic nerve head.

Another common manifestation is chronic endophthalmitis.[113] These children often present with anterior uveitis, hypopyn, posterior synechiae, cyclitic membrane, vitritis, and retinal detachment. Leukocoria may be noted in some children

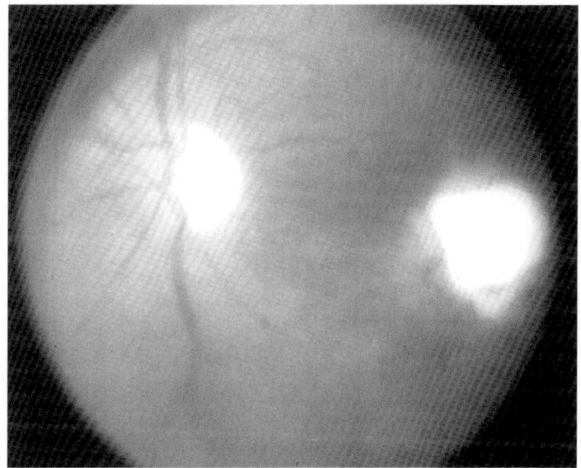

FIGURE 9-2. Ocular toxocariasis with posterior pole granuloma.

because of the severe inflammatory reaction. The inflammation may resolve without treatment in some cases revealing a more typical posterior pole or peripheral granuloma.

Children may also present to the ophthalmologist with no active inflammatory disease but instead with decreased visual acuity, amblyopia, or strabismus as a result of damage to the macula. These children may be detected during school screening examinations or as part of a routine examination.

CLINICAL ASSESSMENT

Ocular toxocariasis is a clinical diagnosis; however, serological tests are often useful when evaluating children with possible toxocariasis. Currently, ELISA tests for *Toxocara* spp. are the most accurate and widely used serological methods. Many laboratories report ELISA results as the number of standard deviations above a normal population. High serum titers are not common in children with ocular toxocariasis unless testing occurs during the acute phase of the disease.[92] On the other hand, vitreous specimens in ocular toxocariasis have higher ELISA titers compared to serum titers.[12]

SYSTEMIC ASSOCIATIONS AND NATURAL HISTORY

Systemic infection with *T. canis* or *T. catis* is known as *visceral larval migrans* (VLM). VLM occurs most commonly in children less than 6 years of age and is characterized by eosinophilia, fever, and hepatosplenomegaly.[44,45] Most infections are asymptomatic although some children may develop fulminant disease that may result in death. However, most children with ocular toxocariasis do not have VLM. In those cases where ocular disease and VLM are both present, children often present with flu-like symptoms such as cough, wheezing, fever, malaise, and weight loss.

The diagnosis of VLM should be considered in young children with eosinophilia and/or leukocytosis, and hepatomegaly. Less common manifestations include pulmonary symptoms, splenomegaly, and seizures. In most cases, a history of exposure to puppies and pica can be elicited. A definitive diagnosis requires identification of larvae in histological sections from affected tissues. Unfortunately, larvae are not apparent in many histological specimens and therefore serum ELISA tests are useful in confirming the diagnosis.

INHERITANCE

No inheritance pattern.

TREATMENT

The treatment of ocular toxocariasis must be individualized based on several factors including the severity of inflammation, macular involvement, and the visual potential of the eye. For children with active vitritis, periocular or systemic corticosteroids are useful to decrease the inflammatory response. In general, systemic corticosteroids may be the preferred therapy in children less than 10 years of age because multiple periocular corticosteroid injections are the rule in most cases. Systemic corticosteroids should be used at the lowest dosage to achieve the desired response and slowly tapered before discontinuation to avoid recurrence of inflammation. In children with associated anterior uveitis, topical corticosteroids and cycloplegic agents are useful. Thiabendazole at 50 mg/kg/day for 7 days may be considered in children who fail to respond to systemic corticosteroid therapy.[34]

The role of antihelminthic therapy for ocular toxocariasis remains uncertain. A number of reports have described improvement in ocular toxocariasis treated with several different anti-helminthic drugs including thiabendazole, diethylcarbamazine, albendazole, and mebendazole.[35,72] If antihelminthic therapy is considered, consultation with a pediatric infectious disease specialist should be considered because of the potential toxicity associated with several of these agents.

Surgical procedures may be necessary in some children with ocular toxocariasis. Pars plana vitrectomy may be useful in children with refractory vitritis, vitreous membranes, epiretinal membrane, and traction or rhegmatogenous retinal detachment.[49,100,115] Early vitrectomy has been advocated to reduce long-term visual morbidity in selected children.[9]

PROGNOSIS

The visual prognosis for children with ocular toxocariasis is dependent a number of factors. In children with inactive disease, direct damage to the retina may be evident as a macular scar, macular traction detachment, macular heterotopia, rhegmatogenous retinal detachment, and epiretinal membrane. Depending on the location, these lesions may be associated with severe visual loss, amblyopia, and strabismus. Loss of vision can also occur as a result of active posterior segment disease that is dependent on the location, severity, and duration of inflammation. The visual prognosis is also affected by complications resulting from the intraocular inflammation including glaucoma, cataract, cyclitic membrane, and phthisis.

Toxoplasmosis

Toxoplasmosis is the most common form of posterior uveitis in children and adults. In the past, most cases were thought to be caused by congenital infection, but there is increasing evidence that the acquired form of the disease is more common than previously reported.

INCIDENCE

Up to 3000 infants are born with congenital toxoplasmosis each year in the United States, and retinochoroiditic occurs in 70% to 90% of cases.[77] The incidence of ocular disease in children with acquired toxoplasmosis is uncertain although recent reports have suggested that as many as 21% of all patients with acquired disease may develop retinochoroiditis.[15,17]

ETIOLOGY

Toxoplasma gondii is a obligate intracellular protozoan parasite found throughout the world and the etiological agent of toxoplasmosis. Cats are the definitive host for *T. gondii* and are initially infected by eating contaminated meat. Within the cat's intestine, the parasite produces large numbers of oocysts that are shed in feces, thereby contaminating soil and water.[96] Humans and other animals such as pigs, cattle, sheep, and poultry are infected after ingestion of contaminated food or water. The oocysts are then broken down within the intestines and sporozoites and bradyzoites are released into the cells of the intestines. Once inside the epithelial cells of the intestinal tract, these organisms are transformed into tachyzoites. Free tachyzoites are released from the epithelial cells and enter the bloodstream and lymphatic system from where they can infect any tissue or organ.

Most human infections are probably the result of ingestion of undercooked or raw meat containing tissue cysts. Other sources of human infection include contact with contaminated soil or cat litter, contact with raw meat containing tissue cysts, ingestion of unwashed fruits and vegetables, ingestion of raw eggs or unpasteurized milk, and rarely as a result of blood transfusion.[54,114] Transplacental transmission occurs in women who are infected for the first time just before or during pregnancy.[25]

CLINICAL FEATURES

Ocular toxoplasmosis can develop following congenital or acquired infection. The most common ocular manifestation is a focal necrotizing retinitis with underlying choroiditis, vitritis, and retinal vasculitis. Toxoplasmosis retinochoroiditis is typically a recurrent disease, and most recurrent lesions develop adjacent to the border of an inactive scar. Healed toxoplasmosis scars are characterized by well-defined borders with peripheral retinal pigment epithelial hyperplasia and central chorioretinal atrophy (Fig. 9-3). Recurrent lesions may also develop in areas without chorioretinal scars as well as in the fellow eye (Fig. 9-4). A granulomatous or nongranulomatous anterior uveitis is common. Less common findings include punctate outer retinal toxoplasmosis, neuroretinitis, and papillitis.

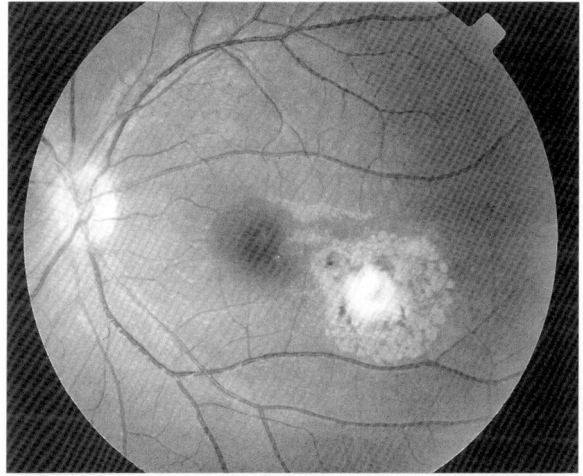

FIGURE 9-3. Resolving retinochoroiditis in the left eye of a 12-year-old Brazilian girl with acquired toxoplasmosis.

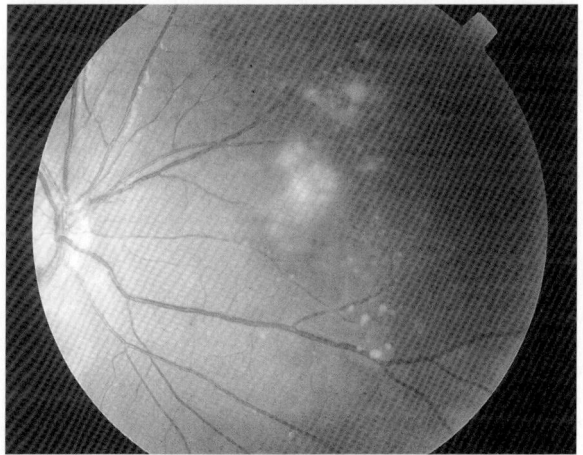

FIGURE 9-4. Recurrent toxoplasmosis in the right eye of the same child as in Figure 9-3. Punctate foci of retinitis affecting the nasal retina occurring 18 months following resolution of macular lesion in the left eye. Multiple small white-gray deposits of inflammatory cells are also visible above the inner retinal surface.

CLINICAL ASSESSMENT

In the newborn, the clinical manifestations and serology are used to establish the diagnosis of congenital toxoplasmosis. Congenital infection is confirmed by elevated serum IgM and IgA titers in the infant. In children with recently acquired toxoplasmosis, elevated titers of IgM, IgA, and IgE are present. Follow-up serology 2 to 4 weeks later often reveals a rising IgG titer, thereby indicating a recent infection. Serum serology is less useful in recurrent disease but can be useful to confirm previous exposure to toxoplasmosis; however, serological tests should not be used in isolation to establish the diagnosis.

SYSTEMIC ASSOCIATIONS AND NATURAL HISTORY

Approximately 10% of infants with congenital infection have clinical manifestations at birth. The clinical manifestations of congenital toxoplasmosis include intracranial calcifications, hydrocephalus, microcephaly, hepatosplenomegaly, jaundice, and retinochoroiditis. Some infants may have severe disability while others are asymptomatic and may not be diagnosed until later in life.

Less information is available about children with acquired toxoplasmosis. Acquired toxoplasmosis is typically asymptomatic or results in a transient lymphadenopathic syndrome in healthy children.[54] Up to 20% of all patients with acquired infections may develop ocular lesions either simultaneously with the systemic manifestations or at a later time.[17,43,78]

INHERITANCE

No inheritance pattern.

TREATMENT

The treatment of ocular toxoplasmosis remains somewhat controversial. However, most authorities would recommend treatment for the following: reduction in visual acuity greater than two Snellen lines, lesions within the macula, lesions near the optic nerve, lesions with severe vitritis, lesions associated with a significant hemorrhage, and any episode of retino-choroiditis during the first year of life. The most commonly used therapy for ocular toxoplasmosis is the combination of pyrimethamine with sulfonamides. Folinic acid is often used in conjunction with pyri-methamine to prevent bone marrow suppression.

Other antibiotics have also been used, including clindamycin, atovaquone, azithromycin, and combination trimethoprim and sulfamethoxazole.[88,93,102,103] Systemic corticosteroids may be useful in children with significant visual loss associated with severe vitritis, macular lesions, optic nerve involvement, or macular edema. Corticosteroids can be started after 48 h of antimicrobial therapy and should be discontinued before the antibiotics. Topical corticosteroids and cycloplegics may be useful for anterior uveitis. Periocular corticosteroid injections should never be used in toxoplasmosis.

PROGNOSIS

The visual prognosis is dependent on a number of factors including the presence of macular lesions, optic nerve involvement, and other complications. Children with retinochoroiditis involving the central macula or large lesions, papillitis, or neuroretinitis may develop marked visual loss. Additionally, some children may develop long-term complications such as glaucoma, choroidal neovascularization, epiretinal membrane, chronic vitreous haze, or retinal detachment that may limit their visual potential. On the other hand, children with peripheral retinochoroiditis or small lesions not involving the fovea may retain excellent visual acuity.

VIRAL DISEASES

Herpes Simplex

Herpes simplex (HSV) is a ubiquitous virus with a worldwide distribution. Infection with HSV results in a spectrum of congenital and neonatal infections as well as primary and recurrent infections. Ocular involvement also includes a spectrum of manifestations ranging from adnexal lesions to recurrent sight-threatening keratitis. HSV is probably one of the most common causes of infectious blindness in developing countries due to the recurrent nature of the disease.

Incidence

The prevalence of antibodies to type 1 herpes simplex virus (HSV-1) increases during the childhood years, whereas the major period of infection with type 2 herpes simplex (HSV-2) occurs following puberty. Epidemiologic studies suggest that 50% to 90% of adults in the United States have antibodies to HSV-1. Following primary infections, HSV becomes latent in the ganglia of the nerves that supply the infected area. For HSV-1, the trigeminal ganglion is most commonly involved. During periods of latency, no active virus is found in the involved areas. Recurrent infections are the hallmark of HSV and occur frequently with both HSV-1 and HSV-2. The cause of these recurrences is unknown but may be triggered by a number of factors such as stress, sunlight, fever, and local trauma. Approximately 0.15% of the U.S. population has a history of ocular infection related to HSV.

ETIOLOGY

Herpes simplex virus is a double-stranded DNA virus. The two types of HSV are classified based upon their clinical and epidemiologic patterns as well as biological and biochemical characteristics. HSV-1 is most commonly found in lesions of the oral cavity, the eye, and on the skin of the face and upper trunk. Transmission occurs by direct contact with infected oral secretions. HSV-2 is found in lesions on the genitalia and the skin of the thighs and buttocks and is spread by contact with genital secretions. However, either type of HSV may infect the mouth, eyes, skin, or the genital area. In most cases, the disease is transmitted during periods of asymptomatic shedding of the virus by infected persons.

CLINICAL FEATURES

Ocular involvement with congenital or neonatal HSV infection is not uncommon and includes conjunctivitis, keratitis, and chorioretinitis.[83] Other less common ocular manifestations include optic atrophy, cataract, and microphthalmia.

Primary ocular HSV infection typically presents with a unilateral blepharoconjunctivitis. Vesicles occur on the eyelid skin or on the eyelid margin with an associated follicular conjunctivitis in most children. Preauricular lymphadenopathy is also a common finding in primary disease. In most cases the vesicles clear within 7 to 10 days without scarring. The majority of patients with primary ocular infection also develop an epithelial keratitis, either superficial punctate keratitis, geographic keratitis, or the more classic dendritic keratitis.

Children with recurrent ocular herpes infections are less likely to develop skin and conjunctival involvement. Ocular findings in recurrent ocular HSV include stromal keratitis, endotheliitis or disciform keratitis, iridocyclitis, elevated intraocular pressure, and rarely retinitis.[8] Complications of recurrent HSV keratitis such as stromal scar formation and induced astigmatism may lead to amblyopia in some children.[10,95] The retinitis seen in HSV-1 and HSV-2 infections is a full-thickness necrotizing retinitis that may present as the acute retinal necrosis syndrome.

CLINICAL ASSESSMENT

In most cases, the diagnosis of HSV infection is based upon the clinical characteristics. However, laboratory testing may be useful in some patients with atypical manifestations. Cell culture is the most sensitive and specific method and can lead to a rapid diagnosis, typically within 3 days. Also, specimens can be examined directly using immunofluorescence, ELISA, and immunoperoxidase assays. Morphological tests such as the Tzanck smear can be used to identify syncytial giant cells and intranuclear inclusions, although similar findings may be present in the ocular lesions of varicella-zoster. Finally, serological tests may be useful in primary HSV infection although recurrent disease does not typically result in an increase in antibody titers.

SYSTEMIC ASSOCIATIONS AND NATURAL HISTORY

Congenital or neonatal herpes infections can be caused by either HSV-1 or HSV-2, although most cases are due to HSV-2 exposure. These infections are acquired either in utero or as the infant passes through an infected birth canal. Approximately 15% to 20% of infants with neonatal infection have ocular involvement.

Primary infections with HSV-1 are usually asymptomatic but may occasionally cause a gingivostomatitis or pharyngitis. After an incubation period of 2 to 12 days, fever and sore throat develop along with vesicles affecting the oral mucosa. Cervical adenopathy is relatively common in these patients. Symptoms and signs resolve spontaneously over the next 1 to 3 weeks in most children. Recurrent herpes labialis is a milder disease and presents with a mild tingling sensation that is followed by the development of painful vesicles. The vesicles crust during the ensuing 3 to 4 days and completely heal within 10 days.

HSV-2 infections are also typically asymptomatic. Primary infection develops after an incubation period of up to 1 week. Initial symptoms and signs include fever, malaise, inguinal lymphadenopathy, and vesicle formation. In most patients, the vesicles are confined to the genital areas; however, extragenital sites may occur. Eventually the vesicles ulcerate and heal completely, after several weeks in most cases. Recurrent HSV-2 infections, like HSV-1 infections, are typically milder than the initial episode. Recurrent disease often presents with itching or tenderness and is quickly followed by the development of vesicles. Complete healing of the lesions occurs in most patients during the next 7 to 10 days.

INHERITANCE

Not inherited.

TREATMENT

Therapy for congenital herpes infections mostly falls within the realm of the pediatric infectious disease specialist, but consultation with the ophthalmologist is essential. For systemic or posterior ocular disease, the mainstay of therapy is intravenous acyclovir. Conjunctival or corneal involvement should be managed with the use of topical trifluridine 1%.

Herpes simplex epithelial keratitis is treated with topical antiviral therapy, trifluridine solution every 2h or vidarabine ointment every 3h. HSV keratitis may also be treated by local debridement of the dendritic lesions, although this may not be well tolerated by younger children. Topical corticosteroids are also beneficial for children with stromal keratitis or uveitis.[129]

Oral acyclovir can be utilized in the treatment of herpes simplex keratitis or keratouveitis. Schwartz and Holland recently reported that oral acyclovir was useful for treating infectious HSV epithelial keratitis in children.[107] Dosages of oral acyclovir used in this study were 20mg/kg per dose four times daily in children up to 40kg and 800mg four times daily in children more than 40kg. Additionally, the Herpetic Eye Disease Study Group has shown that oral acyclovir is effective in the prevention of recurrent herpetic eye disease and concluded that long-term suppressive oral acyclovir therapy reduces the rate of recurrent HSV epithelial keratitis and stromal keratitis.[52]

PROGNOSIS

The prognosis is good for HSV ocular disease confined to the eyelids or conjunctiva. Unfortunately, children with stromal keratitis have a guarded prognosis owing to the recurrent nature of the disease. HSV epithelial keratitis can resolve completely without sequelae in some patients whereas in others it can lead to stromal scarring or the development of stromal keratitis. Increased use of oral acyclovir in selected patients may prove useful in preventing some of these sight-threatening complications of HSV keratitis. The prognosis for patients with HSV iridocyclitis is often dependent on the associated keratitis. For children who develop acute retinal necrosis associated with HSV, the prognosis is similar to adults and dependent on the extent of retina involved and ocular complications such as optic neuropathy or rhegmatogenous retinal detachment.

Lymphocytic Choriomeningitis Virus

Lymphocytic choriomeningitis virus (LCMV) is a human zoonosis that can result in congenital or acquired disease. Congenital infection is an underdiagnosed cause of chorioretinitis in affected children.

INCIDENCE

Worldwide, 49 cases of congenital LCMV infection have been reported. Of these, 21 have occurred in the United States.[5]

ETIOLOGY

LCMV is a member of the arenavirus family of single-stranded RNA viruses. Rodents, including common household and laboratory mice as well as pet hamsters, are the major reservoirs.[7] Infections from house mice have been associated with areas of substandard housing such as inner city dwellings as well as cleaning of rodent-infested farm buildings.[76] Laboratory workers handling mice and hamsters are also at increased risk for infection.[57]

Human infection occurs by inhalation of aerosolized virus, direct contact with rodents, rodent bites, or contact with fomites contaminated by LCMV.[53] Acquired LCMV infection can occur in all age groups and manifests as an asymptomatic infection or an acute febrile illness with meningeal signs.[76] Intrauterine infection occurs by transplacental transmission of the virus during maternal viremia.

CLINICAL FEATURES

The most common ocular manifestation in children born with congenital LCMV infection is chorioretinitis with peripheral or macular chorioretinal scarring. Additional ocular manifestations include optic atrophy, nystagmus, strabismus, cataract, and microphthalmos.[5]

CLINICAL ASSESSMENT

The differential diagnosis of congenital LCMV infection includes the infectious agents associated with the TORCH complex; specifically, toxoplasmosis, rubella, cytomegalovirus (CMV), herpes simplex virus, and syphilis. Clinical findings that may help distinguish between one of the TORCH infections and LCMV include hepatosplenomegaly, deafness, salt-and-pepper retinopathy, and skeletal abnormalities. Hepatosplenomegaly is common in children with neonatal CMV infection while deafness is common in children infected with rubella. Salt-and-pepper retinopathy is common in children with rubella and syphilis but is not seen in congenital LCMV infection.[5] However, the congenital infection most difficult to distinguish clinically from LCMV is toxoplasmosis. The pattern of intra-cerebral calcifications may be useful to distinguish the two diseases. Diffuse intracerebral calcifications are associated with congenital toxoplasmosis whereas periventricular calcifications are associated with LCMV infection. The presence of LCMV antibodies detected by the immunofluorescent antibody test is useful to confirm the diagnosis of congenital LCMV infection.

SYSTEMIC ASSOCIATIONS AND NATURAL HISTORY

Intrauterine infection with LCMV may result in spontaneous abortion or cause congenital hydrocephalus and chorioretinitis in newborns. Systemic findings in children with congenital LCMV infection include hydrocephaly, microcephaly or macro-cephaly, and intracranial calcifications. Long-term neurological sequelae are common including seizures, cerebral palsy, and mental retardation.[5]

INHERITANCE

No inheritance pattern.

TREATMENT

No specific therapy is indicated for intrauterine infection with LCMV; however, preventive measures to reduce the risk of transmission may be useful. Community and household rodent control, elimination of infected laboratory rodents, and avoidance of rodents during pregnancy can reduce the risk of infection.

PROGNOSIS

The visual prognosis for children with chorioretinal scars located in the macula is guarded because they often have decreased visual acuity and may develop nystagmus and strabismus. On the other hand, children with peripheral chorioretinal scarring have a much better visual prognosis.

Measles

Measles is a highly contagious infection that is typically seen in children. The acute infection is caused by the rubeola virus and is characterized by fever, cough, coryza, and conjunctivitis. Although the incidence of measles has markedly decreased in the United States, it continues to be a significant public health problem in developing countries.

INCIDENCE

Measles is no longer endemic in the United States; however, imported measles remains a potential source of transmission. In 1999, a total of 100 cases of confirmed measles was reported to the Centers for Disease Control and Prevention.[21] Approximately one-third of these cases were imported cases from either international visitors or U.S. residents exposed while traveling abroad.

ETIOLOGY

Measles is a single-stranded RNA virus that primarily affects the respiratory epithelium of the nasopharynx. The virus is spread by contact with aerosolized droplets from respiratory secretions of infected persons.

CLINICAL FEATURES

Ocular involvement in developed countries is relatively mild and self-limited as compared to underdeveloped countries where it is a major cause of ocular morbidity. Prodromal measles infection is characterized by a mild catarrhal conjunctivitis, a nonpurulent conjunctivitis with occasional pseudomembrane formation. The conjunctivitis persists for 5 to 7 days after the appearance of the rash. An associated epithelial keratitis may also develop during the prodromal phase and is the most common ocular manifestation, affecting up to 76% of all patients with measles.[30] The keratitis is bilateral and begins in the peripheral cornea adjacent to the limbus but eventually progresses to involve the central cornea. These corneal lesions heal without scarring in the majority of patients. However, in developing countries with high rates of malnutrition and vitamin A and protein deficiency, the keratitis can result in sight-threatening complications. In these situations, keratitis may progress to corneal leucoma, corneal ulceration, perforation, endophthalmitis, and phthisis.[80,81]

Patients with acquired measles may rarely develop sudden vision loss due to retinopathy. When this occurs, patients present with bilateral visual loss 1 to 2 weeks following the onset of the rash. This acquired measles retinitis is characterized by macular edema, neuroretinitis, disc edema, attenuated arterioles, and retinal hemorrhages.[106]

The most severe complication of measles is *subacute sclerosing panencephiltis* (SSPE). Ocular findings are apparent in 50% of all patients who develop SSPE, and often the first clinical manifestation of SSPE is visual loss.[32] Ocular manifestations usually precede the neurological findings by weeks to several years and can occur in one or both eyes. Typically, patients with SSPE develop a maculopathy with retinal pigment epithelial changes and focal retinitis.[19] Other common ocular findings include disc edema, papillitis, and optic atrophy. Additional ocular manifestations of SSPE include serous retinal detachment, chorioretinitis, retinal hemorrhage, retinal folds, hemianopsia, nystagmus, and cortical blindness.[38,100]

CLINICAL ASSESSMENT

The diagnosis of measles is based upon the typical clinical findings. Isolation of the measles virus is not routinely performed to establish the diagnosis. Immunofluorescent staining of secretions from respiratory smears can provide a relatively quick diagnosis if required. Serological tests including ELISA may also be useful, but require acute and convalescent titers, thereby necessitating a delay of 10 to 30 days before the diagnosis can be established.

SYSTEMIC ASSOCIATIONS AND NATURAL HISTORY

Acquired measles normally affects young children and is characterized by catarrhal conjunctivitis, coryza, and cough. Ten to 14 days following exposure, Koplik spots appear on the buccal mucosa and other mucous membranes. These lesions are 1- to 2-mm, bluish-white dots on a red background. Several days later, a characteristic erythematous maculopapular rash develops from the face to the trunk and extremities.[30] The rash lasts approximately 10 days, followed by spontaneous resolution without sequelae in most children. Other manifestations include vomiting, diarrhea, lymphadenopathy, and splenomegaly.

SSPE is a rare progressive neurological disease possibly caused by persistent central nervous system infection. On average, SSPE develops 7 years after measles infection and is characterized by an insidious change in personality such as inappropriate behavior and mental deterioration followed by ataxia, seizures, and eventual death within 1 to 2 years following onset.[79]

INHERITANCE

Not an inherited disease.

TREATMENT

In most cases of acquired measles, the disease is self-limited and requires only supportive therapy. In developing countries, administration of vitamin A to persons with vitamin A deficiency can reduce mortality.[58] Symptomatic treatment may be necessary for some patients with ocular manifestations. Topical antibiotics may also be useful to prevent secondary infections in patients with conjunctivitis or keratitis.

PROGNOSIS

Most children in the United States have an excellent visual prognosis following acquired measles. The conjunctival and corneal manifestations resolve in most children with no long-term sequelae. Children with acquired measles retinitis also have a good visual prognosis in most cases. On the other hand, the prognosis is guarded in developing countries. Up to 1% of children in developing countries will develop permanent ocular damage as a consequence of acquired measles.[31,80,81]

The prognosis for patients with SSPE is poor, with progression to death in 1 to 3 years in almost all patients. However, up to 5% of patients with SSPE may experience a spontaneous remission.

Rubella

Rubella is an acute viral infection of children and adults characterized by low-grade fever, rash, and lymphadenopathy. In many cases, rubella infection causes a mild self-limited illness. Unfortunately, infection during pregnancy can result in fetal infection with severe congenital defects.

INCIDENCE

The incidence of rubella in the United States has continued to decline over the past 30 years. In 1999, only 271 cases of postnatal rubella infection were reported in the United States. The number of cases of congenital rubella syndrome has also dramatically decreased, with 26 cases reported in the United States from 1997 to 1999.[20]

ETIOLOGY

Rubella is a single-stranded RNA virus and a member of the Togavirus family. Before widespread vaccination with rubella vaccine, rubella was responsible for epidemics every 6 to 9 years.[27] Humans are the only known host for rubella, and transmission occurs by droplets from respiratory secretions. Rubella infection is often categorized according to the period that the infection is acquired, postnatal or congenital.

CLINICAL FEATURES

The ocular manifestations of acquired rubella are limited and included conjunctivitis, keratitis, and rarely retinitis. Nonpurulent conjunctivitis occurs in up to two-thirds of patients. Epithelial keratitis is less common and in most cases is transient and self-limited. Retinitis occurs rarely and presents with visual loss associated with dark atrophic lesions visible at the level of the retinal pigment epithelium and exudative retinal detachment.[51]

Ocular complications are a common occurrence in the congenital rubella syndrome, affecting approximately 45% of children. The characteristic "salt-and-pepper" retinopathy typically appears in the macula or periphery of both eyes in 24% to 62% of children with congenital infection.[1,14,75] Often, the retinopathy results in loss of the foveal reflex that is due to atrophy and hyperplasia of the retinal pigment epithelium. Vision is rarely affected unless choroidal neovascularization develops; this can cause a sudden decrease in vision in one or both eyes and ultimately leads to disciform scar formation, typically later in life.

Other ocular manifestations of the congenital rubella syndrome include cataracts, microphthalmia, glaucoma, anterior uveitis, and corneal haze. Cataracts occur in up to 30% of children with congenital rubella and are bilateral in 75% of cases. These nuclear cataracts are often described as pearly, dense, and possibly surrounded by a clear zone or totally opaque. Complete liquefaction of the cortex may eventually occur if the cataract continues to develop.[87] However, some lens opacities that are present at birth are found to be transient. Of all the ophthalmic manifestations of congenital rubella, cataracts account for the greatest ocular morbidity and visual loss.[86] Mild microphthalmia with hypermetropia occurs commonly in children with cataracts.[42,87] In children with congenital rubella, the lens can contain infectious virus up to 30 months of age and must be handled with caution during cataract extraction.

Glaucoma occurs in 9% of all children with congenital rubella and appears to develop by several mechanisms. A hypermature lens may cause a relative pupillary block or a phacolytic response.[1,42] Another mechanism includes an immature anterior chamber angle with abnormal insertion of the longitudinal muscle of the ciliary body into the trabecular meshwork and incomplete maturation of trabecular meshwork.[13]

Corneal haze may also occur as a result of several mechanisms. In some children it may be transient and resolve spontaneously several days following birth. However, it can also be due to glaucoma or as a result of corneal decompensation in eyes with microphthalmos and lens contact with the cornea.

Iris and ciliary body abnormalities have also been described in congenital rubella. These manifestations include a mild nongranulomatous iridocyclitis with posterior synechiae, iris atrophy, hypoplasia of the ciliary body, and hypoplasia of the iris dilator muscle.[13] A decreased response in the affected iris is found with the use of mydriatics and cycloplegics because of the abnormal muscles.

CLINICAL ASSESSMENT

The diagnosis of congenital rubella requires isolation of the rubella virus, the presence of serum IgM antibodies, or the persistence of serum antibodies beyond the first year of age. Isolation of rubella virus is often difficult and requires culture of the nasopharynx, urine, or cerebrospinal fluid. Serum ELISA is the most commonly used serological test for congenital rubella. Additionally, rubella antigens can be detected in blood, cerebrospinal fluid, and tissue specimens by using specific monoclonal antibodies.

The diagnosis of postnatal rubella is often difficult because it is commonly a subclinical infection. Nonspecific findings include leukopenia and atypical lymphocytes. Acute infection is confirmed by a fourfold or greater increase in the titer of serum IgG antibodies obtained during the acute and convalescent phase of the infection.

SYSTEMIC ASSOCIATIONS AND NATURAL HISTORY

Postnatal rubella infections are typically seen in children 5 to 14 years of age and are typically mild. After a 2- to 3-week incubation period, postauricular and occipital adenopathy develops with a nondescript maculopapular rash and a low-grade fever. The rash develops on the face and extends over the trunk and extremities and typically resolves spontaneously in 1 to 4 days. The most common complication of postnatal rubella infection is a transient arthritis affecting the small and medium-sized joints.[59] In rare cases, rubella infection can lead to severe complications including encephalitis, necrotizing vasculitis, and thrombocytopenic purpura.[14,27]

Unlike postnatal infections, congenital rubella infections are associated with significant morbidity. Early descriptions of the congenital rubella syndrome included hearing loss, heart malformations, and cataracts. Currently, the syndrome includes a comprehensive spectrum of findings, and the severity of manifestations is dependent on the gestational age of the fetus at the time of infection. Approximately 80% to 90% of children infected during the first 8 weeks of gestation have one or more malformations; this percentage decreases to 52% if the child is infected during weeks 9 to 12 of gestation. If infection occurs during the second trimester, approximately 25% to 30% of children will develop malformations, whereas third-trimester infections rarely manifest abnormalities.[94] Congenital rubella can also result in spontaneous abortion or stillbirth, low birth weight, or, in some cases, normal-appearing infants.[27]

Children with congenital rubella may develop transient thrombocytopenia, purpura, hepatitis, and hemolytic anemia. The most common permanent manifestation of congenital rubella is unilateral or bilateral sensorineural deafness, although mental retardation and cardiac anomalies are relatively common.[118] Additionally, children with congenital rubella appear to be at increased risk for progressive endocrine complications, including insulin-dependent diabetes mellitus, hypothyroidism, and hyperthyroidism.[75,118]

INHERITANCE

Not inherited.

TREATMENT

Treatment of children with rubella is primarily supportive. Cataract surgery can be performed for children with cataracts but may be complicated by a severe inflammatory response. This severe postoperative inflammatory response may be associated with retained rubella virus within the lens. Complete removal of all lens material and aggressive postoperative topical corticosteroids and cycloplegics is essential in these children. Medical therapy is the initial treatment for rubella-associated glaucoma. Surgical therapy may be necessary when the intraocular pressure cannot be controlled by medications.[108]

PROGNOSIS

The prognosis for children with rubella retinopathy is generally good. Visual loss secondary to choroidal neovascularization is uncommon and typically occurs later in life. Glaucoma associated with rubella is often difficult to control; therefore, the visual prognosis for these children is guarded. In some children with keratitis, glaucoma, and cataract, severe visual loss may occur.

Varicella-Zoster

Varicella or chickenpox is an extremely contagious disease of childhood characterized by a generalized exanthematous rash. It is a disseminated disease resulting from primary infection with varicella-zoster virus (VZV). The virus eventually spreads from the peripheral lesions to the dorsal root ganglia of the corresponding dermatome, where it becomes latent in virtually all patients. Reactivation of the latent virus results in a focal infection affecting one or two dermatomes, herpes zoster.[47,48] Ocular involvement can occur in both varicella and herpes zoster; however, the complications associated with herpes zoster ophthalmicus (HZO) have a greater potential for significant ocular morbidity.

INCIDENCE

Before 1995, approximately 4 million cases of varicella occurred in the United States each year. In 1995, a varicella vaccine was licensed in the United States for routine use in children, and increasing use of this vaccine will reduce the annual incidence of varicella. Current information concerning the incidence of herpes zoster is lacking. However, previous reports indicate an annual incidence of herpes zoster in children of 0.74 per 1000 in children from 0 to 9 years of age and 1.38 per 1000 from ages 10 to 19.[56]

ETIOLOGY

The virus responsible for varicella and herpes zoster is the varicella-zoster virus. This virus is a member of the herpes family of viruses and is spread by airborne droplets and by direct contact with infected lesions.[40,66] It is highly contagious to those individuals who are not immune. Varicella is communicable 1 to 2 days before the onset of vesicles and up until all the lesions have crusted over; however, the disease is most communicable during the prodromal phase. Congenital varicella results from transplacental spread of the virus by an infected mother.

Reactivation of latent virus results in herpes zoster with a characteristic unilateral vesicular rash affecting one to two dermatomes. Reactivation of varicella zoster virus latent in the trigeminal ganglion results in HZO. The mechanisms for reactivation of varicella-zoster are unknown but are probably related to both the host and virus. Herpes zoster is very uncommon in healthy children and is usually encountered in children with cancer or those who are immunocompromised, as well as children who developed primary varicella during the first year of life.[2,47,50,123] Additionally, a recent report suggests that the psychological stress of severe child abuse might result in the development of herpes zoster.[48]

CLINICAL FEATURES

Ocular complications of varicella are not uncommon. The most common manifestations are papillary conjunctivitis and conjunctival vesicle formation. Other less-frequent manifestations include epithelial keratitis that may be punctate or dendritic, subepithelial infiltrates, stromal keratitis, disciform keratitis, or mild nongranulomatous anterior uveitis.[61] The keratitis associated with varicella infection is not recurrent and only rarely leads to permanent scarring. There are isolated reports of neuro-ophthalmic manifestations of varicella including internuclear ophthalmoplegia and oculomotor palsy.[85,111] In children with congenital varicella, chorioretinitis is the major ophthalmic manifestation.

The onset of HZO is heralded by the development of a maculopapular eruption followed by the development of vesicles over the forehead, eyelids, and along the side of the nose. Ocular involvement may occur with the involvement of any branch of the trigeminal nerve but is most likely to occur if the nasociliary branch is involved. Inflammation from herpes zoster has the potential to affect virtually any orbital, adnexal, or ocular tissue. Cranial nerve palsies have been reported during the first week following the onset of the rash. Dermatitis of the eyelids may lead to secondary bacterial infections, as well as lid notching, loss of cilia, entropion, trichiasis, and stenosis of the lacrimal puncta. Follicular conjunctivitis, episcleritis, and scleritis may also occur in children with HZO. Corneal manifestations include superficial or stromal keratitis that can include pseudodendrites, punctate epithelial keratitis, anterior stromal infiltrates, endotheliitis, and neurotrophic keratitis. Corneal hypesthesia often develops in conjunction with HZO-associated keratitis. Iridocyclitis is not uncommon and can be severe in some patients. Elevated intraocular pressure is often present and may lead to glaucoma in some children. Posterior segment manifestations include optic neuritis and the acute retinal necrosis syndrome. Rarely, patients who are severely immunocompromised, such as those with advanced AIDS, may develop the *progressive outer retinal necrosis syndrome* (PORN).

CLINICAL ASSESSMENT

Infection with herpes simplex can resemble herpes zoster; therefore, it may be difficult to distinguish between the two. Tissue culture methods can be used to obtain a specific diagnosis of varicella-zoster virus. Fluorescent antibody staining of cells in scrapings from vesicles may also be useful. Serological tests may be useful in some patients, although they are less timely than other methods because acute and convalescent serum is required to establish the diagnosis.

SYSTEMIC ASSOCIATIONS AND NATURAL HISTORY

Varicella is primarily a disease of childhood, although adults are infected uncommonly. In most patients, the first manifestations include a prodrome of fever, malaise, and anorexia. The characteristic cutaneous exanthem appears 1 to 2 days later and lasts for about 10 to 14 days. The exanthem is characterized by maculopapules with vesicles and scabs in various stages of evolution (Fig. 9-5). Following the onset of the rash, patients develop pruritus, malaise, and anorexia.

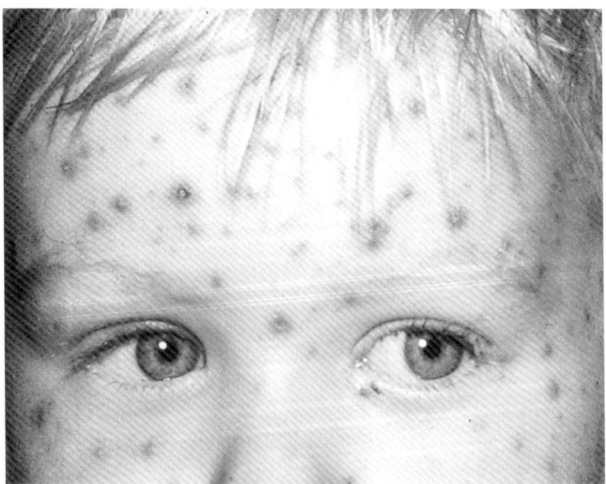

FIGURE 9-5. Child with varicella and multiple facial lesions in various stages of development. Numerous lesions are present on the eyelids of the left eye.

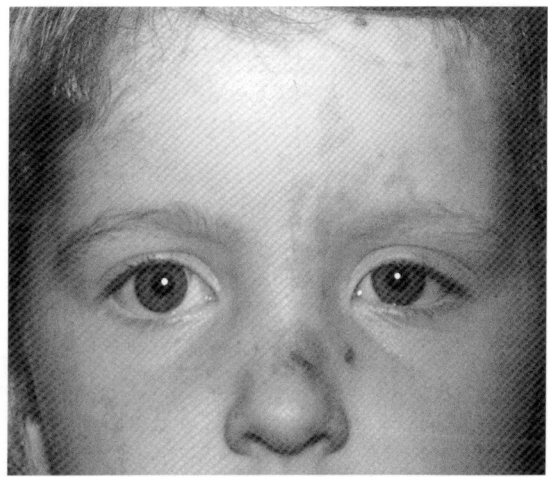

FIGURE 9-6. Eight-year-old girl with leukemia and herpes zoster ophthalmicus of the left eye. Crusted vesicles are visible along the nose and upper forehead. Early scarring is also present along the bridge of the nose and above the brow.

Herpes zoster ophthalmicus is characterized by a vesicular rash affecting the ophthalmic division of the trigeminal nerve. Some patients may experience prodromal symptoms for 2 to 3 days before the onset of the rash, including dermatomal pain, headache, fever, malaise, and chills. In children, pain is not typically a part of the disease as compared to adults. These symptoms are followed by the development of erythematous maculopapular lesions within the affected dermatome that quickly evolve into vesicles and bullous lesions. The lesions continue to develop over a 3- to 5-day period and resolve over the ensuing 3 to 4 weeks (Fig. 9-6). As with herpes zoster in general, HZO in children typically follows a more benign course as compared to adults.

INHERITANCE

Not inherited.

TREATMENT

Most of the ocular complications associated with primary varicella infection are self-limited and require no therapy. However, anterior uveitis or stromal keratitis with decreased visual acuity may require therapy with topical corticosteroids; this is especially important in children who are susceptible to the development of amblyopia. Systemic acyclovir should be considered in immunocompromised children who develop varicella infection.

The treatment of herpes zoster in children is similar to that in the adult population. The cutaneous lesions can be treated with moist compresses and antibiotic ointments to help loosen lid crusting and to prevent secondary infection. Topical corticosteroids may be necessary to treat associated uveitis, stromal keratitis, or disciform keratitis. Systemic administration of corticosteroids may be indicated for either optic nerve or cranial nerve involvement and have been utilized in the treatment of adult patients with these complications.[74] Topical antiviral agents are not effective for any of the ocular manifestations of HZO. Oral acyclovir should be considered for children with involvement of the ophthalmic branch of the trigeminal nerve if treatment can be initiated within 72 h following the onset of the rash. The recommended dosage is 80 mg/kg/day in four or five divided doses to a maximum of 4 g/day for both children and adolescents.[101] Intravenous acyclovir is typically not used in healthy children but may be utilized in the treatment of immunosuppressed patients.

PROGNOSIS

The prognosis for children with varicella-associated ocular disease is generally good. Most of the ocular complications are transient or treatable with topical corticosteroids. However, the prognosis is somewhat guarded for children who develop acute retinal necrosis associated with VZV infection. Overall, the visual prognosis is most dependent on the extent of the retinitis and the severity of the intraocular inflammation. Early aggressive systemic therapy is probably the key to a better visual outcome in children with this syndrome.

References

1. Alfano JE. Ocular aspects of the maternal rubella syndrome. Trans Am Acad Ophthalmol Otolaryngol 1966;70:235–266.
2. Baba K, Yabuuchi H, Takahashi M, et al. Increased incidence of herpes zoster in normal children infected with varicella zoster virus

during infancy: community-based follow up study. J Pediatr 1986; 108:372–377.

3. Bakken LL, Case KL, Callister SM, et al. Performance of 45 laboratories participating in a proficiency testing program for Lyme disease serology. JAMA 1992;268:891–895.

4. Barclay AJ, Foster A, Sommer A. Vitamin A supplements and mortality related to measles: a randomised clinical trial. Br Med J (Clin Res Ed) 1987;294:294–296.

5. Barton LL, Mets MB. Congenital lymphocytic choriomeningitis virus infection: decade of rediscovery. Clin Infect Dis 2001;33:370–374.

6. Baum J, Barza M, Weinstein P, et al. Bilateral keratitis as a manifestation of Lyme disease. Am J Ophthalmol 1988;105:75–77.

7. Bechtel RT, Haught KA, Mets MB. Lymphocytic choriomeningitis virus: a new addition to the TORCH evaluation. Arch Ophthalmol 1996;115:680–681.

8. Beigi B, Algawi K, Foley-Nolan A, et al. Herpes simplex keratitis in children. Br J Ophthalmol 1994;78:458–460.

9. Belmont JB, Irvine A, Benson WE, et al. Vitrectomy in ocular toxocariasis. Arch Ophthalmol 1982;100:1912–1915.

10. Beneish RG, Williams FR, Polomeno RC, et al. Herpes simplex keratitis and amblyopia. J Pediatr Ophthalmol Strabismus 1987;24: 94–96.

11. Berger BW, Johnson RC, Kodner C, et al. Cultivation of *Borrelia burgdorferi* from erythema migrans lesions and perilesional skin. J Clin Microbiol 1992;30:359–361.

12. Biglan AW, Glickman LT, Lobes LA Jr. Serum and vitreous *Toxocara* antibody in nematode endophthalmitis. Am J Ophthalmol 1979;88: 898–901.

13. Boniuk M, Zimmerman LE. Ocular pathology in the rubella syndrome. Arch Ophthalmol 1967;7:455–473.

14. Boniuk V. Systemic and ocular manifestations of the rubella syndrome. Int Ophthalmol Clin 1973;12:67–76.

15. Bowie WR, King AS, Werker DH, et al. Outbreak of toxoplasmosis associated with municipal drinking water. The BC Toxoplasma Investigation Team. Lancet 1997;350:173–177.

16. Breeveld J, Rothova A, Kuiper H. Intermediate uveitis and Lyme borreliosis. Br J Ophthalmol 1992;76:181–182.

17. Burnett AJ, Shortt SG, Issac-Renton J, et al. Multiple cases of acquired toxoplasmosis retinitis presenting as an outbreak. Ophthalmology 1998;105:1032–1037.

18. Carithers HA. Cat scratch disease: an overview based on a study of 1,200 patients. Am J Dis Child 1985;139:1124–1133.

19. Caruso JM, Robbins-Tien D, Brown WD, et al. Atypical chorioretinitis as an early presentation of subacute sclerosing panencephalitis. J Pediatr Ophthalmol Strabismus 2000;37:119–122.

20. Centers for Disease Control and Prevention. Control and prevention of rubella: evaluation and management of suspected outbreaks, rubella in pregnant women, and surveillance for congenital rubella

syndrome. MMWR Morb Mortal Wkly Rep 2001;50(RR-12):1–23.

21. Centers for Disease Control and Prevention. Measles—United States 1999. MWWR Morb Mortal Wkly Rep 2000;49:557–560.

22. Centers for Disease Control and Prevention. Recommendations for test performance and interpretation from the Second National Conference on Serologic Diagnosis of Lyme Disease. MMWR Morb Mortal Wkly Rep 1995;44:590–591.

23. Centers for Disease Control and Prevention. 1998 guidelines for the treatment of sexually transmitted diseases. MWWR Morb Mortal Wkly Rep 1998;47:1–118.

24. Centers for Disease Control and Prevention. Congenital syphilis—United States, 2000. MMWR Morb Mortal Wkly Rep 2000;50:573–577.

25. Chowdhury MN. Toxoplasmosis. A review. J Med 1986;17:373–396.

26. Clark JR, Carlson RD, Sasaki CT, et al. Facial paralysis in Lyme disease. Laryngoscope 1985;95:1341–1345.

27. Cooper LZ. The history and medical consequences of rubella. Rev Infect Dis 1985;7(suppl 1):S2–S10.

28. Cunningham ET, Koehler JE. Ocular bartonellosis. Am J Ophthalmol 2000;130:340–349.

29. Cunningham ET Jr, McDonald HR, Schatz H, et al. Inflammatory mass of the optic nerve head associated with *Bartonella henselae* infection. Arch Ophthalmol 1997;115:1596–1597.

30. Dekkers NW. The cornea in measles. Doc Ophthalmol 1981;52:1–119.

31. Dekkers NW. Post measles blindness. Doc Ophthalmol 1983;56:137–141.

32. De Laey JJ, Hanssens M, Colette P, et al. Subacute sclerosing panencephalitis: fundus changes and histopathologic correlations. Doc Ophthalmol 1983;56:11–21.

33. Deschenes J, Seamone C, Baines M. The ocular manifestations of sexually transmitted diseases. Can J Ophthalmol 1990;25:177–185.

34. Dinning WJ, Gillespie SH, Cooling RJ, et al. Toxocariasis: a practical approach to management of ocular disease. Eye 1988;2:580–582.

35. Dietrich A, Auer H, Titti M, et al. Ocular toxocariasis in Austria. Dtsch Med Wochenschr 1998;123:626–630.

36. Elliot DL, Tolle SW, Goldberg L, et al. Pet-associated illness. N Engl J Med 1985;313:985–995.

37. Flach AJ, Lavoie PE. Episcleritis, conjunctivitis, and keratitis as ocular manifestations of Lyme disease. Ophthalmology 1990;97:973–975.

38. Francois J. Ocular manifestations in demyelinating diseases. Adv Ophthalmol 1979;39:1–36.

39. Gass JDM. Disease of the optic nerve that may simulate macular disease. Trans Am Acad Ophthalmol Otolaryngol 1977;83:76–9.

40. Gershon AA. Chickenpox, measles and mumps. In: Remington JS, Klein JO (eds) Infectious diseases of the fetus and newborn infant, 3rd edn. Philadelphia: Saunders, 1990.

41. Ginsberg CM. Acquired syphilis in prepubertal children. Pediatr Infect Dis 1983;2:232–234.

42. Givens KT, Lee DA, Jones T, et al. Congenital rubella syndrome: ophthalmic manifestations and associated systemic disorders. Br J Ophthalmol 1993;77:358–363.

43. Glasner PD, Silveira C, Kruszon Moran D, et al. An unusually high prevalence of ocular toxoplasmosis in Southern Brazil. Am J Ophthalmol 1992;114:136–144.

44. Glickman LT, Magnaval J. Zoonotic roundworm infections. Infect Dis Clin North Am 1993;7:717–732.

45. Glickman LT, Schantz PM. Epidemiology and pathogenesis of zoonotic toxocariasis. Epidemiol Rev 1981;3:230–250.

46. Golnik KC, Marotto ME, Fanous MM, et al. Ophthalmic manifestations of *Rochalimaea* species. Am J Ophthalmol 1994;118:145–151.

47. Guess HA, Broughton DD, Melton LJ III, et al. Epidemiology of herpes zoster in children and adolescents: a population-based study. Pediatrics 1985;76:512–517.

48. Gupta MA, Gupta AK. Herpes zoster in the medically healthy child and covert severe child abuse. Cutis 2000;66:221–223.

49. Hagler WH, Pollard ZF, Jarrett WH, et al. Results of surgery for ocular *Toxocara canis*. Ophthalmology 1981;88:1081–1086.

50. Hartley W, Mandal B. Herpes zoster in childhood. Practitioner 1982;226:766–770.

51. Hayashi M, Yoshimura N, Kondo T. Acute rubella retinal pigment epitheliitis in an adult. Am J Ophthalmol 1992;93:285–288.

52. Herpetic Eye Disease Study Group. Oral acyclovir for herpes simplex virus eye disease: effect on prevention of epithelial keratitis and stromal keratitis. Arch Ophthalmol 2000;118:1030–1036.

53. Hinman AR, Fraser DW, Douglas RG, et al. Outbreak of lymphocytic choriomeningitis virus infection in medical center personnel. Am J Epidemiol 1975;101:103–110.

54. Holland GN. Reconsidering the pathogenesis of ocular toxoplasmosis. Am J Ophthalmol 1999;128:502–505.

55. Holley HP Jr. Successful treatment of cat scratch disease with ciprofloxacin. JAMA 1991;265:1563–1565.

56. Hope-Simpson RE. The nature of herpes zoster: a long-term study and a new hypothesis. Proc R Soc Med 1965;58:9–20.

57. Hotchin J. The contamination of laboratory animals with lymphocytic choriomeningitis virus. Am J Pathol 1971;64:747–769.

58. Hussey GD, Klein M. A randomized, controlled trial of vitamin A in children with severe measles. N Engl J Med 1990;323:160–164.

59. Ingalls TH, Babbott FL Jr, Hampson KW. Rubella: its epidemiology and teratology. Am J Med Sci 1960;239:363–383.

60. Jackson LA, Perkins BA, Wenger JD. Cat scratch disease in the United States: an analysis of three national databases. Am J Public Health 1993;83:1707–1711.

61. Kachmer ML, Annable WL, DiMarco M. Iritis in children with varicella. J Pediatr Ophthalmol Strabismus 1990;27:221–222.

62. Karma A, Seppälä IJT, Mikkilä HO, et al. Diagnosis and clinical characteristics of ocular Lyme borreliosis. Am J Ophthalmol 1995;119: 127–135.

63. Kerkhoff FT, Ossewaarde JM, de Loos WS, et al. Presumed ocular bartonellosis. Br J Ophthalmol 1999;83:270–275.

64. Koehler JE, Glaser CA, Tappero JW. *Rochalimaea henselae* infection: a new zoonosis with the domestic cat as reservoir. JAMA 1994;271: 531–535.

65. Kornmehl EW, Lesser RL, Jaros P, et al. Bilateral keratitis in Lyme disease. Ophthalmology 1989;96:1194–1197.

66. Leclair JM, Zaia JA, Levin MJ, et al. Airborne transmission of chickenpox in a hospital. N Engl J Med 1980;302:450–453.

67. Lesser RL, Kornmehl EW, Pachner AR, et al. Neuro-ophthalmologic manifestations of Lyme disease. Ophthalmology 1990;97:699–706.

68. Lewis DE, Wallace MR. Treatment of adult systemic cat scratch disease with gentamicin sulfate. West J Med 1991;154:330–331.

69. Litwin CM, Martins TB, Hill HR. Immunologic response to *Bartonella henselae* as determined by enzyme immunoassay and Western blot analysis. Am J Clin Pathol 1997;108:202–209.

70. Luger SW, Krauss E. Serologic tests for Lyme disease: interlaboratory variability. Arch Intern Med 1990;150:761–763.

71. Margileth AM. Antibiotic therapy for cat scratch disease: clinical study of therapeutic outcome in 268 patients and a review of the literature. Pediatr Infect Dis J 1992;11:474–478.

72. Maguire AM, Zarbin MA, Connor TB, et al. Ocular penetration of thiabendazole. Arch Ophthalmol 1990;108:1675.

73. Margo CE, Hamed LM. Ocular syphilis. Surv Ophthalmol 1992;37: 203–220.

74. Marsh RJ. Current management of ophthalmic zoster. Aust NZ J Ophthalmol 1990;18:273–279.

75. Menser MA, Dods L, Harley JD. A twenty-five year follow-up of congenital rubella. Lancet 1967;2:1347–1350.

76. Mets MB, Barton LL, Khan AS, et al. Lymphocytic choriomeningitis virus: an underdiagnosed cause of congenital chorioretinitis. Am J Ophthalmol 2000;130:209–215.

77. Mets MB, Holfels E, Boyer KM, et al. Eye manifestations of congenital toxoplasmosis. JAMA 1996;2:249–256.

78. Montoya JG, Remington JS. Toxoplasmic chorioretinitis in the setting of acute acquired toxoplasmosis. Clin Infect Dis 1996;23: 277–282.

79. Morgan B, Cohen DN, Rothner AD, et al. Ocular manifestations of subacute sclerosing panencephalitis. Am J Dis Child 1976;130:1019–1021.

80. Morley D. Severe measles in the tropics. II. Br Med J 1969;1:297–300.

81. Morley D. Severe measles in the tropics. I. Br Med J 1969;1:363–365.

82. Murph JR. Rubella and syphilis: continuing causes of congenital infection in the 1990s. Semin Pediatr Neurol 1994;1:26–35.

83. Nahmias AJ, Roizman B. Infection with herpes simplex viruses 1–2. N Engl J Med 1973;289:667–674.

84. Nichol G, Dennis DT, Steere AC, et al. Test-treatment strategies for patients suspected of having Lyme disease: a cost-effectiveness analysis. Ann Intern Med 1998;128:37–48.

85. Noel LP, Watson AG. Internal ophthalmoplegia following chicken pox. Can J Ophthalmol 1976;11:267–269.

86. O'Neill JF. Strabismus in congenital rubella. Management in the presence of brain damage. Arch Ophthalmol 1967;77:450–454.

87. O'Neill JF. The ocular manifestations of congenital infection: a study of the early effect and long-term outcome of maternally transmitted rubella and toxoplasmosis. Trans Am Ophthalmol 1998;96:813–879.

88. Opremcak EM, Scales DK, Sharpe MR. Trimethoprim-sulfamethoxazole therapy for ocular toxoplasmosis. Ophthalmology 1992;99:920–925.

89. Ormerod LD, Dailey JP. Ocular manifestations of cat-scratch disease. Curr Opin Ophthalmol 1999;10:209–216.

90. Ormerod LD, Skolnick KA, Menosky MM, et al. Retinal and choroidal manifestations of cat-scratch disease. Ophthalmology 1998;105:1024–1031.

91. Parish JL. Treponemal infections in the pediatric population. Clin Dermatol 2000;18:687–700.

92. Parke DW II, Shaver RP. Toxocariasis. In: Pepose JS, Halland GN, Wilhelmus KR (eds) Ocular infection and immunity. St. Louis: Mosby, 1996:1225–1235.

93. Pearson PA, Piracha AR, Sen HA, et al. Atovaquone for the treatment of toxoplasma retinochoroiditis in immunocompetent patients. Ophthalmology 1999;106:148–153.

94. Peckham C. Congenital rubella in the United Kingdom before 1970: the prevaccine era. Rev Infect Dis 1985;7(suppl 1):S11–S16.

95. Poirier RH. Herpetic ocular infections of childhood. Arch Ophthalmol 1980;98:704–706.

96. Rathinam SR, Cunningham ET Jr. Infectious causes of uveitis in the developing world. Int Ophthalmol Clin 2000;40:137–152.

97. Rawston SA, Bromberg K, Hammerschlag MR. STD in children: syphilis and gonorrhoea. Genitourin Med 1993;69:66–75.

98. Reed JB, Scales DK, Wong MT, et al. *Bartonella henselae* neuroretinitis in cat scratch disease. Diagnosis, management, and sequelae. Ophthalmology 1998;105:459–466.

99. Robb RM, Watters GV. Ophthalmic manifestations of subacute sclerosing panencephalitis. Arch Ophthalmol 1970;83:426–435.

100. Rodriguez A. Early pars plana vitrectomy in chronic endophthalmitis of toxocariasis. Graefe's Arch Clin Exp Ophthalmol 1986;224:18–220.

101. Rothe M, Feder HM Jr, Grant-Kels JM. Oral acyclovir therapy for varicella and zoster infections in pediatric and pregnant patients: a brief review. Pediatr Dermatol 1991;8:236–242.

102. Rothova A, Bosch-Driessen LEH, van Loon NH, et al. Azithromycin for ocular toxoplasmosis. Br J Ophthalmol 1998;83:1306–1308.

103. Rothova A, Meenken C, Buitenhuis HJ, et al. Therapy for ocular toxoplasmosis. Am J Ophthalmol 1993;115:517–523.

104. Rubins S, Janniger CK, Schwartz RA. Congenital and acquired early childhood syphilis. Cutis 1995;56:132–136.

105. Sakai R, Kawashima H, Shibui H, et al. *Toxocara cati*-induced ocular toxocariasis. Arch Ophthalmol 1998;116:1686–1687.

106. Scheie HG, Morse PH. Rubeola retinopathy. Arch Ophthalmol 1972; 88:341–344.

107. Schwartz GS, Holland EJ. Oral acyclovir for the management of herpes simplex virus keratitis in childhood. Ophthalmology 2000; 107:278–282.

108. Sears ML. Congenital glaucoma in neonatal rubella. Br J Ophthalmol 1967;51:744–748.

109. Seltzer EB, Shapiro ED. Misdiagnosis of Lyme disease: when not to order serologic tests. Pediatr Infect Dis J 1996;15:761–763.

110. Shapiro ED, Gerber MA. Lyme disease. Clin Infect Dis 2000;31:533–542.

111. Sharf B, Hyams S. Oculomotor palsy following varicella. J Pediatr Ophthalmol 1972;9:245–247.

112. Sherman MD, Nozik RA. Other infections of the choroid and retina. Toxoplasmosis, histoplasmosis, Lyme disease, syphilis, tuberculosis, and ocular toxocariasis. Infect Dis Clin North Am 1992;6:893–908.

113. Shields JA. Ocular toxocariasis: a review. Surv Ophthalmol 1984;28: 361–381.

114. Siegel SE, Lunde MN, Gelderman AH, et al. Transmission of toxoplasmosis by leukocyte tranfusion. Blood 1971;37:388–394.

115. Small KW, McCuen BW, deJuan E, et al. Surgical management of retina traction caused by toxocariasis. Am J Ophthalmology 1989; 108:10–14.

116. Smith JL. Neuro-ocular Lyme borreliosis. Neurol Clin 1991;9:35–53.

117. Solley WA, Martin DF, Newman NJ, et al. Cat scratch disease. Posterior segment manifestations. Ophthalmology 1999;106:1546–1553.

118. South MA, Sever JL. Teratogen update: the congenital rubella syndrome. Teratology 1985;31:297–307.

119. Spach DH, Koehler JE. Bartonella-associated infections. Infect Dis Clin North Am 1998;12:137–155.

120. Steere AC. Medical progress—Lyme disease. N Engl J Med 1989;321: 586–596.

121. Stoll BJ, Lee FK, Larsen S, et al. Clinical and serological evaluation of neonates for congenital syphilis: a continuing diagnostic dilemma. J Infect Dis 1993;167:1093–1099.

122. Suttorp-Schulten MSA, Kuiper H, Kijlsta A, et al. Long-term effects of ceftriaxone treatment on intraocular lyme borreliosis. Am J Ophthalmol 1993;116:571–575.

123. Takayama N, Yamada H, Kaku H. Herpes zoster in immunocompetent and immunocompromised Japanese children. Pediatr Int 2000; 42:275–279.

124. Vila-Coro A, DelCotero JF, et al. Pediatric herpes simplex masquerading as varicella-zoster. Ann Ophthalmol 1989;21:47–48.

125. Voorhoeve AM, Muller AS, Schulpen TW, et al. Agents affecting health of mother and child in a rural area of Kenya. III. The epidemiology of measles. Trop Geogr Med 1977;29:428–440.

126. Wade NK, Levi L, Jones MR, et al. Optic disc edema associated with peripapillary serous retinal detachment: an early sign of systemic *Bartonella henselae* infection. Am J Ophthalmol 2000;130:321–328.

127. Wade NK, Po S, Wong IG, et al. Bilateral *Bartonella*-associated neuroretinitis. Retina 1999;19:355–356.

128. Weiss AH, Beck RW. Neuroretinitis in childhood. J Pediatr Ophthalmol Strabismus 1989;93:96–101.

129. Wilhelmus KR, Gee L, Hauck WW, et al. Herpetic eye disease study: a controlled trial of topical corticosteroids for herpes simplex stromal keratitis. Ophthalmology 1994;101:1883–1896.

130. Winward KE, Smith JL, Culbertson WW, et al. Ocular Lyme borreliosis. Am J Ophthalmol 1989;108:651–657.

10

Ocular Manifestations of Inherited Diseases

Maya Eibschitz-Tsimhoni

Recognizing an ocular abnormality may be the first step in identifying an inherited condition or syndrome. Identifying an inherited condition may corroborate a presumptive diagnosis, guide subsequent management, provide valuable prognostic information for the patient, and determine if genetic counseling is needed.

Syndromes with prominent ocular findings are listed in Table 10-1, along with their alternative names. By no means is this a complete listing. Two-hundred and thirty-five of approximately 1900 syndromes associated with ocular or periocular manifestations (both inherited and noninherited) identified in the medical literature were chosen for this chapter. These syndromes were selected on the basis of their frequency, the characteristic or unique systemic or ocular findings present, as well as their recognition within the medical literature. The boldfaced terms are discussed further in Table 10-2.

Table 10-2 provides a brief overview of the common ocular and systemic findings for these syndromes. The table is organized alphabetically; the boldface name of a syndrome is followed by a common alternative name when appropriate. Next, the Online Mendelian Inheritance in Man (OMIM™) index number is listed. By accessing the OMIM™ website maintained by the National Center for Biotechnology Information at http://www.ncbi.nlm.nih.gov, the reader can supplement the material in the chapter with the latest research available on that syndrome. A *MIM* number without a prefix means that the mode of inheritance has not been proven. The prefix (*) in front of a *MIM* number means that the phenotype determined by the gene at a given locus is separate from those represented by other asterisked entries and that the mode of inheritance of the phenotype has been proven. The prefix (#) indicates that the same phenotype can be caused by mutation in any of two or more genes. After the *MIM* number, the affected gene location is indicated, when known, followed by the mode of inheritance and the incidence or number of cases reported.

A general description of the syndrome featuring systemic manifestations is then provided, followed by pertinent ocular findings. Ocular findings are separated between "common" and "less common." Under "less common" abnormalities, reported sporadic abnormalities are listed that are not necessarily related to the disease. Findings that are in quotation marks are listed as they were originally described (often not in ophthalmologic nomenclature). A glossary of terms associated with inherited diseases precedes the tables.

Jablonski's Multiple Congenital Abnormality/Mental Retardation website at http://www.nlm.nih.gov/mesh/jablonski/syndrome_title.html is another fine resource for additional information.

Glossary

The following terms are associated with inherited diseases.

Acanthocytosis   a rare condition in which the majority of erythrocytes are acanthocytes; a thorny or peculiarly spiny erythrocyte characterized by multiple spiny cytoplasmic projections. Commonly seen in abetaliproproteinemia.

Acrocephaly   see oxycephaly.

Anencephaly   congenital absence of most of the brain and spinal cord.

Aplasia cutis congenita   congenital absence or deficiency of a localized area of skin, with the base of the defect covered by a thin translucent membrane.

Arachnodactyly   a hereditary condition characterized by excessive length of the fingers and toes.

Argyria   permanent dark discoloration of skin caused by overuse of medicinal silver preparations.

Arhinencephaly   an absence or rudimentary state of the rhino-encephalon, or olfactory lobe of the brain, on one or both sides, with a corresponding lack of development of the external olfactory organs.

Arthrogryposis   the permanent fixation of a joint in a contracted position. A congenital disorder marked by generalized stiffness of the joints, often accompanied by muscle and nerve degeneration, which results in severely impaired mobility of the limbs.

Bathocephaly   craniosynostosis involving the posterior sagittal suture.

Brachycephaly   having a short, broad head with a cephalic index over 80.

Brachydactyly   having abnormally short fingers or toes.

Camptodactyly   permanent flexion of one or more finger joints.

Clinodactyly   a deformity of the hand marked by deviation or deflection of the fingers.

Craniosynostosis   premature fusion of the sutures of the skull.

Cutis marorata   marble-like mottling of the skin on exposure to cold, common in children and some adults.

Dandy–Walker Syndrome   hydrocephalus in infants associated with atresia of the foramen of Magendie.

Ectrodactyly   congenital complete or partial absence of one or more digits.

Holoprosencephaly   failure of the forebrain to divide into hemispheres or lobes.

Hypodactyly   small fingers and/or toes.

Klippel–Feil Syndrome   congenital fusion of the cervical vertebrae resulting in a short and relatively immobile neck.

Metaphysis   the transitional zone at which the diaphysis and epiphysis of a bone come together.

Micrognathia   abnormal smallness of jaw.

Omphalocele   protrusion of abdominal contents through an opening at the navel, occurring especially as a congenital defect.

Oxycephaly   a congenital abnormality of the skull in which the top of the head assumes a conical or pointed shape. *Also called:* acrocephaly, turricephaly.

Polydactyly   the condition of having more than the normal number of toes or fingers.

Prognathism   a jaw that projects forward to a marked degree.

Scaphocephaly   a congenital deformity of the skull in which the vault is narrow, elongated, and boat-shaped because of premature ossification of the sagittal suture.

Symphalangism   ankylosis of the joints of one or more digits.

Syndactyly   a congenital anomaly in humans characterized by two or more fused fingers or toes.

Synostosis   the fusion of normally separate skeletal bones.

Tapetoretinal   of, relating to, or involving both tapetum and retina.

Tapetum   a membranous layer or region, especially the iridescent membrane of the choroid.

Trigonocephaly   congenital deformity in which the head is somewhat triangular and flat.

Turricephaly   see oxycephaly.

TABLE 10-1. Syndromes with Prominent Ocular Findings and Their Alternative Names.

2q− Syndrome—see Deletion 2q Syndrome (2q33.3–q34)
3p− Syndrome—see Deletion 3p Syndrome
3q+ Syndrome—see Duplication 3q Syndrome
4p− Syndrome—see Deletion 4p Syndrome
4q− Syndrome—see Deletion 4q Syndrome
5p− Syndrome—see Deletion 5p Syndrome
9p− Syndrome—see Deletion 9p Syndrome
10q+ Syndrome—see Duplication 10q Syndrome
11p− Syndrome—see Deletion 11p Syndrome
13q− Syndrome—see Deletion 13q Syndrome
15q− Syndrome—see Deletion 15q Syndrome
18p− Syndrome—see Deletion 18p Syndrome
18q− Syndrome—see Deletion 18q Syndrome

A
Aarskog Syndrome
Aase Syndrome
Aase–Smith Syndrome
Abetalipoproteinemia
Ablepharon–Macrostomia Syndrome
Abruzzo–Erickson Syndrome
Acrocallosal Syndrome, Schinzel Type
Acrocephalopolydactylous Dysplasia
Acrocephalopolysyndactyly Type 2—see Carpenter Syndrome
Acrocephalopolysyndactyly Type 4—see Goodman Syndrome
Acrocephaloysyndactyly Type 1—see Apert Syndrome
Acrocephaloysyndactyly Type 5—see Pfeiffer Syndrome
Acrodysostosis
Acrofacial Dysostosis 1, Nager Type—see Nager Syndrome
Acrofacial Dysplasia—see Geleophysic Dysplasia
Acro-Fronto-Facio-Nasal Dysostosis Syndrome
Acromegaloid Facial Appearance Syndrome
Acromegaloid Phenotype–Cutis Verticis Gyrata–Corneal Leukoma
Acromesomelic Dwarfism—see Acromesomelic Dysplasia,
   Maroteaux–Martinelli–Campailla Type
Acromesomelic Dysplasia, Maroteaux–Martinelli–Campailla Type
Acromicric Dysplasia
Acro-Osteolysis Syndrome—see Hajdu–Cheney Syndrome
Acro-Reno-Ocular Syndrome
Adams–Oliver Syndrome
AEC Syndrome—see Hay–Wells Syndrome of Ectodermal Dysplasia
Aglossia-Adactyly Syndrome—see Oromandibular-Limb Hypogenesis Spectrum
Aicardi's Syndrome
Alagille Syndrome—see Arteriohepatic Dysplasia
Albright Hereditary Osteodystrophy
Angelman Syndrome—see Deletion 15q (deletion of maternal allele)
Angio-Osteohypertrophy Syndrome—see Klippel–Trenaunay–Weber Syndrome
   (KTW Syndrome)
Ankyloblepharon-Ectodermal Dysplasia-Clefting Syndrome—see Hay–Wells
   Syndrome of Ectodermal Dysplasia

TABLE 10-1. (continued).

Anophthalmia with Limb Anomalies

Antley–Bixler Syndrome

Apert Syndrome

Arteriohepatic Dysplasia

Arthro-Ophthalmopathy, Hereditary, Progressive, Stickler Type (AOM),
Membranous Vitreous Type—see Stickler Syndrome

Asphyxiating Thoracic Dystrophy—see Jeune Thoracic Dystrophy

Ataxia-Telangiectasia Syndrome

ATR-X Syndrome—see X-Linked Alpha-Thalassemia/Mental Retardation
Syndrome

Axenfeld–Rieger Anomaly with Atrial Septal Defect and Sensorineural Hearing
Loss

Axenfeld–Rieger Anomaly with Partially Absent Eye Muscles, Distinctive Face,
Hydrocephaly, and Skeletal Abnormalities

B

Baller–Gerold Syndrome

Bannayan Syndrome—see Bannayan–Riley–Ruvalcaba Syndrome

Bannayan–Riley–Ruvalcaba Syndrome

Bardet–Biedl Syndrome Type I–VI

Bassen–Kornzweig disease—see Abetalipoproteinemia

Beals' Syndrome

Beckwith–Wiedemann Syndrome

Berardinelli–Lipodystrophy Syndrome

Berardinelli–Seip Congenital Lipodystrophy Syndrome—see
Berardinelli–Lipodystrophy Syndrome

Berman's Syndrome—see Sialolipidosis Syndrome

Bernheimer–Seiteberger disease—see Gangliosidosis Syndrome (GM₂), Type III

Beta-Glucuronidase Deficiency—see Mucopolysaccharidosis Type VII Syndrome

Bird-Headed Dwarfism—see Seckel's Syndrome

Blepharophimosis Syndrome (BPS) Type I, II, III

Bloch–Sulzberger Syndrome—see Incontinentia Pigmenti Syndrome

Borjeson–Forssman–Lehmann Syndrome

Boston-Type Cranisynostosis

Brachmann–de Lange Syndrome

Brachydactyly-Spherophakia Syndrome—see Weill–Marchesani Syndrome

Branchio-Oculo-Facial Syndrome

Branchio-Oto-Renal (BOR) Syndrome—see Melnick–Fraser Syndrome

C

Caffey Pseudo-Hurler Syndrome—see Generalized Gangliosidosis Syndrome
(GM₁), Type I (Severe Infantile Type)

Campomelic Dysplasia

Camptodactyly-Cleft-Palate-Club Foot, Gordon Type—see Distal Arthrogryposis
Syndrome, Type II

Camurati–Engelmann Syndrome

Cardiac-Limb Syndrome—see Holt–Oram Syndrome

Cardio-Facio-Cutaneous Syndrome

Carpenter Syndrome

Cat-Eye Syndrome (CES)

Cerebellar Parenchymal Disorder, Type IV—see Joubert Syndrome

(continued)

TABLE 10-1. Syndromes with Prominent Ocular Findings and Their Alternative Names (continued).

Cerebral Gigantism Syndrome—see Sotos Syndrome
Cerebro-Hepato-Renal Syndrome—see Zellweger Syndrome
Cerebro-Oculo-Facio-Skeletal (COFS) Syndrome
Cervico-Oculo-Acoustic Syndrome
CFC Syndrome—see Cardio-Facio-Cutaneous Syndrome
CHARGE Association
CHARGE-Like Syndrome—see Abruzzo–Erickson Syndrome
Cheney Syndrome—see Hajdu–Cheney Syndrome
Chondrodysplasia Punctata, Autosomal Recessive Type
Chondrodysplasia Punctata, X-Linked Dominant Type
Chondrodysplasia Punctata, X-Linked Recessive Type
Chondrodystrophica Myotonia Syndrome—see Schwart–Jampel Syndrome, Type 1
Cleft Lip Sequence
Cleidocranial Dysostosis
Cleidocranial Dysplasia—see Cleidocranial Dysostosis
Clouston's Syndrome
Cockayne's Syndrome, Type I
Coffin–Lowry Syndrome
Coffin–Siris Syndrome
Cohen Syndrome
Coloboma of Iris-Anal Atresia Syndrome—see Cat-Eye Syndrome (CES)
Conradi–Hunermann Syndrome—see Chondrodysplasia Punctata, X-Linked Dominant Type
Contractual Arachnodactyly, Congenital—see Beals Syndrome
Cornelia de Lange Syndrome—see Brachmann–de Lange Syndrome
Craniodiaphyseal Dysplasia-Lenz–Majewski Type—see Lenz–Majewski Hyperostotic Dwarfism
Craniofacial Dysostosis—see Crouzon Syndrome
Craniofrontonasal Dysostosis—see Craniofrontonasal Dysplasia (CFND)
Craniofrontonasal Dysplasia (CFND)
Craniometaphyseal Dysplasia
Craniosynostosis-Foot Defects, Jackson–Weiss Type—see Jackson–Weiss Syndrome
Craniosynostosis-Radial Aplasia Syndrome—see Baller–Gerold Syndrome
Cri-du-Chat Syndrome—see Deletion 5p Syndrome
Crouzon Syndrome
Cryptophthalmos Syndrome—see Fraser Syndrome

D
De Grouchy Syndrome—see Deletion 18q Syndrome
De Morsier Syndrome—see Septo-Optic Dysplasia Sequence
Deafness-Myopia-Cataract-Saddle Nose, Marshall Type—see Marshall Syndrome
Deletion 2q Syndrome (2q33.3–q34)
Deletion 3p Syndrome
Deletion 4p Syndrome
Deletion 4q Syndrome
Deletion 5p Syndrome
Deletion 9p Syndrome
Deletion 11p Syndrome
Deletion 11q Syndrome

TABLE 10-1. (continued).

Deletion 13q Syndrome Group 1, 2, and 3
Deletion 15q (deletion of maternal allele)
Deletion 15q (deletion of paternal allele)
Deletion 18p Syndrome
Deletion 18q Syndrome
Derry disease—see Generalized Gangliosidosis Syndrome (GM₁), Type II (Juvenile Type)
Desbuquois Syndrome—see Larsen's Syndrome
DiGeorge Sequence
Distal Arthrogryposis Syndrome, Type II
Distichiasis Syndrome
Distichiasis-Lymphedema Syndrome
Donohue's Syndrome—see Leprechaunism
Down Syndrome—see Trisomy 21
Duane Retraction Syndrome 1 (DURS1)—see Duane/Radial Dysplasia Syndrome
Duane/Radial Dysplasia Syndrome
Dubowitz Syndrome
Duplication 3q Syndrome
Duplication 4p Syndrome
Duplication 9p Syndrome
Duplication 10q Syndrome
Duplication 15q Syndrome
Dwarfism-Mulibrey Type—see Mulibrey Nanism Syndrome
Dyskeratosis Congenita Syndrome
Dysmorphic Sialidosis Syndrome—see Mucolipidosis Type I, Subtypes I, II
Dystrophia Myotonica Syndrome—see Steinert Myotonic Dystrophy Syndrome

E
Ectodermal Dysplasia 1—see Hypohidrotic Ectodermal Dysplasia Syndrome
Ectodermal Dysplasia 2—see Clouston Syndrome
Ectodermal Dysplasia-Hidrotic—see Clouston Syndrome
Ectopia Lentis et Pupillae
Ectrodactyly-Ectodermal Dysplasia-Clefting Syndrome I
Edwards' Syndrome—see Trisomy 18 Syndrome
Ehlers–Danlos Syndrome Type I, II, III, IV, V, VI, VII, VIII, IX, X
Elejalde Syndrome—see Acrocephalopolydactylous Dysplasia
Encephalofacial Angiomatosis Syndrome—see Sturge–Weber Syndrome (SWS)
Escobar Syndrome
Exomphalos-Macroglossia-Gigantism Syndrome—see Beckwith–Wiedemann Syndrome

F
Facial Diplegia, Congenital—see Möbius Syndrome I, II, III
Facio-Digito-Genital Dysplasia Syndrome—see Aarskog Syndrome
Facio-Oculo-Auriculo-Vertebral (FOAV) Dysplasia—see Goldenhar Syndrome
Familial Blepharophimosis Syndrome—see Blepharophimosis Syndrome (BPS)
Familial Neurovisceral Lipidosis—see Generalized Gangliosidosis Syndrome (GM₁), Type I (Severe Infantile Type)
Fanconi Pancytopenia Syndrome, Complementation Group A,B,C,D1,D2,E,F
Femoral Hypoplasia-Unusual Facies Syndrome
Femoral-Facial Syndrome—see Femoral Hypoplasia-Unusual Facies Syndrome

(continued)

TABLE 10-1. Syndromes with Prominent Ocular Findings and Their Alternative Names (continued).

Fetal Akinesia Sequence—see Pena–Shokeir Syndrome, Type 1
Fetal Face Syndrome—see Robinow's Syndrome
FG Syndrome
Fifth Digit Syndrome—see Coffin–Siris Syndrome
Focal Dermal Hypoplasia—see Goltz Syndrome
Fragile X Syndrome
Franceschetti–Klein Syndrome—see Treacher Collins Syndrome
Francois Dyscephalic Syndrome—see Hallermann–Streiff Syndrome
Fraser Syndrome
Freeman–Sheldon Syndrome
Frontometaphyseal Dysplasia
Frontonasal Dysplasia Sequence

G
Gangliosidosis Syndrome (GM$_2$), Type I
Gangliosidosis Syndrome (GM$_2$), Type II
Gangliosidosis Syndrome (GM$_2$), Type III
Geleophysic Dwarfism—see Geleophysic Dysplasia
Geleophysic Dysplasia
Genee–Wiedemann Syndrome—see Miller Syndrome
Generalized Gangliosidosis Syndrome (GM$_1$), Type I (Severe Infantile Type)
Generalized Gangliosidosis Syndrome (GM$_1$), Type II (Juvenile Type)
Gillespie Syndrome
Goldenhar's Syndrome
Goldenhar–Gorlin Syndrome—see Goldenhar's Syndrome
Goltz Syndrome
Goltz–Gorlin Syndrome—see Goltz Syndrome
Goodman Syndrome
Gorlin's Syndrome
Greig Cephalopolysyndactyly Syndrome

H
Hajdu–Cheney Syndrome
Hallermann–Streiff Syndrome
Hay–Wells Syndrome of Ectodermal Dysplasia
Hirschsprung Disease-Pigmentary Anomaly—see Waardenburg Syndrome
Holt–Oram Syndrome
Homocystinuria
Hunter's Syndrome
Hurler Syndrome
Hurler–Scheie Syndrome
Hutchinson–Gilford Syndrome—see Progeria Syndrome
Hypochondroplasia
Hypohidrotic Ectodermal Dysplasia Syndrome
Hypohidrotic Ectodermal Dysplasia, Autosomal Dominant Type—see Rapp–Hodgkin Ectodermal Dysplasia Syndrome
Hypomelanosis of Ito
Hypophosphatasia

I
Incontinentia Pigmenti Syndrome
Incontinentia Pigmentosa Achromians—see Hypomelanosis of Ito

TABLE 10-1. (continued).

J
Jackson–Weiss Syndrome
Jacobsen Syndrome—see Deletion 11q Syndrome
Jarcho–Levin Syndrome
Jeune Thoracic Dystrophy
Johanson–Blizzard Syndrome
Joubert Syndrome

K
Kabuki Syndrome
Keratitis-Ichthyosis-Deafness Syndrome, Autosomal Dominant—see Kid Syndrome, Autosomal Dominant
Keratitis-Ichthyosis-Deafness Syndrome, Autosomal Recessive—see Kid Syndrome, Autosomal Recessive
Kid Syndrome, Autosomal Dominant
Kid Syndrome, Autosomal Recessive
Killian/Teschler–Nicola Syndrome
Kivlin–Krause Syndrome—see Peters' Anomaly with Short-Limb Dwarfism
Klippel–Trenaunay–Weber Syndrome (KTW Syndrome)
Kniest Dysplasia

L
Lacrimo-Auriculo-Dento-Digital Syndrome, LADD Syndrome—see Levy–Hollister Syndrome
Langer–Giedion Syndrome
Larsen's Syndrome
Laurence–Moon–Bardet–Biedl Syndrome—see Bardet–Biedl Syndrome
Leber's Congenital Amaurosis, Type I, II, III, IV, V
Lenz–Majewski Hyperostotic Dwarfism
Leopard Syndrome—see Multiple Lentigines Syndrome
Leprechaunism Donohue Syndrome
Leroy I-Cell Syndrome—see Mucolipidosis Type II
Levy–Hollister Syndrome
Linear Nevus Sebaceous of Jadassohn
Lipodystrophy, Partial, with Rieger Anomaly, Short Stature, and Insulinopenic Diabetes Mellitus
Louis–Bar Syndrome—see Ataxia-Telangiectasia Syndrome
Lowe Syndrome—see Oculocerebrorenal Syndrome

M
Mandibulofacial Dysostosis—see Treacher Collins Syndrome
Marden–Walker Syndrome
Marfan Syndrome
Marfanoid Craniosynostoisis Syndrome—see Shprintzen–Goldberg Craniosynostosis Syndrome
Marker X Syndrome—see Fragile X Syndrome
Maroteaux–Lamy Syndrome
Marshall Syndrome
Marshall–Smith Syndrome
Martin-Bell Syndrome—see Fragile X Syndrome
Median Cleft Face Syndrome—see Frontonasal Dysplasia Sequence

(continued)

TABLE 10-1. Syndromes with Prominent Ocular Findings and Their Alternative Names (continued).

Melnick–Fraser Syndrome
Melnick–Needles Osteodysplasty
Metatropic Dwarfism II—see Kniest Dysplasia
Microphthalmia with Linear Skin Defects Syndrome
Midas Syndrome—see Microphthalmia with Linear Skin Defects Syndrome
Miller Syndrome
Miller–Dieker Lissencephaly Syndrome
Möbius Syndrome I, II, III
Mohr Syndrome
Monosomy 9p Syndrome—see Deletion 9p Syndrome
Morquio Syndrome
Mucolipidosis IV—see Sialolipidosis Syndrome
Mucolipidosis Type I, Subtypes I, II
Mucolipidosis Type II
Mucolipidosis Type III—see Pseudo-Hurler Polydystrophy Syndrome
Mucolipidosis Type IV—see Sialopidosis
Mucopolysaccharidosis III Type A, B, C, D—see Sanfilippo Syndrome
Mucopolysaccharidosis Type I H, MPS 1 H—see Hurler Syndrome
Mucopolysaccharidosis Type I H/S, MPS 1H/S—see Hurler–Scheie Syndrome
Mucopolysaccharidosis Type II—see Hunter's Syndrome
Mucopolysaccharidosis Type IS—see Scheie Syndrome
Mucopolysaccharidosis Type IV Subtypes A and B—see Morquio Syndrome
Mucopolysaccharidosis Type VII Syndrome
Mucopolysaccharidosis VI Mild, Moderate and Severe Types—see Maroteaux–Lamy Syndrome
Mulibrey Nanism Syndrome
Multiple Lentigines Syndrome
Multiple Pterygium Syndrome—see Escobar Syndrome
Multiple Synostosis Syndrome

N
Nager Syndrome
Nail-Patella Syndrome
Neurofibromatosis Type II
Neurofibromatosis, Type I (NF1)
Nevoid Basal Cell Carcinoma Syndrome—see Gorlin's Syndrome
Niikawa–Kuroki Syndrome—see Kabuki Syndrome
Noonan Syndrome 1
Norrie's Disease

O
Ocephaloysyndactyly Type 3—see Saethre–Chotzen Syndrome Acr
Oculocerebrorenal Syndrome
Oculodentodigital Syndrome
Oculodentoosseous Dysplasia (ODOD)—see Oculodentodigital Syndrome
Oculomandibulodyscephaly—see Hallermann–Streiff Syndrome
OFD Syndrome Type II—see Mohr Syndrome
Onychoosteodysplasia—see Nail-Patella Syndrome
Opitz Syndrome Type I, II
Opitz–Frias Syndrome—see Opitz Syndrome
Opitz–Kaveggia FG Syndrome—see FG Syndrome

TABLE 10-1. (continued).

Oral-Facial-Digital Syndrome 1
Oromandibular-Limb Hypogenesis Spectrum
Osteogenesis Imperfecta Syndrome, Type I
Oto-Palato-Digital Syndrome, Type I

P
Pachyonychia Congenita Syndrome, Type 1
Pallister–Hall Syndrome
Pallister–Killian Syndrome—see Killian/Teschler–Nicola Syndrome
Pancytopenia Syndrome, Fanconi Type—see Fanconi Pancytopenia Syndrome,
  Complementation Group A,B,C,D1,D2,E,F
Patau Syndrome—see Trisomy 13 Syndrome
Pena–Shokeir Syndrome, Type 1
Pena–Shokeir Syndrome, Type II—see Cerebro-Oculo-Facio-Skeletal (COFS)
  Syndrome
Penta X Syndrome—see XXXXX Syndrome
Peppe Syndrome—see Cohen Syndrome
Perheentupa Syndrome—see Mulibrey Nanism Syndrome
Perinatal Lethal Hypophosphatasia—see Hypophosphatasia
Peters' Anomaly—Associated with Other Ocular Defects
Peters' Anomaly—Isolated Ocular Abnormality
Peters' Anomaly with Short-Limb Dwarfism
Peters'-Plus Syndrome
Pfeiffer's Syndrome, Type I, II, III
Pitt–Rogers–Danks Syndrome (PRDS)—see Deletion 4p Syndrome
Poikiloderma Congenitale Syndrome—see Rothmund–Thomson Syndrome
Postaxial Acrofacial Dysostosis—see Miller Syndrome
Prader–Willi Syndrome—see Deletion 15q (deletion of paternal allele)
Progeria Syndrome
Progressive Diaphyseal Dysplasia—see Camurati–Engelmann Syndrome
Proteus Syndrome
Pseudoglioma—see Norrie's Disease
Pseudo-Hurler Polydystrophy Syndrome

R
Radial Aplasia-Thrombocytopenia Syndrome
Rapp–Hodgkin Ectodermal Dysplasia Syndrome
Renal Tubular Acidosis II
Renal Tubular Acidosis, Proximal, with Bilateral Glaucoma, Cataract, and Band
  Keratopathy—see Renal Tubular Acidosis II
Retinoblastoma, RB1
Rhizomelic Chondrodysplasia Punctata, Type II—see Chondrodysplasia
  Punctata, Autosomal Recessive Type
Rieger's Syndrome, Type I, II
Riley–Smith Syndrome—see Bannayan–Riley–Ruvalcaba Syndrome
Robinow's Syndrome
Rosenthal–Kloepfer Syndrome—see Acromegaloid Phenotype-Cutis Verticis
  Gyrata-Corneal Leukoma
Rothmund–Thomson Syndrome
Rubinstein–Taybi Syndrome
Ruvalcaba–Myhre Syndrome—see Bannayan–Riley–Ruvalcaba Syndrome

(continued)

TABLE 10-1. Syndromes with Prominent Ocular Findings and Their Alternative Names (continued).

S

Saethre–Chotzen Syndrome

Sandhoff disease—see Gangliosidosis Syndrome (GM₂), Type II

Sanfilippo's Syndrome

Scheie's Syndrome

Schinzel–Giedion Midface-Retraction Syndrome

Schmid–Fraccaro Syndrome—see Cat-Eye Syndrome (CES)

Schwart–Jampel Syndrome, Type 1

Sclerosteosis

Seckel's Syndrome

Septo-Optic Dysplasia Sequence

SHORT Syndrome

Shprintzen Syndrome

Shprintzen–Goldberg Craniosynostosis Syndrome

Sialidosis Syndrome Type II—see Mucolipidosis Type I, Subtypes I, II

Sialolipidosis Syndrome

Simple Ectopia Lentis

Simpson–Golabi–Behmel Syndrome Type I, II

Sly Syndrome—see Mucopolysaccharidosis Type VII Syndrome

Smith–Lemli–Opitz Syndrome, Type 1

Sotos' Syndrome

Spondylocarpotarsal Synostosis Syndrome

Spondyloepiphyseal Dysplasia Congenita

Spondyloepiphyseal Dysplasia Tarda

Spondylothoracic Dysplasia Syndrome—see Jarcho–Levin Syndrome

Spranger's Syndrome—see Mucolipidosis Type I, Subtypes I, II

Steinert Myotonic Dystrophy Syndrome

Stickler Syndrome Type I

Stickler Syndrome, Beaded Vitreous Type—see Stickler Syndrome

Sturge–Weber Syndrome (SWS)

Symphalangism Syndrome—see Multiple Synostosis Syndrome

T

TAR Syndrome—see Radial Aplasia-Thrombocytopenia Syndrome

Taybi Syndrome—see Oto-Palato-Digital Syndrome, Type I

Tay–Sachs disease—see Gangliosidosis Syndrome (GM₂), Type I

Trapezoidocephaly-Synostosis Syndrome—see Antley–Bixler Syndrome

Treacher Collins Syndrome

Tricho-Rhino-Phalangeal Syndrome Type II, TRP II—see Langer–Giedion Syndrome

Triploidy Type II

Trisomy 13 Syndrome

Trisomy 18 Syndrome

Trisomy 21, Down Syndrome

Trisomy 4p Syndrome—see Duplication 4p Syndrome

Trisomy 8 Syndrome

Trisomy 9 Syndrome

Trisomy 9p Syndrome—see Duplication 9p Syndrome

Turner's Syndrome—see XO Syndrome

Turner-like Syndrome—see Noonan Syndrome 1

TABLE 10-1. (continued).

U
Usher Syndrome Type I (A to F), II (A, B, C), Type III

V
VATER Association
Velo-Cardio-Facial Syndrome—see Shprintzen Syndrome
von Hippel–Lindau Disease
Von Recklinghausen Disease—see Neurofibromatosis, Type I (NF-1)

W
Waardenburg Anophthalmia Syndrome—see Anophthalmia with Limb Anomalies
Waardenburg's Syndrome, Types I, IIA, IIB, III, and IV
Waardenburg-Ocular Albinism—see Waardenburg's Syndrome
WAGR Syndrome—see Deletion 11p Syndrome
Walker–Warburg Syndrome
Warburg Syndrome—see Walker–Warburg Syndrome
Warkany Syndrome—see Trisomy 8 Syndrome
Weaver Syndrome
Weill–Marchesani Syndrome
Werner Syndrome
Whistling Face Syndrome—see Freeman–Sheldon Syndrome
Wildervanck Syndrome—see Cervico-Oculo-Acoustic Syndrome
Williams Syndrome
Williams–Beuren Syndrome—see Williams Syndrome
Wolf-Hirschhorn Syndrome (WHS)—see Deletion 4p Syndrome

X
Xeroderma Pigmentosum Syndrome (Group A through I plus a variant)
X-Linked Alpha-Thalassemia/Mental Retardation Syndrome
X-Linked Spondyloepiphyseal Dysplasia—see Spondyloepiphyseal Dysplasia Tarda
XO Syndrome
XXX and XXXX Syndrome
XXXXX Syndrome
XXXY and XXXXY Syndromes

Y
Yunis–Varon Syndrome

Z
Zellweger Syndrome
Zinsser–Cole–Engman Syndrome—see Dyskeratosis Congenita Syndrome

TABLE 10-2. Ocular and Systemic Findings in Selected Inherited Syndromes.

Aarskog Syndrome *Facio-Digito-Genital Dysplasia Syndrome* MIM 100050, *305400

Gene map locus: Xp11.21. Inheritance: X-linked recessive, with carrier females showing some minor manifestations of the disorder. One hundred cases reported.

General Description: short stature, brachydactyly, shawl scrotum

Ocular Findings
Common: hypertelorism (90%), variable ptosis of eyelids (50%), slight downslanting palpebral fissures
Less common: strabismus, hyperopic astigmatism, latent nystagmus, blue sclera, posterior embryotoxon, corneal enlargement

Aase Syndrome MIM 205600 Inheritance: most likely autosomal recessive. Over 10 cases reported.

General Description: triphalangeal (finger-like) thumbs, congenital hypoplastic anemia

Ocular Findings: occasional downslanting palpebral fissures, occasional retinopathy

Aase–Smith Syndrome MIM *147800 Inheritance: autosomal dominant. Five cases reported.

General Description: cleft palate, joint contractures, Dandy–Walker malformation

Ocular Findings
Common: short palpebral fissures, ptosis in adulthood
Less common: oculomotor palsy

Abetalipoproteinemia *Bassen–Kornzweig disease* MIM #200100 Gene map locus: 4q22–q24. Inheritance: autosomal recessive. Rare.

General Description: intestinal fat malabsorption with poor absorption of vitamins A and E, progressive ataxia, peripheral neuropathy, acanthocytosis, anemia, congestive heart failure, cardiac dysarrhythmias, abnormal levels of plasma lipids. Onset occurs between 5 and 15 years of age with ataxia, steatorrhea, hepatosplenomegaly, and psychomotor retardation. Results from absence of plasma apolipoproteins, plasma apolipoprotein B-containing lipoproteins, and microsomal triglyceride transfer protein from the endoplasmic reticulum of hepatocytes and enterocytes.

Ocular Findings
Common: pigmentary degeneration of the retina usually develops in the early teens but may present at any age (50%). Electroretinographic findings often are subnormal before the appearance of ophthalmoscopic changes. Funduscopic changes are similar to retinitis pigmentosa in some and to retinitis punctata albescens in others. The macula may or may not be affected. Patients complain of decreased vision and nyctalopia. Vitamin A and E supplementation have been reported to have beneficial retinal effects.
Less common: strabismus, nystagmus, angioid streaks, subretinal neovascularization, cataract, ptosis

TABLE 10-2. (continued).

Ablepharon-Macrostomia Syndrome MIM 200110 Inheritance: possibly autosomal recessive or X-linked recessive. Three cases reported.

General Description: macrostomia, sparse hair, thickened skin, absent or small nipples, genital anomalies, absent zygomatic arches

Ocular Findings: absent eyebrows, absent upper and lower eyelids and eyelashes, corneal irritation and dryness due to lack of eyelids

Abruzzo–Erickson Syndrome *CHARGE-Like Syndrome* MIM 302905 Inheritance: X-linked inheritance or autosomal dominant with milder expression in females. Four cases reported.

General Description: cleft palate, coloboma of iris and/or retina, deafness, hypospadias, radial synostosis, short stature

Ocular Findings: coloboma of iris and/or retina, anterior segment dysgenesis, epicanthal folds, esotropia

Acrocallosal Syndrome, Schinzel Type MIM *200990 Gene map locus: 12p13.3–p11.2. Inheritance: autosomal recessive. Fifteen cases reported.

General Description: hypoplastic or absent corpus callosum, seizures, hypotonia, severe mental retardation, hydrocephaly, postaxial polydactyly of hands and feet, hallux duplication. Neonatal respiratory distress and intercurrent infections lead to early death in approximately 15% of patients.

Ocular Findings
Common: optic atrophy, decreased retinal pigmentation, hypertelorism, epicanthal folds, down-slanting palpebral fissures, strabismus
Less common: nystagmus

Acrocephalopolydactylous Dysplasia *Elejalde Syndrome* MIM 200995 Inheritance: probably autosomal recessive. Fifteen cases reported.

General Description: craniosynostosis producing turricephaly, macrosomia, thick skin, severe lung hypoplasia, renal dysplasia, short limbs, polydactyly. Diagnosis by histological demonstration of overgrowth of connective tissue in different organs.

Ocular Findings
Common: hypertelorism, epicanthal folds
Less common: microcornea, corneal opacity, optic atrophy, nystagmus, foveal hypoplasia, posterior embryotoxon

Acrodysostosis MIM *101800 Inheritance: autosomal dominant. Over 20 cases reported.

General Description: short hands with peripheral dysostosis, short stature, vertebral defects, small nose, mental deficiency

Ocular Findings: epicanthal folds (39%), hypertelorism (35%). Optic atrophy has been reported.

Acro-Fronto-Facio-Nasal Dysostosis Syndrome MIM 201180, 239710 Inheritance: autosomal recessive suggested. Eight cases reported.

General Description: frontonasal dysplasia with skeletal anomalies and polydactyly in a severely retarded child

(continued)

TABLE 10-2. Ocular and Systemic Findings in Selected Inherited Syndromes (continued).

Ocular Findings: hypertelorism, S-shaped palpebral fissures, ptosis, long eyelashes

Acromegaloid Facial Appearance Syndrome MIM *102150 Inheritance: autosomal dominant with complete penetrance. One family described.

General Description: progressive acromegaloid facial appearance

Ocular Findings: progressively thickened periorbital skin, narrow palpebral fissures secondary to thickened skin around the eyes, blepharophimosis, hypertelorism, synophrys, highly arched eyebrows

Acromegaloid Phenotype-Cutis Verticis Gyrata-Corneal Leukoma
Rosenthal–Kloepfer Syndrome MIM *102100 Inheritance: autosomal dominant. One family described.

General Description: progressive leukoma formation and gyrate convolutions of the scalp in association with acromegaly-like features including large hands and feet, large chin, tall stature. Soft skin, "split ridge" dermal ridge pattern, cutis verticis gyrata with longitudinal folding.

Ocular Findings: unilateral or bilateral progressive opacification of the cornea occurs during the first decade of life. It characteristically begins in the inferonasal quadrant of the corneal epithelium as a flat leukoma, which subsequently becomes slightly elevated (about 0.5 mm) and considerably more widespread, leading to blindness. The peripheral 1 mm of the cornea is usually spared. The lateral half of the supraorbital arch of the frontal bone is enlarged.

Acromesomelic Dysplasia, Maroteaux–Martinelli–Campailla Type
Acromesomelic Dwarfism MIM *602875 Gene map locus: 9p13–p12. Inheritance: autosomal recessive. Approximately 30 cases reported.

General Description: disproportionate short stature with relatively large head, short forearms, small hands and feet, short fingers, general joint laxity except at elbows, radial head dislocation, characteristic skeletal X-rays

Ocular Findings: corneal opacities have been reported

Acromicric Dysplasia MIM 102370 Inheritance: probably autosomal dominant. Fewer than 10 cases reported.

General Description: dwarfism, with markedly shortened hands and feet. Mild facial anomalies including short, stubby nose with anteverted nostrils

Ocular Findings: narrow palpebral fissures

Acro-Reno-Ocular Syndrome MIM 102490 Inheritance: autosomal dominant. A three-generation family has been reported.

General Description: Duane syndrome, radial ray anomalies such as thenar hypoplasia and thumb anomalies, kidney malformations including malrotation, ectopia, hypoplasia, or ureterovesicular reflux

Ocular Findings
Common: Duane syndrome
Less common: Optic nerve coloboma, iris coloboma, ptosis, microcornea, cataract, strabismus, and nystagmus have been reported.

TABLE 10-2. (continued).

Adams–Oliver Syndrome MIM *100300 Inheritance: autosomal dominant. More than 80 cases reported.

General Description: aplasia cutis congenita over the posterior parietal region of the scalp, with or without underlying defect of bone (the skull and scalp defects usually heal spontaneously), terminal transverse defects of limbs, short fingers, small toenails, mild growth deficiency, cutis marmorata

Ocular Findings: occasional esotropia, microphthalmia

Aicardi's Syndrome MIM *304050 Gene map locus: Xp22. Inheritance: X-linked dominant (lethal in the hemizygous male). Over 200 cases, all females, with the exception of one male with XXY karyotype.

General Description: a definite diagnosis requires presence of the three following major features: infantile spasms or seizure activity, absent corpus callosum (usually with other brain malformations), and characteristic chorioretinal "lacunar" lesions. Most patients with Aicardi syndrome die in the first decade of life, usually from recurrent pneumonia.

Ocular Findings
Common: the chorioretinal lesions of Aicardi syndrome are characteristic. The lesions are discrete yellow-white, round, well-defined, excavated (lacunar) lesions with sharp borders and minimal pigmentation along their edges. They are bilateral and most frequently found around the optic nerve head and in the posterior pole. The lesions decrease in size and number toward the peripheral fundus. The sensory retina may be completely absent in the "lacuna."
Less common: unilateral or bilateral microphthalmia, retrobulbar cysts, diminished size of optic nerves and chiasma, gliosis at the nerve head, persistence of the hyaloid system of blood vessels, persistence of the pupillary membrane, posterior synechiae, chorioretinal colobomata at the disc or in the inferior fundus, retinal detachment, sixth cranial nerve palsy, nystagmus.

Albright Hereditary Osteodystrophy MIM #103580, 203330, 300800 Gene map locus: 20q13.2. Inheritance: autosomal dominant, autosomal recessive, and X-linked respectively. Over 50 kindreds (2:1 female-to-male ratio).

General Description: short stature, obesity, mental deficiency, brachydactyly with short metacarpals, rounded facies, hypocalcemia, mineralization in subcutaneous tissues and basal ganglia (pseudohypoparathyroidism)

Ocular Findings: cataract (peripheral lenticular opacities), corneal opacities, macular degeneration, nystagmus, anisocoria, optic nerve swelling, optic atrophy, tortuosity of vessels, diplopia, microphthalmia, hypertelorism

Anophthalmia with Limb Anomalies *Waardenburg Anophthalmia Syndrome* MIM *206920 Inheritance: autosomal recessive. Twenty-one cases reported.

General Description: distal limb abnormalities such as syndactyly, camptodactyly, hypodactyly, or other deformities of the hands and/or feet. Mental retardation may occur. Occasionally, widely spaced nipples and genitourinary malformations.

Ocular Findings: unilateral or bilateral clinical anophthalmia

Antley–Bixler Syndrome *Trapezoidocephaly-Synostosis Syndrome* MIM *207410 Inheritance: autosomal recessive. Approximately 12 cases.

(continued)

TABLE 10-2. Ocular and Systemic Findings in Selected Inherited Syndromes (continued).

General Description: craniosynostosis, brachycephaly, frontal bossing, severe midface hypoplasia, dysplastic ears, camptodactyly, radiohumeral synostosis, femoral bowing/fractures, choanal stenosis/atresia

Ocular Findings: proptosis (100%)

Apert Syndrome *Acrocephaloysyndactyly Type 1* MIM #101200 Gene map locus: 10q26. Inheritance: autosomal dominant. Incidence 1:100,000–160,000 births.

General Description: craniosynostosis: acrocephalic skull (a wide midline calvarial defect, which is gradually filled by islands of bone in the 2 to 4 years after birth until the gap is obliterated. No true sagittal or metopic sutures are ever formed. The coronal sutures are generally fused at birth). The brain is typically megalocephalic. A significant proportion of patients are mentally retarded. High forehead with depressed nasal bridge, beaked nose, hypoplastic midface, asymmetrical face, downturned mouth, prominent mandible, narrow and high-arched palate, lateral palatal swellings, clefting of the soft palate (30%), crowded upper teeth. Symmetrical mitten-type partial to complete syndactyly of digits, most often digits 2, 3, and 4, in hands and feet. Brachydactyly, aplasia, or ankyloses of joints, most commonly the shoulder, hip, and elbow. Cardiovascular defects (10%), genitourinary defects (10%), respiratory defects (1.5%), and gastrointestinal defects (1.5%).

Ocular Findings
Common: shallow bony orbits that lead to significant ocular proptosis, hypertelorism, down-slanting palpebral fissures, a horizontal groove above the supraorbital ridges, V-pattern exotropia, abnormal origins, size or insertion of ocular muscles

Less common: absence of superior rectus muscle, albinotic appearance of the fundus including depigmentation of the fundus and absence of foveal reflexes although vision is not markedly impaired and pendular nystagmus is absent. Optic atrophy, keratoconus, glaucoma, and subluxation of the globe are occasionally seen.

Arteriohepatic Dysplasia *Alagille Syndrome* MIM #118450 Gene map locus: 20p12. Inheritance: autosomal dominant. More than 100 cases reported.

General Description: at least three of the following five primary clinical criteria should be present: 1, cholestasis (91%) due to paucity of intrahepatic interlobular bile ducts; 2, characteristic facies (95%) consisting of triangular chin, prominent forehead, long straight nose with flat tip, and flat midface; 3, posterior embryotoxon; 4, butterfly vertebrae (hemivertebrae); and 5, cardiac findings, most often pulmonary artery stenosis (85%)

Ocular Findings
Common: Anterior segment dysgenesis including prominent posterior embryotoxon (88%), or Axenfeld–Rieger anomaly. Up to 90% of patients have unilateral optic nerve head drusen and as many as 65% have bilateral drusen. If patients have elevated serum cholesterol levels, arcus juvenilis may develop.

Less common: retinal pigment clumping, chorioretinal atrophy (when retinal changes are present, the electroretinogram findings are consistent with rod-cone dystrophy), choroidal folds, marked tortuosity of the retinal vessels, strabismus, myopia. Keratoconus is a rare associated finding.

TABLE 10-2. (continued).

Ataxia-Telangiectasia Syndrome *Louis–Bar Syndrome* MIM *208900, 208910
Gene map locus: 11q22.3. Inheritance: autosomal recessive. Incidence
1:30,000–100,000 live births.

General Description: onset of rapidly progressive cerebellar ataxia at 1 to 2 years
of age, with subsequent development of choreoathetosis, dysarthrai, and
dystomia. Slow regression of intellectual milestones may occur. Bilateral
conjunctival telangiectasia develop between 3 to 7 years of age followed by
cutaneous telangiectasia. Deficiency in cellular immunity with thymic
hypoplasia, low or absent serum and secretory IgA serum IgE, and IgG, normal
to elevated levels of low-molecular-weight IgM. Frequent sinusitis, pneumonia,
bronchiectasis, and skin infections. Increased rate of lymphoma, leukemia, and
other neoplasms. Drying of skin and loss of hair, particularly when exposed to
ultraviolet radiation. Endocrine dysfunction with glucose intolerance, hypogonadism with delayed sexual maturation, and growth retardation is often
found. Sinopulmonary infection is a major cause of mortality. Death occurs
during the second decade of life.

Ocular Findings: telangiectasia of the conjunctiva develops in all patients
beginning between the ages of 3 and 7 years. Involvement is initially
interpalpebral away from the limbus, eventually becoming generalized. Ocular
motor abnormalities are common. Characteristically, the ability to initiate
saccades is poor, very similar to the findings of congenital ocular motor
apraxia. Strabismus and nystagmus may also be present.

**Axenfeld–Rieger Anomaly with Atrial Septal Defect and Sensorineural Hearing
Loss** MIM *602482. Inheritance: autosomal dominant. One family.

General Description: atrial septal defect and sensorineural hearing loss.

Ocular Findings: Axenfeld's–Reiger anomaly (consists of anterior segment
dysgenesis resulting in hypoplasia of the anterior iris stroma, posterior
embryotoxon, abnormal iris strands crossing the anterior chamber angle to
attach to a prominent Schwalbe's line), glaucoma (60%)

**Axenfeld–Rieger Anomaly with Partially Absent Eye Muscles, Distinctive Face,
Hydrocephaly, and Skeletal Abnormalities** MIM 109120. Inheritance:
autosomal dominant. One family.

General Description: prominent forehead, flat midface, mild sensorineural
deafness, communicating hydrocephalus, psychomotor retardation, flat femoral
epiphyses.

Ocular Findings: Axenfeld's-Reiger anomaly (consists of anterior segment
dysgenesis resulting in hypoplasia of the anterior iris stroma, posterior
embryotoxon, abnormal iris strands crossing the anterior chamber angle to
attach to a prominent Schwalbe's line), glaucoma (60%), absent eye muscles,
proptosis, hypertelorism

Baller–Gerold Syndrome *Craniosynostosis-Radial Aplasia Syndrome* MIM
218600 Inheritance: autosomal recessive. Over 20 cases reported.

General Description: craniosynostosis of one or more sutures (any of the cranial
sutures may be affected). Preaxial upper limb abnormalities: aplasia or
hypoplasia of the thumb, aplasia or hypoplasia of the radius (bilateral in over
90% of cases), short curved ulna, missing carpals, metacarpals, and phalanges,

(continued)

TABLE 10-2. Ocular and Systemic Findings in Selected Inherited Syndromes (continued).

fused carpals. Prenatal and postnatal growth deficiency. Vertebral anomalies (30%). A wide variety of internal malformations most frequently affect the anus, urogenital system, heart, and central nervous system.

Ocular Findings
Common: down-slanting palpebral fissures, epicanthal folds, hypertelorism
Less common: exotropia, ectropion, nystagmus, high myopia, optic atrophy

Bannayan–Riley–Ruvalcaba Syndrome *Ruvalcaba–Myhre Syndrome, Riley–Smith Syndrome, Bannayan Syndrome* MIM #153480 Gene map locus: 10q23.3. Inheritance: autosomal dominant. Fifteen kinships reported.

General Description: macrocephaly with ventricles of normal size, ileal and colonic hamartomatous polyps (45%), subcutaneous/cranial (20%)/osseous (10%) hamartomas that are lipomas (75%), hemangiomas (10%), or mixed type (20%). Cutis marmorata, skin telangiectases, enlarged penis, hemangiomas, or mixed pigmentary changes of the penis.

Ocular Findings
Common: down-slanting palpebral fissures (60%), pseudo-papilledema
Less common: prominent Schwalbe lines and prominent corneal nerves (35%), hypertelorism may be associated with midfacial hypoplasia, strabismus (15%), anisometropia

Bardet–Biedl Syndrome type I–VI *Laurence–Moon–Bardet–Biedl Syndrome* MIM *209901, *209900, *600151, *600374, *603650, #605231 Gene map loci include: 11q13, 16q21, 3p13–p12, 15q22.3–q23, 2q31, and 20p12, respectively. Inheritance: autosomal recessive. Incidence: 1:100,000.

General Description: truncal obesity, short stature, polydactyly, hypogenitalism, hypogonadism, mental retardation, renal anomalies, dental anomalies, occasional congenital heart disease. *(In Laurence–Moon syndrome, there is spastic paraplegia, and absence of obesity and polydactyly. In Alstrom syndrome (*203800) there is retinitis pigmentosa, obesity, diabetes mellitus and perceptive deafness. In Biemond syndrome II (210350) there is iris coloboma, hypogenitalism, obesity, polydactyly, and mental retardation).*

Ocular Findings
Common: Progressive cone-rod retinal dystrophy begins in childhood and progresses to severe visual loss and a marked constriction of visual fields usually by age 30 years (90–100%). The retinal degeneration is not a typical retinitis pigmentosa in that hyperpigmentation is not a prominent feature, rather, there is coarse granularity of the periphery. The macula is often involved early with atropic and pigmentary changes, sometimes in a bull's-eye configuration. Optic nerve pallor and arteriolar narrowing occur. The electroretinogram is nonrecordable in early childhood. Myopia (75%), astigmation (63%), nystagmus (52%). By age twenty, 73% of patients are blind.
Less common: glaucoma (22%), posterior capsular cataract (44%), mature cataract (30%), typical retinitis pigmentosa (8%).

Beals' Syndrome *Contractual Arachnodactyly, Congenital* MIM *121050 Gene map locus: 5q23–q31. Inheritance: autosomal dominant. Twenty families and over 13 isolated cases reported.

TABLE 10-2. (continued).

General Description: long slim limbs (dolichostenomlia) with arachnodactyly (86%), camptodactyly (78%), joint contractures especially of knees, elbows, and hips, "crumpled" ears with poorly defined conchas and prominent crura from the root of the helix (75%).

Ocular Findings: ectopia lentis, iris coloboma, keratoconus, and myopia have been reported

Beckwith–Wiedemann Syndrome *Exomphalos-Macroglossia-Gigantism Syndrome* MIM #130650, *602631, *603240 Gene map locus: 11p15.5. Inheritance: autosomal dominant, many sporadic. Approximately 200 cases reported.

General Description: macroglossia, capillary nevus flammeus of central forehead and eyelids, macrosomia, ear creases, accelerated osseous maturation, omphalocele, neonatal polycythemia, hypoglycemia in early infancy, cardiovascular defects, large kidneys with renal medullary dysplasia, pancreatic hyperplasia, fetal adrenocortical cytomegaly, occasional hemihypertrophy. An increased risk of malignancy seems to be associated with those who have hemihypertrophy.

Ocular Findings: prominent eyes with relative infraorbital hypoplasia, capillary nevus flammeus of central forehead and eyelids

Berardinelli–Lipodystrophy Syndrome *Berardinelli–Seip Congenital Lipodystrophy Syndrome* MIM *269700 Gene map locus: 9q34. Inheritance: autosomal recessive. Rare disorder.

General Description: accelerated growth and maturation, enlargement of hands and feet, phallic enlargement, hypertrophy of muscles, lack of metabolically active adipose tissue from early life with sparing of mechanical adipose tissue such as in the orbits, palms, tongue, and scalp. Coarse skin with hyperpigmentation, hepatomegaly, hyperlipidemia, hypertriglyceridemia, insulin-resistant diabetes mellitus.

Ocular Findings: occasional corneal opacities

Blepharophimosis Syndrome (BPS) Type I, II, III *Familial Blepharophimosis Syndrome* MIM #110100, *601649 Gene map loci: 3q23 (types I and II), 7p21–p13 (type III). Inheritance: autosomal dominant. More than 150 families reported.

General Description: Type I is associated with infertility in affected females whereas type II is not. Both may be associated with incomplete development of the ears, malar hypoplasia, poorly developed nasal bridge, and variable hypotonia in early life.

Ocular Findings

Common: blepharophimosis (reduction of the palpebral fissure in the horizontal axis from the normal of 25–30 mm to 20–22 mm). Ptosis of the upper eyelid, and epicanthus inversus. In most patients there is an increased length of the medial canthal ligament resulting in telecanthus. Ptosis is present at birth and is typically associated with absent or poor levator function and no eyelid fold. To compensate for the ptosis, patients assume a characteristic head posture with chin elevation and furrowing of the eyebrows. The upper eyelid margin is characteristically S-shaped while the lower eyelid margin has abnormal downward concavity, with or without slight ectropion. The eyelids are smooth

TABLE 10-2. Ocular and Systemic Findings in Selected Inherited Syndromes (continued).

and inelastic with skin deficiency in both the upper and lower lids and there is often hypoplasia of the tarsal plates of the upper eyelids. Trichiasis and hypoplastic appearance of the caruncle and plica semilunaris are common. Of the four types of epicanthal folds, epicanthus inversus is the most common form associated with BPS. The eyebrows are increased in their vertical height and are arched.

Less common: microphthalmia, anophthalmia, microcornea, cataract, angle dysgenesis, optic disc coloboma, optic nerve hypoplasia, optic atrophy, superior rectus underaction with limitation of upgaze, divergent strabismus, nystagmus, hypermetropia

---

Borjeson–Forssman–Lehmann Syndrome MIM *301900 Gene map locus: Xq26.3. Inheritance: X-linked recessive. Five families reported.

General Description: large ears, hypogonadism, severe mental deficiency, seizures, marked obesity, hypometabolism, swollen subcutaneous facial tissue

Ocular Findings: nystagmus, ptosis, poor vision, retinal and/or optic nerve abnormalities, narrow palpebral fissures, deep-set eyes

---

Boston-Type Cranisynostosis MIM #604757 Gene map locus: 5q34–q35. Inheritance: autosomal dominant. Nineteen cases reported.

General Description: frontal bossing, frontoorbital recession, turribrachycephaly, and cloverleaf skull. Intelligence is normal. Short but not broad, first metatarsals. Cleft of soft palate and triphalangeal thumb each occurred in only one individual.

Ocular Findings
Common: myopia, hyperopia
Less common: visual field defects

Brachmann–de Lange Syndrome *Cornelia de Lange Syndrome* MIM 122470 Gene map locus: 3q26.3. Inheritance: most cases are sporadic. Incidence: 1:10,000 live births.

General Description: physical and mental retardation, hirsutism, synophrys, microcephaly, long or protruding philtrum, anteverted nostrils, small or grossly malformed hands, cutis marmorata

Ocular Findings: bushy eyebrows and synophrys (98%), long curly eyelashes (99%), myopia, ptosis, and nystagmus.

Branchio-Oculo-Facial Syndrome MIM *113620 Inheritance: autosomal dominant. Over 30 cases reported.

General Description: characteristic cervical/infra-auricular skin defects including aplastic/hemangiomatous lesions and sinus/fistulous tracts (45%). Abnormal upper lip (90%) (pseudocleft, incomplete or complete cleft lip), dental anomalies, micrognathia, conductive hearing loss (71%), low-set/posteriorly rotated/overfolded and/or malformed ears, premature graying of hair (70%), renal malformations, developmental delay (25%), hypotonia, growth deficiency (50%)

Ocular Findings
Common: nasolacrimal duct obstruction with recurrent dacryocystitis (75%), telecanthus (58%), coloboma (47%), microphthalmia/anophthalmia (44%), up-slanting palpebral fissures (48%), myopia (46%)

TABLE 10-2. (continued).

Less common: ptosis, orbital hemangiomatous cyst, cataract, strabismus, orbital dermoids

Campomelic Dysplasia MIM *114290 Gene map locus: 17q24.3–q25.1. Inheritance: autosomal dominant. Over 100 cases reported. Most patients die in infancy.

General Description: short limb dwarfism of prenatal onset with retarded osseous maturation, large head, large brain with gross cellular disorganization, flat facies, cleft palate, malformed and/or low-set ears, bowed tibiae, hypoplastic scapula, XY gonadal dysgenesis (ovarian, mullerian duct, and vaginal development in some of the affected XY individuals)

Ocular Findings: short palpebral fissures, hypertelorism

Camurati–Engelmann Syndrome *Progressive Diaphyseal Dysplasia* MIM #131300 Gene map locus: 19q13.1. Inheritance: autosomal dominant. More than 100 cases reported.

General Description: progressive diaphyseal dysplasia, thickening of the bone, and narrowing of the medullary canal. Sclerosis of skull base, weakness, leg pain

Ocular Findings: occasional exophthalmos. Hyperostosis may progress to cause optic nerve compression.

Cardio-Facio-Cutaneous Syndrome *CFC Syndrome* MIM #115150 Gene map locus: 12q24. Inheritance: autosomal dominant. More than 35 cases reported.

General Description: congenital heart defects (77%), sparse, curly, and slow-growing hair (100%), abnormalities of skin (95%) varying from severe atopic dermatitis to hyperkeratosis, frontal bossing, mental retardation, hypotonia, postnatal growth deficiency, relative macrocephaly with large prominent forehead and bitemporal narrowing

Ocular Findings: lack of eyebrows and eyelashes, nystagmus, strabismus, shallow orbital ridges (100%), down-slanting palpebral fissures (71%), hypertelorism (84%), ptosis (53%), exophthalmos (55%)

Carpenter Syndrome *Acrocephalopolysyndactyly Type 2* MIM *201000 Inheritance: autosomal recessive. More than 40 cases reported.

General Description: craniosynostosis (multiple sutures are usually involved, often beginning with the sagittal and lambdoid sutures, causing marked asymmetry and acrocephaly). Intellectual impairment (75%). The fingers are typically short, with varying degree of soft tissue syndactyly. The feet often have preaxial polydactyly, and each toe has only two phalanges. Congenital heart defects (33%) including atrial and ventricular septal defects, patent ductus arteriosus, pulmonic stenosis, and tetralogy of Fallot. The ears are low-set and may have minor abnormalities such as preauricular pits.

Ocular Findings
Common: hypoplastic supraorbital ridges, hypertelorism, shallow orbits, lateral displacement of the inner canthi, down-slanting palpebral fissures, epicanthal folds
Less common: corneal opacity, microcornea optic nerve atrophy, blurring of disc margins. Conjugate downward movements alternating with horizontal and vertical nystagmus, foveal hypoplasia, and posterior embryotoxon have been reported.

(continued)

TABLE 10-2. Ocular and Systemic Findings in Selected Inherited Syndromes (continued).

Cat-Eye Syndrome (CES) *Schmid–Fraccaro Syndrome, Coloboma of Iris-Anal Atresia Syndrome* MIM #115470 Gene map locus: 22q11. Inheritance: autosomal dominant. Over 40 cases reported.

General Description: mild mental deficiency, preauricular pits or tags, micrognathia, cleft palate, cardiac defects (33%), hearing impairment, anal atresia with rectovestibular fistula, renal agenesis, cryptorchidism, hemivertebrae, and failure to thrive. Anal atresia and coloboma of iris, initially considered the hallmarks of this disorder, are present in combination in only a minority of patients.

Ocular Findings
Common: inferior coloboma of iris (common but not obligate), choroid and/or retina. The coloboma can involve the posterior segment with or without iris involvement. Mild hypertelorism, down-slanting palpebral fissures, epicanthal folds.
Less common: microphthalmia. Various forms of Duane syndrome have been reported. Poor vision has been reported.

Cerebro-Oculo-Facio-Skeletal (COFS) Syndrome *Pena–Shokeir Syndrome, Type II* MIM #214150 Gene map locus: 10q11. Inheritance: autosomal recessive. Rare disorder.

General Description: brain degenerative disorder with reduced white matter, microgyria, agenesis of corpus callosum, microcephaly, hypotonia, hyporeflexia or areflexia, neurogenic arthrogryposis (persistent flexure or contracture of a joint) especially in the elbows and knees. Rocker-bottom feet, camptodactyly, hirsutism, wide-set nipples, micrognathia, upper lip overlapping lower lip. The course of the disorder is progressive deterioration, with little growth and cachexia, ending in death. Survival is usually under 5 years.

Ocular Findings: hypoplasia of optic tracts and chiasm, microphthalmia, nystagmus, cataract (may be infantile), blepharophimosis with deep-set eyes

Cervico-Oculo-Acoustic Syndrome *Wildervanck Syndrome* MIM 314600 Inheritance: unknown (sporadic cases). The frequency among children with hearing loss is 1%. The vast majority of affected individuals have been females.

General Description: Klippel–Feil anomaly (fusion of two or more cervical and sometimes thoracic vertebrae), short neck, facial asymmetry, low hairline, malformed vestibular labyrinth, preauricular tags and pits, sensorineural, conductive or mixed hearing loss

Ocular Findings: Duane syndrome, epibulbar dermoids. Occasionally, pseudopapilledema.

CHARGE Association MIM 214800 Inheritance: sporadic in most cases (familial recurrence has been reported). Over 50 cases reported.

General Description: the acronym CHARGE has been used to represent the major features of this condition: Coloboma of the eye or eye defects, Heart disease, choanal Atresia, Retarded growth and development with or without central nervous system anomalies, Genital hypoplasia, and Ear anomalies with or without deafness. Four of the six major findings are generally required for diagnosis. Additional abnormalities include seventh cranial nerve palsy (up to 45%), and facial clefts.

TABLE 10-2. (continued).

Ocular Findings
Common: microphthalmia and colobomatous malformation sequence (80%): unilateral or bilateral colobomas of the iris, choroids, retina, or optic nerve. Visual impairment and retinal detachment can occur. It is estimated that 15%–30% of patients with microphthalmia/coloboma have CHARGE association.
Less common: strabismus, seventh cranial nerve palsy (up to 45%). Clinical anophthalmia, persistent hyperplastic primary vitreous, congenital cataract, Marcus Gunn jaw-winking, ptosis, and delayed visual maturation have been reported.

Chondrodysplasia Punctata, Autosomal Recessive Type *Rhizomelic Chondrodysplasia Punctata, Type II* MIM #215100 Gene map locus: 6q22–q24. Inheritance: autosomal recessive. Over 40 cases reported.

General Description: severe problem in growth and mental deficiency, cortical atrophy, seizures, spasticity, microcephaly, low nasal bridge and flat facies, frontal bossing, microganthia, sensorineural deafness, symmetric proximal shortening of humeri and femora, coronal cleft in vertebrae, punctate epiphyseal mineralization, ichthyosis (30%), alopecia. Patients usually die before 1 to 2 years of age.

Ocular Findings
Common: congenital cataract (72%)
Less common: up-slanting palpebral fissures

Chondrodysplasia Punctata, X-Linked Dominant Type *Conradi–Hunermann Syndrome* MIM #302960 Gene map locus: Xp11.23–p11.22. Inheritance: X-linked dominant (lethal in hemizygous males). Over 50 cases reported.

General Description: mild to moderate growth deficiency, variable low nasal bridge with flat facies, frontal bossing, hypoplasia of malar eminences, deafness, asymmetrical limb shortness related to areas of punctate mineralization in epiphyses, scoliosis related to early punctate mineralization, erythema and thick adherent scales in the newborn period. In older children, variable follicular atrophoderma with large pores resembling "orange peel" and ichthyosis, sparse, coarse hair, patchy areas of alopecia.

Ocular Findings
Common: cataract, down-slanting palpebral fissures
Less common: nystagmus, hazy cornea, microphthalmus, glaucoma, atrophy of retina and optic nerve

Chondrodysplasia Punctata, X-Linked Recessive Type MIM #302950 Gene map locus: Xp22.3. Inheritance: X-linked recessive. Rare.

General Description: chondrodysplasia punctata, ichthyosis, short stature, hypoplastic distal phalanges, microcephaly, developmental delay, hearing loss, linear or whorled atrophic and pigmentary skin lesions, striated ichthyosiform hyper-keratosis, follicular atrophoderma, cicatricial alopecia. Occasional anosmia and hypogonadism in males (Kallmann syndrome).

Ocular Findings: cataract

(continued)

TABLE 10-2. Ocular and Systemic Findings in Selected Inherited Syndromes (continued).

Cleft Lip Sequence MIM *119530 Gene map locus: 6p24.3. Inheritance: autosomal dominant (isolated cases (75%–80%), familial (10%–15%), and syndromal (1%–5%). Incidence: 1:1,000.

General Description: cleft lip frequently associated with cleft palate. Other secondary anomalies include defects of tooth development in the area of the cleft lip and incomplete growth of the ala nasi on the side of the cleft. Tertiary abnormalities can include poor speech, repeated otitis media, and conductive hearing loss.

Ocular Findings: occasional mild hypertelorism

Cleidocranial Dysostosis *Cleidocranial Dysplasia* MIM #119600 Gene map locus: 6p21. Inheritance: autosomal dominant. Over 500 cases reported.

General Description: partial to complete aplasia of clavicles with associated muscle defects, small thorax, late ossification of cranial sutures, late eruption of teeth, hand anomalies. Occasional deafness.

Ocular Findings: hypertelorism

Clouston's Syndrome *Ectodermal Dysplasia-Hidrotic, Ectodermal Dysplasia 2* MIM #129500 Gene map locus: 13q12. Inheritance: autosomal dominant. Over 200 cases reported.

General Description: nail hypoplasia to aplasia, nail dysplasia, hair hypoplasia to alopecia, thick dyskeratotic palms and soles

Ocular Findings
Common: deficiency of eyelashes and eyebrows, strabismus
Less common: cataract, photophobia

Cockayne's Syndrome, Type I MIM *216400 Gene map locus: chromosome 5. Inheritance: autosomal recessive. Over 60 cases reported.

General Description: senile-like changes beginning in infancy. Profound postnatal growth deficiency, impaired hearing, photosensitive dermatitis.

Ocular Findings: cataract, salt-and-pepper retinal pigmentation, optic atrophy, strabismus, hyperopia, corneal opacity, decreased lacrimation, nystagmus, moderately sunken eyes, poor pupillary dilation secondary to hypoplasia of the dilator muscle, iris transillumination

Coffin–Lowry Syndrome MIM #303600 Gene map locus: Xp22.2–p22.1. Inheritance: X-linked dominant. Over 40 cases reported.

General Description: mild to moderate growth deficiency, severe mental deficiency, hypotonia, coarse facies, bullous nose, maxillary hypoplasia, large open mouth with thick everted lower lip, prominent ears, hypodontia, vertebral defects, large soft hands with tapering fingers

Ocular Findings: down-slanting palpebral fissures, mild hypertelorism, prominent eyebrows

Coffin–Siris Syndrome *Fifth Digit Syndrome* MIM 135900 Inheritance: autosomal dominant. Over 30 cases reported.

TABLE 10-2. (continued).

General Description: hypoplastic to absent fifth fingers and toenails, coarse facies, generalized hirsutism with tendency to have sparse scalp hair, mild to moderate growth deficiency, mental deficiency

Ocular Findings
Common: bushy eyebrows, long eyelashes
Less common: ptosis, hypotelorism

Cohen Syndrome *Peppe Syndrome* MIM *216550 Gene map locus: 8q22–q23. Inheritance: autosomal recessive. Over 80 cases reported.

General Description: hypotonia and weakness, microcephaly, mental deficiency, truncal obesity, short stature, prominent incisors, high nasal bridge, maxillary hypoplasia, micrognathia, large ears, long and narrow hands and feet, hypermobility of the joints, delayed puberty

Ocular Findings
Common: pigmentary retinopathy with night blindness, constricted visual fields, decreased visual acuity, and a nonrecordable ERG. Ophthalmoscopic findings include macular atrophic and pigmentary changes (sometimes in a bull's-eye configuration) and optic nerve pallor with arteriolar narrowing. Myopia, strabismus, mild down-slanting palpebral fissures.
Less common: microphthalmia, coloboma

Craniofrontonasal Dysplasia (CFND) *Craniofrontonasal Dysostosis* MIM #304110, 122920 Gene map locus: Xp22. Inheritance: X-linked with metabolic interference. Over 50 cases reported.

General Description: There is a difference in the clinical phenotype between males and females with females more severely affected. Females: craniosynostosis, brachycephaly, frontal bossing, syndactyly of fingers. Males: increased bony interorbital distance. Females and males: hypertelorism, facial asymmetry, broad nasal root, bifid nasal tip, longitudinal splitting of nails, syndactyly of toes, broad first toe, clinodactyly.

Ocular Findings
Common: females and males: hypertelorism, down-slanting palpebral fissures
Less common: females: telecanthus, exotropia, nystagmus

Craniometaphyseal Dysplasia MIM #123000, *218400 Gene map loci: 5p15.2–p14.1 (Jackson Type, autosomal dominant), 6q21–q22 (autosomal recessive type). Inheritance: autosomal dominant and autosomal recessive types. Over 50 cases reported.

General Description: cranial hyperostosis with thick calvarium, increased density of cranial vault, facial bones, and mandible, variable absence of pneumatization, and bony wedge over bridge of nose and supraorbital area (leonine facies). Macrocephaly. Mild splaying of metaphyses. Compression of the brain and cranial nerves particularly II, VII, and VIII may lead to facial palsy, deafness and blindness.

Ocular Findings: hypertelorism, compression of cranial nerves II, and VII may lead to blindness.

Crouzon Syndrome *Craniofacial Dysostosis* MIM #123500 Gene map locus: 10q26. Inheritance: autosomal dominant with variable expression. Incidence: 1 : 25,000.

(continued)

TABLE 10-2. Ocular and Systemic Findings in Selected Inherited Syndromes (continued).

General Description: craniosynostosis, especially of the coronal, lambdoid, and sagittal sutures. The head is most commonly brachycephalic, secondary to synostosis of the coronal sutures. Intelligence is generally normal. Conductive hearing loss, midfacial hypoplasia, "beaked" (parrot-like) nose, relative mandibular prognathism, short upper lip, lateral palatal swellings, dental problems such as malocclusion and crowding of teeth secondary to the hypoplastic maxilla, calcification of the stylohyoid ligament (88%), cervical spine anomalies (30%) (most frequently C2–C3 fusion). Occasionally acanthosis nigricans.

Ocular Findings

Common: proptosis secondary to shallow bony orbits, hypertelorism. The proptosis may lead to exposure keratitis, and in extreme cases to spontaneous subluxation of the globe. Exotropia (77%) typically a V-pattern exotropia. Some degree of optic nerve involvement reported to occur in 80% of patients, and optic atrophy reported in 22% of patients.

Less common: acanthosis nigricans involving eyelids. Nystagmus, iris coloboma, aniridia, anisocoria, corectopia, micro- or megalocornea, keratoconus with acute hydrops, cataract, ectopia lentis, blue sclera, and glaucoma, have been reported.

Deletion 2q Syndrome *(2q33.3–q34) 2q– Syndrome (deletion of 2q33 may be associated with the Seckel Syndrome phenotype (bird-headed dwarfism) for which the inheritance is autosomal recessive).* Over 50 cases reported.

General Description: growth retardation, developmental delay, microcephaly, large beaked nose, micrognathia, radial head dislocation, clinodactyly, absent ear lobes

Ocular Findings: down-slanting palpebral fissures, epicanthus, narrow palpebral fissures, thick eyebrows and lashes, ptosis, blepharophimosis, corneal opacities, cataract, optic nerve hypoplasia, nystagmus, hypertelorism, colobomatous microphthalmia

Deletion 3p Syndrome *3p– Syndrome* Gene map locus: partial deletion of the short arm of chromosome 3 del(3p25-pter). Inheritance: In all but one reported case the deletion has occurred de novo. Fifteen cases reported.

General Description: mental and growth deficiency, microcephaly with flat occiput, postaxial polydactyly, malformed ears, downward corners of mouth, micrognathia

Ocular Findings: synophrys, epicanthal folds, ptosis, up-slanting palpebral fissures, hypertelorism, iris coloboma

Deletion 4p Syndrome *4p– Syndrome, Wolf–Hirschhorn Syndrome (WHS), Pitt–Rogers–Danks Syndrome (PRDS)* MIM #194190 Gene map locus: partial deletion of the short arm of chromosome 4 at 4p16.3. Inheritance: In most cases the deletion occurs de novo. Incidence: 1 : 50,000 live births.

General Description: developmental delay (100%), growth retardation (90%), microcephaly (90%), cranial asymmetry, prominent glabella (50%), broad or beaked nose, down-turned "fishlike" mouth, cleft-lip and/or palate (60%), micrognathism (70%), low-set posteriorly rotated ears with preauricular tags, genital abnormalities (65%), cardiac anomalies (50%), hearing loss, hypotonia, abnormalities of the corpus callosum

TABLE 10-2. (continued).

Ocular Findings

Common: hypertelorism (65%), arched eyebrows with medial thinning/flare (55%), epicanthus (25%–50%), ptosis (25%), unilateral or bilateral coloboma or corectopia, with or without microphthalmia (over 30%), cataract (25%), strabismus (33%–66%)

Less common: up-slanting or down-slanting palpebral fissures (5%), inferior scleral show, periorbital swelling, proptosis, shallow orbits, blue sclera. Atypical "Brushfield" spots on the iris (more centrally located than those commonly seen in trisomy 21), iris heterochromia, nasolacrimal duct obstruction, Rieger anomaly, and nystagmus have been reported.

Deletion 4q Syndrome *4q− Syndrome* Gene map locus: partial deletion of the long arm of chromosome 4 del4q31–qter, del4q27–31, del4q12–q13.1. Inheritance: In all cases the deletion occurred de novo. Approximately 40 cases reported.

General Description: del 4q31–qter: growth deficiency, mild mental retardation, dental anomalies, hypotonia, high forehead, posteriorly rotated ears, flat nasal bridge, micrognathia, cardiac defects (60%), hand anomalies (50%). Uncommon malformations may include renal malformations, seizures, deafness, and cleft palate. Fifty percent of patients died before 15 months of age. del 4q27–31: mild mental retardation, micrognathia, dental malocclusion. del 4q12–q13.1: mild mental retartdation and dental anomalies.

Ocular Findings

Common: del 4q31–qter: hypertelorism (60%), epicanthal folds (40%), up-slanting palpebral fissures (20%). del 4q12–q13.1: hypopigmentation of eyebrows, anomalies of iris color

Less common: del 4q12–q13.1: esotropia, refractive error, epicanthus, dystopia canthorum, colobomatous microphthalmia, pigmentary retinopathy, and exotropia have been reported. del 4q27–31: bilateral type II Duane syndrome with ptosis has been reported.

Deletion 5p Syndrome 5p− Syndrome, *Cri-du-Chat Syndrome* MIM #123450 Gene map locus: partial deletion of the short arm of chromosome 5. Although the size of the deletion is variable, a critical region for the high-pitched cry maps to 5p15.3, while the chromosomal region involved in the remaining features maps to 5p15.2. Inheritance: In most cases the deletion occurs de novo. Over 100 cases reported.

General Description: cat-like cry in infancy (100%) due to an abnormality in structure of the larynx, microcephaly (100%), round face (68%), micrognathia, low-set ears, cardiac malformations (30%), low birth weight (72%), hypotonia (78%), slow neonatal growth rate (100%), simian crease (81%)

Ocular Findings: hypertelorism (94%), epicanthal folds (85%), down-slanting palpebral fissures (81%), strabismus (often divergent, 61%)

Deletion 9p Syndrome 9p− Syndrome, *Monosomy 9p Syndrome* MIM #158170 Gene map locus: deletion of the distal portion of the short arm of chromosome 9. In most cases, the breakpoint is located at band 9p22. Inheritance: In most cases the deletion is de novo. Over 40 cases reported.

General Description: craniostenosis with trigonocephaly, mental retardation, delayed motor development, high arched palate, long middle phalanges of the

(continued)

TABLE 10-2. Ocular and Systemic Findings in Selected Inherited Syndromes (continued).

fingers with extra flexion creases. Ventricular septal defects, patent ductus arteriosus, and/or pulmonic stenosis (30%–50%).

Ocular Findings: up-slanting palpebral fissures, epicanthal folds, prominent eyes secondary to hypoplastic supraorbital ridges, highly arched eyebrows. One report of a child with congenital glaucoma and monosomy 9p23-pter (the child had also trisomy 1q41–qter).

Deletion 11p Syndrome *11p– Syndrome, WAGR Syndrome* MIM #194072 Gene map locus: contiguous gene deletion syndrome involving *PAX6* at 11p11.3 and extending distally into the Wilms' tumor gene, WT1 at 11p13. Inheritance: most cases represent de novo deletion. Over 50 cases reported.

General Description: the acronym WAGR has been used to represent the major features of this condition: Wilms' tumor, Aniridia, Genitourinary anomalies, and retardation. Hypotonia, trigonocephaly, hearing deficits, midline brain anomalies, and minor abnormalities of fingers are also seen. It is estimated that 33% of patients with sporadic aniridia develop Wilms' tumor. The risk of Wilms' tumor in patients with aniridia, genitourinary anomalies, and mental retadation is estimated to be 50%. The risk of Wilms' tumor in patients with aniridia who have a cytogenetically detectable deletion of 11p13 increases to 60%.

Ocular Findings: aniridia, congenital cataract, macular hypoplasia, ptosis, glaucoma, keratopathy, nystagmus, Peters' anomaly

Deletion 11q Syndrome *11q– Syndrome, Jacobsen Syndrome* MIM #147791 Gene map locus: terminal 11q deletion with a breakpoint including or distal to 11q23. It has been suggested that deletion of 11q24.1 is critical. Inheritance: most cases arise de novo. Incidence: less than 1:100,000.

General Description: mental deficiency (96%), trigonocephaly (90%), depressed nasal bridge (93%), short nose with upturned nasal tip (91%), large, carp-shaped mouth (78%), cardiac defects (60%), joint contractures (65%)

Ocular Findings: strabismus (75%), hypertelorism (70%), ptosis (67%), epicanthal folds (60%). Ocular colobomas with or without microphthalmia, correctopia, nuclear cataract, persistent pupillary membrane, "circular white spots" in the iris stroma, optic atrophy, juvenile glaucoma, lid colobomas, ectropion, short/long eyelashes, retinal vasculopathy, and retinal dysplasia have been reported.

Deletion 13q Syndrome Group 1, 2, and 3 *13q– Syndrome* MIM *180200 (for del 13q14.1–q14.2), *603073, 602553, respectively. Gene map loci: Group 1: Proximal deletions not extending into q32 (13q14.1–q14.2 may be involved). Group 2: 13q32. Group 3: 13q32.2–q34. Well over 100 cases reported.

General Description: Group 1: mild to moderate mental retardation, growth retardation, hypotonia and variable minor anomalies, with or without microcephaly. When the q14 region in involved, there is a significant risk for retinoblastoma. Group 2: microcephaly, brain malformations such as anencephaly or encephalocele, cardiac malformations, thumb/big toe hypoplasia, Hirschprung disease. Group 3: severe mental retardation.

TABLE 10-2. (continued).

Ocular Findings
Common: Group 1: The majority of patients with deletions of chromosome 13 involving q14 region develop retinoblastoma usually bilateral (13%–20% remain unaffected). Hypertelorism, iris heterochromia. Group 2: ptosis, epicanthal folds, down-slanting palpebral fissures, "fixed pupils," microphthalmia, colobomas. Group 3: hypertelorism, iris heterochromia.
Less common: Group 1: retinal calcification, retinoma (translucent grayish retinal mass protruding into the vitreous), optic nerve and retinal dysplasia

Deletion 15q (deletion of maternal allele) *15p-Syndrome, Angelman Syndrome (the previous name for Angelman Syndrome, "Happy Puppet Syndrome," has been abandoned)* MIM #105830 Gene map locus: approximately 70% of cases are due to deletion of maternally derived 15q11–q13. Inheritance: sporadic. Over 80 cases reported.

General Description: severe mental retardation with absence of speech, characteristic ataxia and jerky arm movement ("puppet-like") (100%), paroxysms of inappropriate laughter, microbrachiocephaly, mandibular prognathism, protruding tongue, EEG abnormalities (92%), seizures beginning usually between 18 and 24 months (86%), blond hair (65%), hypopigmentation

Ocular Findings
Common: decreased pigmentation of the choroid and iris, the latter resulting in pale blue eyes (88%), deep set eyes
Less common: strabismus (42%), myopia, hypermetropia, nystagmus, oculocutaneous albinism (1%)

Deletion 15q (deletion of paternal allele) *15p− Syndrome, Prader–Willi Syndrome* MIM #176270 Gene map locus: approximately 70% of cases are due to deletion of paternally derived 15q11–q13. Inheritance: sporadic. Incidence: 1:15,000.

General Description: neonatal hypotonia and feeding difficulties followed later by obesity, developmental delay, and in some children, hyperphagia that may be associated with behavior problems. Other features include small hands and feet, narrow bifrontal skull, primary hypogonadism with cryptorchidism, and small genitals.

Ocular Findings
Common: palpebral fissures are often described as "almond shaped," which may be up-slanting, strabismus, blue eyes, myopia
Less common: oculocutaneous albinism (1%)

Deletion 18p Syndrome *18p− Syndrome* Gene map locus: deletion of short arm of chromosome 18. Inheritance: sporadic. Over 100 cases reported.

General Description: mild to moderate growth deficiency, mental deficiency, microcephaly (30%), prominent auricles, rounded facies, low nasal bridge, wide mouth, downturning corners of mouth, relatively small hands and feet

Ocular Findings: hypertelorism (41%), epicanthal folds (40%), ptosis (38%), strabismus, cataract, ulerythema ophryogenes (atrophy, reticular erythema, small papules, and permanent loss of hair in outer halves of eyebrows)

Deletion 18q Syndrome *18q− Syndrome, De Grouchy Syndrome* MIM #601808 Gene map locus: terminal deletion of the long arm of chromosome 18. Inheritance: sporadic. Over 100 cases reported.

(continued)

TABLE 10-2. Ocular and Systemic Findings in Selected Inherited Syndromes (continued).

General Description: severe mental and motor retardation, hypotonia, seizures, failure to thrive, short stature, conductive deafness, prominent auricular antihelix, narrow or atretic external ear canal, long hands, whorl digital pattern, midfacial hypoplasia, carp-shaped mouth, narrow palate, IgA deficiency, growth hormone deficiency

Ocular Findings: deep-set eyes, nystagmus (35%), optic atrophy (28%), abnormal optic disc, "retinal abnormalities" (29%), tapetoretinal degeneration. Epicanthal folds, slanted palpebral fissures, hypertelorism, microphthalmia, "corneal opacification", microcornea, cataract, iris hypoplasia, retinal detachment, strabismus, exophthalmos, and myopia have been reported.

Digeorge Sequence MIM ˙188400, ˙600594 Gene map locus: microdeletion of 22q11.2. Inheritance: autosomal dominant. Incidence: 1:80,000

General Description: hypoplasia to aplasia of the thymus, hypocalcemia due to hypoparathyroidism, aortic arch anomalies, other heart defects, short philtrum, micrognathia, ear anomalies. Patients may have juvenile rheumatoid arthritis (JRA). *(second most common cause of congenital heart disease to Down syndrome).*

Ocular Findings: lateral displacement of outer canthi with short palpebral fissures. Patients may have JRA but the risk for iritis is unknown.

Distal Arthrogryposis Syndrome, Type II *Camptodactyly-Cleft-Palate-Club Foot, Gordon Type* MIM ˙114300 Gene map locus: pericentromeric region of chromosome 9. Inheritance: autosomal dominant. Five families with 38 members have been reported.

General Description: distal congenital contractures, clenched hands with medial overlapping of the fingers at birth, ulnar deviation and camptodactyly in adult, cleft palate, cleft lip, small tongue, short stature, scoliosis, dull–normal intelligence

Ocular Findings: ptosis, mild epicanthal folds

Distichiasis Syndrome MIM ˙126300 Inheritance: autosomal dominant. Several families have been reported.

Ocular Findings: distichiasis

Distichiasis-Lymphedema Syndrome MIM #153400 Gene map locus: 16q22–q24. Inheritance: autosomal dominant. Approximately 20 cases reported.

General Description: distichiasis (100%), lymphedema causing painless swelling of the extremities predominantly below the knee (66%). The lymphedema first becomes evident between 5 and 20 years of age. Vertebral anomalies (62%), epidural spinal cysts (46%), cardiac defects (38%), webbed neck.

Ocular Findings
Common: distichiasis, corneal irritation, corneal ulceration, photophobia
Less common: microphthalmia, ptosis, strabismus, partial ectropion of the lateral third of the lower lid, epicanthal folds, apparent deficiency of inferior tarsus

TABLE 10-2. (continued).

Duane/Radial Dysplasia Syndrome *Duane Retraction Syndrome 1 (DURS1)* MIM
*126800 Gene map locus: 8q13. Inheritance: autosomal dominant. Incidence:
eight families reported.

General Description: Duane syndrome, deafness, radial dysplasia that can range
from hypoplasia of the thenar eminence to an absent forearm, renal dysplasia.
Variably expressed vertebral anomalies (fusion of C2 and C3), cardiac and facial
anomalies.

Ocular Findings: Duane syndrome

Dubowitz Syndrome MIM *223370 Inheritance: autosomal recessive. More than
50 cases reported.

General Description: short stature, mild microcephaly, small facies, shallow
supraorbital ridge, prominent or mildly dysplastic ears, eczema-like skin
disorders on face and flexural area, sparse scalp hair, missing teeth, lag in
eruption of teeth, hand abnormalities, cryptorchidism. Occasionally, cardiac
defects, bone marrow hypoplasia, malignancies including lymphoma,
neuroblastoma, leukemia, and fatal aplastic anemia.

Ocular Findings
Common: sparse lateral eyebrows, shallow supraorbital ridge, short palpebral
fissures, telecanthus, appearance of hypertelorism, variable ptosis and
blepharophimosis, epicanthal folds
Less common: strabismus, microphthalmia, hyperopia, megalocornea, hypoplasia
of iris, coloboma, ocular albinism, abnormalities of the fundus including
abnormal veins, tapetoretinal degeneration

Duplication 3q Syndrome *3q Plus Syndrome* Gene map locus: Duplication for
3q21-qter. More than 40 cases reported.

General Description: mental and growth deficiency, craniosynostosis,
micrognathia, broad nasal root, short webbed neck, malformed ears,
downturned corners of mouth, hypertrichosis, limb abnormalities, cardiac
defects, renal and urinary tract anomalies, chest deformities

Ocular Findings
Common: synophrys, hypertelorism, epicanthal folds, up-slanting palpebral
fissures
Less common: microphthalmia, glaucoma, cataract, coloboma, strabismus

---

Duplication 4p Syndrome *trisomy 4p Syndrome* Gene map locus: Trisomy for
part or most of the short arm of chromosome 4. More than 85 cases reported.

General Description: microcephaly, small flat forehead, flat nasal bridge with
bulbous tip, macroglossia, irregular teeth, severe mental deficiency, growth
deficiency

Ocular Findings
Common: synophrys, prominent supraorbital ridges
Less common: microphthalmia, coloboma of uveal tract (15%)

Duplication 9p Syndrome *Trisomy 9p Syndrome.* Approximately 100 patients
have been reported.

(continued)

TABLE 10-2. Ocular and Systemic Findings in Selected Inherited Syndromes (continued).

General Description: severe mental deficiency. Partial trisomy 9pter-p21 is associated with mild craniofacial features and rare skeletal or visceral defects. Partial trisomy 9pter-p11 is associated with typical craniofacial features. Partial trisomy 9pter-q11–13 is associated with typical craniofacial features, skeletal and cardiac defects. Partial trisomy 9pter-q22–32 is associated with typical craniofacial features, intrauterine growth deficiency, cleft lip/palate, micrognathia, cardiac defects, and congenital hip dislocation. Skeletal defects may include: short fingers and toes with small nails and short terminal phalanges. Craniofacial defects include delayed closure of anterior fontanel, microcephaly and the abnormalities listed under ocular findings. Most affected individuals do not survive beyond the neonatal period.

Ocular Findings
Common: microphthalmia (61%), hypertelorism, down-slanting palpebral fissures, "deep-set eyes" (45%).
Less common: epicanthal folds. Cataract and corneal clouding have been reported.

Duplication 10q Syndrome *10q Plus Syndrome* Gene map locus: trisomy 10q11–q22. More than 35 cases reported.

General Description: growth deficiency, mild to moderate developmental delay, microcephaly, prominent forehead, anteverted nares, micrognathia, flat thick ear helices with/without hearing loss, long slender limbs

Ocular Findings: small deep-set eyes, epicanthus. Down-slanting palpebral fissures, blepharophimosis, iris coloboma, and retinal dysplasia have been reported.

Duplication 15q Syndrome Gene map locus: Duplication of Distal 15q. More than 30 cases reported.

General Description: prominent nose with broad nasal bridge, camptodactyly, cardiac defects, growth deficiency, severe mental deficiency, microcephaly, micrognathia

Ocular Findings: short palpebral fissures (78%), down-slanting palpebral fissures (71%), ptosis (56%)

Dyskeratosis Congenita Syndrome *Zinsser–Cole–Engman Syndrome* MIM #305000 Gene map locus: Xq28. Inheritance: X-linked recessive. Over 100 cases reported.

General Description: mental retardation, irregular reticular brownish-gray pigmentation of skin (which may be telangiectatic), hyperkeratosis and hyperhidrosis of palms and soles, premalignant leukoplakia (frequent cancer in leukoplakia of anus, mouth, or skin), nail dystrophy, osteoporosis, pancytopenia, testicular hypoplasia. Esophageal, nasopharyngeal, anal, urethral, and vaginal strictures. Deafness and opportunistic infections may occur.

Ocular Findings: blepharitis, conjunctivitis, ectropion, nasolacrimal obstruction, lacrimal duct atresia. Premalignant leukoplakia may be found on conjunctiva.

Ectopia Lentis et Pupillae MIM *225200 Inheritance: autosomal recessive. Twenty cases reported.

TABLE 10-2. (continued).

Ocular Findings

Common: congenital subluxation of the crystalline lens, which may be progressive. The lens can be displaced in any direction. Zonules are generally stretched but may be disrupted. The lens may become totally loose with age and may cause pupillary block. Eccentric, miotic, difficult to dilate pupil (60%). The lens and pupil are usually displaced in opposite directions. Remnants of the pupillary membrane (88%), prominent iris processes in the angle (80%), axial elongation of the globe (78%).

Less common: enlarged corneal diameter (44%), cataract (34%), iridohyaloid adhesions (29%), open-angle glaucoma (15%), retinal detachment (9%)

Ectrodactyly-Ectodermal Dysplasia-Clefting Syndrome I *EEC 1 Syndrome* MIM ⋆129900 Gene map locus: 7q11.2–q21.3. Inheritance: autosomal dominant. Over 100 cases reported.

General Description: syndactyly, ectrodactyly, ectodermal dysplasia, fair and thin skin with mild hyperkeratosis, hypoplastic nipples, light-colored, sparse, thin wiry hair, distortion of the hair bulbs, partial anodontia, microdontia, caries, cleft lip with or without cleft palate (72%), genitourinary anomalies (52%)

Ocular Findings: blue irides, photophobia, blepharophimosis, blepharitis, defects of lacrimal duct system (84%), dacryocystitis, keratitis

Ehlers–Danlos Syndrome Type I, II, III, IV, V, VI, VII, VIII, IX, X MIM #130000, #130010, #130020, #130050, ⋆305200 #225400, #130060, #225410, ⋆130080, #304150, 225310, ⋆147900, 130090, 225320 Gene map loci: 2q31, 17q21.31–q22, 9q34.2–q34.3, Xq12–q13, 1p36.3–p36.2, 5q23. Inheritance: autosomal dominant and autosomal recessive (see below). More than 100 cases reported.

General Description: a heterogeneous group of connective tissue disorders that share hyperextensibility of joints, hyperextensibility of skin, poor wound healing with thin scar. Ten distinct entities are recognized:

Type I—*Gravis Type:* velvety, hyperextensible and fragile skin; poor wound healing, hyperextensible joints with tendency for dislocation, easy bruisability of blood vessels, mitral valve prolapse, aortic root and/or sinus of valsalva dilatation. Occasionally: short stature, kyphoscoliosis, long neck, slim skeletal build, small irregularly placed teeth, dissecting aneurysm, intracranial aneurysm, hemorrhage, atrial septal defect, tricuspid valve prolapse, other heart defects, inguinal hernia, diaphragmatic hernia, ectasia of intestine, intestinal diverticuli, ureteropelvic anomaly, renal tubular acidosis, mental deficiency, autism. Autosomal dominant with wide variance in expression. There is evidence that at least some cases of the syndrome are caused by mutation in the collagen alpha-1(V) gene (COL5A1), the collagen alpha-2(V) gene (COL5A2), or the collagen alpha-1(I) gene (COL1A1).

Type II: *Mitis Type:* similar to Type I but milder. Autosomal dominant. There is evidence that this form of EDS is caused by mutations in the COL5A1 and COL5A2 genes. Since other mutations in these genes cause type I Ehlers–Danlos syndrome, the two syndromes are allelic.

Type III—*Benign Hypermobile Type:* joint hypermobility with frequent joint dislocation, normal skin. Autosomal dominant. It is likely that mutations in more than 1 gene can lead to this phenotype. One such gene is the COL3A1 gene, mutations in which typically cause type IV EDS.

(continued)

TABLE 10-2. Ocular and Systemic Findings in Selected Inherited Syndromes (continued).

Type IV—*Arterial, Ecchymotic, or Sack Type:* neurovascular manifestations including spontaneous carotid-cavernous fistulae, intracranial aneurysms, carotid artery aneurysms, easy bruising, thin skin with easily visible veins, normal joint mobility with the exception of the small joints of the hands, bowel and/or arterial rupture leading to death, uterine rupture during pregnancy. Autosomal dominant. There is evidence that a defect in the gene for type III collagen (COL3A1) is usually, perhaps always, the basis of this phenotype.

Type V—*X-linked Type:* similar to type II. Female carriers are asymptomatic.

Type VI—*Ocular-Scoliotic Type:* severe scoliosis, ocular fragility, keratoconus, soft hyperextensible skin with moderate scarring and easy bruising, joint laxity, muscle hypotonia. Autosomal recessive. Some patients with EDS VI have molecular defects in the gene for lysyl hydroxylase (PLOD). However, it appears that the EDS VI phenotype sometimes occurs with normal lysyl hydroxylase activity.

Type VII (Type A, B, C)—*Arthrochalasis Multiplex Congenital:* hyperextensible and easy bruising skin, marked joint hyperextensibility, congenital hip dislocation, short stature; type A and type B are autosomal dominant and type C is autosomal recessive. Mutation at one of at least two loci, COL1A1 and COL1A2, can produce this phenotype. There is evidence that mutations in the ADAMTS2 gene result in this disorder.

Type VIII—*Periodontitis Type:* severe periodontitis leading to premature loss of teeth, marked bruising, mild or no joint hypermobility, thin skin with hyperextensibility, poor wound healing. Autosomal dominant.

Type IX—*Occipital Horn Syndrome:* occipital hornlike exostosis, short humeri, short clavicles, chronic diarrhea, bladder diverticula with tendency to bladder rupture, soft and mildly extensible skin. X-linked recessive.

Type X—*Fibronectin Abnormalities:* joint hypermobility and dislocation, mildly hyperextensible, fragile skin with poor wound healing, platelet aggregation defect that corrects with addition of fibrinectin. Autosomal recessive.

Ocular Findings: occasionally, epicanthal folds, blue sclera, myopia, microcornea, keratoconus, glaucoma, ectopia lentis, retinal detachment. Type IV: characteristic face with large eyes. Type VI: ocular fragility, rupture of the sclera and cornea or retinal detachment often result from minor trauma.

Escobar Syndrome *Multiple Pterygium Syndrome* MIM *265000, 178110, *253290 (lethal), *263650 (lethal). Inheritance: autosomal recessive, autosomal dominant, and X-linked. Approximately 50 cases reported.

General Description: short stature, micrognathia, downturning corners of mouth, cleft palate, low-set ears, pterygia of neck, axillae, antecubital, popliteal, intercrural area, and limbs; camptodactyly, syndactyly, rocker-bottom feet, cryptochidism, absence of labia majora, scoliosis, kyphosis, absent or dysplastic patella

Ocular Findings: ptosis, down-slanting palpebral fissures, inner canthal folds, hypertelorism. Absent eyebrows and absent eyelashes reported in *263650.

Fanconi Pancytopenia Syndrome, Complementation Group A,B,C,D1,D2,E,F *Pancytopenia Syndrome, Fanconi Type* MIM *227650, *227660, *227645, *605724, *227646, *600901, *603467 Gene map loci: 16q24.3(A), 9q22.3(C), 3p25.3(D2), 6p22–p21(E), 11p15(F). Autosomal recessive. Incidence: heterozygote frequency estimated at 1:300 to 1:600.

TABLE 10-2. (continued).

General Description: pancytopenia, leukemia, myelodysplastic syndrome, short stature, hyperpigmentation (60%), radial hypoplasia (50%), renal and urogenitary anomalies (30%), mental deficiency (25%), other skeletal defects (20%), gastrointestinal anomalies (14%), cardiac defect (13%), deafness (11%), central nervous system anomalies (8%)

Ocular Findings: anomalies in 40% of patients including: ptosis, strabismus, nystagmus, microphthalmus

---

Femoral Hypoplasia-Unusual Facies Syndrome *Femoral-Facial Syndrome* MIM 134780 Inheritance: sporadic (possibly autosomal dominant). Approximately 50 cases reported.

General Description: short stature (short lower limbs), hypoplastic to absent femora, short nose with hypoplastic alae nasi, long philtrum, thin upper lip, micrognathia, cleft palate, dysplastic sacrum, genitourinary abnormalities

Ocular Findings
Common: up-slanting palpebral fissures
Less common: esotropia, astigmatism

FG Syndrome *Opitz–Kaveggia FG Syndrome* MIM *305450, *300321 Gene map locus: Xq12–q21.31, Xq28 respectively. Inheritance: X-linked recessive. Over 50 cases reported.

General Description: mental deficiency, delayed motor development, hypotonia, postnatal onset of short stature and of macrocephaly, prominent forehead, small ears, facial skin wrinkling, fine, sparse hair, imperforate anus, broad thumbs and great toes. Occasionally, craniosynostosis.

Ocular Findings
Common: hypertelorism (83%), epicanthal folds, short down-slanting palpebral fissures (85%), large-appearing cornea (75%), strabismus
Less common: craniosynostosis

Fragile X Syndrome *Martin–Bell Syndrome, Marker X Syndrome* MIM *309550 Gene map locus: Xq27.3. Inheritance: X-linked. Incidence: 1:2,000 male births.

General Description: mental deficiency, mild connective tissue dysplasia, macro-orchidism, macrocephaly in early childhood, prognathism after puberty, thickening of nasal bridge extending down to the nasal tip, large ears with soft cartilage, dental crowding, 50% of females with learning disability or mild mental retardation

Ocular Findings
Common: epicanthal folds, pale blue irides.
Less common: strabismus, nystagmus, myopia

Fraser Syndrome *Cryptophthalmos Syndrome* MIM *219000 Inheritance: autosomal recessive. Over 100 cases reported.

General Description: partial cutaneous syndactyly (57%), mental deficiency (50%), genital anomalies (49%), ear anomalies, most commonly atresia of external auditory canal and cupped ears (44%), laryngeal stenosis or atresia (21%), renal hypoplasia or agenesis (37%). Twenty-five percent of affected babies are stillborn. An additional 20% die before age 1 (usually secondary to renal or laryngeal defects).

(continued)

TABLE 10-2. Ocular and Systemic Findings in Selected Inherited Syndromes (continued).

Ocular Findings
Common: cryptophthalmos (93%) usually bilateral. The eyelid defect is frequently accompanied by ocular anomaly; thus, the likelihood of achieving adequate vision is small.
Less common: hair growth on lateral forehead extending to lateral eyebrow (34%). Occasionally, hypertelorism, lacrimal duct defect (9%), coloboma of upper lid (6%).

Freeman–Sheldon Syndrome *Whistling Face Syndrome* MIM *193700, 277720 Inheritance: autosomal dominant and autosomal recessive. More than 60 cases reported.

General Description: masklike "whistling" facies, hypoplastic alae nasi with coloboma, small nose, long philtrum, microstomia, H-shaped cutaneous dimpling on chin, talipes equinovarus, ulnar deviation of hands, normal stature. Most of the features are secondary to increased muscle tone.

Ocular Findings
Common: deep-set eyes, prominent supraorbital ridge, telecanthus, hypertelorism, epicanthal folds, strabismus, blepharophimosis, down-slanting palpebral fissures
Less common: ptosis

Frontometaphyseal Dysplasia MIM *305620 Inheritance: X-linked with severely affected males and mildly affected females. Over 20 cases reported.

General Description: coarse facies, wide nasal bridge, prominent supraorbital ridges, incomplete sinus development, partial anodontia, high palate, small mandible; flexion contracture of fingers, wrists, elbows, knees, and ankles; arachnodactyly with wide and elongated phalanges, partial fusion of carpal and tarsal bones, Erlenmeyer-flask appearance to femur and tibia, wide foramen magnum with various cervical vertebral anomalies, mixed conductive and sensorineural hearing loss, wasting of muscles in arms and legs

Ocular Findings
Common: prominent supraorbital ridges
Less common: hypertelorism, down-slanting palpebral fissures

Frontonasal Dysplasia Sequence *Median Cleft Face Syndrome* MIM 136760, 305645 Inheritance: sporadic, X-linked dominant, autosomal recessive, and autosomal dominant reported. Rare disorder.

General Description: defect in midfacial development with incomplete anterior appositional alignment of eyes. Widow's peak, deficit in midline frontal bone, nose abnormalities. Occasionally, tetralogy of Fallot, conductive deafness, preauricular tags, low-set ears, mental deficiency, agenesis of corpus callosum.

Ocular Findings
Common: hypertelorism, lateral displacement of inner canthi
Less common: microphthalmia, anomalies of optic disc, optic nerve, retina, iris

Gangliosidosis Syndrome (GM₁), Type I (Severe Infantile Type) *Caffey Pseudo-Hurler Syndrome, Familial Neurovisceral Lipidosis* MIM *230500 Gene map locus: 3p21.33. Inheritance: autosomal recessive. Over 30 cases reported.

TABLE 10-2. (continued).

General Description: growth deficiency, psychomotor retardation, Hurler-like coarse facial features, facial and peripheral edema in early infancy, hirsutism, kyphosis in early infancy, moderate joint limitation, thick wrists, contractures at the elbows and knees, development of claw-hand, short broad hands. Congestive heart failure, variable hepatosplenomegaly with some foamy histiocytes, vacuolation in glomerular epithelial cells and within cytoplasm of leukocytes, foam cells in marrow. Mucopolysaccharides occasionally may be increased in the urine with the excretion of keratan sulfate-like materials. Usually death occurs during early infancy (by 2 years of age). The diagnosis can be confirmed by assay of beta-galactosidase in the peripheral leukocytes or in cultured skin fibroblasts. Prenatal diagnosis based on cultured amniotic fluid cells. All three beta-galactosidase isoenzymes (hexosaminidase A, B, and C) are missing.

Ocular Findings: cherry-red macular spot (50%), clear cornea, wide-spaced eyes, pendular nystagmus, tortuous conjunctival vessels with saccular microaneurysms, optic atrophy, occasional corneal clouding, papilledema, high myopia.

Gangliosidosis Syndrome (GM₁), Type II (Juvenile Type) *Derry disease* MIM #230600 Gene map locus: 3p21.33. Inheritance: autosomal recessive. Incidence: unknown.

General Description: the first sign is locomotor ataxia followed by progressive psychomotor deterioration and seizures. Affected children are decerebrate and rigid by the end of their second year of life. Death occurs between the ages of 3 and 10. Beta-galactosidase isoenzymes B and C are lacking.

Ocular Findings: nystagmus, esotropia, pigmentary retinopathy, optic atrophy

---

Gangliosidosis Syndrome (GM₂), Type I *Tay–Sachs disease* MIM *272800 Gene map locus: 15q23–q24. Inheritance: autosomal recessive. Incidence of carrier state is 1 in 300 for non-Jews and 1 in 30–40 among European Jews living in the United States and Canada. Birth incidence among Ashkenazi Jews is approximately 1 in 4000.

General Description: affected children become apathetic, hypotonic, and abnormally sensitive to sound. Seizures and progressive neurologic deterioration ensue, and patients usually die by 24 to 30 months of age. There is a deficiency in isoenzyme hexosaminidase A. A very effective genetic screening has reduced the number of cases. The disease used to occur most often in individuals of eastern European Jewish descent. French Canadians can also be affected more often than the general population.

Ocular Findings: A cherry-red macular spot is characteristic by 6 months of age and vision is reduced by 12 to 18 months of age. The abnormal finding is the white ring resulting from accumulation of storage material in the ganglion cells around the normally pigmented macula. Nystagmus, optic atrophy, and narrowing of the retinal vessels develop. As the ganglion cells of the retina die, the white ring can disappear.

Gangliosidosis Syndrome (GM₂), Type II *Sandhoff disease* MIM *268800 Gene map locus: 5q13. Inheritance: autosomal recessive. Approximately 50 cases reported.

(continued)

TABLE 10-2. Ocular and Systemic Findings in Selected Inherited Syndromes (continued).

General Description: most affected children die as a result of progressive psychomotor deterioration by the age of 2 to 12 years. The disorder has an ocular and systemic course similar to that of Tay–Sachs disease. Hexosaminidase A and B are absent.

Ocular Findings: decreased visual acuity, strabismus, corneal clouding, a prominent cherry-red spot, normal-appearing optic nerves

Gangliosidosis Syndrome (GM$_2$), Type III *Bernheimer–Seiteberger disease* MIM *230700 Inheritance: autosomal recessive. Six cases reported.

General Description: the disorder begins in early childhood with progressive psychomotor retardation, locomotor ataxia, speech loss, and spasticity. It leads to death before the age of 15 years. There is partial deficiency of hexosaminidase A.

Ocular Findings: late-onset visual loss, optic atrophy, and pigmentary retinopathy. No cherry-red spot appears.

Geleophysic Dysplasia *Geleophysic Dwarfism, Acrofacial Dysplasia* MIM *231050 Inheritance: autosomal recessive. Twelve cases reported.

General Description: short stature, round full face, short nose with anteverted nares, wide mouth, long philtrum, thickened helix of ear, "pleasant, happy-natured" appearance, short hands and feet with markedly short tubular bones and relatively normal epiphyses, progressive contractures of joints, progressive thickening of heart valves with incompetence, hepatomegaly, thickened tight skin

Ocular Findings: up-slanting palpebral fissures, hypertelorism, superior oblique muscle abnormality

Gillespie Syndrome *Aniridia-Cerebellar Ataxia-Mental Deficiency* MIM *206700 Inheritance: autosomal recessive. Nine cases reported.

General Description: aniridia or partial aniridia (irides reduced to a stump), cerebellar ataxia, moderate mental deficiency. Fusion of vertebrae C1 and C2, valvular pulmonary stenosis, cardiac malformations, and transpalmar crease have been reported.

Ocular Findings
Common: aniridia or partial aniridia (irides reduced to a stump)
Less common: ptosis, telecanthus, strabismus, hypermetropia, congenital glaucoma, photophobia, partial remains of the Wachendorf membrane have been reported.

Goldenhar Syndrome *Goldenhar–Gorlin Syndrome, Facio-Oculo-Auriculo-Vertebral (FOAV) Dysplasia* MIM 164210 Inheritance: most cases are sporadic although autosomal dominant and presumed autosomal recessive reported. Incidence: 1:5,000–1:45,000 births with a slight male predominance (3:2).

General Description: facial anomalies are usually unilateral, and when bilateral they are markedly asymmetrical. The facial anomalies include: hemifacial microsomia with maxillary and sometimes mandibular hypoplasia, facial palsy, microtia, preauricular appendages and/or pits most commonly in a line from the tragus to the corner of the mouth. Middle ear anomalies with variable deafness,

TABLE 10-2. (continued).

diminished to absent parotid secretion, anomalies in function or structure of the tongue, vertebral abnormalities occur most commonly in the cervical region but may also be thoracic or lumbar. Cardiac anomalies, genitourinary anomalies, and mental deficiency have been reported. *The presence of epibulbar dermoids is necessary for the designation of Goldenhar's syndrome (Vs FOAV association).*

Ocular Findings
Common: colobomas of the upper lid (the coloboma usually overlies an epibulbar dermoid), epibulbar dermolipomas, limbal dermoids predisposing to astigmatism, anisometropic amblyopia and strabismus, Duane syndrome
Less common: colobomatous microphthalmia (20%), blepharophimosis, anophthalmia, cataract, "iris abnormalities", decreased corneal sensitivity.

Goltz Syndrome *Focal Dermal Hypoplasia, Goltz–Gorlin Syndrome* MIM *305600 Inheritance: X-linked dominant. Over 175 cases reported.

General Description: streaks of dermal hypoplasia—pink or red atrophic macules, may be slightly raised or depressed, have a linear and asymmetrical distribution mainly on thighs, forearms, and cheeks. Telangiectasis and lipomatous nodules herniating through localized areas of skin atrophy. Angiofibromatous nodules around lips, in vulval area, perianal area, around the eyes, the ears, the fingers and toes, the groin, umbilicus, inside the mouth, and in esophagus. Sparse hair with local areas of alopecia, dystrophic nails, hypoplasia of teeth. Asymmetrical syndactyly, absence or hypoplasia of digits, absence of extremity, polydactyly of hands and feet (60%). Asymmetrical face with mild hemihypertrophy, renal anomalies.

Ocular Findings
Common: angiofibromatous nodules around the eyes, strabismus, iris and/or choroidoretinal coloboma, aniridia, microphthalmia, anophthalmia. Involvement is frequently unilateral.
Less common: bulbar angiofibroma, ectopia lentis. Nystagmus, esotropia, choroidal sclerosis, optic atrophy, and lack of retinal pigmentation have been reported.

Goodman Syndrome *Acrocephalopolysyndactyly Type 4* MIM *201020 Inheritance: autosomal recessive. Three cases reported.

General Description: craniosynostosis, acrocephaly, postaxial polydactyly, soft tissue syndactyly of the hands, syndactyly of the feet, clinodactyly and camptodactyly of the fifth digits, ulnar deviation of the fingers, genu valgum, prominent nose, large protruding ears, congenital heart disease

Ocular Findings: high-arched eyebrows, epicanthal folds, mild up-slanting palpebral fissures

---

Gorlin's Syndrome *Nevoid Basal Cell Carcinoma Syndrome* MIM #109400 Gene map loci: 9q31, 9q22.3, 1p32. Inheritance: autosomal dominant. Over 500 cases reported.

General Description: multiple basal cell epitheliomas usually appear between puberty and 35 years of age. Nevoid basal cell carcinomas characteristically occur on the eyelids, periorbital areas, and face and, less commonly, on the neck, upper arms, malar region, and trunk. Epidermal cysts, punctate dyskeratotic pits on palms and/or soles, milia (especially facial), odontogenic keratocysts of jaws,

(continued)

TABLE 10-2. Ocular and Systemic Findings in Selected Inherited Syndromes (continued).

ovarian calcification or fibromas, cardiac fibromas, medulloblastomas, lipomas. Macrocephaly, broad nasal bridge and face, bifid, synostotic, and partially missing ribs.

Ocular Findings
Common: basal cell carcinoma of eyelids and periorbital areas, tumor involvement of the orbit. Prominent supraorbital ridges, synophrys with heavy eyebrows, hypertelorism.
Less common: telecanthus, inner epicanthal folds, highly arched eyebrows, subconjunctival epithelial cysts, cataract, corneal opacity, glaucoma, coloboma of iris, choroid, and optic nerve, prominent medullated retinal nerve fibers, retinal atrophy, retinal hamartomas, chalazion, strabismus

Greig Cephalopolysyndactyly Syndrome MIM #175700 Gene map locus: 7p13. Inheritance: autosomal dominant. Over 50 cases reported.

General Description: broad nasal root (80%), high forehead (70%), frontal bossing (60%), macrocephaly (52%), postaxial polydactyly (80%), broad thumbs (90%), syndactyly primarily of fingers 3 and 4 (80%), preaxial polydactyly of feet (80%), broad halluces (90%), syndactyly of toes primarily of 1 to 3 (90%). Occasional craniosynostosis.

Ocular Findings
Common: apparent hypertelorism
Less common: down-slanting palpebral fissures

Hajdu–Cheney Syndrome *Cheney Syndrome, Acro-Osteolysis Syndrome* MIM *102500 Inheritance: autosomal dominant. Over 30 cases reported.

General Description: short stature, which is increased by osseous compression, failure of ossification of cranial sutures, bathrocephaly, absence of frontal sinus, elongated sella turcica, hydrocephalus, foramen magnum impaction, early loss of teeth, short distal fingers and nails, acro-osteolysis, pseudoclubbing, lax joints, thick straight hair. Basilar skull compression can be life threatening.

Ocular Findings: prominent eyebrows and eyelashes, synophrys, down-slanting palpebral fissures, epicanthal folds, exophthalmos, hypertelorism, cataract, nystagmus, abducent palsy, disc pallor, optic atrophy

Hallermann–Streiff Syndrome *Francois Dyscephalic Syndrome, Oculomandibulodyscephaly* MIM 234100 Inheritance: most cases are sporadic, autosomal recessive and autosomal dominant reported. Over 100 cases reported.

General Description: short stature (proportionate), brachycephaly with frontal and parietal bossing, delayed ossification of cranial sutures, malar hypoplasia, micrognathia, thin small and pinpoint nose with hypoplasia of cartilage, becoming parrot-like with age. Narrow and high arched palate, hypoplasia of teeth, atrophy of the skin, thin and light hair with hypotrichosis, tracheomalacia, upper airway obstruction. Anesthetic risk due to micrognathia, microstomia, upper airway compromise.

Ocular Findings
Common: bilateral microphthalmia (80%), congenital cataract (94%) which are white, liquefied, and often resorb spontaneously, nystagmus, strabismus, hypotrichosis of the eyebrows and eyelashes

TABLE 10-2. (continued).

Less common: blue sclera, down-slanting palpebral fissures, optic disc coloboma, glaucoma, aniridia, sclerocornea, persistence of pupillary membrane, various chorioretinal pigment alterations with degeneration, retinal folds, Coats' disease.

The major handicap is the ocular defect, which usually culminates in blindness despite surgery.

Hay–Wells Syndrome of Ectodermal Dysplasia *Ankyloblepharon-Ectodermal Dysplasia-Clefting Syndrome, AEC Syndrome* MIM #106260 Inheritance: autosomal dominant. Twelve cases reported.

General Description: cleft lip-palate, oval face, broadened nasal bridge, maxillary hypoplasia, conical widely spaced teeth, hypodontia or partial anodontia, palmar and plantar keratoderma, peeling erythematous eroded skin at birth, hyperpigmentation, hyperkeratosis, patchy partial deficiency of sweat glands, absent or dystrophic nails, sparse hair to alopecia

Ocular Findings
Common: ankyloblepharon filiforme adnatum (areas of fusion between the upper and lower lids by strands of fibrovascular tissue, muscle fibers may be observed as well). Anomalies of the eye are not associated with these tissue bands. Photophobia is common.

Less common: lacrimal duct atresia (early ophthalmologic evaluation of the lacrimal duct system is needed)

Holt–Oram Syndrome *Cardiac-Limb Syndrome* MIM #142900 Gene map locus: 12q24.1 in some families. Inheritance: autosomal dominant. Over 200 cases reported.

General Description: congenital cardiac anomalies most commonly ostium secundum atrial septal defect and ventricular septal defect, spectrum of upper limb anomalies such as absent thumb, bifid thumb, radial ulnar anomalies. Vertebral anomalies, thoracic scoliosis, absent pectoralis major, pectus excavatum or carinatum.

Ocular Findings: hypertelorism, Duane's syndrome has been reported

Homocystinuria MIM ⋅236200 Gene map locus: 21q22.3, Inheritance: autosomal recessive. Incidence: 1:60,000–1:146,000

General Description: mental retardation (50%), dry, fine, sparse, fair hair, hypopigmentation, normal to tall stature, slim skeletal build, arachnodactyly, kyphoscoliosis, deformed sternum, joint laxity or stiffness, and generalized osteoporosis with vertebral collapse, a thromboembolic diathesis with associated increased anesthetic risk, medial degeneration of the aorta and elastic arteries with intimal hyperplasia and fibrosis. Homocystinuria is caused by a defect in methionine metabolism. The disease results from cystathionine-beta-synthetase deficiency. Fifty percent of patients with cystathionine-beta-synthase deficiency respond to vitamin B_6 supplementation.

Ocular Findings: progressive bilateral lens dislocation (90%) (occurs in about 40% of patients by the age of 5 years). The lens dislocation is most typically in the inferior or inferonasal direction. The lenses move initially in an inferior direction behind the iris but may later occlude the pupil, which may lead to pupillary block and glaucoma or dislocate into the anterior chamber. The zonules are

(continued)

TABLE 10-2. Ocular and Systemic Findings in Selected Inherited Syndromes (continued).

broken in homocystinuria (which is in contradistinction to the elongated but intact zonules in Marfan syndrome). Zonular remnants are present in the equatorial zone. When zonules are disrupted, the lens becomes globular, its diameter is reduced (microspherophakia), and high myopia develops. The patients often have blue irides. Cystic and pigmentary changes in the retinal periphery have been reported.

Hunter's Syndrome *Mucopolysaccharidosis Type II* MIM *309900 Gene map locus: Xq28. Inheritance: X-linked recessive. Incidence: 1:100,000 live births.

General Description: an inborn mucopolysccharide metabolism disorder with iduronate-2-sulfatase deficiency. Clinically distinguishable by the dermatological findings of ivory-white papules or nodules that can be found on the upper trunk. Clinical characteristics are similar to those in MPS I, except for the absence of corneal clouding and slower progression of the disease. Two types are recognized. A severe form (MPS IIA) is characterized by onset at 2 to 4 years of age, growth deficiency, neurodegeneration leading to profound mental retardation and neurological deterioration, communicating hydrocephalus with increased intracranial pressure, aggressive hyperactive behavior, spasticity, coarsening of facial features, full lips, macroglossia, macrocephaly, short neck, stiff joints with partial contractures, valvular heart disease, ischemic heart disease, congestive heart failure, obstructive airway disease, hepatosplenomegaly, chronic diarrhea, inguinal hernias, recurrent ear infections, progressive deafness, mucoid nasal discharge, delayed tooth eruption, widely spaced teeth, hoarse voice, hypertrichosis, and death at about 10 to 15 years of age. A milder form (MPS IIB) is marked by preservation of intelligence, hearing impairment, carpal tunnel syndrome, joint stiffness, survival into the fifth and sixth decades.

Ocular Findings: *clear corneas* clinically, or very subtle corneal opacities (however, mucopolysaccharides have been shown histologically in corneas that appeared clear clinically). Pigmentary retinopathy with an extinguished electroretinogram may lead to severe visual impairment. Optic nerve swelling and optic atrophy are partly due to the hydrocephalus. Glaucoma and ptosis have been reported. In MPS IIB optic nerve swelling and optic atrophy can still occur, even though the majority of patients do not have hydrocephalus. Retinal dysfunction occurs at a much slower progression than in MPS IIA.

Hurler Syndrome *Mucopolysaccharidosis Type I H, MPS 1 H* MIM *252800 Gene map locus: 4p16.3. Inheritance: autosomal recessive. Incidence: 1:100,000 live births.

General Description: an inborn mucopolysccharide metabolism disorder with alpha-iduronidase deficiency resulting in progressive multisystem involvement leading to death within the first decade. At birth, patients appear normal except for umbilical or inguinal hernias, but by 6 to 18 months of age, they may present with deceleration of growth, and by 2 years of age, with mental deficiency, communicating hydrocephalus, macrocephaly with frontal prominence, coarse facies with full lips, flared nostrils, low nasal bridge, hypertrophied alveolar ridge and gums with small malaligned teeth, enlarged tongue, stiff joints, cardiac failure, hepatosplenomegaly, upper airway obstruction, hearing loss, and hirsutism. Skeletal dysmorphism includes dwarfism, claw-shaped hand, stubby fingers, chest deformity, large skull, and synostosis of the cranial sutures.

TABLE 10-2. (continued).

Ocular Findings: on histological examination, inclusions are noted in cornea epithelium, keratocytes, stroma, Descemet's membrane, iris pigment epithelium, trabecular endothelium, ciliary epithelium and smooth muscle, pericytes, fibrocytes, lens epithelium, RPE, ganglion cells, sclerocytes, Schwann's cells, optic nerve pericytes, and vascular endothelium. Diffuse severe progressive corneal opacification appears by 6 months of age (may present with photophobia). The fine punctate corneal opacities are usually distributed throughout the stroma, although they are most pronounced centrally. Late retinal degeneration includes arteriolar attenuation, decreased foveal reflex, pigmentary changes, and abnormal electroretinogram (the electroretinogram is abolished by age 5–6 years). Optic nerve swelling and optic atrophy may be present. In some cases megalocornea and/or glaucoma (glaucoma may occur, presumably as a result of accumulation of mucopolysaccharides in the trabecular meshwork). Shallow orbits with proptosis may occur as a result of premature closure of cranial sutures. Prominent supraorbital ridges, heavy eyebrows, puffy lids, inner epicanthal folds, hypertelorism.

Hurler–Scheie Syndrome *Mucopolysaccharidosis Type I H/S, MPS 1H/S* MIM *252800 Gene map locus: 4p16.3. Inheritance: autosomal recessive. Rare disorder.

General Description: an inborn mucopolysaccharide metabolism disorder with alpha-iduronidase deficiency, an intermediate form between Hurler and Scheie syndromes. The signs and symptoms usually become apparent by the age of 2 years. Patients generally survive into the twenties. Generally normal mental development with psychotic symptoms later in life. Growth deficiency, dysostosis multiplex, hepatosplenomegaly, umbilical and inguinal hernia, macrocephaly, low nasal bridge, prominent lips, micrognathia, thickened skin with fine hirsutism, moderate joint limitation, chronic rhinorrhea, middle ear fluid, deafness, possible cardiac valvular changes. Most do not have hydrocephalus but can have cervical cord compression. Patients typically die of upper airway obstruction or cardiac sequelae.

Ocular Findings
Common: diffuse progressive corneal clouding with an onset by 1 to 2 years of age, retinal pigmentary degeneration
Less common: glaucoma, optic nerve swelling, optic atrophy

Hypochondroplasia MIM #146000 Gene map locus: 4p16.3. Inheritance: autosomal dominant. Incidence: 1:180,000

General Description: short stature, short limbs, caudal narrowing of spine, macrocephaly, mild frontal bossing, normal/mild midface hypoplasia, brachydactyly, stubby hands and feet. Occasional mental deficiency.

Ocular Findings: occasionally cataract, esotropia, ptosis

Hypohidrotic Ectodermal Dysplasia Syndrome *Ectodermal Dysplasia 1* MIM *305100 Gene map locus: Xq12–13.1. Inheritance: X-linked recessive. Over 130 cases reported.

General Description: hypoplasia of sweat glands, hypoplasia to absence of eccrine glands, apocrine glands more normally represented, hypoplasia to absence of sebaceous glands, hypoplasia with absence of mucous glands in oral and nasal

(continued)

TABLE 10-2. Ocular and Systemic Findings in Selected Inherited Syndromes (continued).

membranes. Thin and hypoplastic skin with decreased pigment and tendency toward papular changes on face, scaling or peeling of skin in immediate newborn period, sparse to absent hair, hypodontia to anodontia. Hyperthermia as a consequence of inadequate sweating is a threat to life and may be a cause of mental deficiency.

Ocular Findings: periorbital wrinkling and hyperpigmentaion, corneal dystrophy, lacrimal gland hypoplasia, alacrima

---

Hypomelanosis of Ito *Incontinentia Pigmentosa Achromians* MIM *300337 Inheritance: autosomal dominant has been demonstrated in some. Incidence: 1:8,000–1:10,000.

General Description: streaked, whorled, or mottled areas of hypopigmentaion on the limbs and/or trunk usually evident in infancy. With time, there is a tendency of the area of hypopigmentation to darken. Approximately 70% of reported cases have associated anomalies. With the exception of mental retardation (67%), seizures (35%), and cerebral atrophy (16%), all other abnormalities have occurred in less than 8%.

Ocular Findings: occasional iridial heterochromia, abnormal retinal pigmentation, strabismus, iris coloboma, cataract

---

Hypophosphatasia *Perinatal Lethal Hypophosphatasia* MIM #146300 (adult type), #241500 (infantile type), #241510 (childhood type) Gene map locus: 1p36.1–p34. Inheritance: autosomal dominant for the adult type, autosomal recessive for the infantile and childhood types. Over 30 cases reported.

General Description: deficiency in bone, liver, and kidney alkaline phosphatase. Infantile type presents within the first 6 months of life and is associated with growth deficiency, rachitic-like skeletal defects, recurrent respiratory infections, increased intracranial pressure, and death in about 50% of patients. Childhood type that presents after 6 months of age is associated with short limb dwarfism, generalized lack of ossification, rachitic-like skeletal defects, poorly mineralized cranium, craniosynostosis, microcephaly, poorly formed teeth, hypoplastic fragile bones, and short ribs. Adult type presents later in life with premature loss of adult teeth, recurrent fractures, and pseudofractures.

Ocular Findings: blue sclera

Incontinentia Pigmenti Syndrome *Bloch–Sulzberger Syndrome* MIM #308300 Gene locus: Xq28 Inheritance: X-linked dominant (lethal for males). Incidence: Approximately 700 cases reported.

General Description: a generalized ectodermal dysplasia. Irregular pigmented skin lesions. Initially the skin lesions appear as bullous eruptions, which develop into characteristic pigmented streaks and flecks along the limbs and around the trunk within the first few weeks of life. As the blisters begin to heal, hyperkeratotic lesions develop on the distal limbs and scalp and rarely on the face. Pale, hairless patches or streaks most evident on lower legs develop when the hyperpigmentation disappears. Other manifestations include hypodontia (80%), atrophic patchy alopecia (50%), nail abnormalities (40%), eosinophilia, mental deficiency (30%), hemivertebrae, kyphoscoliosis (20%).

TABLE 10-2. (continued).

Ocular Findings
Common: vascular retinal abnormalities and retinal pigment epithelial cell abnormalities may lead to retinal ischemia, new vessel proliferation, bleeding, and fibrosis (40%), strabismus (30%), refractive errors
Less common: retinal detachment (may be congenital), uveitis, keratitis, cataract, microphthalmia, optic atrophy

Jackson–Weiss Syndrome *Craniosynostosis-Foot Defects, Jackson–Weiss Type* MIM #123150 Gene map locus: 10q26, 8p11.2–p11.1. Inheritance: autosomal dominant. Three families reported.

General Description: craniosynostosis, prominent forehead, maxillary hypoplasia, bony abnormalities of the feet, cutaneous syndactyly of second and third toes. Intelligence is generally normal.

Ocular Findings: ocular proptosis, hypertelorism, strabismus

Jarcho–Levin Syndrome *Spondylothoracic Dysplasia Syndrome* MIM #277300 Gene map locus: 19q13. Inheritance: autosomal recessive. Over 21 cases reported.

General Description: short stature, short trunk, short neck, normal length limbs, prominent occiput, broad forehead, wide nasal bridge, short thorax with "crablike" rib cage, other rib anomalies, multiple vertebral defects, protuberant abdomen. The majority of patients die in early infancy as a result of recurrent respiratory infections.

Ocular Findings: up-slanting palpebral fissures

Jeune Thoracic Dystrophy *Asphyxiating Thoracic Dystrophy* MIM *208500 Inheritance: autosomal recessive. Over 100 cases reported.

General Description: short stature, small thorax, short limbs, hypoplastic iliac wings; lung hypoplasia is a major cause of death in early infancy; renal cystic tubular dysplasia and/or glomerular sclerosis, biliary dysgenesis with portal fibrosis and bile duct proliferation

Ocular Findings: retinal degeneration with predominantly cone-type cells remaining

Johanson–Blizzard Syndrome MIM *243800 Inheritance: autosomal recessive. Over 28 cases reported.

General Description: short stature, mental deficiency (70%), sensorineural deafness (75%), hypotonia (80%), variable sparse hair with frontal upsweep (96%), hypoplastic ala nasi, imperforate anus, genitourinary abnormalities, hypothyroidism (30%), pancreatic insufficiency with malabsorption (100%)

Ocular Findings
Common: nasolacrimal duct cutaneous fistula (66%)
Less common: strabismus

Joubert Syndrome *Cerebellar Parenchymal Disorder, Type IV* MIM *213300, 243910 Gene map locus: 9q34.3. Inheritance: autosomal recessive. Over 45 cases reported.

(continued)

TABLE 10-2. Ocular and Systemic Findings in Selected Inherited Syndromes (continued).

General Description: neonatal episodes of tachypnea and apnea, hypotonia, ataxia, tremor, mental retardation, cerebellar vermis hypoplasia, in some patients renal cysts are present

Ocular Findings
Common: nystagmus, oculomotor apraxia, retinal dystrophy in patients with renal cysts
Less common: bilateral chorioretinal colobomas, optic nerve colobomas. Rarely, congenital fibrosis of the extraocular muscles.

Kabuki Syndrome *Niikawa–Kuroki Syndrome* MIM 147920 Inheritance: sporadic. Over 100 cases reported.

General Description: postnatal growth deficiency, mental retardation, hypotonia, short incurved fifth finger, brachydactyly, rib anomalies, scoliosis, cardiac defects (50%), craniofacial abnormalities such as short nasal septum, large protuberant ears, preauricular pit, cleft palate, tooth abnormalities, open mouth with tented upper lip.

Ocular Findings
Common: long palpebral fissures with eversion of the lateral portion of the lower eyelid (often difficult to appreciate in the neonatal period), ptosis, epicanthal folds, arched eyebrows with sparse or dispersed lateral one third, strabismus
Less common: blue sclera

Kid Syndrome, Autosomal Dominant *Keratitis-Ichthyosis-Deafness Syndrome, Autosomal Dominant* MIM 148210. Inheritance: autosomal dominant. Approximately 8 cases reported.

General Description: ichthyosiform erythroderma with mild lamellar ichthyosis and hyperkeratosis of the skin of the palms, soles, elbows, and knees. Variable alopecia, nail dystrophy, and malformations of teeth. Sensorineural deafness. Recurrent skin infections (>50%). One patient reported of having a "fatal skin cancer."

Ocular Findings: progressive keratitis with neovascularization of the cornea (95%), which may lead to blindness

---

Kid Syndrome, Autosomal Recessive *Keratitis-Ichthyosis-Deafness Syndrome, Autosomal Recessive* MIM 242150. Inheritance: autosomal recessive. Approximately 15 cases reported.

General Description: short stature, mental retardation, neuropathy, hepatic cirrhosis, hepatomegaly, hepatic glycogen storage, sensorineural deafness, cryptochidism, inguinal hernia, ichthyosiform erythroderma with mild lamellar ichthyosis and hyperkeratosis of the skin of the palms, soles, elbows, and knees. Variable alopecia, nail dystrophy, and malformations of teeth. Recurrent skin infections (>50%).

Ocular Findings: progressive keratitis with neovascularization of the cornea (95%), which may lead to blindness

---

Killian/Teschler–Nicola Syndrome *Pallister-Killian Syndrome* MIM #601803 Gene map locus: mosaic tetrasomy 12p due to extra metacentric isochromosome. Over 30 cases reported.

TABLE 10-2. (continued).

General Description: profound mental deficiency, seizures, sparse anterior scalp hair, prominent forehead, coarsening of face over time, streaks of hyper- and hypopigmentation, broad hands with short digits, accessory nipples, disproportionate shortening of arms and legs

Ocular Findings
Common: sparse eyebrows and eyelashes, up-slanting palpebral fissures, hypertelorism, ptosis, strabismus, epicanthal folds
Less common: cataract

Klippel–Trenaunay–Weber Syndrome (KTW Syndrome) *Angio-Osteohypertrophy Syndrome* MIM 149000 Inheritance: sporadic. Over 800 cases reported.

General Description: congenital or early childhood hypertrophy of soft tissues and bone of limbs (the condition involves one leg in 75% of cases). Vascular skin lesions including: capillary and cavernous hemangiomas, phlebectasia, and varicosities, which are more common on the legs, buttocks, abdomen, and lower trunk. Unilateral distribution predominates but bilateral involvement is not uncommon. The hypertrophy may or may not coincide with the area of hemangiomatous involvement. Occasional abnormalities include facial nevus flammeus, asymmetrical facial hypertrophy, hyperpigmented nevi and streaks, skin ulcers and vesicles, cutis marmorata, telangiectasia, arteriovenous fistula, lymphangiomatous anomalies, macrodactyly, syndactyly, polydactlyly, microcephaly, macrocephaly, intracranial calcifications, visceromegaly, mental deficiency, seizures, small or tall stature, aberrant major blood vessels, hemangiomata of the intestinal tract, urinary system, mesentery, and pleura.

Ocular Findings: Port-wine nevus (nevus flammeus) in the distribution of the first and second divisions of the trigeminal nerve (these patients are at risk for neuro-ocular involvement). (See Sturge-Weber Syndrome.)

Kniest Dysplasia *Metatropic Dwarfism II* MIM #156550 Inheritance: autosomal dominant. Fifteen cases reported. There is evidence that the causative mutation resides in the COL2A1 gene (*120140 Gene map locus: 12q13.11–q13.2). An autosomal recessive lethal form of Kniest-like dysplasia was reported in male and female offspring of nonconsanguineous parents (245190). A Kniest-like dysplasia with microstomia, pursed lips, and ectopia lentis was described in two siblings, a male and a female (245160).

General Description: disproportionate short stature with short extremities and a short, barrel-shaped chest; enlarged joints with limited joint mobility and variable pain and stiffness, bowing and flexion contractures in hips, kyphoscoliosis; flat facies, low nasal bridge, cleft palate, hearing loss. Radiographically: dumbbell-shaped femurs, hypoplastic pelvic bones, platyspondyly, vertical clefts of vertebrae in the newborn period. By age 3 years, the pelvis becomes "dessert-cup" shaped.

Ocular Findings
Common: congenital severe myopia and vitreoretinal degeneration in all patients. Rhegmatogenous retinal detachment (60%).
Less common: cataract (30%), ectopia lentis

Langer–Giedion Syndrome *Tricho-Rhino-Phalangeal Syndrome Type II, TRP II* MIM #150230 Gene map locus: 8q24.11–q24.13 Inheritance: autosomal dominant. Over 30 cases reported.

(continued)

TABLE 10-2. Ocular and Systemic Findings in Selected Inherited Syndromes (continued).

General Description: postnatal onset of mild growth deficiency, mild to severe mental deficiency, hearing loss, microcephaly, large laterally protruding ears, large bulbous nose, sparse scalp hair, loose redundant skin in infancy, maculopapular skin nevi, cone-shaped epiphyses, multiple exostoses of long tubular bones

Ocular Findings
Common: heavy eyebrows, deep-set eyes, exotropia
Less common: hypotelorism, ptosis, prominent eyes, epicanthal folds, iris coloboma, abducens palsy

Larsen's Syndrome *Desbuquois Syndrome* MIM *150250, *245600 Gene map locus: 3p21.1–p14.1. Inheritance: autosomal dominant and autosomal recessive respectively. Six cases reported.

General Description: multiple joint dislocations with dysplastic epiphyseal centers developing in childhood, flat facies with depressed nasal bridge and prominent forehead, cleft palate, long nontapering fingers with spatulate thumbs, short fingernails, talipes equinovalgus or varus, dysraphism of spine

Ocular Findings
Common: hypertelorism
Less common: entropion of lower eyelids, anterior cortical cataract

Leber's Congenital Amaurosis, Type I, II, III, IV, V MIM #204000, #204100, *604232, #604393, *604537, Gene map locus: 19q13.3, 17p13.1, 1p31, 14q24, 6q11–q16. Inheritance: autosomal recessive. Incidence: 1:33,000.

General Description: in some patients: mental retardation, retarded growth, neurological disorders, hearing loss, midfacial hypoplasia, renal disorders, hyperthreoninemia

Ocular Findings: most common cause of congenital visual impairment in infants and children, vision ranges from 20/200 to bare light perception in most patients. The disease affects both rods and cones.
Common: nystagmus beginning in the second or third month of life, sluggish pupillary response, hyperopic refraction, vision of 20/200 to bare light perception. Ophthalmoscopic findings range from a normal appearance, particularly in infancy, to classic retinitis pigmentosa with bone spicules, attenuation of arterioles, and disc pallor. Other ocular abnormalities include cataract, keratoconus, keratoglobus, photophobia, oculodigital reflex (eye poking). Given the variability in fundus appearance, the diagnosis of Leber's congenital amaurosis cannot be based on fundus appearace alone and requires an electroretinogram. Because both Refsum's disease (infantile phytanic acid storage disease) and Bassen–Kornzweig syndrome (abetalipoproteinemia), which are treatable, have been reported to present as Leber's congenital amaurosis, they should be ruled out.
Less common: irregularity of the retinal pigment epithelium, extensive chorioretinal atrophy, macular "coloboma," white dots (similar to retinitis punctata albescens), marbleized retinal appearance, disc edema

Lenz–Majewski Hyperostotic Dwarfism *Craniodiaphyseal Dysplasia-Lenz Majewski Type* MIM 151050 Inheritance: autosomal dominant. Seven cases reported.

TABLE 10-2. (continued).

General Description: early failure to thrive, short stature, mental retardation, dense thick bone, proximal symphalangism, short or absent middle phalanges, delayed closure of fontanel, progeroid appearance. Cutis laxa in infancy, later skin becomes hypotrophic and thin with prominent subcutaneous veins, especially over the scalp, cutaneous syndactyly of the digits, absence of elastic fibers on skin biopsy. Sparse hair in infancy, dysplastic enamel of teeth. No affected patient has yet survived to adulthood.

Ocular Findings: hypertelorism with protuberant eyes, nasolacrimal duct stenosis

Leprechaunism *Donohue's Syndrome* MIM #246200 Gene map locus: 19p13.2. Inheritance: autosomal recessive. Over 30 cases reported.

General Description: prenatal adipose deficiency, severe failure to thrive, small facies with full lips and large ears, islet cell hyperplasia, hyperglycemia, hyperinsulinemia. Death often occurs in early infancy.

Ocular Findings: prominent eyes, hypertelorism

Levy–Hollister Syndrome *Lacrimo-Auriculo-Dento-Digital Syndrome, LADD Syndrome* MIM *149730 Inheritance: autosomal dominant. Over 20 cases reported.

General Description: cup-shaped ears, mild to severe mixed conductive and sensorineural hearing loss, hypodontia, enamel hypoplasia, poor saliva production, digital abnormalities including digitalization of thumb, preaxial polydactyly, syndactyly between index and middle fingers, clinodactyly of third and fifth fingers, absent radius and thumb, shortening of radius and ulna

Ocular Findings
Common: nasolacrimal duct obstruction, aplasia or hypoplasia of lacrimal puncta (45%), alacrima due to hypoplasia or aplasia of lacrimal glands (40%)
Less common: nasolacrimal fistulae, hypertelorism, telecanthus, down-slanting palpebral fissures

Linear Nevus Sebaceous of Jadassohn MIM 163200 Inheritance: sporadic. Over 450 cases reported.

General Description: nevus sebaceous with hyperpigmentation and hyperkeratosis. The lesions, which are present at birth, are yellowish-orange or tan and brownish raised linear skin lesions on the face, head, and neck, or thorax, usually distributed along the midline. The nevi become verrucous and nodular at puberty, and malignant transformation may occur in the postpubertal period (15%–20%) especially into basal cell carcinoma; therefore, early surgical removal should be considered. Patients frequently have convulsions, developmental delay, and asymmetrical overgrowth. Vitamin D-resistant rickets sometimes occurs.

Ocular Findings: occasionally, the nevus may involve the eyelids extensively, and a large vascularized choriostomatous mass may comprise the lids, conjunctiva, and cornea. The conjunctival lesions are choriostomas and consist of hyperplastic sebaceous glands, apocrine glands, and immature hair follicles. Patients may have scarring and vascularization of the cornea. Other manifestations include nystagmus, strabismus, ptosis, short palpebral fissures, esotropia, optic nerve atrophy, subretinal neovascularization, cortical

(continued)

TABLE 10-2. Ocular and Systemic Findings in Selected Inherited Syndromes (continued).

blindness. Colobomatous microphthalmia, iris and choroidal colobomas, corectopia, limbal dermoids (which may enlarge during the first decade of life), lipodermoids, and intrascleral cartilage and bone have been reported.

Lipodystrophy, Partial, with Rieger Anomaly, Short Stature, and Insulinopenic Diabetes Mellitus MIM 151680. Inheritance: autosomal dominant. One family reported.

General Description: lipodystrophy (especially of the face and buttocks), short stature, insulinopenic diabetes mellitus, midface hypoplasia, hypotrichosis, joint hypermobility, retarded bone age

Ocular Findings: Reiger anomaly consists of anterior segment dysgenesis, resulting in hypoplasia of the anterior iris stroma in addition to the changes typical of Axenfeld's anomaly (posterior embryotoxon accompanied by abnormal iris strands crossing the anterior chamber angle to attach to a prominent Schwalbe's line). Other abnormalities may include glaucoma, microcornea, and corneal opacity. Glaucoma occurs in about 60% of patients by age 20 years.

Marden–Walker Syndrome MIM *248700, 600920 Inheritance: autosomal recessive. Twenty cases reported.

General Description: blepharophimosis (100%), multiple joint contractures present at birth, immobile facies with fixed facial expression (100%), micrognathia (100%), severe growth deficiency (90%), severe mental retardation (90%), hypotonia (85%), microcephaly (56%), cleft palate (40%). Death occurred at about 3 months of age in 19% of affected individuals.

Ocular Findings
Common: blepharophimosis (100%), strabismus (70%), ptosis, hypertelorism, "abnormal eyelashes"
Less common: microphthalmia

Marfan Syndrome MIM #154700 Gene map locus: 15q21.1. Inheritance: autosomal dominant. About 25% of cases arise as new mutations. Incidence: 1:10,000.

General Description: common and major manifestations of the disease include subluxation of the crystalline lens, dilation of the aortic root, aneurysm of the ascending aorta, and skeletal abnormalities such as kyphoscoliosis, an upper segment/lower segment ratio that is 2 standard deviations below the mean for age, and pectus excavatum. Myopia, mitral valve prolapse, arachnodactyly, joint laxity, tall stature, pes planus, striae atrophicae, pneumothorax, obstructive sleep apnea, and dural ectasia may also be present.

Ocular Findings
Common: subluxation of the lens (70%) is usually bilateral, slowly progressive in the first two decades of life, and varies in severity. Superior and temporal displacement of the lens is most common. The zonular fibers are stretched and may be reduced in number. Other common findings include flat cornea (average keratometric values are 41.38 ± 2.04 D), increased axial length of the globe, miosis, and hypoplastic ciliary muscle.
Less common: cataracts (typically the nuclear sclerotic type) develop 10–20 years earlier than in the general population, a deep anterior chamber, prominent iris

TABLE 10-2. (continued).

processes to Schwalbe's line, thin and velvety iris, with absent crypts and convolutions, iridodonesis. The pupil may be difficult to dilate. Strabismus (20%). Retinal detachment. Open-angle glaucoma is significantly more common in all age groups compared to the general population. Total dislocation of the lens into the vitreous cavity occurs rarely and may be complicated by phacolytic glaucoma and uveitis. Anterior dislocation of the lens into the pupil or anterior chamber is rare and may be complicated by pupillary block glaucoma. Microspherophakia has also been reported.

Maroteaux–Lamy Syndrome *Mucopolysaccharidosis VI Mild, Moderate and Severe Types* MIM *253200 Gene map locus: 5q11–q13. Inheritance: autosomal recessive. Rare disorder.

General Description: arylsulfatase B deficiency. Growth deficiency, coarse facies, mild stiffness of joints, thick and tight skin, small widely spaced teeth, hepatosplenomegaly, aortic valve dysfunction, varying degrees of deafness. No mental retardation. Most die of cardiopulmonary complications by the second or third decade.

Ocular Findings
Common: corneal clouding is marked (mucopolysaccharides are within the corneal epithelium), Bowman's layer, and keratocytes
Less common: glaucoma, optic nerve swelling, optic atrophy, thickened and/or enlarged cornea, scleral thickening

Marshall Syndrome *Deafness-Myopia-Cataract-Saddle Nose, Marshall Type* MIM #154780 Gene map locus: 1p21. Can be caused by mutations in the COL11A1 gene, located on chromosome 1p21. Inheritance: autosomal dominant. Over 20 cases reported. (There remains debate as to whether Marshall syndrome and Stickler syndrome represent separate entities.)

General Description: short stature (relative to unaffected family members) and a stocky build. Flat and retracted midface with a saddle, short and depressed nose with a flat nasal bridge and anteverted nares. Prominent protruding upper incisors, thick lips. Sensorineural hearing loss noted as early as 3 years of age, with gradual progression to moderate or severe levels by adulthood. Calvarial thickening, absent frontal sinuses, congenital occipital cutis aplasia. Falx, tentorial, and meningeal calcifications. Spondyloephiphyseal abnormalities including mild platyspondyly, slightly small and irregular distal femoral and proximal tibial epiphyses, outward bowing of radius and ulna, and wide tufts of distal phalanges. Occasionally, mental deficiency, cleft palate.

Ocular Findings: high axial myopia, which becomes apparent during the first decade of life, infantile and juvenile cataracts, shallow orbits and appearance of large eyes, hypertelorism, esotropia, hypertropia, glaucoma, vitreoretinal degeneration, retinal breaks, retinal detachment.

Marshall–Smith Syndrome MIM 602535 Inheritance: sporadic. Over 20 cases reported.

General Description: accelerated growth and maturation, broad middle phalanges, motor and mental deficiency, long cranium with prominent forehead, upturned nose. Most patients die of respiratory infections in early infancy.

Ocular Findings: shallow orbits with prominent eyes, bluish sclera

(continued)

TABLE 10-2. Ocular and Systemic Findings in Selected Inherited Syndromes (continued).

Melnick–Fraser Syndrome *Branchio-Oto-Renal (BOR) Syndrome* MIM #113650
Gene map locus: 8q13.3. Inheritance: autosomal dominant. Incidence: 1:40,000 (the syndrome occurs in about 2% of profoundly deaf children).

General Description: the association of branchial arch anomalies (preauricular pits, branchial fistulas), hearing loss, and renal hypoplasia.

Ocular Findings
Common: lacrimal duct stenosis or aplasia
Less common: gustatory lacrimation (the shedding of tears during eating due to misdirected growth of seventh cranial nerve fibers)

Melnick–Needles Osteodysplasty MIM 309350, 249420 Inheritance: X-linked dominant form (autosomal recessive and autosomal dominant suggested). Over 30 cases reported.

General Description: small facies with prominent forehead, full cheeks, small mandible, micrognathia, malaligned teeth, late closure of fontanels. Short upper arms and distal phalanges, bowing of humerus, radius, ulna, and tibia. Relatively small thoracic cage with irregular ribbon-like ribs and short clavicles with wide medial ends and narrow shoulders, short scapulae, and pectus excavatum.

Ocular Findings
Common: exophthalmos, hypertelorism
Less common: strabismus, glaucoma

Microphthalmia with Linear Skin Defects Syndrome *Midas Syndrome* MIM *309801 Gene map locus: Xp22.31. Inheritance: X-linked (presumably lethal in hemizygous males). Over 10 cases reported.

General Description: dermal aplasia, without herniation of fatty tissue, usually involving face, scalp, and neck but occasionally upper part of the thorax. Occasional abnormalities include microcephaly, central nervous system defects including agenesis of corpus callosum and absence of septum pellucidum, cardiac defects, diaphragmatic hernia. Death occurred in the first year of life in two children, presumably secondary to cardiac arrhythmias.

Ocular Findings
Common: microphthalmia, sclerocornea
Less common: anterior chamber defects, cataract, iris coloboma, pigmentary retinopathy, orbital cysts

Miller Syndrome *Genee–Wiedemann Syndrome, Postaxial Acrofacial Dysostosis* MIM *263750 Inheritance: autosomal recessive. Over 24 cases reported.

General Description: Treacher Collins-like facies, hypoplasia or aplasia of the fifth digital ray, abnormalities may extend to the radius and ulna, which can be shortened or even fused

Ocular Findings (as in Treacher Collins syndrome)
Common: lack of lateral canthal fixation causing drooping of the lower eyelid in an S-shaped contour. Colobomas or pseudocolobomas of the lateral third of the lower eyelid (75%). The medial part of the lower eyelid may be thin, absent of tarsal plate, and devoid of all marginal structures, including eyelashes and

TABLE 10-2. (continued).

meibomian glands (50%). "Egg-shaped" orbit caused by deformities of the temporal orbital wall. The relative protrusion of the nose may produce an enophthalmic appearance.

Less common: atresia of the lower lacrimal punctum and canaliculus, ptosis, distichiasis, trichiasis, ectropion, entropion, upper eyelid coloboma, microphthalmia, anophthalmos, pupillary ectopia, iris coloboma, cataract, corneal guttae

---

Miller–Dieker Lissencephaly Syndrome MIM #247200 Gene map locus: 17p13.3. Inheritance: autosomal dominant. Approximately a dozen kinships as well as sporadic cases have been reported.

General Description: cerebral dysgenesis, absent or hypoplastic corpus callosum (74%), large cavum septi pellucidi (77%), type I lissencephaly (incomplete development of the brain, often with a smooth surface, thickened cortex with four rather than six cell layers), infantile spasms. Characteristic craniofacial features: microcephaly with bitemporal narrowing. Variable high forehead, and vertical forehead, soft tissue ridging and furrowing, especially when crying. Small nose with anteverted nostrils, protuberant upper lip, thin vermilion border of upper lip, and micrognathia. Appearance of "low-set" and/or posteriorly angulated auricles. Death usually occurs before 2 years of age.

Ocular Findings
Common: up-slanting palpebral fissures
Less common: cataract

Möbius' Syndrome I, II, III *Facial Diplegia, Congenital* MIM *157900, *601471, *604185 Gene map locus: 13q12.2–q13, 3q21–q22, 10q21.3–q22.1 Inheritance: autosomal dominant. Over 100 cases reported.

General Description: mask-like facies with sixth and seventh nerve palsy. Some patients have more extensive cranial nerve involvement, including the third, fourth, fifth, eighth, ninth, tenth, and twelfth nerves. Patients with Möbius' syndrome usually present with congenital deafness, nonprogressive facial paralysis, and inability to abduct the eyes beyond the midline. About 15% have mental deficiency. Non-CNS defects may include limb reduction defects, syndactyly, the Poland sequence, and, occasionally, the Klippel–Feil anomaly.

Ocular Findings: sixth (causing inability to abduct the eyes beyond the midline) and seventh nerve palsy, variable fifth nerve palsy, absent blink reflex in type 2. On forced abduction, pupils usually become miotic, indicating that convergence is substituting for abduction. Bell's phenomenon is not usually present, predisposing the patient to exposure keratopathy during sleep.

Mohr Syndrome *OFD Syndrome Type II* MIM *252100 Inheritance: autosomal recessive. Approximately 25 cases reported.

General Description: short stature, cerebellar atrophy, midline partial cleft of lip, cleft palate, cleft tongue, papilliform tongue protuberances, hypoplasia of zygomatic arch, maxilla, and body of mandible, conductive hearing loss, partial reduplication of hallux and first metatarsal, polydactyly, syndactyly

Ocular Findings: lateral displacement of inner canthi

(continued)

TABLE 10-2. Ocular and Systemic Findings in Selected Inherited Syndromes (continued).

Morquio Syndrome *Mucopolysaccharidosis Type IV Subtypes A and B* MIM *253000, #253010 Gene map locus: Type A, 16q24.3. Inheritance: autosomal recessive. Incidence: probably less than 1:100,000.

General Description: keratan sulfate degradation is abnormal. Two subtypes: A (more severe type), *N*-acetylgalactosamine-6-sulfatase deficiency, subtype B (milder type), beta-galactosidase deficiency. The distinctive feature in this disorder is the skeletal dysplasia. Onset at 1 to 3 years of age, severe limitation of growth, marked vertebral defects, instability of the first cervical articulation can lead to life-threatening subluxation, severe kyphosis and knock-knees, mild coarsening of facial features, late onset of aortic regurgitation, hearing loss, hepatomegaly, inguinal hernia, widely spaced teeth with thin enamel that tends to become grayish, normal intelligence.

Ocular Findings: corneal stromal clouding (mild, fine haze), evident usually after 5 to 10 years of age. Rare: retinal pigmentary changes, glaucoma, optic atrophy.

Mucolipidosis Type I Subtypes I, II *Dysmorphic Sialidosis Syndrome, Sialidosis Syndrome Type II, Spranger's Syndrome* MIM *256550 Gene map locus: 6p21.3. Inheritance: autosomal recessive. Approximately 20 cases reported.

General Description: deficiency of glycoprotein sialidase (alpha-*N*-acetyl-neuroaminidase). Myoclonus, gait abnormalities, dysmorphic Hurler-like facies (prominent brow, hypertrichosis, frontal bossing, and saddle nose), organomegaly, mental retardation, dysostosis multiplex, sensorineural hearing loss, and progressive neurological decline. Most patients do not survive past adolescence or early adulthood. Subtype II has an infantile onset and is more severe.

Ocular Findings: macular cherry-red spot with or without optic atrophy and decreased visual acuity, nystagmus, spokelike lenticular opacities, tortuous retinal and conjunctival vessels, pigmentary degeneration of the retina, fine corneal epithelial and stromal opacities (can occur but do not typically produce significant corneal clouding)

Mucolipidosis Type II *Leroy I-Cell Syndrome* MIM *252500 Gene map locus: 4q21–q23. Inheritance: autosomal recessive. Incidence: undetermined.

General Description: abnormality of *N*-acetylglucosamine phosphotransferase. Marked, early-onset growth deficiency and developmental deficiency, Hurler-type phenotype, coarse facies, progressive early alveolar ridge hypertrophy, high narrow forehead, low nasal bridge, anteverted nostrils, long philtrum, gingival hyperplasia, short neck, moderate joint limitation, kyphosis, thick tight skin during early infancy, cavernous skin hemangiomas, minimal hepatomegaly, valvular heart disease, hearing loss. Death usually occurs by 5 years of age from pneumonia or congestive heart failure. Caused by failure of incorporation of acid hydrolase into lysosomes (see pseudo-Hurler polydystrophy syndrome).

Ocular Findings: hypoplastic orbits with hypoplasia of the supraorbital ridges and prominence of the globes, thin eyebrows, puffy eyelids, inner epicanthal folds, cavernous skin hemangiomas. Corneal clouding (the cornea usually remains clear in early life, but approximately 40% of patients later develop abnormal stromal granularity and mild opacity). Glaucoma and megalocornea have been reported. Normal funduscopic examination.

TABLE 10-2. (continued).

Mucopolysaccharidosis Type VII Syndrome *Sly Syndrome, Beta-Glucuronidase Deficiency* MIM *253220 Gene map locus: 7q21.11. Inheritance: autosomal recessive. Over 20 cases reported.

General Description: beta-glucuronidase deficiency. Mild, intermediate, and severe forms. Growth deficiency, moderately severe mental deficiency, macrocephaly, coarse facies, short neck, joint contractures, radiologic signs of dysostosis multiplex, J-shaped sella turcica, thoracolumbar gibbus, hepatosplenomegaly, valvular hear disease, frequent respiratory infections, hearing loss, hydrocephalus, neurodegeneration (the neurological decline generally does not present until 3–4 years of age). Death may occur in the first few months of life. In the milder forms there is survival into adolescence.

Ocular Findings: hypertelorism, corneal clouding (in the severe form). Pigment retinopathy, optic nerve swelling, and optic atrophy have been reported.

Mulibrey Nanism Syndrome *Perheentupa Syndrome, Dwarfism-Mulibrey Type* MIM #253250 Gene map locus: 17q22–q23. Inheritance: autosomal recessive. Over 40 cases reported.

General Description: short stature, triangular facies with frontal bossing, relatively small tongue, dental crowding, dolichocephaly with J-shaped sella turcica, thick adherent pericardium with pericardial constriction, hepatomegaly, prominent neck veins, muscle hypotonia, high-pitched voice

Ocular Findings: decreased retinal pigmentation with dispersion and clusters of pigment and "yellowish dots" in the midperipheral region, choroid hypoplasia

Multiple Lentigines Syndrome *Leopard Syndrome* MIM *151100 Inheritance: autosomal dominant. Over 70 cases reported.

General Description: multiple lentigines, mild pulmonic stenosis, hypertrophic obstructive cardiomyopathy, mild growth deficiency, mild to moderate sensorineural deafness, prominent ears, cryptorchidism

Ocular Findings: mild hypertelorism

Multiple Synostosis Syndrome *Symphalangism Syndrome* MIM 185650, *185700, 185750, #185800, *186400, #186500 Gene map locus: 17q22 (for #185800 and #186500). Inheritance: autosomal dominant. Fifty cases reported.

General Description: multiple fusion of midphalangeal joints, elbows, carpal and tarsal bones, multiple hand abnormalities, vertebral anomalies, fusion of middle ear ossicles with conductive deafness, hypoplasia of alae nasi

Ocular Findings: strabismus

Nager Syndrome *Acrofacial Dysostosis 1, Nager Type* MIM 154400 Gene map locus: 9q32. Inheritance: autosomal dominant. Over 75 cases reported.

General Description: Treacher Collins craniofacial abnormalities, with preaxial upper limb defects, hypoplastic thumbs, absent thumbs

Ocular Findings (as in Treacher Collins syndrome)
Common: lack of lateral canthal fixation causing drooping of the lower eyelid in an S-shaped contour. Colobomas or pseudocolobomas of the lateral third of the lower eyelid (75%). The medial part of the lower eyelid may be thin, absent of tarsal plate, and devoid of all marginal structures, including eyelashes and

(continued)

TABLE 10-2. Ocular and Systemic Findings in Selected Inherited Syndromes (continued).

meibomian glands (50%). "Egg-shaped" orbit caused by deformities of the temporal orbital wall. The relative protrusion of the nose may produce an enophthalmic appearance.

Less common: atresia of the lower lacrimal punctum and canaliculus, ptosis, distichiasis, trichiasis, ectropion, entropion, upper eyelid coloboma, microphthalmia, anophthalmos, pupillary ectopia, iris coloboma, cataract, corneal guttae

---

Nail-Patella Syndrome *Onychoosteodysplasia* MIM #161200 Gene map locus: 9q34.1. Inheritance: autosomal dominant. Over 400 cases reported. The disorder is caused by mutations in the LIM-homedomain protein LMX1B (*602575).

General Description: dysplasia of the nails and absent or hypoplastic patellae are the cardinal features of the syndrome. Abnormalities of nails include slow nail growth, hypoplastic to absent nails, longitudinal ridging, splitting (most commonly of thumbnail), discoloration, poorly formed and triangular (a unique finding) or absent lunulae (98%). The severity of the nail involvement is worse radial to ulnar. Toenails are involved in 1 of 7 individuals. Hypoplastic to absent patellae (60%–90%), patellar dislocation, hypoplasia of lateral femoral condyle and small head of fibula (92%), elbow deformities (60%–90%) with limited range of motion, hypoplasia of head of radius (90%), fifth finger clinodactyly, absence of distal phalangeal joints, talipes equinovarus, spur in midposterior ilium (iliac horn) (81%), hypoplasia of scapula (44%). Glomerulonephritis, nephrotic syndrome, renal insufficiency (48%). Occasionally, other musculoskeletal abnormalities, short stature, mental deficiency, psychosis, cleft lip/palate, hearing loss.

Ocular Findings
Common: open-angle glaucoma (reported in 9 of 28 families with the nail-patella syndrome). In most cases the glaucoma occurs in adulthood, but it can occur at any age.

Less common: keratoconus, microcornea, microphakia, cataract, ptosis. (These are sporadic abnormalities reported, not proven to be related to the disease.)

Neurofibromatosis, Type I (NF1) *Von Recklinghausen Disease* MIM *162200 Gene map locus: 17q11.2. Inheritance: autosomal dominant. Incidence: 1:2000–1:4000.

General Description: the disease is diagnosed when two or more of the following criteria are met: (1) six or more café au lait spots, measuring at least 1.5 cm in diameter in postpubescent individuals or 0.5 cm in diameter in prepubescent individuals; (2) two or more neurofibromas of any type or one plexiform neurofibroma; (3) freckling of axillary, inguinal, or other intertriginous areas; (4) two or more iris hamartomas (Lisch nodules); (5) optic glioma; (6) distinctive osseous lesions, such as sphenoid dysplasia or thinning of long bone cortex, with or without pseudoartharoses, and (7) a first-degree relative with NF1 (according to the above criteria).Every system in the body may be affected by complications arising from NF1, and patients are at higher risk for malignancies.

TABLE 10-2. (continued).

Ocular Findings

Common: iris hamartomas (Lisch nodules) rarely seen before age 2 years, found in 92% over age 5 years, and in nearly 100% of patients over age 20 years. Lisch nodules are usually no larger than 1 mm, sharply demarcated, dome-shaped excrescences. They consist primarily of uniform spindle-shaped melanin-containing cells.

Less common: chiasmal or optic nerve gliomas (optic glioma) (15%–19%). Symptomatic optic gliomas (producing complications such as visual loss, proptosis) occur in 1% to 5% of patients with NF1 and usually become symptomatic before the age of 10 years. Tumors confined to the optic nerve at the time of clinical presentation infrequently extend into the chiasm and very rarely develop metastases. There is almost no mortality with these tumors. Tumors primarily involving the chiasm may cause bilateral visual loss, hydrocephalus, and hypothalamic dysfunction. Mortality of 50% or higher has been reported with these tumors. Plexiform neurofibromas (30%) appear as extensive subcutaneous swellings with indistinct margins, and feel like a "bag of worms." Approximately 10% of plexiform neurofibromas involve the face, commonly the upper eyelid and orbit causing ptosis, and an S-shaped configuration of the eyelid margin. Rarely malignant degeneration occurs within the lesion, producing a neurofibrosarcoma capable of metastasis. Glaucoma in the ipsilateral eye is found in as many as 50% of cases. Choroidal lesions (30%–50% of adults with NF1) are flat with indistinct borders, yellow-white to dark brown. NF1 patients are believed to be predisposed to developing uveal melanoma and other malignant neoplasms; however, the incidence of iris or choroidal tumors is low. Glaucoma (1%–2%) is associated in most cases with ipsilateral plexiform neurofibroma of the upper eyelid or with iris ectropion (ectropion uvea). Buphthalmos, enlargement of the cornea, corneal edema, and high myopia may result.

Neurofibromatosis Type II MIM *101000 Gene map locus: 22q12.2. Inheritance: autosomal dominant. Incidence: 1:33,000–40,000.

General Description: diagnostic criteria include bilateral vestibular schwannomas (called acoustic neuromas, although arising from the vestibular nerve rather than the acoustic nerve) (85%), or a first-degree relative with neurofibromatosis type II and either unilateral eighth nerve mass or two of the following: neurofibroma, meningioma, glioma, schwannoma, posterior capsular cataract, or other lens opacities at a young age.

Ocular Findings

Common: lens opacities (69%–80%): posterior subcapsular cataracts are the most common and usually develop during adolescence or young adulthood, peripheral cortical cataracts and other lens opacities have been associated with NF2, retinal astrocytic hamartomas (23%), juvenile-onset ocular motor paresis (12%)

Less common: small retinal scars, epiretinal membranes, juvenile-onset vitreoretinal degeneration (6%), retinal detachment, combined pigment epithelial and retinal astrocytic hamartomas, optic nerve sheath meningioma, Mittendorf dot, embryonal cataract, persistent hyperplastic primary vitreous, anisocoria, uveal melanoma, optic nerve head gliomas, myelinated nerve fibers, choroidal hamartoma, choroidal nevus, and choroidal hemangioma have been reported

(continued)

TABLE 10-2. Ocular and Systemic Findings in Selected Inherited Syndromes (continued).

Visual loss in NF2 is more commonly due to intracranial and optic nerve sheath meningioma than to cataract. Other causes of visual loss include combined pigment epithelial and retinal hamartomas, epiretinal membranes, chronic papilledema, and amblyopia due to ocular motor paresis.

Noonan Syndrome 1 *Turner-Like Syndrome* MIM *163950 Gene map locus: 12q24. Inheritance: autosomal dominant. Incidence: 1:1000–1:2500 live births.

General Description: short or webbed neck, low posterior hairline, shield chest and pectus excavatum or pectus carinatum or both, pulmonary valve stenosis, cryptorchidism, coagulation defects, postnatal growth deficiency (50%), mental retardation (25%), low-set and/or abnormal auricles, anterior dental malocclusion, increased width of mouth, prominent protruding upper lip, moderate retrognathia

Ocular Findings: epicanthal folds, ptosis, hypertelorism, down-slanting palpebral fissures, myopia, keratoconus, strabismus, nystagmus, blue-green irides

Norrie's Disease *Pseudoglioma* MIM *310600 Gene map locus: Xp11.4–p11.3. Inheritance: X-linked. Over 200 cases reported.

General Description: microcephaly, severe and progressive mental retardation, psychosis, seizures, progressive sensorineural deafness (25%), which has its onset in the second or third decade of life, hypogonadism, cryptochidism

Ocular Findings: ocular signs are present at birth and include bilateral retinal folds, or retinal detachment and bilateral retrolental masses formed by dysplastic detached retinas. Shallow anterior chambers with dilated pupils, hypoplastic irides, posterior synechiae, and ectropion uvea. The ciliary processes are elongated and often visible through the pupil. The globes usually become phthisical. Other reported manifestations include pseudoglioma, cataract, and band-shaped corneal degeneration.

Oculocerebrorenal Syndrome *Lowe Syndrome* MIM *309000 Gene map locus: Xq26.1. Inheritance: X-linked recessive. Incidence: unknown.

General Description: growth retardation, fair skin, chubby cheeks, frontal bossing, severe mental retardation, areflexia, hypotonia, seizures, noninflammatory joint swelling, generalized proximal renal tubular dysfunction (renal Fanconi's syndrome) develop during the first year of life producing renal wasting of water, bicarbonate, glucose, and amino acids. Patients present with polyuria and polydipsia. Calcium and phosphorus loss may result in bone resorption. Proteinuria may develop as renal failure ensues.

Ocular Findings: congenital cataracts of the nuclear, polar or complete type are characteristic and essential to the diagnosis. The lens tends to be small, thick, opaque, and disc shaped, with no demarcation between the nucleus and cortex. Posterior lenticonus may be demonstrated. The anterior capsule tends to be irregularly thickened, often with fibrous anterior subcapsular plaques. The posterior capsule is extremely thinned. The peripheral lens may show vacuolization, clefting, and focal opacifications. Congenital glaucoma (65%) is thought to be due to goniodysgenesis. Miotic pupils due to hypoplastic dilator muscle and hypertrophied sphincter muscle. Corneal keloids are common after 6 years of age and may contribute to visual impairment. Obligate carriers have characteristic multiple gray-white opacities in the cortex of the lens.

TABLE 10-2. (continued).

Oculodentodigital Syndrome *Oculodentoosseous Dysplasia (ODOD)* MIM *164200 Gene map locus: 6q22–q24. Inheritance: autosomal dominant. Approximately 85 cases reported.

General Description: enamel hypoplasia, microdontia or hypodontia, camptodactyly of fifth fingers, bilateral syndactyly of fourth and fifth fingers and third and fourth toes, midphalangeal hypoplasia or aplasia of one or more fingers and/or toes, thin nose with hypoplastic alae nasi and small nares, fine dry and/or sparse and slow-growing hair, broad tubular bones, and mandible with wide alveolar ridge. Occasionally cleft lip and palate, conductive hearing loss, and osteoporosis.

Ocular Findings
Common: "small eyes," microcornea with otherwise normal ocular dimensions, microphthalmia, scarce eyebrows, narrow and short palpebral fissures, telecanthus, epicanthal folds, bony orbital hypotelorism with normal inner canthal distance
Less common: open-angle glaucoma or angle-closure glaucoma, various degrees of iris hypoplasia, cataract, strabismus
Glaucoma is the major cause of visual loss, with an onset ranging from infancy to adulthood; therefore, periodic ophthalmic evaluation is recommended.

Opitz Syndrome Type I, II *Opitz–Frias Syndrome* MIM *300000, *145410 Gene map locus: Type I, Xp22; Type II, 22q11.2. Inheritance: Type I, X-linked recessive; Type II, autosomal dominant. Over 30 cases reported.

General Description: mild to moderate mental deficiency, hypotonia, hypospadias, laryngotracheal abnormalities, swallowing difficulties with recurrent aspiration, stridorous respirations. Initial failure to thrive is followed by normal growth in survivors. Broad flat nasal bridge with anteverted nostrils, cleft lip with or without cleft palate, short frenulum of tongue, micrognathia, posterior rotation of auricles, congenital heart defects.

Ocular Findings
Common: hypertelorism, upward- or downward-slanting palpebral fissures, epicanthal folds
Less common: strabismus

Oral-Facial-Digital Syndrome 1 *OFD Syndrome, Type I* MIM #311200 Gene map locus: Xp22.3–p22.2. Inheritance: X-linked dominant. Over 160 cases reported.

General Description: corpus callosum agenesis on CT scan, mental retardation, clumsy gait, dysarthria, broad nasal root, small nostrils, hypoplasia of alae nasi, cleft jaw, midline cleft of upper lip, aberrant hyperplastic oral frenula, lobulate tongue, tongue hamartomas, irregular asymmetrical cleft palate, digital asymmetry, syndactyly, brachydactyly, facial milia, spotty alopecia, polycystic kidneys, renal failure. Lethal in hemizygotes.

Ocular Findings: lateral displacement of inner canthi

Oromandibular-Limb Hypogenesis Spectrum *Aglossia-Adactyly Syndrome* MIM 103300 Inheritance: autosomal dominant. Incidence: less than 1:20,000 births.

(continued)

TABLE 10-2. Ocular and Systemic Findings in Selected Inherited Syndromes (continued).

General Description: brain defect, especially of cranial nerve nuclei, causing Möbius sequence, small mouth, micrognathia, hypoglossia, variable clefting or aberrant attachments of tongue, mandibular hypodontia, cleft palate, facial asymmetry, limb hypoplasia of varying degrees to the point of limb deficiency, syndactyly, adactyly, splenogonadal fusion. Problems with hyperthermia can occur in children with four-limb amputation.

Ocular Findings: cranial nerve palsies including Möbius sequence, telecanthus, lower eyelid defect

Osteogenesis Imperfecta Syndrome, Type I MIM #166200 Gene map locus: 17q21.31–q22, 7q22.1. Inheritance: autosomal dominant. Incidence: 3.5:100,000 live births.

General Description: hyperextensibile joints (100%), bone fractures (92%), postnatal onset growth deficiency (50%). Hypoplasia of dentin and pulp of teeth with translucency and yellowish or bluish-gray coloration, susceptibility to caries, irregular placement and late eruption of teeth, thin skin, easy bruising (75%), postnatal onset of mild limb deformity, primarily anterior or lateral bowing of femora, hearing impairment (35%) secondary to otosclerosis (usually first noted in third decade)

Ocular Findings
Common: partial visualization of the choroid gives the sclera a blue appearance
Less common: ectopia lentis is rare, embryotoxon, keratoconus, megalocornea

Oto-Palato-Digital Syndrome, Type I *Taybi Syndrome* MIM ˙311300 Gene map locus: Xq28. Inheritance: X-linked. Approximately 30 cases reported.

General Description: moderate conductive deafness, frontal and occipital prominence, absence of frontal and sphenoid sinuses, facial bone hypoplasia, cleft palate, partial anodontia, broad distal digits with short nails, mild mental deficiency, short stature

Ocular Findings: hypertelorism with lateral fullness of the supraorbital ridges

Pachyonychia Congenita Syndrome, Type 1 MIM #167200 Gene map locus: 17q12–q21, 12q13. Inheritance: autosomal dominant. Several kindreds reported. (Pachyonychia congenita, recessive, MIM 260130, has been described in 3 cases.)

General Description: progressive thickening of nails with yellow-brown discoloration, pinched margins, and an upward angulation of distal tips (the nails may eventually become hypoplastic or absent), patchy to complete hyperkeratosis of palms and soles, callosities of feet, palmar and plantar bullae formation in areas of pressure, keratosis pilaris, epidermal cysts filled with loose keratin on face, neck, and upper chest, verrucous lesions on the elbows, knees and lower legs, leukokeratosis of mouth and tongue, scalloped tongue edge, erupted teeth at birth, lost by 4 to 6 months, early loss of secondary teeth, other teeth anomalies, hair anomalies, alopecia. An abnormality of cell-mediated immunity with tendency to oral and cutaneous candidiasis. Occasionally mental retardation. Areas of chronic bullous formation should be followed for development of skin malignancy.

Ocular Findings: occasionally "corneal thickening," cataract, bushy eyebrows

TABLE 10-2. (continued).

Pallister–Hall Syndrome MIM #146510 Gene map locus: 7p13. Inheritance: autosomal dominant. Sixteen cases reported.

General Description: holoprosencephaly with midline cleft lip and palate, arrhinencephaly, hypothalamic hamartoblastoma, panhypopituitarism, imperforate anus, postaxial polydactyly. The majority of patients have died by 3 years of age, usually of hypoadrenalism.

Ocular Findings: microphthalmia, coloboma

Pena–Shokeir Syndrome, Type 1 *Fetal Akinesia Sequence* MIM *208150 Inheritance: autosomal recessive. Several dozen cases reported.

General Description: neurogenic arthrogryposis, pulmonary hypoplasia, prenatal onset of growth deficiency, rigid expressionless face, poorly folded ears. Approximately 30% are stillborn.

Ocular Findings: hypertelorism, prominent eyes, telecanthus, epicanthal folds

Peters' Anomaly–Associated with Other Ocular Defects MIM 603807, *116150 Gene map locus: 11p13 (603807). Inheritance: autosomal dominant (*116150). Incidence: unknown.

Ocular Findings: Peters' anomaly consists of a central corneal leukoma, with corresponding defects in the posterior corneal stroma Descemet's membrane, and endothelium and a variable degree of iris and lenticular attachments to the central aspect of the posterior cornea. The condition is bilateral in 60%–80% of cases. Associated ocular defects may include: microcornea, microphthalmia, anterior polar cataract, dysgenesis of the angle and iris, glaucoma, spontaneous corneal perforation, cornea plana, sclerocornea, colobomas, aniridia, congenital aphakia, persistence of the hyaloid system, and total posterior coloboma of the retina and choroids.

Peters' Anomaly–Isolated Ocular Abnormality MIM #604229 Inheritance: autosomal recessive (can be caused by mutation in the PAX6 gene and in the PITX2 gene), occasional autosomal dominant transmission has been reported. Many of the cases are sporadic. Incidence: unknown.

Ocular Findings: Peters' anomaly is a congenital central corneal leukoma, with corresponding defects in the posterior corneal stroma Descemet's membrane, and endothelium and a variable degree of iris and lenticular attachments to the central aspect of the posterior cornea. The condition is bilateral in 60%–80% of cases. The visual prognosis depends on the degree of corneal opacification and on the severity of associated ocular malformations. Unilateral cases are usually associated with deep amblyopia. Congenital or postsurgical glaucoma is a major cause of visual loss in many cases. As many as 50% of patients with Peters' anomaly eventually lose light perception.

Peters' Anomaly with Short-Limb Dwarfism *Kivlin-Krause Syndrome* MIM *261540 Inheritance: autosomal recessive. Incidence: several reports of familial cases.

General Description: short stature, short hands, tapering brachydactyly, short fifth finger, fifth finger clinodactyly

(continued)

TABLE 10-2. Ocular and Systemic Findings in Selected Inherited Syndromes (continued).

Ocular Findings: Peters' anomaly consists of a central corneal leukoma, absence of the posterior corneal stroma and Descemet's membrane, and a variable degree of iris and lenticular attachments to the central aspect of the posterior cornea (see Peters' Anomaly—Isolated Ocular Abnormality, above)

Peters'-Plus Syndrome MIM *261540 Inheritance: autosomal recessive. Over 40 cases reported.

General Description: Peters' anomaly occurs in association with cleft lip/palate, round face, depressed nasal bridge, anteverted nostrils, thin upper lip, mental retardation, abnormal ears, hearing loss, cerebral atrophy on CT scan, macrocephaly, hydrocephaly, hypoplastic female genitalia, cryptorchidism, cardiovascular anomalies, midline defects. Sixty percent of patients with Peters' anomaly have systemic malformations or developmental delay. Patients with unilateral disease are as likely to have systemic malformations as patients with bilateral disease. Chromosomal studies should be obtained in those patients with multiple congenital malformations and Peters' anomaly.

Ocular Findings: Peters' anomaly consists of a central corneal leukoma, absence of the posterior corneal stroma and Descemet's membrane, and a variable degree of iris and lenticular attachments to the central aspect of the posterior cornea (see Peters' anomaly—Isolated Ocular Abnormality, above). Narrow palpebral fissures.

Pfeiffer's Syndrome, Type I, II, III *Acrocephaloysyndactyly Type 5* MIM #101600 Gene map locus: 10q26, 8p11.2–p11.1. Inheritance: Type I is autosomal dominant. Types II and III are sporadic. Over 30 cases reported.

General Description: craniosynostosis results in turribrachycephalic skull, broad, short thumbs and great toes with radial deviation are characteristic, malformed proximal phalanx. Various internal organ anomalies have been reported, more frequent in type II and type III. Type I patients usually have normal intelligence and generally good outcome, whereas patients with Types II and III often have neurological involvement and shortened life expectancy.

Ocular Findings
Common: shallow orbits, proptosis, down-slanting palpebral fissures, hypertelorism, strabismus
Less common: ptosis, scleralization of the cornea, optic nerve hypoplasia, anterior chamber defects including Peters' anomaly, bilateral superior iris coloboma (reported in one affected patient)

Progeria Syndrome *Hutchinson–Gilford Syndrome* MIM 176670 Inheritance: likely autosomal dominant. Incidence: 1:4,000,000–1:8,000,000.

General Description: precocious senility of striking degree is characteristic, death from coronary heart disease is frequent and can occur before 10 years of age, alopecia, atrophy of subcutaneous fat, skeletal hypoplasia and dysplasia, short stature

Ocular Findings: congenital or acquired cataract, microphthalmia

Proteus Syndrome MIM 176920 Inheritance: sporadic. Several dozen cases reported.

TABLE 10-2. (continued).

General Description: overgrowth that may involve the whole body, may be unilateral, may involve one limb or may be localized involving a digit or any combination of the above, macrocephaly, generalized thickening of skin, hyperpigmented areas that appear to represent epidermal nevi, lipomata, lymphangiomata, and hemangiomata, hemihypertrophy, bony prominences over skull, angulation defects of knees, scoliosis, kyphosis, vertebrae anomalies, hip dislocation, macrodactyly, soft tissue hypertrophy of hands and feet, cardiac and renal abnormalities

Ocular Findings: ptosis, strabismus, epibulbar dermoid, "enlarged eyes," microphthalmia, myopia, cataract, nystagmus

Pseudo-Hurler Polydystrophy Syndrome *Mucolipidosis Type III* MIM *252600 Inheritance: autosomal recessive. Incidence: Unknown.

General Description: decreased growth rate in early childhood, mild mental deficiency, development of mildly coarse facies by 6 years, joint stiffness by 2 to 4 years, aortic valve disease, no mucopolysacchariduria. Some patients live into the fourth or fifth decade. A disorder similar to mucolipidosis II but milder (see mucolipidosis II). Lysosomal disorder resulting from deficiency of *N*-acetylglucosamine-1-phosphtransferase.

Ocular Findings: fine opacities of the corneal stroma, evident by 6 to 8 years of age (do not significantly affect vision), hyperopic astigmatism. epiretinal membranes, retinal vascular tortuosity and optic nerve head swelling have been reported

Radial Aplasia-Thrombocytopenia Syndrome *TAR Syndrome* MIM *274000 Inheritance: autosomal recessive. Over 100 cases reported.

General Description: thrombocytopenia, bilateral absence of radius, hypoplasia of ulna

Ocular Findings: nevus flammeus of forehead, strabismus, ptosis

Rapp–Hodgkin Ectodermal Dysplasia Syndrome *Hypohidrotic Ectodermal Dysplasia, Autosomal Dominant Type* MIM *129400 Inheritance: autosomal dominant. Approximately 25 cases reported.

General Description: hypohidrosis; thin skin with decreased number of sweat pores, sparse, fine hair, small dysplastic nails, hypodontia with small conical teeth, low nasal bridge, high forehead, small mouth with oral clefts, hypospadias. Occasional abnormalities include short stature, atretic ear canals, hearing loss, syndactyly. Predisposed to hyperthermia in early childhood, and frequent occurrence of otitis media.

Ocular Findings
Common: frequent occurrence of purulent conjunctivitis
Less common: ptosis, absent lacrimal puncta

Renal Tubular Acidosis II *Renal Tubular Acidosis, Proximal, with Bilateral Glaucoma, Cataract, and Band Keratopathy* MIM #604278 Gene map locus: 4q21. Inheritance: autosomal recessive. Over 8 cases reported.

General Description: mental retardation, growth deficiency, dental anomalies, renal tubular acidosis, hyperchloremic acidosis

(continued)

TABLE 10-2. Ocular and Systemic Findings in Selected Inherited Syndromes (continued).

Ocular Findings: bilateral cataract, bilateral glaucoma, band keratopathy, nystagmus, corneal opacities

Retinoblastoma, RB1 MIM *180200 Gene map locus: 13q14.1–q14.2. Inheritance: Inheritance of the predisposition to retinoblastoma is an autosomal dominant trait because the presence of a single mutant allele renders the cell susceptible to tumorgenesis. Tumor formation, however, is a recessive trait and requires the additional loss or inactivation of the remaining wild-type, or normal allele. Inactivation of the tumor suppressor genes plays a major role in the etiology or progression of the malignancy. A germline loss of function (LOF) mutation at the RB1 locus can be heritable or spontaneous, but it always results in a genetic predisposition to retinoblastoma because of its presence in every cell in the body. The clinical result of a germline LOF mutation is bilateral/multifocal retinoblastoma. Somatic or nongenetic RB, caused by two spontaneous LOF mutations in the same retinoblast, is a rare event. Statistically, such a rare double hit in one cell would never occur more than once. The clinical result is a unilateral, unifocal nature of nongenetic retinoblastoma and an older age of onset (average 24 months for somatic RB, versus 12 months for genetic RB). Approximately 15% of sporadic unilaterally affected individuals are heterozygous at the RB1 allele and possibly did not receive the second LOF mutation in one or both eyes by chance alone. Incidence: 1:15,000–20,000. *Retinoblastoma is the most common malignant ocular tumor of childhood.*

General Description: In children with the hereditary disease there is a high rate of second malignancies (up to 90% at 30 years of age with a peak incidence at age 13 years) including osteogenic sarcoma, leukemia, lymphoma, and Ewing sarcoma. Cleft palate has been reported. Trilateral retinoblastoma (3% of cases) is the association of bilateral retinoblastoma with midline brain tumors, especially pinealoblastoma.

Ocular Findings: retinoblastoma, retinomas, retinal calcifications. Leukocoria is the presenting feature in nearly 50% of cases and strabismus in 20%. Less common presentations include vitreous hemorrhage, hyphema, ocular or periocular inflammation, glaucoma, proptosis, and hypopyon. Growth patterns of retinoblastoma are endophytic and exophytic. Endophytic retinoblastoma arises from the inner retina and seeds the vitreous. Exophytic retinoblastoma arises from outer retinal layers and causes a solid retinal detachment. A variant of endophytic retinoblastoma is the diffuse infiltrating retinoblastoma.

Rieger's Syndrome, Type I, II MIM #180500, *601499 Gene map locus: Type I, 4q25–q26; Type II, 13q14. Inheritance: autosomal dominant. Incidence: 1:200,000.

General Description: Type I is accompanied by facial, dental, umbilical, and skeletal abnormalities. Facial features include broad nasal root with maxillary hypoplasia, mild prognathism, and protruding lower lip. Dental anomalies include hypodontia and partial anodontia, most commonly absence of the central and lateral maxillary incisors. The remaining teeth have small crowns. Failure of involution of the periumbilical skin, umbilical hernia, inguinal hernia, hypospadias, anal stenosis. Rare associated findings include empty or enlarged sella turcica, growth hormone deficiency, and growth hormone deficiency with congenital parasellar arachnoid cyst, myotonic dystrophy. There is a rare association of Rieger anomaly with psychomotor retardation. Type II is accompanied by congenital hip anomalies, congenital heart defects, anal stenosis,

TABLE 10-2. (continued).

maxillary hypoplasia, mild prognathism, broad nasal root, short philtrum, protruding lower lip, dental anomalies as in type I, abnormal ear, hearing defect, umbilical hernia, inguinal hernia, hypospadias, fetal lobulations of kidney, cryptorchidism, hydrocephaly. There is no involution of periumbilical skin.

Ocular Findings: Reiger anomaly consists of anterior segment dysgenesis resulting in hypoplasia of the anterior iris stroma with the changes typical of Axenfeld's anomaly (posterior embryotoxon accompanied by abnormal iris strands crossing the anterior chamber angle to attach to a prominent Schwalbe's line). Other abnormalities may include glaucoma (60%), microcornea, corneal opacity, hypertelorism, and telecanthus.

Robinow's Syndrome *Fetal Face Syndrome* MIM *180700 Inheritance: autosomal dominant and autosomal recessive. Incidence: 1:500,000.

General Description: flat facial profile, frontal bossing, small upturned nose, triangular mouth with downturned angles, micrognathia, crowded teeth, short forearms, hypoplastic genitalia, postnatal growth deficiency

Ocular Findings
Common: hypertelorism (100%), prominent eyes (86%), down-slanting palpebral fissures (80%)
Less common: epicanthal folds, nevus flammeus (23%)

Rothmund–Thomson Syndrome *Poikiloderma Congenitale Syndrome* MIM #268400 Gene map locus: 8q24.3. Inheritance: autosomal recessive. Over 200 cases reported.

General Description: short stature of prenatal onset, irregular erythema progressing to poikiloderma (telangiectasia, scarring, irregular pigmentation and depigmentation, skin atrophy), sparse hair, prematurely gray hair, hypodontia

Ocular Findings
Common: juvenile bilateral zonular cataract (52%), thinning of brows and eyelashes
Less common: corneal dystrophy

Rubinstein–Taybi Syndrome MIM #180849 Gene map locus: 16p13.3. Inheritance: autosomal dominant. Over 500 cases reported.

General Description: mental deficiency, speech difficulties, broad thumbs and toes with radial angulation, hypoplastic maxilla with narrow palate, prominent and/or beaked nose

Ocular Findings
Common: down-slanting palpebral fissures (88%), heavy eyebrows (76%), highly arched eyebrows (73%), long eyelashes (87%), epicanthal folds (55%), strabismus (69%)
Less common: stenosis of nasolacrimal duct (43%), ptosis (36%), enophthalmia (22%), glaucoma, iris colomba

Saethre-Chotzen Syndrome *Acrocephalosyndactyly Type 3* MIM #101400 Gene map locus: 7p21. Inheritance: autosomal dominant. Over 30 cases reported.

General Description: craniosynostosis, brachycephaly or acrocephaly with maxillary hypoplasia, plagiocephaly with facial asymmetry, prominent ear crus, soft tissue syndactyly (usually digits 2 and 3) of hands and feet, low-set frontal hairline

(continued)

TABLE 10-2.   Ocular and Systemic Findings in Selected Inherited Syndromes (continued).

Ocular Findings

Common: hypertelorism, ptosis of the eyelids is usually unilateral or asymmetric, strabismus, shallow orbits, plagiocephaly with asymmetry of orbits

Less common: blepharophimosis, dacryostenosis, epicanthal folds, optic atrophy, down-slanting palpebral fissures, anomalies of the eyelids and eyebrows, and glaucoma have been reported.

Sanfilippo Syndrome *Mucopolysaccharidosis III Type A, B, C, D* MIM #252900, ⁎252920, ⁎252930, ⁎252940 Gene map locus: Type A, 17q25.3, Type B, 17q21, Type C, chromosome 14, Type D, 12q14. Inheritance: autosomal recessive. Incidence: 1:25,000.

General Description: abnormal degradation of heparan sulfate resulting from four distinct enzymatic abnormalities: Type A, heparan *N*-sulfatase deficiency; Type B, *N*-acetyl-alpha-glucosaminidase deficiency; Type C, acetyl coenzyme A:alpha-glucosaminide *N*-acetyltransferase deficiency; Type D, *N*-acetylglucosamine-6-sulfatase deficiency. This disorder is unique among the mucopolysaccharidoses because of their severe neurological sequelae with little somatic involvement. Type A is the most severe. Onset in early childhood (between 1 and 4 years of age), normal to accelerated growth for 1 to 3 years followed by slow growth, mild stiff joints, mild hearing loss, mildly coarse facies. The neurological degeneration is severe with cortical atrophy progressing to severe dementia. Many die of pneumonia by 10 to 20 years of age.

Ocular Findings: clear cornea, patients usually do not have glaucoma or swelling of the optic nerve. Optic atrophy develops rarely. Pigmentary retinopathy may appear similar to that in retinitis pigmentosa with marked photoreceptor loss. Synophrys.

Scheie's Syndrome *Mucopolysaccharidosis Type IS* MIM ⁎252800 Gene map locus: 4p16.3. Inheritance: autosomal recessive. Rare disorder.

General Description: an inborn mucopolysccharide metabolism disorder with alpha-iduronidase deficiency. Scheie's syndrome is the mildest form of the mucopolysaccharidosis. Normal intelligence, normal stature, broad mouth with full lips by 5 to 8 years of age, prognathism, joint stiffness but only limited deformities of the hand, hearing loss, aortic valve defect, body hirsutism. Onset of symptoms usually after 5 years of age. Lifespan is nearly normal, depending on cardiac complications.

Ocular Findings

Common: uniform progressive clouding of the cornea in the early stage, diffusely involving the stroma (onset after 4 years of age), becoming most dense in the periphery

Less common: pigmentary retinal degeneration (late finding). Occasionally, optic nerve swelling or late optic atrophy. Glaucoma (occurs more frequently than in Hurler syndrome).

Schinzel–Giedion Midface-Retraction Syndrome MIM 269150 Inheritance: possibly autosomal recessive, although autosomal dominant cannot be excluded. Sixteen cases have been reported.

TABLE 10-2. (continued).

General Description: postnatal growth deficiency, profound mental deficiency, spasticity, ventriculomegaly secondary to cerebral atrophy, coarse face, high protruding forehead (100%), widely patent fontanels and sutures (100%) with metopic suture extending anteriorly to nasal root, genital anomalies (100%), renal anomalies (92%), hypertrichosis (91%). High early mortality.

Ocular Findings: shallow orbits with apparent proptosis (100%), hypertelorism

Schwart–Jampel Syndrome, Type 1 *Chondrodystrophica Myotonia Syndrome* MIM #255800 Gene map locus: 1p36.1. Inheritance: autosomal recessive. Over 50 cases reported.

General Description: myotonia, joint contractures, short stature, high-pitched voice, low hairline, flat facies, fixed facial expression, small mouth, small chin, short neck, epiphyseal dysplasia, kyphoscoliosis, pectus carinatum, umbilical hernia, inguinal hernia

Ocular Findings
Common: blepharophimosis, intermittent ptosis, telecanthus, myopia, medial displacement of outer canthi, long eyelashes in irregular rows
Less common: microcornea, microphthalmia, pseudoptosis, juvenile cataract

Sclerosteosis MIM #269500 Gene map locus: 17q12–q21. Inheritance: autosomal recessive. Over 60 cases reported.

General Description: progressive thickening and overgrowth of bone, leading to mild or moderate gigantism. Prominent, sometimes asymmetrical mandible. Cranial hyperostosis leads to occlusion of cranial foramina resulting in deafness and facial palsy. Syndactyly of second to third fingers, nail dysplasia. The progression of the dense thickening of bone leads to severe distortion of the face, dental malocclusion, proptosis, midfacial hypoplasia, and occlusion of multiple cranial foramina and increased intracranial pressure. Sudden death may occur from impaction of medulla oblongata in the foramen magnum.

Ocular Findings: proptosis (in adulthood). The progression of the dense thickening of bone leads to occlusion of multiple cranial foramina and increased intracranial pressure. Optic nerve atrophy, strabismus, and blindness may be a consequence.

Seckel's Syndrome *Bird-Headed Dwarfism* MIM *210600, 210700 Gene map locus: 3q22.1–q24. Inheritance: autosomal recessive. Incidence: 1:10,000

General Description: severe short stature, mental deficiency, microcephaly with secondary premature synostosis, micrognathia, prominent nose, low-set malformed ears with lack of lobules

Ocular Findings
Common: down-slanting palpebral fissures, large eyes
Less common: strabismus, ptosis

Septo-Optic Dysplasia Sequence *De Morsier Syndrome* MIM #182230 Gene map locus: 3p21.2–p21.1. Inheritance: unknown. Incidence: the majority of cases are sporadic, although over 30 familial cases have been reported.

General Description: small anterior visual pathways with associated midline central nervous system anomalies consisting of absence of the septum pellucidum and agenesis or thinning of the corpus callosum, often accompanied by manifestations of hypothalamic and pituitary (15%–62%)

(continued)

TABLE 10-2. Ocular and Systemic Findings in Selected Inherited Syndromes (continued).

dysfunction. Growth hormone deficiency is more common, but hypocortisolism, diabetes insipidus, hyperprolactinemia, hypothyroidism, and panhypopituitarism are also seen. Growth hormone deficiency may not be clinically apparent within the first 3 to 4 years of life because of high prolactin levels, which can stimulate normal growth over this period. Children with septo-optic dysplasia and corticotropin deficiency are at risk for sudden death during febrile illness. These children may have coexistent diabetes insipidus that contributes to dehydration. Some also have hypothalamic thermoregulatory disturbances. Subclinical hypopituitarism can manifest as acute adrenal insufficiency following surgery under general anesthesia. Neurodevelopmental defects, when present, are usually the result of associated cerebral hemispheric abnormalities.

Ocular Findings: hypoplastic optic nerves, chiasm, and infundibulum. Ophthalmoscopically, the hypoplastic disc appears as an abnormally small optic nerve head. It may be gray or pale in color and is often surrounded by a yellowish mottled peripapillary halo, bordered by a ring of increased or decreased pigmentation (the "double-ring" sign). Care should be taken to avoid mistaking the entire hypoplastic disc/ring complex for a normal-sized disc. There may be too few or too many disc vessels. Retinal vascular tortuosity is common. Visual acuity ranges from normal to no light perception. Affected eyes show localized visual field defects often combined with generalized constriction. Patients may have pendular nystagmus, occasionally a "see-saw" nystagmus, astigmatism, and strabismus.

SHORT Syndrome MIM 269880 Inheritance: autosomal recessive. Ten cases reported.

General Description: "SHORT" is an acronym for this syndrome: S = short stature, H = hyperextensibility of joints, and/or hernia (inguinal), O = ocular depression (sunken eyes), R = Rieger anomaly, and T = teething delay. Other features include lipoatrophy, congenital hip dislocation, triangular face, downturned corners of mouth, deafness, clinodactyly, developmental delay, delayed bone age.

Ocular Findings: sunken eyes; Reiger anomaly consists of anterior segment dysgenesis resulting in hypoplasia of the anterior iris stroma with the changes typical of Axenfeld's anomaly (posterior embryotoxon accompanied by abnormal iris strands crossing the anterior chamber angle to attach to a prominent Schwalbe's line). Other abnormalities may include glaucoma, microcornea, corneal opacity.

Shprintzen Syndrome *Velo-Cardio-Facial Syndrome* MIM #192430 Gene map locus: 22q11. Inheritance: autosomal dominant. Over 100 cases reported.

General Description: cleft of the secondary palate (either overt or submucous), velopharyngeal incompetence, small or absent adenoids, prominent nose with squared nasal root and narrow alar base, abundant scalp hair, deficient malar area, vertical maxillary excess with long face, retruded mandible with chin deficiency, microcephaly (40%–50%), minor auricular anomalies. Cardiac defects (85%), the most common being ventricular septal defect (62%), right aortic arch (52%), tetralogy of Fallot (21%). Internal carotid artery abnormalities. Slender and hypotonic limbs with hyperextensible hands and fingers (63%). Conductive hearing loss secondary to cleft palate. Postnatal

TABLE 10-2. (continued).

onset of short stature (33%). Learning disabilities (40%), psychiatric disorders (10%). Rarely T-lymphocyte dysfunction with frequent infections and neonatal hypocalcemia.

Ocular Findings
Common: narrow palpebral fissures, tortuosity of retinal vessels (30%)
Less common: small optic discs, ocular coloboma, cataract, posterior embryotoxon

Shprintzen–Goldberg Craniosynostosis Syndrome *Marfanoid Craniosynostoisis Syndrome* MIM #182212 Gene map locus: 15q21.1 Inheritance: autosomal dominant. Twelve cases reported.

General Description: Phenotypically similar to Marfan syndrome with mutations in many cases occurring at the same gene locus, 15q21.1. There is, however, no ectopia lentis, and craniosynostosis is present. Features include mental retardation, hypotonia, craniosynostosis, mandibular and maxillary hypoplasia, low-set anomalous ears, multiple large abdominal hernia, hyperelastic skin, arachnodactyly, obstructive apnea, dilated aortic root, aortic dissection.

Ocular Findings: NO ectopia lentis, shallow orbits, exopthalmos

Sialolipidosis Syndrome *Mucolipidosis IV, Berman's Syndrome* MIM #252650 Gene map locus: 19p13.3–p13.2. Inheritance: autosomal recessive. Over 70 cases reported.

General Description: progressive psychomotor regression and hypotonia become apparent during the first year of life. There are no facial or skeletal changes. The defect may concern ganglioside sialidase (neuraminidase).

Ocular Findings: prominent diffuse corneal clouding secondary to epithelial opacities is apparent at birth or during the first year of life. Pigmentary retinopathy with depression of the electroretinographic signals, optic atrophy, attenuated retinal vasculature, cataract, strabismus, nystagmus, myopia, puffy eyelids, photophobia.

Simple Ectopia Lentis MIM *129600 Inheritance: autosomal dominant. Incidence: unknown

Ocular Findings: ectopia lentis. The characteristics of lens subluxation are indistinguishable from those of patients with Marfan syndrome. The lens most often moves superotemporally, and stretched zonules may be visible before or after pupillary dilation. Congenital lens dislocation has been reported.

Simpson–Golabi–Behmel Syndrome Type I, II MIM # 312870, *300209 Gene map locus: Type I, Xq26, Type II, Xp22. Inheritance: X-linked recessive. Six families and one sporadic case reported.

General Description: prenatal onset of overgrowth, macrocephaly, coarse facies, broad flat nasal bridge with short nose, macrostomia, macroglossia, midline groove of lower lip, postaxial polydactyly of hands, syndactyly of second and third fingers and toes, nail hypoplasia, broad thumb and great toe, vertebral segmentation defects, cardiac conduction defects

Ocular Findings
Common: up-slanting palpebral fissures, hypertelorism
Less common: coloboma of optic disc, cataract, retinal detachment

(continued)

TABLE 10-2. Ocular and Systemic Findings in Selected Inherited Syndromes (continued).

Smith–Lemli–Opitz Syndrome, Type 1 MIM #270400 Gene map locus: 11q12–q13. Inheritance: autosomal recessive. Incidence: 1:40,000

General Description: microcephaly, anteverted nostrils, slanted or low-set auricles, syndactyly of second and third toes, hypospadias and cryptorchidism in males. Moderate to severe mental deficiency, with variable altered muscle tone. Failure to thrive.

Ocular Findings
Common: ptosis, inner epicanthal folds, strabismus
Less common: cataract, demyelination of optic nerves, sclerosis of lateral geniculate bodies, opsoclonus

Sotos Syndrome *Cerebral Gigantism Syndrome* MIM *117550 Inheritance: autosomal dominant. Over 150 cases reported.

General Description: prenatal onset of excessive size. Length increases during childhood and early adolescence. Final height often within normal range. Macrocephaly, prominent forehead, large hands and feet, poor coordination, variable mental deficiency, hypotonia.

Ocular Findings
Common: down-slanting palpebral fissures, apparent hypertelorism not always confirmed by measurement
Less common: strabismus

Spondylocarpotarsal Synostosis Syndrome MIM *272460 Inheritance: autosomal recessive. Twelve cases reported.

General Description: disproportionate short stature with short trunk, failure of spinal segmentation leading to block vertebrae when symmetrical, and to scoliosis or lordosis when asymmetrical. Carpal synostosis.

Ocular Findings: occasionally, hypertelorism

Spondyloepiphyseal Dysplasia Congenita MIM #183900 Inheritance: autosomal dominant. Approximately 14 cases reported. Caused by mutations in COL2A1 gene located on chromosome 12q13.11–q13.2 and accordingly shares features with Stickler syndrome and Kniest's dysplasia.

General Description: prenatal onset of growth deficiency, short trunk, lag in epiphyseal mineralization, diminished joint mobility at elbows, knees and hips, short spine including neck with ovoid flattened vertebrae and narrow intervertebral disk spaces, odontoid hypoplasia, kyphoscoliosis, lumbar lordosis, barrel chest with pectus carinatum, muscle weakness, hypoplasia of abdominal muscles, variable flat facies, cleft palate, malar hypoplasia

Ocular Findings
Common: vitreous degeneration, varying degrees of myopia (up to −20 D), retinal detachment (50%)
Less common: ectopia lentis is rare

Spondyloepiphyseal Dysplasia Tarda *X-Linked Spondyloepiphyseal Dysplasia* MIM #313400, *271600, *271630, *184100 Gene map locus: Xp22.2–p22.1. Inheritance: X-linked recessive. Autosomal dominant and autosomal recessive described. Incidence: 1:100,000

TABLE 10-2. (continued).

General Description: onset between 5 and 10 years of age. Short stature. Flattened vertebrae with hump-shaped mound of bone in central and posterior portions of vertebral endplate, narrowing of disc spaces, kyphosis, mild scoliosis, short neck. Small iliac wings, short femoral neck. Eventual pain and stiffness in hips, shoulders, cervical and lumbar spine. Vague back pain in adolescence is frequently the initial symptom.

Ocular Findings: occasionally, corneal opacities

Steinert Myotonic Dystrophy Syndrome *Dystrophia Myotonica Syndrome* MIM #160900 Gene map locus: 19q13.2–q13.3 Inheritance: autosomal dominant. Incidence: 1:8000.

General Description: myotonia, degeneration of swollen muscle cells with muscle atrophy and weakness, hypogonadism, conduction heart defects with arrhythmias

Ocular Findings
Common: cataract (often evident only as "myotonic dust"), ptosis
Less common: "macular abnormalities," blepharitis, keratitis sicca

Stickler Syndrome Type I *Arthro-Ophthalmopathy, Hereditary, Progressive, Stickler Type (AOM), Membranous Vitreous Type* MIM #108300 Gene map locus: caused by mutations in the type II collagen gene, COL2A1, located on chromosome 12q13.11–q13.2. Inheritance: autosomal dominant. Incidence: 1:20,000. There is evidence of **Stickler Syndrome Type II** *Stickler Syndrome, Beaded Vitreous Type* MIM #604841. Gene map locus: caused by mutations in the COL11A1 gene, located on chromosome 1p21 (type I is the most frequent form). (There remains debate as to whether Marshall syndrome and Stickler syndrome represent separate entities.)

General Description: flat facies with depressed nasal bridge, sensorineural (usually) and conductive (occasionally) hearing loss (slight hearing loss in type I and early-onset severe hearing loss in type II). Pierre–Robin sequence of cleft palate, glossoptosis, and micrognathia. Musculoskeletal abnormalities such as marfanoid habitus, kyphosis, scoliosis, arachnodactyly, hypotonia, hyperextensible joints. Prominence of large joints may be present at birth and severe progressive arthropathy may occur in childhood. Roentgenographic findings beginning in childhood include mild to moderate spondyloepiphyseal dysplasia (flat vertebrae with anterior wedging, flat irregular femoral epiphyses, underdevelopment of the distal tibial epiphyses). Mitral valve prolapse (46%). The diagnosis should be considered in a neonate with the Pierre–Robin sequence, particularly in those with a family history of cleft palate and in patients with dominantly inherited myopia, nontraumatic retinal detachment, and/or mild spondyloepiphyseal dysplasia.

Ocular Findings
Common: optically empty vitreous. Fibrillar vitreous degeneration and liquefaction by the second decade. Sheets of vitreous may condense behind the lens, forming a veil. Anterior and posterior vitreous membranes are seen in type I and a "beaded" appearance is seen in type II. Posterior vitreous detachment is common. Perivascular and peripheral retinal pigment deposition is seen associated with chorioretinal atrophy. Retinal breaks most commonly in the superotemporal quadrant (75%), retinal detachments by the second

(continued)

TABLE 10-2. Ocular and Systemic Findings in Selected Inherited Syndromes (continued).

decade (50%), almost half are bilateral, myopia in the range of 8–18 diopters associated with increased axial length by age 10 years in 40%, and by age 20 years in 75%. Progressive, presenile, lenticular changes with anterior and posterior cortical fleck and wedge-shaped opacities (>50%). Prominent eyes, epicanthal folds.

Less common: staphylomata, choroidal neovascularization, lacquer cracks, glaucoma, uveitis secondary to chronic retinal detachment, ptosis, strabismus. Ectopia lentis is rare.

Sturge–Weber Syndrome (SWS) *Encephalofacial Angiomatosis Syndrome* MIM 185300 Inheritance: sporadic. Incidence: Unknown.

General Description: SWS belongs to the phakomatoses. It consists of congenital hamartomatous malformations that may affect the eyes, skin, and central nervous system at different times. The primary defect is a developmental insult affecting precursors of tissues that originate in the pro- and mesencephalic neural crest. The hallmark of SWS is a facial pink to purplish red nonelevated cutaneous hemangioma of irregular outline, most commonly in a trigeminal facial distribution, referred to as nevus flammeus or port-wine stain. It occurs in as many as 96% of patients and is visible at birth. Involvement is usually unilateral but can be bilateral. A leptomeningeal congenital venous angiomatosis, usually ipsilateral to the facial lesion is located most commonly in the meninges overlying the occipital and posterior parietal lobes, with characteristic progressive "double contour" convolutional calcification in the external layers of the cerebral cortex beneath the angiomatosis, associated with cortical atrophy can be demonstrated on CT. Focal or generalized motor seizures occur in up to 85% of patients. They usually begin in the first year of life and may become profound, resulting in further neurologic and developmental deterioration. Some degree of mental retardation is seen in about 60% of patients, as well as neurologic deficits such as hemiplegia and homonymous hemianopsia. Occasional abnormalities include: hemangiomatosis in nonfacial areas, macrocephaly, coarctation of aorta, abnormal external ears.

Ocular Findings

Common: Port-wine nevus (nevus flammeus) in the distribution of the first and second divisions of the trigeminal nerve (these patients are at risk for neuro-ocular involvement), hemangiomas of the choroid, conjunctiva, and episclera. Glaucoma (in 30%–70% of patients) is almost always unilateral and ipsilateral to the port-wine stain, although contralateral or bilateral glaucoma with unilateral skin lesions has been reported. Prominent tortuous conjunctival and episcleral vascular plexi (in up to 70% of patients) often correlate with increased episcleral venous pressure. Diffuse choroidal hemangioma (in up to 50% of patients) are flat, commonly cover more than half the fundus, involve the posterior pole, extend into the equatorial zone, may show diffuse involvement of the entire uvea, and can have a striking reddish "tomato ketchup fundus" appearance. Choroidal angiomas grow slowly and are usually asymptomatic in childhood, but during adolescence or adulthood marked thickening of the choroid may become evident with secondary changes to overlying ocular structures.

Less common: retinal vascular tortuosity with occasional arteriovenous communications, iris heterochromia, retinal detachment, strabismus, coloboma of iris (reported)

TABLE 10-2. (continued).

Treacher Collins Syndrome *Mandibulofacial Dysostosis, Franceschetti–Klein Syndrome* MIM *154500 Gene map locus: 5q32–q33.1. Inheritance: autosomal dominant. Incidence: 1:25,000–50,000 live births

General Description: abnormal development of branchial arch derivatives. The primary features include severe hypoplasia of the malar bone and zygomatic process of the temporal bone, with retrusion of the malar region. Frequently there is also maxillary hypoplasia. Maldevelopment of the mandible causes micrognathia and receding chin. There are deformities of the medial pterygoid plates and hypoplasia of the pterygoid muscles. Malformation of the external and middle ear occur that may result in conductive hearing loss (50%). There is macrostomia, abnormal highly arched palate/cleft palate, and anomalies of dentition (30%). The hair growth patterns are unusual, often showing tonguelike extension of hair onto the cheeks. Blind fistulas are located between the ears and the angles of the mouth. Abnormalities are bilateral and symmetrical.

Ocular Findings *(the ophthalmic features are among the most consistent and diagnostic in this syndrome)*
Common: lack of lateral canthal fixation causing drooping of the lower eyelid in an S-shaped contour. Colobomas or pseudocolobomas of the lateral third of the lower eyelid (75%). The medial part of the lower eyelid may be thin, absent of tarsal plate, and devoid of all marginal structures, including eyelashes and meibomian glands (50%). "Egg-shaped" orbit caused by deformities of the temporal orbital wall. The relative protrusion of the nose may produce an enophthalmic appearance.
Less common: atresia of the lower lacrimal punctum and canaliculus, ptosis, distichiasis, trichiasis, ectropion, entropion, upper eyelid coloboma, microphthalmia, anophthalmos, pupillary ectopia, iris coloboma, cataract, corneal guttae

Triploidy Type II

General Description: in Type I triploidy, fetal death usually occurs before 8 weeks. Type II triploidy results in intrauterine growth retardation, macrocephaly, hydrocephalus, agenesis of the corpus callosum, congenital heart disease, myelomeningocele, adrenal hypoplasia, cryptorchidism, hypogonadism and intestinal malrotation. Facial dysmorphism may be characterized by malformed, low-set ears, a large bulbous nose, and micrognathia (with or without cleft lip and palate). Minor skeletal abnormalities such as vertebral malformations, clubfoot and syndactyly of the third and fourth fingers may occur. In most cases, the extra set of chromosomes is paternally derived.

Ocular Findings: hypertelorism, coloboma, and microphthalmia. Iris heterochromia may occur.

Trisomy 8 Syndrome *Warkany Syndrome.* Trisomy for chromosome 8, the majority of patients being mosaics. Over 100 cases reported.

General Description: mental retardation, a dysmorphic facies with prominent anterverted nasal tip, prominent lower jaw, mouth held open, absent or dysplastic patella, joint contractures (in particular limited supination/pronation), vertebral defects, urinary anomalies, a distinctive toe posture (flexed and turned toward the midline of foot, with digits 2 and 3 having equal length), deep furrows in the palms and soles. Features seen in 50% or more include cleft or high palate,

(continued)

TABLE 10-2. Ocular and Systemic Findings in Selected Inherited Syndromes (continued).

sacral dimple/spina bifida occulta, congenital heart disease, clinodactyly/long fingers, slender pelvis, abnormal ears, hip dysplasia, everted lower lip, sternum abnormalities, abnormal nails.

Ocular Findings: deep-set eyes, canthal abnormalities, strabismus (50%), abnormal palpebral slanting (30%), pseudo-hypertelorism/hypertelorism, microphthalmia, corneal opacity, cataract, iris heterochromia. Rarely, myopia.

Trisomy 9 Syndrome Trisomy for chromosome 9. Trisomy 9 is rare in liveborn infants.

General Description: intrauterine growth retardation, severe mental deficiency, skeletal anomalies, congenital heart disease, congenital kidney disease, and genitourinary malformations. Rocker-bottom feet, joint contractures, overlapping fingers, and hypoplastic nails. Malformed low-set ears with possible absent external canals, cleft/arched palate, micrognathia, bulbous nose, facial asymmetry. The majority of patients die during the early postnatal period.

Ocular Findings
Common: micropthalmia (61%), "deep-set eyes" (45%), up-slanting short palpebral fissures
Less common: cataract, corneal clouding, absence of optic tracts, Peters' anomaly

Trisomy 13 Syndrome *Patau Syndrome.* Complete or near-complete trisomy of chromosome 13. Incidence estimated to be 1 in 20,000 liveborn infants.

General Description: defects of eye, nose, lip and forebrain of holoprosencephaly type, polydactyly, narrow hyperconvex fingernails, skin defects of posterior scalp. Eighty percent of patients die within the first month. Only 5% survive the first 6 months. Trisomy 13 is the most common chromosomal abnormality associated with congenital ocular malformations at birth.

Ocular Findings *(the ocular anomalies are frequently severe, bilateral, and incompatible with vision)*
Common: microphthalmia or anophthalmia (>50%). Trisomy 13 is the most common chromosomal aberration associated with microphthalmia or anophthalmia. Colobomas of the iris and ciliary body (>50%), retina, choroid, and optic nerve. Colobomas of the iris and ciliary body may be associated with cartilage or other choriostomatous tissue in the ciliary body. Dysembryogenesis of the anterior segment with Rieger anomaly or, less commonly, Peters' anomaly, malformed anterior chamber angle, vascularized and hypercellular cornea with dysgenesis of Descemet's or Bowman's membranes, cataract with retention of the cell nuclei within the lens nucleus. There may be lens epithelium beneath the posterior part of the lens capsule. Trisomy 13 is the most common chromosomal aberration found in association with PHPV. Optic nerve hypoplasia and congenital retinal nonattachment or folds due to retinal dysplasia with or without intraocular cartilage may occur.
Less common: shallow supraorbital ridges, slanting palpebral fissures, absent eyebrows, hypertelorism, hypotelorism, synophthalmos, and cyclopia. Congenital unilateral facial paralysis may rarely occur. Nonelevated simple capillary hemangiomata of forehead have been reported.

Trisomy 18 Syndrome *Edwards Syndrome.* Trisomy for all or a large part of chromosome 18. Incidence: 1:6000 births with a female preponderance of 3:1.

TABLE 10-2. (continued).

General Description: only 5%–10% survive the first year of life. Feeble fetal activity, polyhydramnios, growth deficiency, mental deficiency, low-set auricles, small oral opening, clenched hand, short sternum, low arch dermal ridge patterning on fingertips, ventricular septal defect, cryptorchidism, hirsutism.

Ocular Findings

Common: hypoplastic supraorbital ridges, ptosis, blepharophimosis, epicanthus, hypertelorism

Less common: nystagmus, anisocoria, strabismus, corneal opacities, uveal and optic nerve colobomas, optic nerve hypoplasia or gliosis, cataract, ciliary process abnormalities, microphthalmia, anophthalmia, myopia, retinal folds, congenital glaucoma, malformations of the iris pigment, stroma, sphincter, and dilator. Hypopigmentation of the posterior pole retinal pigment epithelium, neural retinal immaturity, focal areas of retinal dysplasia. Trisomy 18 is the second most common chromosomal aberration associated with microphthalmia or anophthalmia. Thickened or bluish sclera, scleral icterus, persistent hyperplastic primary vitreous, congenital aphakia, congenital unilateral facial paralysis, and ankyloblepharon have been described.

Trisomy 21, Down Syndrome MIM #190685 Trisomy for all or a large part of chromosome 21. Incidence: 1:660 live births.

General Description: hypotonia, mental deficiency, brachycephaly with relatively flat occiput and tendency toward midline parietal hair whorl, mild microcephaly, short nose with low nasal bridge, flat facies, a large protruding tongue, up-slanting palpebral fissures ("mongoloid slant"), small ears, short thick neck, loose skin folds in posterior neck in infancy, fine soft hair, cardiac anomalies, primary gonadal deficiency, higher incidence of leukemia, stubby hands with a single palmar crease, clinodactyly of fifth digit with hypoplasia of middigital phalanges, short stubby feet with a wide gap between first and second toes.

Ocular Findings

Common: up-slanting palpebral fissures ("mongoloid slant"), epicanthal folds, chronic xeroderma can affect the periorbital area and eyelids, syringomas which have a predisposition for the periorbital area. Refractive error, mostly myopia (70%), lens opacities in children ranging from visually insignificant fine cortical lens opacities to significant dense total congenital cataract (20%–60%), premature development of nuclear sclerosis (30%–60%), strabismus (45%), nystagmus (35%), Brushfield spots (30%–90%), peripheral hypoplasia of iris, blocked tear duct (20%).

Less common: keratoconus (6%–15%), congenital cataract (3%). Optic nerve hypoplasia, a characteristic "spoke wheel" disc (the vessels radiate out from the disc at multiple "clock" hours), crowded disc, bilateral lens subluxation.

Usher Syndrome Type I (A to F), II (A, B, C), Type III MIM IA *276900, IB *276903, IC #276904, IC *605242, ID #601067, IE *602097, IF *602083, IIA *276901, IIB *276905, IIC *605472, III *276902 Gene map locus: IA, 14q32, IB, 11q13.5, IC, 11p15.1, ID, 10q21–q22, IE, 21q21, IF, chr.10, IIA, 1q41, IIB, 3p24.2–p23, 2C, 5q14–q21, III, 3q21–q25. Inheritance: autosomal recessive. Incidence: 1:33,000. *50% of all patients deaf and blind likely have Usher syndrome.*

(continued)

TABLE 10-2. Ocular and Systemic Findings in Selected Inherited Syndromes (continued).

General Description: Type I, profound congenital sensorineural deafness, speech rarely develops, vestibular functions are abnormal. Ataxia, psychosis, and mental retardation may develop (in IA, IB, IC). In Type II, congenital hearing loss is less severe than in type I, and speech may develop, vestibular and neurological functions are normal. In Type III, there is progressive hearing loss and vestibular hypoactivity. Ataxia, psychosis, and mental retardation may develop.

Ocular Findings: Type I, retinitis pigmentosa with visual symptoms of visual loss, night blindness, and visual field loss apparent by age 10, cataract by age 40. The electroretinogram is markedly diminished or absent. Type II, visual symptoms start in the late teens. The electroretinogram is usually decreased, but a wave is recordable. Type III, visual symptoms start in the late teens.

VATER Association MIM 192350 Inheritance: sporadic. Over 250 cases reported.

General Presentation: the acronym VATER has been used to represent the major manifestations of this disorder: Vertebral anomalies, Atresia of the anus, TracheoEsophageal atresia or fistula, Radial limb defects, and Renal malformations

Ocular Findings: microphthalmia has been reported to occur in patients with hydrocephalus

von Hippel–Lindau Disease MIM *193300 Gene map locus: 3p26–p25. Inheritance: autosomal dominant. Incidence: 1:33,000.

General Description: von Hippel–Lindau (VHL) is an inherited tumor suppressor gene syndrome predisposing affected individuals to hemangioblastomas of the retina and central nervous system, renal cell carcinoma, pheochromocytoma, and renal, pancreatic, and epididymal cysts. Criteria for diagnosis in isolated cases are two or more hemangioblastomas (retinal or central nervous system) or a single hemangioblastoma in association with a visceral manifestation (pancreatic/renal/epididymal cysts, or renal carcinoma). For familial cases, the criteria for diagnosis are a single hemangioblastoma or visceral complication. The most common presenting features are retinal hemangioblastomas, followed by cerebellar hemangioblastomas, renal cell carcinoma (10%), and pheochromocytoma (5%). Retinal hemangioblastoma occur in 57%, cerebellar hemangioblastoma in 55%, spinal cord hemangioblastoma in 14%, renal cell carcinoma in 24%, and pheochromocytoma in 19%. Pancreatic tumors are usually islet cell adenomas or carcinomas. Cerebellar hemangioblastomas and renal cell carcinoma develop at an earlier age than those who develop sporadic forms of the tumor. Renal cell carcinomas are bilateral or multicentric in 50% of patients. Central nervous system hemangioblastomas are often asymptomatic and need to be detected by gadolinium-enhanced MRI. Renal cell carcinoma is the most common cause of death, and median survival is reduced to 49 years.

Ocular Findings: retinal hemangioblastomas (mean age at diagnosis is 25 years). All patients with a retinal hemangioblastoma and their first-degree relatives should be screened for VHL. Multiple retinal hemangioblastomas are diagnostic of VHL, as are single retinal hemangioblastoma and a first-degree family member with any of the manifestations of VHL. There are two types of retinal and optic nerve head hemangioblastomas: endophytic and exophytic.

TABLE 10-2. (continued).

Endophytic lesions are elevated red vascular tumors arising from the superficial retina or optic disc and growing into the vitreous. Larger peripheral tumors often have a feeding arteriole and a draining venule. Smaller tumors consist of a net of dilated capillaries and can be harder to diagnose. Visual loss results from exudative or traction retinal detachment, vitreous hemorrhage, macular edema, epiretinal membrane formation, or macular holes. Exophytic hemangioblastomas are less common and arise from the outer retinal layers, often in the peripapillary area. More posterior optic nerve hemangioblastomas may present as a progressive optic neuropathy or a chiasmal syndrome. Generally, hemangioblastomas progressively enlarge, hence the advantage of early detection and prophylactic treatment.

Waardenburg's Syndrome, Types I, IIA, IIB, III, and IV *Hirschsprung Disease-Pigmentary Anomaly, Waardenburg-Ocular Albinism* MIM *193500, #193510, *600193, #148820, #277580 Gene map locus: Type I, 2q35; Type IIA, 3p14.1–p12.3; Type IIB, 1p21–p13.3; Type IV, 2q35; Type IV, 22q13, 20q13.2–q13.3. Inheritance; Type I, II, III have autosomal dominant transmission; Type IV has autosomal recessive transmission. Incidence: 1:20,000–40,000 live births.

General Description: Partial albinism manifested by hypopigmented ocular fundus, poliosis (white forelock), premature graying of hair, hypopigmented skin lesions (not seen in type IV), hypochromic iridis. Deafness is the most serious feature, and, if present, is usually bilateral and severe. Deafness occurs in 25% of type I cases and in 50% of type II. (Three percent of congenitally deaf children have this syndrome.) Deafness not seen in type IV. Broad and high nasal bridge with hypoplastic alae nasi, medial flare of bushy eyebrows, synophrys. Facial dysmorphism not seen in type IIB. Absent vagina, absent uterine adnexa, spina bifida, lumbosacral myelomeningocele. In type III, there are bilateral defects of the upper limbs, including hypoplasia of musculoskeletal system, carpal bone fusion, syndactyly.

Ocular Findings
Common: lateral displacement of inner canthi (in type I and III). Partial albinism manifested by hypopigmented ocular fundus, heterochromia of irides, isochromic pale blue eyes with hypoplastic iridic stroma sometimes restricted to a single segment of one eye (25%), mottled peripheral pigmentation of the retina. Often premature graying of eyelashes and eyebrows as early as age 7 years. Visual acuity is usually normal.
Less common: poor lacrimal conduction, glaucoma, unilateral ptosis, and the Marcus Gunn phenomenon (type II), anophthalmia, blepharophimosis (type III), esotropia

Walker–Warburg Syndrome *Warburg Syndrome* MIM *236670 Gene map locus: 9q31. Inheritance: autosomal recessive. Approximately 60 cases reported.

General Description: severe brain and eye malformations with death in the neonatal period in the majority of affected individuals. Type II lissencephaly (100%) manifested by widespread argyria with scattered areas of macrogyria and polymicrogyria, abnormally thick cortex with absent or hypoplastic septum pellucidum and corpus callosum, cerebellar malformation (100%), Dandy–Walker malformation (53%), hydrocephalus (53%).

(continued)

TABLE 10-2. Ocular and Systemic Findings in Selected Inherited Syndromes (continued).

Ocular Findings: anterior chamber malformations (91%) including cataract, corneal clouding usually secondary to Peters' anomaly, and narrow iridocorneal angle with or without glaucoma, retinal malformations (100%) including retrolental masses caused by persistent hyperplastic primary vitreous, and retinal detachment secondary to retinal dysplasia, microphthalmia (53%), coloboma (24%), optic nerve hypoplasia, megalocornea

Weaver Syndrome MIM 277590 Inheritance: sporadic. Over 20 cases reported.

General Description: accelerated growth and maturation of prenatal onset, mild developmental delay (80%), mild hypertonia, macrocephaly (80%), flat occiput, camptodactyly, broad thumbs, thin deep-set nails, prominent fingertip pads, relatively loose skin

Ocular Findings: down-slanting palpebral fissures, hypertelorism, epicanthal folds, strabismus

Weill–Marchesani Syndrome *Brachydactyly-Spherophakia Syndrome* MIM *277600 Inheritance: autosomal recessive. Incidence: 1:100,000

General Description: short stature, brachycephaly, short stubby spadelike hands and feet, limited arm overhead extension, depressed nasal bridge, "pug nose," microspherophakia, subluxated lenses, normal intelligence, occasional subvalvular fibromuscular aortic stenosis

Ocular Findings: a microspheroophakic lens (the lens diameter may be as small as 6.75 mm, and the lens may be increased by 25% in thickness), ectopia lentis (50%). The microspheroophakic lens may move into the pupillary area, causing pupillary block and glaucoma. Total dislocation into the anterior chamber is uncommon but may occur. Myopia results from spherophakia, but may be axial. The anterior chamber is usually shallow, predisposing to angle-closure glaucoma.

Werner Syndrome MIM #277700 Gene map locus: 8p12–p11.2. Inheritance: autosomal recessive. Incidence: 1:50,000–1:1,000,000

General Description: early adult appearance, with thin skin and thick fibrous subcutaneous tissue, scleroderma-like skin on face and lower legs, loss of subcutaneous fat, slim extremities with small hands and feet, beaked nose, irregular dental development, gray sparse hair, short stature, osteoporosis, atherosclerosis with calcification, muscle hypoplasia, propensity toward malignancy (10%), especially sarcoma and meningioma

Ocular Findings: cataract, retinal degeneration

Williams Syndrome *Williams–Beuren Syndrome* MIM *194050 Gene map locus: 7q11.2. Inheritance: autosomal dominant. Over 100 cases reported.

General Description: postnatal growth deficiency, mental retardation, friendly personality, prominent lips with open mouth, depressed nasal bridge, anteverted nares, hoarse voice, hypersensitivity to sound, mild spasticity, cardiovascular anomalies, renal anomalies

Ocular Findings
Common: medial eyebrow flare, short palpebral fissures, epicanthal folds, periorbital fullness of subcutaneous tissues, blue eyes, "stellate" pattern of the iris

TABLE 10-2. (continued).

Less common: hypertelorism, strabismus, refractive errors, tortuosity of retinal vessels

Xeroderma Pigmentosum Syndrome (Group A Through I Plus a Variant) MIM *278700, *133510, *278720, #278730, *278740, #278760, #278780, 278810, #278750 Gene map locus: Group A, 9q22.3, Group B, 2q21, Group C, 3p25, Group D,19q13.2–q13.3, Group E, 11p12–p11, Group F, 16p13.3–p13.13, Group G, 13q33, Variant type, 6p21.1–p12. Inheritance: autosomal recessive (a milder autosomal dominant form has been reported). Over 1000 cases.

General Description: the repair of UV light-induced damage to the DNA of epidermal cells is defective. The skin is normal at birth, with the first signs of the disease presenting as increased dryness and freckling on skin areas with the greatest light exposure, particularly the face. Seventy-five percent of patients show the first skin changes between 6 months and 3 years of age. Skin tumors present in the affected areas, usually before 20 years of age. Sunlight sensitivity, freckling, progressive skin atrophy with irregular pigmentation, cutaneous telangiectasia, angiomata, keratoses. Development of basal cell and squamous cell carcinoma, and less often keratocanthoma, adenocarcinoma, melanoma, neuroma, sarcoma, and angiosarcoma, squamous cell carcinoma of tongue tip, gingiva and/or palate. Slowly progressive neurological abnormalities sometimes associated with mental deterioration, microcephaly, cerebral atrophy, choreoathetosis, ataxia, spasticity, impaired hearing, abnormal speech. Occasionally, primary internal neoplasms including brain tumors, lung tumors, and leukemia. Immune abnormalities with frequent infections (33% of deaths are due to cancer and 11% due to infection). The mean age of first nonmelanoma skin cancer is 8 years. Ninety-seven percent of squamous cell and basal cell cancers occur on face, head, or neck.

Ocular Findings
Common: the most common ocular manifestation is progressive atrophy of the lower eyelid, which may lead to loss of the entire eyelid. The resulting exposure leads to inflammation, symblepharon, corneal ulceration, and corneal scarring. Conjunctival involvement begins with hyperemia with serous or mucopurulent discharge and may progress to xerosis, keratinization, and shrinkage that leads to ankyloblepharon. Neoplasms involving conjunctiva, cornea, and eyelids. The limbal zone is a common site for involvement, usually by squamous cell carcinoma. Patients often present with photophobia and conjunctivitis.
Less common: band-shaped nodular corneal dystrophy (reported in African-Americans)

X-Linked Alpha-Thalassemia/Mental Retardation Syndrome *ATR-X Syndrome* MIM #301040 Gene map locus: Xq13. Inheritance: X-linked recessive. Over 40 cases reported.

General Description: severe mental retardation, postnatal growth deficiency, microcephaly, low nasal bridge, small triangular nose with anteverted nares, midface hypoplasia, large "carplike" mouth frequently held open, full lips, large protruding tongue, deformed ears, tapering fingers, fifth finger clinodactyly, genital abnormalities, mild hypochromic microcytic anemia, mild form of hemoglobin H disease

Ocular Findings: telecanthus, epicanthal folds

(continued)

TABLE 10-2. Ocular and Systemic Findings in Selected Inherited Syndromes (continued).

XO Syndrome *Turner's Syndrome* Faulty chromosome distribution. Incidence: 1:5,000 live births.

General Description: short female, delay in motor skills, neuropsychological deficits, broad chest with wide spacing of nipples, congenital lymphedema, ovarian dysgenesis, anomalous auricles, narrow maxilla, low posterior neck hairline, short neck (>80%), webbed posterior neck (50%), elbow and knee anomalies, narrow, hyperconvex and/or deep-set nails, excessive pigmented nevi (50%), loose skin (about the neck in infancy), kidney anomalies (60%), cardiac defects (40%), perceptive hearing impairment (50%)

Ocular Findings
Common: inner epicanthal folds (40%)
Less common: ptosis (16%), strabismus, blue sclera, cataract

XXX and XXXX Syndrome Incidence: XXX occurs in 1:1000 newborn females, XXXX reported in 40 cases.

General Description: mental deficiency, speech and behavioral problems, midfacial hypoplasia, occasional hand abnormalities, seizures

Ocular Findings: mild hypertelorism, up-slanting palpebral fissures, epicanthal folds

XXXXX Syndrome *Penta X Syndrome* Incidence: unknown

General Description: mental deficiency, short stature, microcephaly, low hairline, dental malocclusion, small hands with mild clinodactyly of fifth fingers, congenital heart defects (patent ductus arteriosus or ventricular septal defect)

Ocular Findings
Common: hypertelorism, epicanthal folds, mild up-slanting palpebral fissures
Less common: coloboma of iris

XXXY and XXXXY Syndromes Incidence: unknown

General Description: mental deficiency, hypotonia, joint laxity, short stature, sclerotic cranial sutures, low nasal bridge, wide upturned nasal tip, low-set malformed ears, short neck, thick undersegmented sternum, limited pronation of elbow, clinodactyly of fifth finger, hypogenitalism, low dermal ridge count on fingertips

Ocular Findings
Common: wide-set eyes, up-slanting palpebral fissures, inner epicanthal folds, strabismus
Less common: down-slanting palpebral fissures, Brushfield spots, myopia

Yunis–Varon Syndrome MIM *216340 Inheritance: autosomal recessive. Thirteen reported cases.

General Description: severe developmental delay, severe failure to thrive, microcephaly, enlarged fontanels, dysplastic ears, agenesis/hypoplasia of thumbs and great toes, short tapering fingers and toes with nail hypoplasia, agenesis/hypoplasia of distal and middle phalanges of fingers and toes, absence or hypoplasia of clavicle(s). Death in the neonatal period has occurred in the majority of liveborn infants.

TABLE 10-2. (continued).

Ocular Findings
Common: sparse eyebrows and eyelashes, short up-slanting palpebral fissures
Less common: sclerocornea, cataract, mild hypertelorism

Zellweger Syndrome *Cerebro-Hepato-Renal Syndrome* MIM #214100 Gene map locus: 2p15, 7q21–q22, 6q23–q24, Chromosome 1. Inheritance: autosomal recessive. Rare disorder.

General Description: prenatal and postnatal growth deficiency, hypotonia, seizures, gross defects of early brain development, high forehead with flat facies, hepatomegaly. Most patients die within the first year of life.

Ocular Findings
Common: up-slanting palpebral fissures, congenital cataract, pallid hypoplastic optic disc, retinal pigmentary changes, puffy eyelids, hypertelorism, Brushfield spots, epicanthal folds, cloudy cornea
Less common: glaucoma, nystagmus

References

1. Jablonski's Multiple Congenital Abnormality/Mental Retardation website. http://www.nlm.nih.gov/mesh/jablonski/syndrome_title.html
2. Jones KL: Smith's recognizable patterns of human malformation, 5th edn. Philadelphia: Saunders, 1997.
3. Online Mendelian Inheritance in Man (OMIM™) website. http://www.ncbi.nlm.nih.gov
4. Traboulsi EI: Genetic diseases of the eye. New York: Oxford University Press, 1998.

Index

A

Aarskog syndrome, 527, 537
  differentiated from Opitz G/BBB
    syndrome, 458
Aase-Smith syndrome, 527
Aase syndrome, 527, 537
Abducens nerve. *See* Cranial nerve VI
Abduction, Möbius sequence-related
  impairment of, 197, 198
Abetalipoproteinemia, 527, 537
Ablepharon-macrostomia syndrome,
  527, 538
Abortion, spontaneous, chromosomal
  abnormalities associated with, 83
Abruzzo-Erickson syndrome, 527, 538
Acanthosis, 607
Acanthosis nigricans, Crouzon
  syndrome-related, 169
    Physician-parent interactions,
      69–70
Acetyl-coenzyme A deficiency, 364
N-Acetylcystine, 321
N-Acetyl galactosamine-4-sulfatase
  deficiency, 366
N-Acetyl galactosamine-6-sulfatase
  deficiency, 357, 365
α-*N*-Acetyl glucosaminidase acetyl
  transferase deficiency, 357
α-*N*-Acetyl glucosaminidase deficiency,
  357, 364
Acid sphingomyelinase deficiency,
  379
Acrocallosal syndrome, 527, 538
  Schnizel type, 527
Acrocephalopolydactylous dysplasia,
  527, 538
Acrocephalopolysyndactyly
    type 2, 168
    type 3, 590–591
    type 4, 564

Acrodysostosis, 527, 538
Acrofacial dysostosis 1, 580–581
Acrofacial dysplasia, 563
Acro-fronto-facio-nasal dysostosis
  syndrome, 527, 538–539
Acromegaloid facial appearance
  syndrome, 527, 539
Acromegaloid phenotype-cutis verticis
  gyrata-cornea leukoma, 527, 539
Acromesomelic dysplasia, Maroteaux-
  Martinelli-Campailla type, 527,
  539
Acromicric dysplasia, 527, 539
Acro-osteolysis syndrome, 565
Acro-reno-ocular syndrome, 527,
  539
Acyclovir, 504, 505, 518
Adam complex, 207–209
Adams-Oliver syndrome, 527, 540
Adduction, Möbius sequence-related
  impairment of, 197, 198
Adenoma sebaceum, tuberous sclerosis
  complex-related, 304, 308–309
Adrenocorticotropic hormone, 433
Aging, premature. *See also* Progeria
  ataxia-telangiectasia-related, 320
Aglossia-adactyly syndrome, 584–585
Agnathia-holoprosencephaly, 54
Aicardi's syndrome, 178, 430–434, 527,
  540
    clinical assessment of, 431–433
    clinical features of, 430–431
    etiology of, 430
    genetic factors in, 433
    prognosis for, 434
    systemic associations of, 431–433
    treatment of, 433–434
Alagille syndrome, 527
Albers-Schonberg disease
  (osteopetrosis), 271–272

611